RD
99
.N874
2005

Nursing the Surgical Patient

D1285885

For Elsevier

Senior Commissioning Editor: Ninette Premdas
Project Development Editor: Katrina Mather
Project Manager: Derek Robertson/Emma Riley
Design: George Ajayi

BELL LIBRARY-TAMU-CC

Nursing the Surgical Patient

SECOND EDITION

Edited by

Rosemary Pudner BA(Hons) RGN RCNT DipNEd DipAppSS(Open)

Senior Lecturer, Faculty of Health and Social Care Sciences,
Kingston University and St George's, University of London, UK

Illustrations by
Ian Ramsden

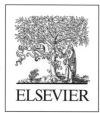

EDINBURGH LONDON NEW YORK OXFORD PHILADELPHIA ST LOUIS SYDNEY TORONTO 2005

ELSEVIER

© Harcourt Publishers Limited 2000
© Elsevier Science Limited 2003
© Elsevier Science Limited 2005. All rights reserved.

The right of Rosemary Pudner to be identified as Editor of this work has been
asserted by her in accordance with the Copyright, Designs and Patents Act 1988

No part of this publication may be reproduced, stored in a retrieval system, or
transmitted in any form or by any means, electronic, mechanical, photocopying,
recording or otherwise, without either the prior permission of the publishers or a
licence permitting restricted copying in the United Kingdom issued by the
Copyright Licensing Agency, 90 Tottenham Court Road, London W1T 4LP.
Permissions may be sought directly from Elsevier's Health Sciences Rights
Department in Philadelphia, USA: phone: (+1) 215 238 7869, fax: (+1) 215 238
2239, e-mail: healthpermissions@elsevier.com. You may also complete your
request on-line via the Elsevier homepage (http://www.elsevier.com), by
selecting 'Customer Support' and then 'Obtaining Permissions'.

First edition 2000
Reprinted 2001, 2003
Second edition 2005

ISBN 0 7020 2757 X
British Library Cataloguing in Publication Data
A catalogue record for this book is available from the British Library

Library of Congress Cataloging in Publication Data
A catalog record for this book is available from the Library of Congress

Note
Knowledge and best practice in this field are constantly changing. As new research
and experience broaden our knowledge, changes in practice, treatment and drug
therapy may become necessary or appropriate. Readers are advised to check the
most current information provided (i) on procedures featured or (ii) by the
manufacturer of each product to be administered, to verify the recommended dose
or formula, the method and duration of administration, and contraindications. It is
the responsibility of the practitioner, relying on their own experience and knowledge of the patient, to make diagnoses, to determine dosages and the best treatment
for each individual patient, and to take all appropriate safety precautions. To the
fullest extent of the law, neither the Publisher nor the editor assumes any liability
for any injury and/or damage to persons or property arising out or related to any
use of the material contained in this book.

The Publisher

Working together to grow libraries in developing countries

www.elsevier.com | www.bookaid.org | www.sabre.org

ELSEVIER   BOOK AID International   Sabre Foundation

your source for books,
journals and multimedia
in the health sciences

www.elsevierhealth.com

The
Publisher's
policy is to use
**paper manufactured
from sustainable forests**

Printed in China

Contents

Contributors

Adèle Atkinson MEd, BA(Hons), RGN, RNT
Senior Lecturer, Faculty of Health and Social Care Sciences, Kingston University & St George's, University of London, UK

Martin Beynon BSc(Hons), PGDip(Ed), RGN
Clinical Development Manager, Coloplast Ltd, UK; Formerly Lecturer Practitioner Urology, South Bank University, London, UK

Emin Carapeti BSc MB BS MD FRCS (Gen)
Consultant Colorectal Surgeon, St Thomas' Hospital, London, UK

Rosie Castle BA(Hons) MSc Nursing Studies, RGN Cert Ed
Senior Lecturer, Faculty of Health and Social Care Sciences, Kingston University & St George's, University of London, UK

Jacky Cotton RGN RM MHS
Head of Nursing – Gynaecology, Birmingham Women's Hospital, Birmingham, UK

Christine Eberhardie MSc RGN RNT ILTM MHSM
Senior Lecturer, Faculty of Health and Social Care Sciences, Kingston University & St George's, University of London, UK

Emma L Gardner BSc(Hons) Health Studies (Nursing) RGN Dip PGCMSCE
Lecturer/Practitioner Cardiac, Brighton University, Institute of Nursing and Midwifery, Brighton, UK

Diane Gilmour RN PGCEA BN DANS Dip Infection Control (RCN)
Clinical Team Leader (Theatres), Surrey and Sussex Healthcare NHS Trust, Crawley Hospital, Crawley, UK

Elisabeth Grimsey RGN RM MSc
Macmillan Nurse Consultant – breast care, East Sussex Hospitals NHS Trust, Eastbourne, UK

Suzanne J Hart RGN OND
Senior Staff Nurse, Ophthalmic Department, Ipswich Hospital NHS Trust, Ipswich, Suffolk, UK

Fiona Hibberts BSc(Hons) RN MSc PGCert
Colo-rectal Nurse Specialist, Department of Colorectal Surgery, St Thomas' Hospital, London

Nicola L Judge MSc BSc(Hons) ANP RN
Senior Practice Educator/Advanced Nurse Practitioner, Matron for Perioperative Care, South West London Elective Orthopaedic Centre, Epsom, UK

Teresa Rooney-Kaymakci RGN SCM NDNCert PWT PGCEA Diploma in Health Promotion
Senior Lecturer, Faculty of Health and Social Care Sciences, Kingston University and St George's, University of London, UK

Sharon Kitcatt RN MSc (Pain Management) ONC
Consultant Nurse, Acute Pain Service, Ashford and St Peter's NHS Trust, Surrey, UK

Biddy Knight MA DA DipN DipNEd RGN OND
Nurse Lecturer

Shelagh Murray BSc(Hons) RN
Vascular Nurse Consultant, Vascular Surgery, St George's Hospital NHS Trust, London, UK; Honorary Senior Lecturer, Faculty of Social Care Sciences, Kingston University & St George's, University of London, UK

Melanie Oakley RN BSc(Hons) MSc PGCE
*Matron for Perioperative Care, South West London,
Elective Orthopaedic Centre, Epsom, UK*

Lindsey Ockenden MSc BSc(Hons) DipN CertEd RGN
*Formerly Senior Lecturer, Faculty of Health and Social
Care Sciences, Kingston University & St George's,
University of London, UK*

Rosemary Pudner BA(Hons) RGN RCNT DipNEd
DipAppSS(Open)
*Senior Lecturer, Faculty of Health and Social Care
Sciences, Kingston University & St George's,
University of London, UK*

Christine Spiers MSc BSc(Hons) PGDip RNT RN
*Senior Lecturer, Institute of Nursing and Midwifery,
University of Brighton, Brighton, UK*

Julie A Wain RN BA MN GradDip Health Counselling
*ENT Perioperative Clinical Nurse Specialist, President
Otolaryngology Head and Neck Nurses Group,
St Vincent's and Mercy Private Hospital, East Melbourne,
Victoria, Australia*

Susanne Wood RGN DipN
*Formerly Nutrition Nurse Specialist, Kingston Hospital,
Surrey, UK*

Preface

It is 5 years since the first edition of this book was published, and I am delighted that so many people, including numerous student nurses, have found it to be of value in their studies and clinical practice. Some aspects of surgical nursing have changed in recent years, and many patients are now undergoing surgery in day surgery units, and those requiring an inpatient stay are being discharged back into the community much earlier than before.

All the chapters in the book have been updated, by either the original authors or new contributors, to reflect any new surgical procedures and changes in clinical practice, although many procedures and nursing care remain the same. As evidence-based practice is part of our everyday lives, the reference lists and further reading have been updated and also include relevant website addresses at the time of writing.

A brand new chapter on preoperative assessment has been included, as the majority of patients now visit a preadmission or preassessment clinic prior to entering hospital for their surgery. Several chapters have been completely rewritten, i.e. perioperative care, concepts of pain and the surgical patient, and care of the patient requiring cardiac interventions and surgery. Many aspects included in the original chapter on minimally invasive surgery have now been incorporated into the chapters on preoperative assessment and perioperative care, as key-hole surgery is now an accepted part of surgical care. A complete glossary is now situated at the beginning of the book rather than at the end of each chapter.

The main aim of the book remains the same, in that it will enable the reader to link the theoretical concepts of surgical nursing to the application of clinical practice.

It is impossible to totally divorce the care required by a surgical patient from other related medical aspects of their care. The reader is therefore directed to other sources of information throughout the book, as well as to other specialist nursing texts and relevant websites.

The intended readership for this book remains the same, i.e. it is written predominantly for nurses caring for surgical patients. It is of value for pre-registration nursing students, especially those undertaking the adult branch of Diploma in Nursing courses. Many students have commented how valuable the book has been to them, as it is clear and easy to understand, and has been a useful resource both for revision and when in clinical practice. The book will also be a valuable resource for newly qualified nurses who have chosen to work in a surgical area.

The book is now divided into two sections. In Section I the chapters relate to aspects of surgical nursing care that are relevant to all patients undergoing a surgical procedure. The first chapter on preoperative assessment outlines the physiological, psychological and sociological considerations that should be considered as part of the assessment process. The second chapter on perioperative care outlines the care patients require from the time they enter the operating theatre to the time they arrive back on the ward. The third chapter on day surgery outlines the journey the patient will take if having surgery in a day surgery unit. The remaining chapters in this section are on wound healing, nutrition, altered body image and pain, which address general aspects of care relating to surgical patients. The final chapter in this section discusses the importance of discharge planning in the surgical patient's journey.

Section II relates to specific areas of surgical nursing. Chapters in this section relate to neurological surgery; ophthalmic surgery; surgery to the ear, nose and throat; thyroid surgery; cardiac and thoracic surgery; surgery on the gastrointestinal tract; surgery for renal and urologic disorders; surgery on the breast and reproductive organs; vascular surgery; orthopaedic surgery; and finally plastic/reconstructive surgery. Some of these chapters are very detailed in relation to the surgical procedures and ensuing nursing care, as the authors feel that detailed information is required by the reader in order to be able to comprehend the complexities of the surgical interventions.

Each of the chapters in Section II follows a similar format, in that a brief review of the related anatomy and physiology and the relevant pathophysiology is discussed, so as to assist the reader in the understanding of the common disorders that require surgical intervention and the surgical procedure itself. Relevant investigations required prior to the surgical intervention are highlighted, and a brief explanation of each surgical intervention is given. Specific issues relating to pre-operative assessment are identified, followed by specific pre- and postoperative care required by the patient and their family/carer. Rationale for nursing interventions and related research findings are also included in the discussion on patient care. At the end of each chapter, any specific health education needs, patient teaching and preparations for discharge are discussed.

The approach adopted in this book is designed to be patient-centred whenever possible, utilizing a problem-solving, evidence-based approach to care. The care required by individuals is discussed with respect to the principles involved, although some specific nursing procedures are included. It is also recognized that the delivery of nursing care may vary between local areas, regions and countries. Various case studies and care plans are included to illustrate the use of the problem-solving approach to patient care. A variety of nursing models have been used to provide a structure within the problem-solving approach to care, although it is recognized that many clinical areas now have integrated care pathways.

It must be remembered that it will often be necessary to adapt the suggested nursing interventions to meet individual patient needs. This may mean that information presented in this book may differ from that seen by practitioners in other clinical areas.

Reference to relevant research findings is considered a vital part of this text, in order to provide an evidence base to clinical practice. References are given at the end of each chapter and a further reading list and relevant websites are provided to encourage the reader to develop knowledge beyond this text.

It is intended that the book should act as a guide to the theoretical and practical aspects of nursing an individual who has undergone a surgical intervention. It is envisaged that the reader will not necessarily read the whole of the book, but will identify the relevant sections within the book as they relate to each individual surgical patient in their care. The chapters are written by nurses working in clinical practice and lecturers who have an active clinical role, so ensuring the link between theory and practice. The contributors are from many regions from within the UK and one author is from Australia, so adding a diversity of experiences which will benefit the reader. As each contributor has a very distinctive professional profile, the reader may encompass a variety of approaches to the delivery of information and patient care.

Finally, I hope you enjoy reading the book and find it a valuable resource for your clinical practice. It has been an interesting and valuable experience in compiling this second edition, as it has given me the opportunity to be in contact with many new people as well as old colleagues. My final thanks go to all the original contributors who have made the book such a success, and the new contributors who have added to the book which will hopefully prove to be a useful resource for many.

Rosemary Pudner
London, 2005

Glossary

Abduction Movement of a limb away from the midline of the body.

Absorption The passing of substances into the surrounding tissue.

Accommodation A process by which the refractive power of the lens is increased by contraction of the ciliary muscle causing an increased thickness and curvature of the lens, allowing near objects to be focused on the retina.

Achlorhydria An abnormal condition where there is absence of hydrochloric acid in the stomach.

Adduction Movement of a limb towards the midline of the body.

Adhesions Following an inflammatory process, two surfaces, not normally joined, unite together.

Adjuvant A substance or treatment that can be used to enhance the action of an analgesic.

Agnosia Inability to recognize objects because of damage to the sensory pathways.

Alignment The state of being arranged in the correct anatomical position.

Altered body image This exists when coping strategies fail to deal with changes in body reality, body ideal and body presentation.

Amblyopia Subnormal vision associated with squints due to a lack of retinal stimulation in the first years of life.

Amenorrhoea Absence of periods (menses).

Anaesthetic Administration of a regime of drugs and/or gases and/or volatile agents to abolish the sensation of feeling.

Anastomosis The joining of two hollow structures, usually by suturing together during a surgical procedure, e.g. two sections of the colon, or stomach to small intestine, or blood vessels.

Aneurysm Local dilatation of a blood vessel, usually an artery, caused by a fault in the wall due to defect, disease or injury, producing a pulsating swelling over which a murmur may be heard.

Angina Pain emanating from the heart, due to inadequate blood supply to the myocardium, that radiates into the chest, jaw and down the left arm.

Angiogenesis The process of new blood vessel formation.

Angiography X-ray of the arterial system by means of injecting a radio-opaque contrast medium.

Ankle brachial pressure index (ABPI) A non-invasive test to assess arterial blood supply to a lower limb by measuring the ankle–brachial systolic pressure ratio using a hand-held Doppler ultrasonic probe.

Anorexia Lack or complete loss of appetite, which may result in malnutrition and/or starvation.

Antacid A substance which buffers, neutralizes or absorbs the effects of hydrochloric acid in the contents of the stomach.

Antiseptics Solutions which are intended to inhibit the proliferation of pathogens.

Aperient Mild laxative medication which stimulates a bowel action.

Aphakia Absence of a lens in the eye, following cataract surgery or trauma.

Apposition Bringing together two opposing structures.

Arrhythmia An abnormal heart rhythm that may be regular or irregular.

Arterial occlusive disease Obstruction of the arteries by embolus, thrombus or atherosclerosis.

Arteriosclerosis/atherosclerosis Degeneration of the artery, with thickening and loss of elasticity of the arterial walls.

Arteriotomy Cutting or opening into an artery.

Arthrodesis An operation to produce bony fusion across a joint.

Arthroplasty Surgical reconstruction of a joint.

Arthroscopy Examination of a joint using an arthroscope.

Asepsis Prevention of wound contamination by using only sterile instruments and solutions.

Astigmatism Irregularity of the cornea in one or more planes.

Atherectomy Removal of obstructing atheroma using high-speed cutters.

Atheroma Deposits of hard yellow plaques of lipoid material in the intimal layer of arteries.

Athetosis Involuntary, slow writhing movements.

Atrophy Degeneration of cells, resulting in wasting of any part of the body.

Bacteraemia Presence of bacteria in the blood.

Bartholin's abscess Localized infection of the Bartholin's duct.

Biopsy Examination of a sample of tissue or organ taken for the purpose of diagnosis.

Bioptome catheter An intravascular catheter device with a small opening and closing capsular mouth that can take tiny tissue samples from the heart.

Bitemporal hemianopia Tunnel vision.

Blepharo Conditions related to the eyelids.

BlomSinger valve A voice prosthesis for a laryngectomy patient; it allows air to enter the oesophagus, and the vibrating tissue, together with oral articulation, enables the patient to produce speech.

Body ideal The picture in our heads of how we would like our body to look and perform.

Body image A psychological experience focusing on conscious and unconscious attitudes and feelings. It is dependent on body ideal, body reality and body presentation.

Body presentation The body as it is presented to the world.

Body reality The physical body as it exists.

Bone scan A radiological examination to assess for metastatic disease.

Bougie A flexible instrument which is used to dilate a tubular organ such as the oesophagus.

Bradyarrhythmia Abnormal regular or irregular heart rhythm with a rate that is less than 60 beats per minute, which may cause hypotension and hypoperfusion.

Bronchopleural fistula Pathological connection between the pleural cavity and one of the bronchi.

Brace A support used in orthopaedics to hold parts of the body in their correct position.

Bronchoscopy Endoscopic examination of the main bronchi.

Bunion Prominence of the head of the metatarsal bone at its junction with the great toe.

Buphthalmos Congenital glaucoma, also referred to as 'ox eye'.

Capillary refill The time taken for the capillaries to refill – usually tested by pressing on area with a finger (to occlude the capillary) and then releasing the pressure.

Carpopedal spasm Cramp in the hands and feet due to a deficiency of ionized calcium in the blood.

Cataract Opacity of the lens.

Chalazion/meibomian cyst/internal hordeolum Enlargement and blockage of the meibomian gland.

Chemosis Oedema of the conjunctiva.

Chemotherapy A systemic cytotoxic drug treatment.

Cheyne–Stokes respiratory pattern A pattern of breathing which includes stertorous breathing with periods of apnoea.

Chorea Involuntary sudden movements which are both flexor and extensor.

Chvostek's sign Spasm of the facial muscles produced by tapping the facial nerve.

Circumcision Surgical removal of the foreskin.

Cirrhosis Damage to an organ, causing fibrosis, which results in dysfunction; often associated with the liver.

Colic Severe spasmodic episodes of pain caused by involuntary muscular contraction.

Compartment syndrome Swelling within the muscle compartments of a limb due to haemorrhage or oedema, resulting in muscle necrosis and nerve damage.

Conjunctivitis Inflammation of the conjunctiva, usually caused by a bacterial or viral infection.

Contraction Drawing together of wound edges.

Contralateral Pertaining to the opposite side.

Coping Process by which a person attempts to manage stressful demands.

Cortical blindness Blindness caused by damage to the occipital lobe.

Counter traction A force applied to oppose traction.

COX-2 inhibitor A new group of non-steroidal anti-inflammatory medicines which selectively block cyclooxygenase 2.

CT scan Computerized tomography scan.

Cyanosis Bluish discoloration of the skin caused by a relative decrease in oxygen saturation levels within the capillaries.

Cycloplegia Paralysis of the ciliary muscle.

Cystectomy Surgical removal of the bladder.

Cystocele Herniation and descent of the bladder through the anterior vaginal wall.

Cystoscopy Endoscopic visualization of the urethra and bladder using a fibreoptic light source.

Cytology Study of cells used in diagnosis of premalignant disease.

Dacrocystorhinostomy Formation of an opening between the lacrimal sac and the nasal cavity.

Decortication Surgery to remove the thick cortex that is formed as a result of empyema within the pleural cavity.

Deep vein thrombosis A blood clot that forms in the deep veins of the legs or pelvic area which can become dislodged and travel via the venous system to the lungs.

Dehiscence Breakdown of a surgically closed wound.

Denervated Lacking nerve endings.

Depolarization A surge of charged particles that bring about muscle contraction.

Dermatome An area of the body corresponding to a particular nerve root.

Digital subtraction angiography (DSA) A computerized method of angiography without background information (e.g. bones, bowel).

Dilatation and curettage Gentle dilatation of the cervix and scraping (curetting) of the endometrium for diagnostic purposes.

Diplopia Double vision.

Dislocation Displacement of a bone from its anatomical position.

Dissection Tearing or splitting, e.g. the inner lining of the coronary artery wall.

Distension Enlargement of the abdomen with a collection of gas or fluid from the intestines.

Donor site Area from which a skin graft or flap has been taken.

Dorsiflexion Bending the ankle upwards.

Drug Tariff A list of products drawn up by the Department of Health which can be dispensed on prescription.

Duct ectasia A benign condition affecting the breast.

Ductal carcinoma in situ A pre-invasive ductal carcinoma of the breast.

Duplex scan A non-invasive ultrasonic scan providing accurate diagnosis of arterial stenosis/occlusion or deep vein thrombosis.

Dysarthria Difficulty with articulating speech.

Dyscalculia Difficulty with calculating.

Dysfunction Reduction or absence of the normal function of a part of the body.

Dysgraphia Difficulty with writing, caused by brain damage.

Dyslexia Difficulty with reading and abstract thinking.

Dysmenorrhoea Painful periods.

Dyspareunia Painful sexual intercourse.

Dyspepsia Symptoms associated with indigestion, nausea, vomiting, discomfort of the abdomen and flatulence.

Dysphagia Difficulty in swallowing.

Dysphasia Difficulty with the processing of language. It can be (a) receptive, in which the individual experiences difficulty understanding language, or (b) expressive, in which the individual has a difficulty in expressing himself in words.

Dyspnoea Difficulty in breathing.

Dyspraxia Difficulty in performing a pattern of movements, e.g. locating and picking up a cup.

Dysuria Painful micturition.

Ectopic pregnancy Pregnancy which implants outside the uterus, most commonly in the Fallopian tubes.

Ectropion Turning out of the lid margin, usually the bottom lid.

Electronic larynx A device which produces mechanical sound; the patient places a probe either inside the mouth or against the neck and then mouths the words, resulting in speech.

Electrosurgery The surgical application of heat to coagulate blood vessels to prevent excessive bleeding, and also to cut tissue.

Embolectomy Surgical removal of an embolism.

Embolism Obstruction of blood vessels by impaction of a solid body (e.g. thrombi, fat or tumour cells).

Empyema Collection of purulent fluid within the pleural space.

Endarterectomy Surgical removal of an atheromatous plug in an artery.

Endometriosis A condition where the endometrium grows in other parts of the body outside the uterus.

Enteral nutrition May refer to food or fluids taken orally or via a tube placed within the gastrointestinal tract.

Entropion Turning in of the lid margin, usually the bottom lid.

Enucleation Removal of the eye.

Epiphora Overflow of tears onto the cheek due to a defective or inadequate drainage system.

Erectile dysfunction/impotence Inability to achieve or maintain an erection.

Euthyroid A normally functioning thyroid gland.

Evisceration Removal of the internal structures of the eye.

Excoriation Superficial breakdown of skin, usually surrounding a wound and caused by fluid containing proteolytic enzymes.

Exenteration Removal of an organ.

Exostosis A bony outgrowth from the surface of the bone.

Exudate Fluid produced in wounds, which consists of serum, leucocytes and wound debris.

Fasciotomy Incision of a fascia to relieve damaging tension in a muscle compartment or prevent compression of arteries or nerves.

Fat necrosis Death of fat tissue, creating a hard craggy lump that often mimics cancer, and often occurs following trauma.

Fibroadenoma A benign tumour of fibrous or glandular tissue.

Fibroids Benign fibrous tumour found in the muscle of the uterus or cervix.

Fine-needle aspiration cytology An investigation where cells are obtained from a lump by passing a small needle into it to obtain cells to enable a cytological diagnosis.

Fistula An abnormal track which may connect one epithelial surface to another, organ to organ, or organ to epithelial surface.

Flap Tissue which is moved from one part of the body to another and takes its own blood supply with it.

Flatus The presence of gas in the stomach or intestines.

Fluoroscope X-ray equipment that allows direct viewing of images without taking or developing X-ray pictures.

Foreign body Material found in the body which does not normally belong, e.g. prosthetic material, sutures, staples.

Gallstone A stone consisting of bile pigments and calcium salts that forms in the biliary tract.

Gastric function tests Tests carried out to establish the levels of hydrochloric acid secretion.

Gastric lavage Stomach contents are washed out through a tube inserted into the stomach.

Gastrostomy Incision into the stomach. A tube is placed within the incision; often used for feeding.

Glaucoma Raised intraocular pressure.

Glucose intolerance The inability to metabolize glucose efficiently as a result of the presence of large quantities of cortisol during the stress response.

Goitre An enlargement of the thyroid gland, which presents as a pronounced swelling in the neck.

Graft bed The wound site on which skin grafting will take place.

Growth factors Proteins which act as cell messengers and are vital for cell proliferation.

Guttae Eyedrops.

H_2 receptor antagonists Drugs which lower the acid secretion by blocking the action of the receptors in the parietal cells of the stomach.

Haematoma A localized collection of blood within the tissues.

Haematuria Blood in the urine.

Haemostasis The cessation of bleeding.

Haemothorax The abnormal presence of blood in the pleural space.

Halitosis Unpleasant or foul-smelling breath which often results from systemic disease.

Heimlich valve A small, portable, one-way valve device for draining air from a pneumothorax, but unsuitable if fluid is draining as well.

Hemiballismus Violent involuntary movements of the limbs.

Histology The study of tissues.

Homonymous hemianopia Loss of vision in the right or left visual fields.

Hormone replacement therapy A treatment used in postmenopausal women to replace oestrogen so as to prevent menopausal symptoms such as hot flushes and to prevent a loss of bone density.

Hydatidiform mole A condition in pregnancy in which the chorionic villi degenerate into clusters of cysts.

Hydrocele Collection of fluid in the tunica vaginalis.

Hydrocephalus Excessive accumulation of cerebrospinal fluid in the ventricles or around the brain.

Hydrophilic A substance that attracts water.

Hypercholesterolaemia Excessive cholesterol in the blood.

Hyperlipidaemia Excessive fat in the blood.

Hyperthyroidism Excessive secretions of thyroid hormones.

Hypertrophic scar An increase in the volume of tissue produced by enlargement of existing cells.

Hyphaema Presence of red blood cells in the anterior chamber of the eye.

Hypocalcaemia Diminished amount of blood calcium.

Hypoparathyroidism Diminished function of the parathyroid glands.

Hypopyon Presence of white blood cells in the anterior chamber of the eye.

Hypothyroidism Insufficiency of thyroid hormone secretion.

Hypoxaemia Low levels of oxygen in the blood.

Hypoxia Lack of oxygen to the tissues and body organs.

Hysterosalpingogram Diagnostic X-ray examination of the uterus and Fallopian tubes following the injection of a radio-opaque dye.

Hysteroscopy A diagnostic procedure examining the uterine cavity via an endoscope.

Inadvertent hypothermia The accidental lowering of the body temperature.

Induction The process of causing unconsciousness by the use of anaesthetic agents.

Infection The presence of microorganisms in sufficient numbers to cause a host reaction.

Infertility Inability to conceive; may be primary or secondary.

Intermenstrual bleeding Bleeding between periods.

Intermittent claudication Sudden, severe pain in the calves, thigh or buttock muscles, occurring after walking a certain distance; caused by an inadequate blood supply to the muscles.

Intra-abdominal pressure Increased pressure within the abdominal cavity.

Intraduct papilloma A wart-like growth in the duct of a breast.

Intramedullary Within the medullary cavity of long bone.

Intraoperative The phase which starts when the patient is transferred to the operating table and ends when the patient is transferred to the recovery room.

Intrathecal antibiotics Antibiotics introduced into the cerebrospinal fluid in the theca of the spinal canal.

Invasive ductal carcinoma An invasive cancer arising from the ducts of the breast.

Invasive lobular carcinoma An invasive cancer arising from the lobules in the breast.

Ipsilateral Pertains to the same side.

Ischaemia Lack of blood supply to a part of the body.

Jaundice The mucous membranes and sclera become yellow due to bile bilirubin in the blood.

Jejunostomy A surgically made fistula between the jejunum and abdominal wall. A fine tube is placed within the fistula, usually for feeding.

Keloid scar A type of scar which results from the formation of large amounts of scar tissue around the wound.

Keratitis Inflammation of the cornea.

Keratoconus Abnormality of the cornea, resulting in apical thinning and bulging.

Keratoplasty Corneal graft.

Ketosis An abnormal amount of ketones in the blood and urine as a result of inefficient metabolism of carbohydrates.

Kirschner wire A thin wire which may be passed through a bone.

Lacrimation Production of tears.

Laminectomy Excision of the posterior arch of the vertebra.

Laparoscopy A surgical procedure to internally examine the abdomen using minimally invasive techniques (keyhole surgery).

Laparotomy A surgical procedure where the abdominal wall is incised either for exploratory procedures or surgery.

Laryngoscopy Examination of the larynx using a laryngoscope.

Laryngospasm Spasm of the larynx.

Latissimus dorsi flap A flap of muscle and skin taken from the latissimus dorsi muscle in the back for reconstructive surgery of the breast, or head and neck.

Lipoma A fatty lump.

Liver ultrasound An ultrasonic scan of the liver used to detect liver disease.

Lobectomy Surgical resection of one or more lobes of a lung.

Lue procedure Operation to straighten the penis.

Lymphadenitis Inflammation of the lymphatic glands.

Lymphoedema Oedema due to the obstruction of lymph vessels.

Magnetic resonance angiography (MRA) A non-invasive scan to accurately detect size and extent of atheromatous lesions in the arteries.

Malnutrition A condition that arises when the body's nutrition becomes depleted. May lead to starvation if not corrected.

Mammogram A radiographic investigation of the breast.

Marsupialization of Bartholin's abscess Drainage of an abscess and suturing the skin edges of the cavity.

Mastectomy Removal of the breast.

Mastitis An infection of the breast.

Meatomy Incision of the urethral meatus.

Meatoplasty Surgical reconstruction of the urethral meatus.

Mediastinoscopy Invasive surgical procedure to visualize and biopsy the lymph glands of the mediastinum.

Mediastinotomy Opening of the mediastinum, allowing insertion of an endoscope.

Melaena Faeces are coloured black with altered blood, as a result of bleeding into the lower part of the digestive system.

Meningitis Inflammation of the meninges.

Menopause The normal cessation of menstruation, commonly occurring at around the age of 50 years.

Menorrhagia Heavy menstrual bleeding.

Mesothelioma A pleural tumour, often associated with contact with asbestos.

Metastases Spread of cancer from a primary tumour, via the blood and lymphatic systems, to other tissue/organs.

Microcalcification Minute chalky deposits in the breast.

Michrodochectomy An operation performed to disconnect a duct in the breast.

Miotic An agent that constricts the pupil.

Morcellated Broken up into small pieces.

Motility The action of spontaneous movement.

Multimodal analgesia The use of different types of analgesics to provide enhanced analgesia while reducing side-effects.

Mydriatic An agent that dilates the pupil.

Myelography A radiological investigation of the spinal cord and subarachnoid space. A contrast medium is introduced through a lumbar puncture in order to identify spinal pathology.

Myomectomy Removal of fibroids, either through laparotomy or laparoscopy.

Myxoedema A syndrome due to hypothyroidism.

Necrotic tissue Localized dead tissue which has a leathery texture and is black/brown in colour.

Needle localization biopsy A mammographically controlled excision biopsy.

Neo-bladder Reconstruction of the whole bladder using bowel.

Nephrectomy Surgical removal of the kidney.

Nephrostomy tube Temporary method of draining the renal pelvis.

Nesbit's procedure Operation which aims to straighten the penis.

Nociception The processing of damaging or potentially damaging stimuli.

Occulentum Ointment.

Occult bloods A specimen of stools obtained for the purpose of detecting small quantities of blood by chemical examination.

Olfaction The sense of smell.

Oophorectomy Surgical removal of one or both ovaries.

Orchidectomy Surgical procedure to remove testes.

Orthoptics Special eye exercises to develop binocular vision.

Ossification The process by which bone is developed.

Osteotomy An operation to cut across bone.

Ototoxicity The degree to which a substance is harmful to the structures of the ear.

Oxygen saturation (SaO$_2$) Measurement of the percentage of oxygen bound to haemoglobin; normal range is 95–99%.

Paget's disease of the nipple A breast cancer involving the nipple and areola.

Palmar Relating to the palm of the hand; also called volar.

Paralytic ileus Reduced peristalsis (motility) in a portion of the bowel, causing the ileum to become obstructed.

Paraphimosis Condition arising from inability to replace foreskin over glans penis.

Parenteral nutrition Nutritional support provided directly into the circulatory system.

Percutaneous An invasive approach through the skin.

Percutaneous transluminal angioplasty (PTA) A balloon catheter is passed into the lumen of the artery at the site of stricture, usually under local anaesthetic, and the balloon inflated, dilating the stricture.

Pericardiocentesis Removal of excess fluid from the pericardial space by needle aspiration.

Perioperative The total surgical journey incorporating pre-, intra- and postoperative phases.

Peripheral vascular disease Impaired circulation to the limbs.

Peristalsis Movement along the wall of a tubular structure.

Pernicious anaemia Anaemia caused by the lack of absorption of vitamin B$_{12}$.

Peyronie's disease Fibrotic process of unknown aetiology, resulting in erectile deformity.

Phacoemulsification A form of cataract removal that uses high-frequency sound waves to emulsify the lens matter, which can then be aspirated more easily.

Phagocytosis The process by which foreign matter is engulfed by phagocytes, e.g. macrophages.

Phasing Regular and frequent measurements of intraocular pressure.

Phimosis Term given to the inability to retract the foreskin over the glans penis.

Phlebitis Inflammation of a vein, which is often associated with clot formation (thrombophlebitis).

Photophobia Sensitivity to light.

Photopsia Sensation of flashing lights.

Pleural effusion (hydrothorax) Collection of fluid within the pleural space.

Pleurectomy Surgical removal of the parietal pleura, in the treatment of pneumothorax.

Pleurodesis Surgical procedure to introduce an irritant substance into the pleural space to cause an inflammatory reaction to adhere the pleural surfaces together.

Pneumonectomy Surgical resection of one lung.

Pneumothorax Abnormal presence of air in the pleural space, causing collapse of the underlying lung.

Postcoital bleeding Bleeding after sexual intercourse.

Postoperative This phase starts when the patient is transferred from the operating theatre to the recovery room.

Potency The dose of a drug required to produce 50% of the maximum response of that drug.

Preoperative Commences either when the patient decides to have surgery and includes the preoperative assessment ensuring that the patient is in optimal health for surgery, or from the moment the patient arrives in the operating theatre. The phase concludes when the patient is transferred onto the operating table.

Presbycusis Progressive deafness that occurs with age.

Priapism A persistent painful erection.

Primary dressing A dressing which is applied directly to the wound surface.

Procidentia Complete prolapse of the uterus so that it extrudes through the vagina.

Proliferation Reproduction of cells.

Proprioception Sensory function which monitors and interprets spatial position and muscle activity.

Proptosis Abnormal protrusion of the eye.

Prostatic stents Implantable device to hold open the prostatic urethra.

Prosthesis Any artificial device attached to the body as a substitute for a missing or non-functional part.

Prosthetic tube An artificial tube fitted into the oesophagus to provide patency to the oesophagus and allow semi-fluid nutritional substances to be taken into the body.

Ptosis Drooping of the upper eyelid.

Pulmonary oedema Accumulation of fluid in the lung tissue, causing prolongation of oxygen transport.

Pulse oximeter An instrument that uses arterial pulsation to detect the level of oxygen saturated on haemoglobin.

Purulent Producing pus.

Pus Fluid containing exudate, bacteria and phagocytes which have completed their work. Is usually seen in infected wounds.

Pyeloplasty Operation to relieve obstruction at the pelviureteric junction in the kidney.

Quadrantectomy Excision of a quadrant of the breast.

Q wave A normal deflection on the ECG that can indicate myocardial necrosis when the Q wave becomes wider than 0.03 seconds and deeper than 1/4 the height of the R wave.

Radiotherapy The treatment of disease with penetrating radiation.

Raised intracranial pressure Pressure within the cranium, resulting from a space-occupying lesion.

Rectocele Hernia and prolapse of the rectum through the posterior vaginal wall.

Reduction Putting a fracture or dislocation in its correct position.

Refraction The convergence of light rays so they focus on the macula.

Regurgitation Backward flow of blood against the normal direction of flow, i.e. blood flows backwards through regurgitant heart valves instead of forwards.

Resection Removal of part of the body by surgery.

Resident flora Microorganisms which reside on the skin and exist in harmony with their host.

Rest pain Severe pain in the leg or foot occurring while the patient is resting, which can prevent the patient from sleeping.

Salpingectomy Surgical removal of one of both Fallopian tubes.

Salpingitis Inflammation and infection of the Fallopian tubes.

Salpingo-oophorectomy Surgical excision of one or both Fallopian tubes and ovaries.

Sclerotherapy A treatment for varicose veins in which the affected veins are injected with a solution that causes inflammation of the vein lining, clotting of the contained blood and adherence and closure of the vein.

Secondary dressing A dressing which holds a primary dressing in place.

Segmentectomy Surgical resection of an anatomical segment of a lobe of lung.

Self-concept An individual's percepts, concepts and evaluations about themselves, including the image they feel others have of them and of the person they would like to be.

Self-esteem The outcome of the process of self-evaluation and self-worth, i.e. thinking favourably of oneself; evaluation of one's self-worth.

Sensory inattention The inability to detect touch or pain in both limbs when the stimulus is applied to both the limbs simultaneously, caused by a lesion in the parietal lobe.

Sentinel node The first lymph node draining the site of a cancer.

Septicaemia Presence of bacteria in the bloodstream, accompanied by symptoms of infection and illness.

Seroma A fluid collection.

Serosanguinous Composed of serum and blood.

Sinus A wound where one end is open to the skin, with a track leading to a blind cavity.

Skin graft A piece of skin that has been totally separated from its blood supply, to be used on another area.

Skin graft take The adherence and healing of a skin graft.

Sloughy tissue Devitalized tissue which contains some exudate, and is yellow, white or grey in colour.

Staging Investigations to detect metastatic disease.

Stenosis An abnormal narrowing of a orifice or opening of a vessel.

Stent A small tubular mesh structure that prevents an artery or other hollow structure from collapsing.

Stoma An artificial opening of a tube that has been brought to the surface.

Strabismus Squint.

Stress A response to a difficult situation, or a set of circumstances which require an unusual response.

Stress incontinence Incontinence caused by increased abdominal pressure, e.g. in coughing.

ST segment A section on the ECG that represents the resting period of the heart, which, when abnormally elevated above the isoelectric line, indicates acute myocardial injury and myocardial infarction. ST depression indicates myocardial ischaemia.

Subarachnoid haemorrhage A haemorrhage from the vessels of the circle of Willis into the subarachnoid space.

Subcuticular Within the subcutaneous tissues.

Subluxation A partial dislocation.

Surgical emphysema Air in the subcutaneous tissue that can result from thoracic surgery and pneumothorax.

Sympathectomy Surgical excision to remove part of the sympathetic nervous system supply to an area in order to limit constriction of the blood vessels and therefore increase blood flow.

Sympathetic ophthalmitis Severe uveitis in one eye following trauma involving the uvea of the other eye.

Synovectomy Excision of diseased synovial membrane.

Tachyarrhythmia Abnormal heart rhythm that may be regular or irregular at a rate greater than 100 beats per minute: e.g. ventricular tachycardia, which may cause hypotension and hypoperfusion.

Tachypnoea Rapid respiratory rate greater than 20 breaths per minute.

Tamponade The abnormal presence of blood or fluid in the pericardial space, which can prevent the heart chambers from filling adequately with blood, and may lead to shock and death.

Tenesmus A painful condition when the faeces will not be expelled from the rectum despite the effort of straining.

Tension pneumothorax Like a pneumothorax, but a flap of tissue allows air to enter but not leave the pleural space, causing increased intrathoracic pressure and is potentially fatal.

Tentorial herniation The herniation of the uncus of the temporal lobe between the brainstem and the tentorium cerebelli when the intracranial pressure is greater above the tentorium cerebelli than below it.

Tetany A condition marked by spasms of the hands and feet, due to a diminished blood calcium level.

Thiersch graft The name given to split skin grafts.

Thoracentesis Aspiration of fluid from the pleural cavity.

Thoracoscopy Endoscopic examination of the pleural surfaces.

Thoracotomy Surgical opening of the chest.

Thrombectomy Surgical removal of a thrombus from within a blood vessel.

Thrombolysis Dissolution of a clot in a vessel using a thrombolysing agent.

Thrombosis Formation of blood clot within a blood vessel.

Thymectomy Resection of the thymus gland.

Thyroidectomy Surgical removal of the thyroid gland.

Thyrotoxicosis A condition produced by overactivity of the thyroid gland.

Tie-over pack A type of pressure dressing used on Wolfe grafts.

Tinnitus Noise in the ear, ringing, rushing or buzzing sound.

Tissue expander An inflatable device which is inserted under the skin and slowly expanded in order to provide enough skin to cover an adjacent defect without the need to use additional donor skin.

Torsion of the testis Twisting of the testis on its mesentery.

Total abdominal hysterectomy Surgical removal of the uterus and cervix, via an incision in the abdomen.

Total parenteral nutrition The provision of full nutritional support via routes (intravenous or subcutaneous) other than the mouth or rectum.

Tracheostomy An opening through the neck into the trachea with an indwelling tube inserted.

Traction A pulling or drawing force.

Transducer A device that converts a physical variable, e.g. pressure, into an electrical waveform: e.g. blood pressure is recorded directly from an artery, and the waveform and pressures are displayed on a monitor.

Transient flora Microorganisms which are transferred onto the skin through contact with other people or objects.

Transluminal Through the space/lumen of a blood vessel.

Transverse rectus abdominus myocutaneous flap A flap of muscle and skin taken from the abdominal muscle to reconstruct the breast.

Trousseau's sign A spasm of the muscles, occurring in tetany, if pressure is applied over large arteries or nerves.

Tru-cut biopsy An incisional biopsy taking a small core of tissue for histological diagnosis.

T-tube A tube placed into the common bile duct following exploration or surgery to keep the common bile duct patent, allowing bile to be passed freely until any oedema subsides.

Ultrasound A radiological investigation using sound waves.

Urethroplasty Open operation to reconstruct the urethra.

Urethrotomy Endoscopic cutting of urethral stricture.

Urgency Overwhelming desire to pass urine immediately.

Urinary flow rate The rate and volume of urine voided in mL.

Urinary frequency Voiding frequency, e.g. up to 10–12 times per day.

Urinary incontinence Absence of voluntary control over the passing of urine.

Vacuum-assisted closure Application of topical negative pressure to a wound, to assist closure in wounds healing by secondary intention and after the application of skin grafts.

Vaginal hysterectomy Removal of the uterus and cervix via the vagina.

Valgus Displacement outwards.

Varicocele Varicose condition of the veins of the spermatic cord.

Varus Displacement inwards.

Vasectomy Surgical procedure for sterilization of the male.

Vasoconstriction Contraction of blood vessels.

Vasodilatation Dilatation of blood vessels.

Vasovasostomy Surgical procedure for reversal of vasectomy.

Venography X-ray examination of venous system by injecting a radio-opaque contrast medium.

Ventricular aneurysm Bulging, thinning and enlargement of part of the ventricle wall due to myocardial infarction.

Vertigo Hallucination of movement; dizziness.

Viscera The internal organs of the body cavities.

Vulvectomy Total or partial excision of the vulva.

Wedge resection Surgical excision of part of a lung without reference to anatomical divisions.

Wide local excision Removal of a lump plus a good margin of healthy tissue surrounding it.

Wolfe graft The name given to full-thickness skin grafts.

Wound An injury which causes tissue damage and may result in the loss of continuity of the skin or tissue.

Xenograft An animal graft.

Acknowledgements

I would like to acknowledge the following authors who contributed chapters to the first edition of *Nursing the Surgical Patient*: Delia Smith, Clare Shaw, Carolyn Galpin, Mary Malone, Karen Dutton, Gobnait Waters, Jan McCabe, Stephanie Chabane, Suzanne Owen, Angela Hallett, Jean Douglas, Imogen Rider and Hilda Bradbury.

Rosemary Pudner 2004

SECTION I

The basis of surgical care

SECTION CONTENTS

Chapter 1

Preoperative assessment

Melanie Oakley

Key objectives of the chapter

At the end of the chapter the reader should be able to:

■ give a definition of preoperative assessment and what is involved

■ discuss the three key components of preoperative assessment and how they interface with each other

■ detail what is involved in the physiological assessment and the criteria for preoperative investigations

■ discuss the psychological component of preoperative assessment

■ identify the sociological considerations needed when preoperatively assessing a patient.

INTRODUCTION

Undergoing anaesthesia and surgery promotes anxiety in most patients. Anxieties will include the amount of pain patients will experience following surgery and whether they will suffer nausea and vomiting. Many patients are highly anxious about the anaesthetic, and common questions are 'Will I be awake during the anaesthetic?' and 'Will I wake up when it is over?' These fears are normal and the nurse caring for the patient must accept them and develop strategies to reassure patients, empowering them with the knowledge to enable them to cope with the forthcoming anaesthesia and surgery.

Traditionally, patients requiring surgery were admitted the day before. Recently, the trend has been to admit the patient on the day of surgery, because financially this is more prudent. This can lead to the patient not being adequately prepared for the surgery both physically and psychologically. Furthermore, they may have social problems that prevent the surgery or lead to an extended stay in hospital. Added to this, patients often do not attend for surgery, or when they do, the surgery is no longer necessary (NHS Modernisation Agency, 2003). This system is not only anxiety provoking for the patient and time consuming but it is also a waste of hospital resources. Thus, a thorough assessment prior to admission should negate all these problems.

This chapter will examine preoperative assessment, how it has evolved and more importantly how it has benefited the patient undergoing anaesthesia and surgery.

WHAT IS PREOPERATIVE ASSESSMENT?

Preoperative assessment establishes that the patient is fully informed and wishes to undergo the procedure. It ensures that the patient is as fit as possible for the surgery and anaesthetic. It minimises the risk of late cancellations by ensuring that all essential resources and discharge requirements are identified and co-ordinated.

(NHS Modernisation Agency, 2003:2)

This definition is multifaceted: the first part implies that the patient consents to the procedure and this involves all the issues around informed consent. The second part examines the physiological considerations that must be taken into account to ensure the patient is as fit as possible to undergo anaesthesia and surgery. The final part incorporates a number of issues. There is acknowledgement that sociological considerations must be taken into account and discharge must be discussed before admission. Late cancellations are also an issue: from August 2001 to November 2002, 52% of inpatient cancellations in the United Kingdom were due to patient cancellations (NHS Modernisation Agency, 2003). It is only by being rigorous in preoperative assessment that there will be a reduction in late cancellations. The nearer the cancellation to the day of surgery the greater the impact, e.g. if the patient cancels their surgery the day before or the day of surgery it is unlikely that theatre time will be able to be reused; this is added to the obvious cost implications of having a vacant bed and wasted theatre time.

AIM OF PREOPERATIVE ASSESSMENT

Preoperative assessment should take into account the physiological, psychological and social needs of the patient undergoing surgery. Dependent upon one's perspective, different emphasis may be put on one aspect to the detriment of the other. Each aspect of preoperative assessment must be given time, because they are of equal importance and are not mutually exclusive (Fig. 1.1). It is laudable to have a patient who is fit for anaesthesia and surgery from a physiological perspective but who on return to their home is the primary carer for their partner (Box 1.1). Practice Exemplar 1 illustrates that the psychological and social aspects of care are just as important as the physiological. It also demonstrates the efficacy of a preoperative assessment.

Thus, preoperative assessment should be multifaceted, and when assessing the patient prior to surgery, the following should be aimed for:

- reduction of fears and anxieties by giving a full explanation of the procedure and making sure the patient understands what is going to happen to them
- assessment of the patient's fitness for the impending anaesthesia and surgery, with interventions as appropriate
- assessment of whether the patient is suitable for day surgery or inpatient surgery
- identification of specialist requirements, e.g. critical care beds
- provision of preoperative instructions
- provision of a contact point
- provision of information about the recovery process postoperatively
- provision of an opportunity for health promotion/ patient teaching
- assessment of the patient's needs post-discharge
- commencement of multidisciplinary preoperative documentation.

Ideally, preoperative assessment should take place following the surgical consultation. The preassessment clinic should always have a consultant anaesthetist available for patient referrals, but there is no reason why the preoperative clinic should not be nurse-led if they work within agreed protocols and have the appropriate training and experience (Association of Anaesthetists of Great Britain and Ireland, 2001). Both inpatient and

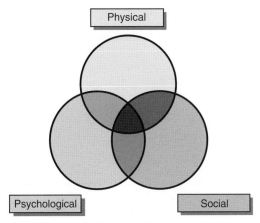

Figure 1.1 Illustration of how the three components of preoperative assessment are inextricably linked: when viewing one, the other two have to be taken into consideration.

Box 1.1   Practice exemplar 1

A fit 70-year-old man was admitted to the day surgery unit for bilateral carpal tunnel syndrome repair; he had not been to the preoperative assessment clinic. On admission the nurse admitting him discovered that he was the primary carer for his disabled wife. The operation was explained to him and the degree to which he would be infirmed following surgery. He agreed that it was going to be a problem but doing the hands one at a time was not an option as leaving his wife for 2 days was a problem. He was adamant about this, and arranging support from the community services rectified the situation. This took time and the operation was delayed until later in the day in order to make sure this was facilitated.

---

day surgery preoperative assessment clinics within the NHS are nurse-led, with the facility to refer patients with multiple problems to the consultant anaesthetist. Once seen, the patient should be given a date for admission (Association of Anaesthetists of Great Britain and Ireland, 2001).

NURSE-LED PREOPERATIVE ASSESSMENT

In day surgery the majority of preoperative assessment is undertaken by nurses and it is this innovation that

has led the way for the development of inpatient preoperative assessment that is nurse-led. Barnes et al (2000) express the view that:

> some aspects of pre-operative preparation can be delegated to trained nurses

> (Barnes et al, 2000:576)

Continuing on from this, Kinley et al (2002) compared the effectiveness of appropriately trained nurses in preoperative assessment with that of pre-registration house officers. They found that the nurses were *'non-inferior'* to house officers; furthermore, it was found that the house officers ordered considerably more unnecessary tests than the nurses. Both these studies were undertaken by members of the medical profession and both appeared to be surprised with the results. However, Clinch (1997) indicated that nurses achieve quality with preoperative assessment clinics. In addition, a number of studies have addressed the issue of improved patient satisfaction with nurse-led preoperative assessment clinics (Muldowney, 1993; Pulliam, 1991).

With the reduction in doctors' working hours, nurses are well placed to run these clinics and have unique skills that enhance the assessment of the patient prior to surgery. However, this should be a collaborative venture. The anaesthetist is responsible for the patient undergoing anaesthesia and thus should make the final decision as to whether that patient is fit for surgery; therefore, the assessment nurse and the anaesthetist should work in partnership to give the best care to the patient. There should be mutual respect for each other's abilities and recognition that each will be viewing the assessment interview from different paradigms. Protocols should be put in place to aid the nurse in this venture. Barnes et al (2000) used a computer-based protocol package to assess orthopaedic patients over 65 years of age and found that the assessment carried out by the nurses was thorough and well thought out.

As mentioned previously, preoperative assessment is divided into three areas and each of these will now be examined in more depth.

PHYSICAL ASSESSMENT

The aim of this assessment is to ensure that the patient is fit for anaesthesia and surgery. To ascertain this, the American Society of Anesthesiologist's (ASA) (1991) fitness for anaesthesia scoring system is utilized (Table 1.1). In day surgery patients generally have to be ASA 1 or 2, but patients who are ASA 3 can and are considered. Inpatient preoperative assessment will also utilize this scoring system, but obviously being ASA 3 onwards

Table 1.1 American Society of Anesthesiologists (ASA) classification of physical status

Class	Description
Class 1	The patient has no organic, physiological, biochemical or psychiatric disturbance. The pathological process for which surgery is to be performed is localized and does not entail systematic disturbance
Class 2	Mild to moderate systematic disturbance caused by either the condition to be treated surgically or by other pathophysiological processes
Class 3	Severe systematic disturbance or disease from whatever cause, even though it may not be possible to define the degree of disability with finality
Class 4	Severe systemic disorders that are already life threatening; not always correctable by operation
Class 5	The moribund patient who has little chance of survival but is submitted to operation in desperation
Class 6	A declared brain-dead patient whose organs are being removed for donor purposes

Source: American Society of Anesthesiologist's (1991) *ASA Classification of Surgical Patients.* Chicago: ASA.

does not exclude the patient from anaesthesia and surgery.

All patients having a preoperative assessment will be categorized as to the urgency of their surgery. The categorization system recommended by the NHS Modernisation Agency (2003) is the National Confidential Enquiry into Peri-operative Deaths (NCEPOD) categories (2002) which gives an indication of the time span until surgery (Table 1.2).

In order to assess health status, a comprehensive questionnaire is given to the patient, which will act as a 'trigger' for further investigations if required (Appendix). It is not necessary to routinely carry out investigations on all patients. Investigations should only be done where indicated: not only does this mean that the patient is not subjected to painful procedures but it also saves time and has considerable financial implications. Investigations are not normally indicated in patients prior to minor surgery who are otherwise healthy. Each hospital should have policies about the investigations to be performed (Table 1.3).

Furthermore, to add clarity to the investigations that should be carried out prior to surgery, the National Institute for Clinical Excellence (2003) have issued guidance on what investigations to carry out dependent upon the grade of surgery and the ASA status of the patient (Table 1.4). For example, a patient who is graded as ASA 1, having grade 1 surgery, and is over 80 years old will require a 12-lead ECG, whereas the patient who is ASA 1, having grade 1 surgery, who is under 80 years old will require no investigations.

Whether the patient is an inpatient or a day surgery patient, information must be given to them about fasting prior to surgery, as the majority will be admitted on the day of surgery and they will be already fasting. The guidelines on fasting prior to surgery are clear – 6 hours for solid food; 4 hours for breast milk and

Table 1.2 NCEPOD categories giving indications for when surgery should be performed

Category	Description	Timing
NCEPOD 1	Resuscitation runs concurrent to surgery	Within 1 hour
NCEPOD 2	Resuscitation can be followed by surgery	Within 24 hours
NCEPOD 3	Not life threatening but need early surgery	Within 3 weeks
NCEPOD 4	Surgery at a time to suit the patient and surgeon	To suit patient and surgeon

Source: adapted from NHS Modernisation Agency (2003:6).

2 hours for clear non-particulate and non-carbonated fluids (Association of Anaesthetists of Great Britain and Ireland, 2001). Obviously, if fasting times are exceeded, particularly in the older or younger patient, supplemental intravenous fluids must be considered.

PSYCHOLOGICAL ASSESSMENT

As seen in Figure 1.1 the three categories of assessment – i.e. physical, psychological and social – are inextricably linked. Determining the perceptions and emotions the patient has about the forthcoming surgery is equally as important as the more concrete components of assessment. The psychological part of preoperative assessment is implicit rather than explicit in the whole process of assessment (Sutherland, 1996).

However, understanding how the patient feels about anaesthesia and surgery is a skilled process. It is about asking relevant questions and listening to the responses given, but also being prompted by things

Table 1.3   A guide to investigations prior to surgery

Test	Description
ECG	Not normally performed in men under 40 years old and women under 50 years old, but indicated in patients with a cardiac or related history
Hb	Only required where the Hb may be low or there may be anticipated significant blood loss during surgery
Biochemistry	Only where medical history indicates
Chest X-ray	Where indicated in accordance with recommendations from the Royal College of Radiologists (1998)

Source: adapted from Association of Anaesthetists of Great Britain and Ireland (2001).

Table 1.4   Surgery grades

Grade	Example
Grade 1 [Minor]	Drainage of a breast abscess
Grade 2 [Intermediate]	Knee arthroscopy
Grade 3 [Major]	Total abdominal hysterectomy
Grade 4 [Major +]	Total hip replacement
Neurosurgery	
Cardiovascular surgery	

Source: adapted from the National Institute for Clinical Excellence – *Preoperative Tests: The use of routine tests for elective surgery* (2003).

the patient is not telling you. Asking a patient if this is his first operation will tell the assessment nurse 'yes' or 'no'. However, this can be built upon by follow-up questions, such as if it is the first operation, 'Do you have anything that is worrying you about it?'. This gives the patient a chance to discuss issues. Remember it is often very small things that will make the patient anxious. The skill of the assessment nurse is to put themselves in the patient's position and forget the knowledge they have as a nurse. Things that seem obvious to healthcare professionals are not obvious to patients who lack nursing and medical knowledge. Family and friends may have told them things, but this may be misinformation.

Whether the patient is having day or inpatient surgery the anxiety will be similar. Just because a patient is having minor surgery or indeed a procedure under local anaesthetic does not preclude them from feeling anxious (Sutherland, 1996). Unfortunately, the assessment process will not address all anxieties or indeed stop the patient being totally without anxiety.

Commonly, the terms stress and anxiety are used interchangeably; however, it is important to look at the concepts individually to understand how the terms are inter-related. In the 1970s and 1980s some of the seminal work on stress and anxiety was carried out, most of which applies today.

Stress can be defined in three ways:

1. **As a stimulus** – meaning that the human condition will have a stressful reaction to any number of stressors in the environment, e.g. meeting new people or hunger (Bond, 1986). Clearly, though, this does not explain stress in its entirety because not everyone will experience a stress response to the same things and the effects of stress will not consistently be the same in each individual.

2. **As a response** – the main proponent of this idea of stress was Selye (1976). This explanation of the stress response is primarily a physiological one and is known as the *general adaptation syndrome*. Whatever the stressor, the processes and systems involved were the same. This neuroendocrine response has three distinct phases: *alarm*, which involves the release of adrenaline (epinephrine) and noradrenaline (norepinephrine) as a reaction to the stressor; *adaptation*, which is characterized by circulating glucocorticoids; and *exhaustion*, where the individual is no longer able to respond to the stressor. If there is prolonged exposure to the stressor from a physiological perspective, it will become life threatening. However, the general adaptation syndrome theory fails to recognize the psychological component of stress.

3. **As a transaction** – this builds upon the work of Selye but takes the view that stress is derived from how we interpret situations and how we cope with the stressor (Lazarus, 1976). Coping involves two processes: primary and secondary appraisal. Primary appraisal looks at the situation and secondary appraisal is when the decision is taken as to how to deal with the situation. This view's strength is the proposition that stress is a necessary function and it results in learning and an improved ability to cope.

Salmon (1993) put forward an interesting hypothesis regarding anxiety, as he suggested that anxiety might serve to reduce the physiological stress response to surgery. He cited studies that demonstrated that patients who had been prepared psychologically prior to surgery, whilst needing less postoperative analgesics, had high levels of urinary adrenaline (epinephrine). Salmon (1993) concluded that rather than take a paternalistic approach to preparing patients for anaesthesia and surgery, perhaps the approach should be to empower the patient. He concludes:

> Rather than countering these (fears) with reassurance the nurse communicates acceptance of these as genuine (as distinct from suggesting that they are realistic).

> (Salmon, 1993:328)

The view that Salmon (1993) puts forward demonstrates the link between the physiological and psychological components of preoperative assessment. It also demonstrates that preoperative assessment should be facilitative and empowering.

REDUCING STRESS DURING THE PREOPERATIVE ASSESSMENT

There are many ways that nurses can help the patient to control anxiety during the preoperative assessment. At this point it must be noted that nurses who carry out preoperative assessment should not be newly qualified or junior staff nurses. It is the experienced nurse that makes the excellent preoperative assessment nurse. By virtue of being more senior, such nurses will have more experiences to draw upon and will probably have undertaken advanced practitioner skills, in order to enhance their role in preoperative assessment.

The main way the nurse can reduce stress in the preoperative assessment is to make sure that patients have all the information they want. This is opposed to giving patients all the information there is to give. This is the skill of the preoperative assessment nurse: to be able to discover by conversation with patients what it is they want to know. The nurse also needs to pick up on the 'cues' that patients will undoubtedly be giving about the information they want to receive.

Mitchell (1997) suggests the anxiety levels can be significantly reduced if the information being given is related to the individuals' coping styles. He looked at internal and external locus of control. Individuals with external locus of control will believe that their life is shaped by others, fate and destiny. Those with internal locus of control will believe that they will be able to influence their future. Applying this to the patient in the preoperative assessment, the individual with an internal locus of control will try and gather as much information as possible in order to feel more in control of the situation. By contrast, the patient with an external locus of control, if given information about the forthcoming anaesthetic and surgery, will only become more anxious and would express the opinion that they would rather not know what is going to happen to them. The skill of the preoperative assessment nurse is being able to differentiate between the two individuals.

INFORMED CONSENT

As alluded to previously, giving information to the patient is key to the psychological component of preoperative assessment. Furthermore, within the information given is the issue of informed consent. One of the fundamental components of informed consent is the concept of information giving, and once the information has been given the patient must consent to treatment (Department of Health, 2001). In order for consent to be valid the patient must understand the information given. Thus, in order to obtain informed consent the patient must understand the information given to them and there must be open communication between the assessment nurse and the patient. As will be seen later in this chapter, there are a number of reasons why a patient may receive the information but may not understand it and this is relevant to the concept of informed consent.

Consent consists of three elements:

1. The capacity of the patient to understand the proposed treatment.
2. The disclosure of information, meaning an understanding of the proposed treatment and an awareness of the potential side effects.
3. Consent should be made on a voluntary basis, which may not apply if the patient has had their premedication (Cahill and Jackson, 1997).

When consent for treatment is gained in the preoperative assessment clinic, it does not guarantee that patients will feel the same way by the time they are admitted for surgery. Wicker (1991) suggests that signing the consent form is only an indication that at that point the individual gives their consent to the operation. Thus, consent should therefore be discussed again on admission.

Thus, gaining informed consent is an integral part of the psychological assessment prior to surgery. The surgeon usually undertakes this role, but the nurse can be an integral part of the process by making sure that the patient understands the treatment to be undertaken.

SOCIAL ASSESSMENT

The aim of this assessment is the same whether the patient will be a day case or an inpatient: i.e. to make sure that discharge is a seamless process but viewed as part of the whole care of the patient. In day surgery, discharge criteria are strictly adhered to (see Ch. 3), and if these criteria are not able to be met the patient will not have their procedure carried out as a day case. The same is applicable to inpatients, but obviously there is more time to make sure the discharge criteria are facilitated.

The social assessment will primarily look at care and support of patients once at home, and having someone to take them home. Obviously, for the day surgery patient it is imperative that they have someone to take them home, as they may only have had a general anaesthetic a matter of hours ago. An assessment will also be made of the dependants at home, the level of input required and the support the patient will get at home: for example, for a mother with small children it may be more viable to have her surgery done as a day case; however, the level of support she will get following surgery needs to be ascertained.

If preoperative assessment takes place, all these issues can be addressed, and often it is useful if the patient's chosen carer is present. This ensures that all the information is heard by two people and the carer is aware of the role they must play, and strategies can be developed to ensure that all discharge criteria are met. It must be noted that it may not always be appropriate to have the patient's chosen carer in the assessment interview, and thus the patient's permission must always be sought.

PATIENT INFORMATION

To supplement the information provided at the preoperative assessment interview, instructional leaflets are given to reinforce the information that has been given to the patient. However, it may be that patients never read this information, or indeed may not have heard or understood the verbal information for a number of reasons. The nurse carrying out the preoperative assessment interview must be aware of how adults learn and also assess whether they understand both verbal and written instructions. To facilitate this, the nurse must look at their practice and the information being given in a critical way.

HOW ADULTS LEARN

We are all individuals and this individuality encompasses physical characteristics such as age and gender, and psychological characteristics which include motivation, personality, intelligence, learning styles and expectations (Quinn, 2000). These must be accepted and incorporated into the preoperative assessment interview.

According to Knowles (1990), adult learners have general characteristics that can be applied to preoperative assessment. The first characteristic is the need to know: it cannot be disputed that all patients undergoing anaesthesia and surgery want to know what is going to happen to them, even if it is only the basic information. The second characteristic is that of self-concept, with patients broadly divided into two categories: some patients will expect information to be given to them, and they will be passive recipients of the information; other patients, while receiving the information actively, will seek answers to their questions and probe further in order to be active in their care. The third characteristic of the adult learner is previous experience. The patient will come with a number of previous experiences that will determine how they receive the information given to them.

What must also be considered in adult patients is their readiness to take in information. There may be many reasons why that information may be listened to but then ignored – this may be anxiety about the forthcoming anaesthesia and surgery and a host of other things. Finally, patients' motivation is integral in their ability to accept and retain the information being given to them. Motivation is based upon perceived need: if patients do not perceive they need the information being given to them, they will not remember it (Box 1. 2).

To summarize, the adult learner must find the information being given to them in the preoperative assessment interview personally meaningful and appreciate the significance of that information (Posel, 1998). Thus,

---

Box 1.2 Practice exemplar 2

A 23-year-old woman attended the preoperative assessment clinic. She was undergoing minor surgery, but had had to take time off work to come to the clinic. She perceived herself as fit and healthy and did not see the need to come to a preassessment interview; consequently, she did not really listen to what was being said, and the nurse conducting the interview did not pick up on this. When she was admitted to the day surgery unit it was found that not only had she come on her own on the bus but also that she had eaten a chocolate bar on the way as she had not had any breakfast. As she said to the nurse admitting her, 'It's not proper food is it?' Obviously, there had been a communication breakdown because of this lady's perceived need.

the preoperative assessment nurse must be aware of this and develop strategies to ensure that the patient listens and understands the information being given. One of the ways of doing this is by giving an information sheet to supplement what has been discussed. However, there may also be problems with giving patients information by this route.

PATIENT INFORMATION SHEETS

Giving a patient an information sheet can never be an effective substitute for verbal communication. However, information sheets do have the advantage of reinforcing verbal information and they can be kept as a reference for the future, which not only the patient can read to remind themselves, but the information can be shared with family and friends (Dixon, 1992; Dixon and Park, 1990).

In 1993 the Audit Commission identified that the quality and content of patient information sheets were a common cause for complaint amongst patients, so when designing an information sheet a number of issues must be considered. Healthcare practices are based upon the evidence available, and that evidence changes regularly in order that practice is moved forward. This means that information sheets will become outdated, so it is important to make sure that they have a date on and are reviewed on a regular basis (Scriven and Tucker, 1997).

Information sheets should be organized in a way that makes sense to the patient. It is useful to pilot the information sheet with patients, in order to check that it has all the information on it they want, which may not be the same as what healthcare professionals think is important (Box 1.3).

Consideration must be given to the format of the information sheet: 'frequently asked questions' is a good way to get the information in an easily understood form. Attention must be paid to the length of the information sheet. One page is ideal, perhaps double-sided, but if more than three or four pages are required, it is useful to have a table of contents so that patients can pick out the salient points (Dixon, 1992).

The writing style is also important, and consideration must be given to the fact that the average reading age of adults in Western countries such as the United Kingdom is between 10 and 14 years old (Vahabi and Ferris, 1995). Therefore, everyday language must be used, without the use of medical words that patients will be unable to understand. Various readability tests have been devised to test how easy information sheets are to read, and take into account sentence construction and the number of words with more than three syllables (Maynard, 1999).

The design of the information sheet must also be well thought out. Probably the size of the font is the most important part of the information sheet: a font no smaller that 12 point should be utilized, and should be larger for elderly and ophthalmic patients. The font should not be too decorative, and commonly used and acceptable fonts are Times New Roman and Arial. The colours of the information sheet are largely a matter of taste, but it should not be so colourful that it detracts from the information being given to the patient. Headings should be in bold, but not underlined (Seker, 1997).

It can be seen from the previous discussion that information sheets are an integral part of the preoperative assessment, but must be used with caution and require thought before being given to patients. Many issues need to be considered and patients need to be consulted as part of the evolution of any information sheet.

In addition, consideration must be given to groups where English is not the first language and so information sheets must be available in other languages based upon the demographics of the area.

Another group requiring special consideration comprises the elderly and patients who are visually impaired. Information sheets should be available in a larger font and preferably in bold. The other end of the age continuum should also be considered and information should be available for children in a form that they will understand and be suitable for the age group. In both these client groups, the information can be supplemented by videos and may even be presented on a compact disc.

BARRIERS TO RECEIVING INFORMATION

Communication and exchange of information become more difficult if time constraints are put on the preoperative assessment interview; therefore, time must be allowed for the interview. The preoperative assessment should always be done, if at all possible, before the day

---

Box 1.3   Practice exemplar 3

A 34-year-old woman was admitted for induction of labour. Prior to this, she had been given an information sheet. She followed the instructions. She eventually went into labour 3 days later, by which time she was highly anxious, because the sheet did not tell her that induction of labour could take a number of days and possibly more then one pessary. The obstetric unit had given her the information they thought she needed to have but had not stopped to consider what a first-time mother would know and the assumptions she would make. She had thought that she would have had the baby the same day and that induction of labour was faster than normal labour!

of surgery. Obviously this is not always possible, but in the majority of cases this can be done ideally following the surgical consultation. The patient will then have time to assimilate the information and an opportunity to ask questions or ring up later in order to clarify any issues. The interview should take place in a quiet room where patients' responses cannot be overheard, so that they feel able to discuss any issues of concern that they may have. Patients should not be made to feel they are being hurried and time should be given to allow them to absorb the facts, which should also be supplemented with written information sheets.

A unique problem to patients having their procedure as a day case is that it may be perceived as 'minor', and not as much value placed on it as a 'major' procedure. They may feel that they should not take up too much time because the time is needed for more 'serious cases'. They may not listen to the information as carefully as they should, and so it is the preoperative assessment nurses' role to assure them that their procedure is just as valid and important as any other, and take as much time to discuss with the patients what they will experience.

RECORD KEEPING

It may be an obvious point to make, but all aspects of the preoperative assessment must be clearly documented. Once the documentation has been written, it becomes a legal document and can be used as evidence in a court of law (Nursing and Midwifery Council, 2002). The Nursing and Midwifery Council (2002) document on standards for records and record keeping details the reasons for keeping records, saying they should provide:

- comprehensive information on the condition and care of the patient
- a record of problems arising and the action taken
- evidence of care and intervention and the response of the patient
- a record of the physical, psychological and social factors which may impact on the patient
- a record of events and decision making
- a baseline against which improvement or deterioration can be measured.

In addition, the following guidelines should be followed when completing any documentation:

- Abbreviations should be avoided. Within the profession we all understand these, but they are open to misinterpretation.
- Nothing should be written that is overtly humorous or false, because these may become defamatory.
- Documentation should be written clearly and grammatically correct, otherwise it may leave the practitioner open to action for negligence.
- Documentation should be factual and concise.

Each preoperative assessment clinic will have its own form of documentation, which will have been scrutinized taking the above factors into account. Furthermore, the NHS Modernisation Agency (2003) has developed templates that can be utilized for a new preoperative assessment clinic, or could be used as a guide to changing existing documentation.

CONCLUSION

This chapter has examined preoperative assessment of the patient prior to anaesthesia and surgery. The advent of day surgery units and the absolute need to assess day surgery patients before the day of their surgery has led the way, and has set the template for assessment of inpatient surgical patients. It has been demonstrated that the preoperative assessment is more than an assessment to determine fitness for anaesthesia and surgery. It has to incorporate the psychological and social aspects of the patient's life in order to make the assessment meaningful. Therefore, preoperative assessment should be viewed as three elements that are not mutually exclusive. Furthermore, assessing the patient prior to surgery gives the patient some knowledge of what to expect and facilitates an empowering experience rather than taking a paternalistic approach. In addition, there are significant financial benefits and hospital time is allocated more appropriately. Finally, this is an ideal opportunity for nurses to develop not only their physical assessment skills but also their time management, organizational and communication skills.

Summary of key points

- Preoperative assessment is vital for all patients who are undergoing surgery.

- The preoperative assessment should be nurse-led, as nurses have unique skills and knowledge they can bring to this process.

- The preoperative assessment comprises three elements – physical, psychological and social – which are not mutually exclusive, and therefore a holistic approach must be taken to preoperative assessment.

References

American Society of Anesthesiologists (1991) *ASA Classification of Surgical Patients.* Chicago: ASA.

Association of Anaesthetists of Great Britain and Ireland (2001) *Pre-operative Assessment. The Role of the Anaesthetist.* London: Association of Anaesthetists of Great Britain and Ireland.

Audit Commission (1993) *What Seems to be the Matter: Communication between Hospitals and Patients.* London: HMSO.

Barnes, P. K., Emerson, P. A., Hajnal, S., et al (2000) Influence of an anaesthetist on nurse-led, computer-based, pre-operative assessment. *Anaesthesia* 55(6): 576–589.

Bond, M. (1986) *Stress and Self Awareness – A Guide for Nurses.* London: Heinemann.

Cahill, H. & Jackson, I. (1997) *Day Surgery Principles and Nursing Practice.* London: Baillière Tindall.

Clinch, C. (1997) Nurses achieve quality with pre-assessment clinics. *Journal of Clinical Nursing* 6(2): 147–151.

Department of Health (2001) *Consent – What Have you a Right to Expect? A Guide for Adults.* London: Department of Health.

Dixon, E. & Park, R. (1990) Do patients understand written health information? *Nursing Outlook* 38(6): 278–281.

Dixon, M. (1992) Please take a leaflet. *Nursing* 5(5): 11–13.

Kinley, H., Czoski-Murray, C., George, S., et al (2002) Effectiveness of appropriately trained nurses in preoperative assessment: randomized controlled equivalence/non-inferiority trial. *British Medical Journal* 325(7376): 1323.

Knowles, M. (1990) *The Adult Learner: A Neglected Species,* 4th edn. Houston: Gulf Publishing.

Lazarus, R. S. (1976) *Psychological Stress and the Coping Process.* New York: McGraw-Hill.

Maynard, A. M. (1999) Preparing readable patient education handouts. *Journal for Nurses in Staff Development* 15(1): 11–18.

Mitchell, M. (1997) Patients' perceptions of pre-operative preparation for day surgery. *Journal of Advanced Nursing* 26(2): 356–363.

Muldowney, E. (1993) Establishing a pre-admission clinic. *AORN Journal* 58(6): 1183–1191.

National Confidential Enquiry into Peri-operative Deaths (2002) *Functioning as a Team?* London: NCEPOD.

National Institute for Clinical Excellence (2003) *Preoperative Tests: The Use of Routine Preoperative Tests for Elective Surgery.* London: National Institute for Clinical Excellence.

NHS Modernisation Agency (2003) *National Good Practice Guidance on Preoperative Assessment for Inpatient Surgery.* London: NHS Modernisation Agency.

Nursing and Midwifery Council (2002) *Guidelines for Records and Record Keeping.* London: Nursing and Midwifery Council.

Posel, N. (1998) Preoperative teaching in the preadmission clinic. *Journal for Nurses in Staff Development* 14(1): 52–56.

Pulliam, L. (1991) Client satisfaction with a nurse-managed clinic. *Journal of Community Health Nursing* 8(2): 97–112.

Quinn, F. M. (2000) *Principles and Practice of Nurse Education,* 4th edn. Cheltenham: Nelson Thornes.

Royal College of Radiologists (1998) *Making the Best Use of a Department of Radiology. Guidelines for Doctors,* 4th edn. London: Royal College of Radiologists.

Salmon, P. (1993) The reduction of anxiety in surgical patients: an important nursing task or the medicalization of preparatory worry? *International Journal of Nursing Studies* 30(4): 323–330.

Scriven, A. & Tucker, C. (1997) The quality and management of written information presented to women undergoing hysterectomy. *Journal of Clinical Nursing* 6(2): 107–113.

Seker, J. (1997) Assessing the quality of patient-education leaflets. *Coronary Health Care* 1(1): 37–41.

Selye, H. (1976) *The Stress of Life.* New York: McGraw-Hill.

Sutherland, E. (1996) *Day Surgery. A Handbook for Nurses.* London: Baillière Tindall.

Vahabi, M. & Ferris, L. (1995) Improving written patient education materials: a review of the evidence. *Health Education Journal* 54(1): 99–106.

Wicker, C. P. (1991) Legal responsibilities of the nurse 3. Assault and consent. *Surgical Nurse* 4(1): 16–17.

Further reading

Basford, L. & Slevin, O. (2003) *Theory and Practice of Nursing. An Integrated Approach to Care in Practice,* 2nd edn. Cheltenham: Nelson Thornes.

Dimond, B. (1995) *Legal Aspects of Nursing,* 2nd edn. London: Prentice Hall.

Jarvis, C. (2004) *Physical Examination and Health Assessment,* 4th edn. St Louis: W. B. Saunders.

NHS Modernisation Agency (2002) *Step Guide to Improving Operating Theatre Performance.* London: NHS Modernisation Agency.

Relevant websites

http://www.nmc-uk.org (accessed 13 April 2004). Nursing and Midwifery Council.

http://www.modern.nhs.uk (accessed 13 April 2004). NHS Modernisation Agency.

http://www.nice.org (accessed 13 April 2004). National Institute for Clinical Excellence.

APPENDIX – Preoperative Assessment Questionnaire

Name:		The South West London **NHS**
Hospital No.:		Elective Orthopaedic Centre
DOB:		ICP for Total Hip Replacement

Day of ICP:	Pre ~ Assessment	Date: ___/___/___

Pre Operative Assessment – Advanced Practitioner

Assessment/Medical History			
Current Symptoms	PMH		
Duration of Symptoms			

Assessment/ Medical History	NO	YES	Outcome
Hypertension			
Diabetes Controlled by			Type 1/Type 2
History of MI			
CVA			
Asthma/COPD Managed by			
Epilepsy Managed by Date of last fit			
TB When Where			
RH fever When			
Jaundice			
DVT/PE			
Anaemia			
Peptic Ulcers Managed by			
Rheumatoid Arthritis			
Long term anti-coagulation therapy Reason			
Recipient of human pituitary hormone			
Recipient of graft of human dura matter			

Day of ICP:			Pre ~ Assessment	Date: ___/___/___

Pre Assessment AP	Family history of CJD			
	Current Smoker			Amount: For how long:
	Previous Smoker			Amount: For how long: Gave up when:
	Alcohol			Units per week
	Allergies			**Antibiotics, Opiates, Latex, Iodine, Elastoplast, Other:**
	Systems enquiry			**Outcome**
	Cardiovascular	NO	YES	Description:
	Chest Pain			
	Palpitations			
	Ankle Oedema			
	Orthopnoea			
	Claudication			
	Respiratory			
	Cough			
	Wheeze			
	Sputum			
	SOB			
	Haemoptysis			
	Abdo			
	Regular			Aperients used:
	Pain			
	Blood PR			
	Dyspepsia			
	Urinary			
	Dysuria			
	Frequency			
	Incontinence			
	Prostatic Symptoms			

	Systems Enquiry	NO	YES	Outcome
	CNS			
	Headaches			
	Dizziness			
	Blackouts			
	Faints			

	Activities of daily living Assessment	NO	YES	Outcome
	Communication English 1st language			
	Interpreter required			
	Problems with vision			Wears glasses/contact lenses/
	Problems with hearing			
	Sleep Problems with sleeping			Usual Pattern / Use of aids to sleeping
	Nutrition Food allergies			
	Difficulty in swallowing			
	Pressure area risk			Waterlow score
	Nutrition state risk			Nutrition score
	Skin intact			Details
	Oral Assessment			
	Teeth			Own / Full dentures / Partial dentures / Caps / Crowns
	Mouth			
	Consenting			
	Preliminary consent for operation obtained			
	Consented to sharing of information for NJR			
	Preliminary consent for anaesthesia obtained			
	Consent for bone donation			

Name:
Hospital No.:
DOB:

The South West London NHS
Elective Orthopaedic Centre
ICP for Total Hip Replacement

Pre Assessment AP

Name:
Hospital No.:
DOB:

The South West London NHS
Elective Orthopaedic Centre
ICP for Total Hip Replacement

Day of ICP:	Pre ~ Assessment-Physical Examination	Date: ___/___/___

Jaundice / Anaemia / Cyanosis / Clubbing / Lymph Nodes / Ankle Oedema

C.V.S: BP: Pulse:

Height   Weight   BMI

Peripheral Pulses		Comments
Heart Sounds:		

Abdomen Soft: Yes / No   Mass: Yes / No   PR   BS

Comments

Respiratory:
Expansion   Rt.   Lt.
Percussion
Auscultation

Signed: Print Name: Date:___/___/___

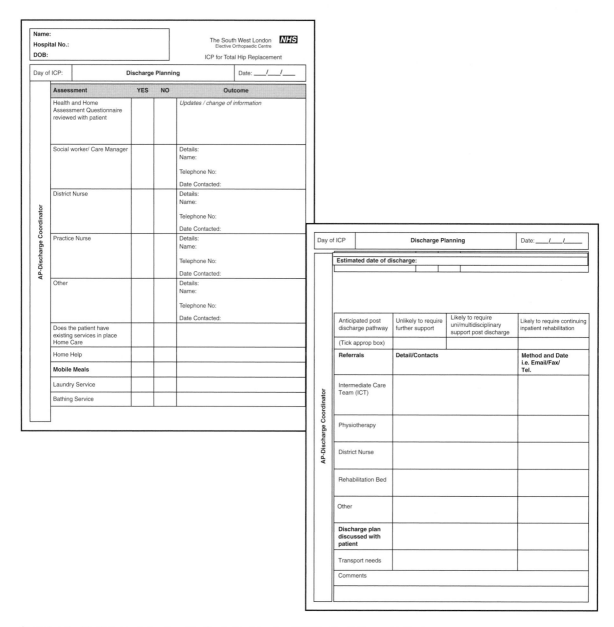

Reproduced with kind permission from The South West London NHS Elective Orthopaedic Centre.

Chapter **2**

Perioperative care

Diane Gilmour

Key objectives of the chapter

The aim of this chapter is to provide a broad introduction to the holistic care given by nurses within the perioperative environment during the patient's immediate preoperative, intraoperative and postoperative phases of their surgical experience.

This chapter will:

- give a definition of the perioperative period

- describe the various roles of the nurses and other healthcare workers within the perioperative environment

- explore in depth the needs of patients during these phases of their surgical experience, and how care for the individual physical and psychological needs can be adapted

- illustrate how technology and innovation has changed perioperative patient care.

INTRODUCTION

Historically, for patients, student nurses and other hospital staff, the perioperative or theatre area has been seen as one of high drama and action, as portrayed regularly by the media, many having preconceived ideas about the roles and contribution made by those within the environment. Yet for many individuals, it is a time when they are most vulnerable or scared. For patients, they are asleep, unsure if they will wake up and what will happen to them; for student nurses, it is a strange experience, which to begin with they feel unable to relate to other environments; and for other hospital staff, they feel as if they are entering an environment where everything is different and goes on behind closed doors. Ensuring that the highest standard of patient care is delivered to each, individual patient throughout their journey within the perioperative environment is fundamental to the perioperative nurse's role. Patient interaction and communication is essential, although covert if the patient is asleep, as perioperative nurses assess, prepare, plan and implement care. This chapter will demonstrate that perioperative nursing care is patient orientated and that nurses must have a thorough knowledge and understanding of the environment. This will enable them to deliver patient care safely, effectively and without harm to that patient.

PERIOPERATIVE PERIOD

'Perioperative' refers to the total surgical experience and includes pre-, intra- and postoperative phases of the patient's surgical journey (Phillips, 2004). For the purpose of this chapter the perioperative period is from the minute the patient arrives in through the operating theatre doors to the moment they leave through those same doors post-procedure.

PREOPERATIVE VISITING

Preoperative visiting is not a new concept and has been around since the 1980s. Researchers have shown that visiting patients in the preoperative period can reduce anxiety, aid recovery and allow the patient the opportunity to express concerns and fears about the impending procedure (Boore, 1978; Copp, 1988; Hayward, 1975). The preoperative visit allows perioperative nurses to learn about their patients, establish a rapport, and develop a plan of care before the patient arrives in the department. In some hospitals preoperative visiting is advocated, particularly for those patients admitted the day before. However, preoperative visiting has met with resistance from staff due to limited staffing, timings of the visits and availability of the patient themselves (Phillips, 2004; Taylor and Campbell, 1998; Torrance and Serginson, 1997).

In modern surgery, the period of hospitalization both before and after surgery is decreasing rapidly and most patients are admitted less than 24 hours before surgery, many on the actual day. Although visits to the patient would broaden the scope of the perioperative nurse's role and contribute to the continuity of care,

the patient may have their anxiety heightened by the continual visits from different multidisciplinary teams immediately prior to surgery and in a relatively short period of time. Pre-admission/assessment clinics are now an essential part of the patient's surgical pathway in preparing the patient for surgery, and are discussed more fully in Chapter 1 (Phillips, 2004; Taylor and Campbell, 1998; Torrance and Serginson, 1997).

Communication between such clinics and perioperative staff is therefore essential to ensure that patient's specific needs are identified at this early stage, and preparation by perioperative staff ensures that the patient's needs are met.

ELECTIVE OR EMERGENCY SURGERY

Surgical procedures can be broadly categorized as either elective (that which is planned) or emergency (that which is unplanned). Elective surgery aims to be performed when the patient is in optimal health but before the surgery affects the quality and threatens their life: e.g. an inguinal hernia can become life threatening if the bowel becomes obstructed within the sac. Clinicians decide if a planned procedure is 'urgent' or can be arranged at a time convenient for the surgeon and patient (Phillips, 2004; Smith, 2000).

Emergency surgery may be as a result of trauma or an accident, gastrointestinal obstruction, or from perforated viscera. The injury may be immediately life threatening, and therefore the procedure will be carried out within 1–2 hours from admission. Other emergencies may require procedures within 24–48 hours following the injury, but in both instances it may not be possible to preoperatively screen these patients. Information may be limited, and therefore it is essential that the perioperative team communicate with each other to coordinate the delivery of safe patient care during this potentially traumatic period in the patient's journey (Smith, 2000).

For this chapter the emphasis will be on the care of the patient for elective surgery, as many of the principles discussed apply to any patient undergoing a surgical procedure.

PATIENT PREPARATION

Preparing the perioperative environment starts before the patient arrives. Turner et al (2000) identified that the perioperative environment is potentially one of the most hazardous of all clinical environments. The only information that may be available for the staff is retrieved from the operating theatre list, which is written daily and produced ideally 48 hours before the scheduled surgery (National Health Service Modernisation Agency, 2002). At a minimum, this should detail the patient's name, age, gender and procedure. This will enable the perioperative nurse to prepare their own area to ensure a safe working environment. For example, knowing the patient's age allows the anaesthetist and recovery nurses to prepare the correct equipment for the management of that patient's airway; the procedure will identify how this patient will be positioned and potentially how long they may be in that position for. However, liaison with the preassessment clinic may also have highlighted specific needs for that patient, such as latex allergy (requiring special preparation of the theatre environment), immobility problems, hearing impairment or medical history requiring additional interventions from the clinicians.

MEETING AND GREETING THE PATIENT

The patient is escorted to the operating theatre either with a porter or ward nurse, or both. Ward staff must check the patient's identity, operating consent form, patient notes, and that all documentation is completed before the patient is transferred to theatres (NATN, AODP, RCN et al, 1998; Taylor and Campbell, 2000a). The patient may be transported by wheelchair or on their bed, or in some hospitals, particularly within a day surgery unit, they are given the choice of walking (Phillips, 2004). Depending on the facilities within each unit, the patient is either admitted to the holding area (this may be part of recovery) or waits in reception. The patient at this time may have their stress and anxiety heightened due to the unknown environment and unfamiliar staff. It is therefore essential that the perioperative nurse communicates effectively with patients, to ensure that they understand the actions being performed, and that they are able to question and challenge these at any time (Reid, 2003). An accurate assessment at this time by the perioperative nurse will form the basis for delivering high standards of patient care tailored to meet their needs (O'Reilly, 2001). An adult or parent may accompany a child to the operating department and therefore the perioperative care extends to the whole family. Parents themselves may be anxious as they relinquish care of their child to strangers and consideration of their needs as well as the child's needs to be defined (NATN, 1996).

Adolescents, too, may have concerns about their surgery but be too embarrassed or scared to articulate those fears and, depending on their age and hospital policy, may be nursed in an adult or paediatric ward (Smith, 2000).

An elderly patient may be confused and require additional explanations and reassurance. The nurse

with experience may assess the patient's skin condition, mobility and general appearance as an indication of the patient's health and well-being (Smith, 2000).

The patient should be greeted by name and then the nurse should introduce themselves to the patient. A preoperative checklist should be completed in accordance with hospital policy (Table 2.1). This documentation ensures that the correct operation is carried out on the correct patient, who has been prepared to enable the safe administration of anaesthesia and continuation of the surgical procedure. At all times the patient must be treated with privacy, dignity and respect. Perioperative nurses also need to provide equitable and appropriate care with respect to cultural, religious, ethnic and racial beliefs (NATN, 1999a).

THE PRINCIPLES OF CARE DURING ANAESTHESIA

The anaesthetic nurse will, based on the information known or relayed by the anaesthetist, prepare the anaesthetic room, anaesthetic machines and all other equipment to ensure the maintenance of a safe environment for the delivery of care during anaesthesia. This will include not only preparing the anaesthetic equipment but also applying knowledge and skills of anaesthesia related to age, medical history and surgical procedure to ensure that the patient's individual needs are met: e.g. if the patient is elderly, then additional precautions are needed when caring for their skin; if the patient has language difficulties, an interpreter may be required.

An anaesthetic nurse must hold an appropriate, recognized qualification as identified by the Royal College of Anaesthetists in 1998. The nurse must also continue to demonstrate continuing knowledge, skills and understanding in the field of anaesthesia (NMC, 2002).

King (1998: p 95) listed those skills required by the anaesthetic nurse and essential to patient care in the anaesthetic room as:

- communication
- comfort and dignity
- reassurance and explanation
- consideration of patient's special needs.

Patients may be frightened or anxious, which can inhibit communication at this point. Barriers, such as the wearing of a mask when greeting the patient, undue background noise such as talking and telephones and lack of explanations when performing tasks, must be removed. It is therefore essential to support and reassure the patient, offer appropriate explanations and provide care based on their needs at the time (Taylor and Campbell, 2000b). Communication is not

Table 2.1 The preoperative checklist

To check	Rationale
Name/date of birth of patient	To ensure that this is the correct patient with the correct notes. The date of birth acts as an additional check, as patients with the same name may be on the same ward
Consent	Written consent is preferred as it provides documentary evidence (NATN, 1999b; Reid, 2003). The consent form should clearly state without abbreviations the operative procedure and should be signed by the patient (exceptions apply such as minors, life-threatening situation, legally or mentally incompetent (Hind, 2000)) and a qualified practitioner competent to carry out the procedure. For consent to be valid the patient must be informed of the procedure, its expected outcomes, benefits, potential risks and alternatives (NATN et al, 1998; Hind, 2000). The perioperative nurse must check the patient's understanding of the procedure to safeguard their autonomy (Reid, 2003)
Procedure site is marked	Side or site is clearly marked with an indelible marker to avoid confusion. This should then be confirmed with the patient's notes, X-rays and the operating list. It is the responsibility of the person performing the procedure to ensure that the correct side/site is marked (NATN et al, 1998)
Last ate or drank	Patients must fast preoperatively to minimize the risk of inhaling gastric contents while under anaesthetic, which could prove fatal (Jester, 1999; Dean and Fawcett, 2002). Dean and Fawcett (2002) recommend that fasting times for fluids should not normally be less than 2 hours or more than 4 hours, and that for solids fasting should be not less than 4 hours or more than 6 hours. Rowe (2000) also identified that prolonged fasting preoperatively can result in dehydration, hypoglycaemia and confusion. Reducing fasting times may improve wound healing, comfort and postoperative outcomes
Allergies	Identify allergies to minimize risk for patient during surgery. These should include elastoplast, specific drugs (antibiotics, suxamethonium, or any that contain eggs or nuts), fluids such as iodine, latex, and also note patients' adverse reactions to anaesthetic or blood transfusions (King, 1998; Phillips, 2004)
State of teeth	Caps, crowns, dentures or loose teeth can become dislodged or damaged during intubation and may compromise the airway (King, 1998). Dentures, if tight fitting, and if the patient does not normally remove them routinely, may be left in place throughout the procedure at the anaesthetist's discretion
Jewellery	Some items of jewellery are worn for religious or cultural reasons and may cause offence if removed, so perioperative nurses must respect patient needs. Some body piercings may interfere with the surgery or compromise the airway and may be removed if required.
	Secure all rings and other jewellery to ensure that they are not lost during positioning or moving of the patient (NATN, 1998)
Wearing of any prosthesis	Hearing aids are essential for the patient to communicate with theatre staff, so can be left in until the patient reaches the anaesthetic room and is about to be anaesthetized. The hearing aid should then be removed and given to recovery staff so that they can insert it once the patient regains consciousness.
	Glasses can also be worn to theatres for the same reason.
	Contact lenses should not be worn, because during the procedure there is a risk that they can become dry and may scratch the cornea.
	Other prostheses such as wigs, false eyes and artificial limbs should be removed prior to surgery and retained on the ward for safe-keeping. However, patients may express anxiety and every effort should be made to preserve a patient's dignity and respect during the perioperative period (King, 1998)
Medical and nursing records	All medical and nursing records should accompany the patient to the operating theatre so that an accurate assessment of the patient's history can be made for the delivery of safe perioperative care.
	Documentation should include results from investigations completed at preoperative assessment, blood tests, X-rays and baseline observations (NATN, 1999b)

always verbal and the use of touch, holding the patient's hand and just being a physical presence can offer additional support for the patient (Hughes, 2002). Continuing with cleaning and decontamination of equipment, and preparation of specialist equipment, may be unavoidable while the patient is in the anaesthetic room, but the anaesthetic nurse must be aware that some patients may be afraid of needles, and find such activities distressing, so the nurse should aim to prepare the room before the patient arrives (King, 1998). The anaesthetic nurse may also need to remove dentures, glasses, prostheses or wigs in preparation for surgery. Reassurance, comfort and sensitivity about the patient's potential loss of dignity are essential in reducing the patient's anxiety further (Hughes, 2002).

'*Anaesthesia*' is a Greek word meaning 'no feeling' and '*analgesia*' means 'without pain' (Simpson and Popat, 2002). The anaesthetist must ensure that both anaesthesia and analgesia are achieved and maintained for the duration of the procedure (Simpson and Popat, 2002; Wheeler, 2002). When making a decision about the type of anaesthesia to be administered – i.e. general, regional or local – the anaesthetist will be influenced by the type and technique of the planned surgery, the patient's risk factors, their personal skills and patient's preference. Most anaesthetists assess their patients preoperatively to decide on the type of anaesthetic and any additional requirements required for each individual.

A general anaesthetic can be divided into three components, called the triad of anaesthesia. These three elements are hypnosis (sleep), analgesia and relaxation (usually of the muscles). Different surgical procedures require differing degrees of each. Surgical stimulation and pain can cause a series of physiological responses such as tachycardia, hypertension, sweating and vomiting. Analgesics reduce the body's response to such stimulation (Hughes, 2002). Anaesthetic techniques and drug therapy have evolved, which allow the anaesthetist to adjust the proportions of each part of the triad of anaesthesia to suit individual requirements. For procedures requiring little or no muscle relaxation, the anaesthetist may induce anaesthesia using an intravenous agent (although a gas induction can be used with patients with a needle phobia), and maintain anaesthesia with a volatile agent, allowing the patient to breathe the gases spontaneously via a mask or a laryngeal mask airway attached to the appropriate breathing system. Where muscle relaxation is required after anaesthesia is induced, a muscle relaxant is given and the patient's airway maintained via an endotracheal tube or a laryngeal mask airway, and the patient is connected to a ventilator. The third part of the triad of anaesthesia is analgesia. This is achieved using differing categories of drugs, which block the stimulation of pain at the nerve impulses (Griffiths, 2000). Opioid analgesics such as fentanyl are used intraoperatively because of its short duration of action and thus it can be titrated to the patient's needs. Side-effects include respiratory depression, nausea and vomiting and sedation (Simpson and Popat, 2002).

Regional and local anaesthesia provide the patient with excellent analgesia and negate the need for rendering the patient unconscious. Such techniques include peripheral nerve blocks (injection of a local anaesthetic agent into a plexus of nerves); central nerve blocks (injection of local anaesthetic into the subarachnoid space or epidural space for surgery on lower abdomen, lower limbs and postoperative analgesia); and infiltration anaesthesia (injection of local anaesthetic around the surgical incision site or prior to cannulation) (Avidan et al, 2003; Simpson and Popat, 2002; Wheeler, 2002). Table 2.2 gives information on agents used for anaesthesia.

During regional anaesthesia the patient is awake or sedated, therefore requiring additional reassurance and support from all perioperative staff. Diligence by clinical staff is essential in maintaining confidentiality of other patients and ensuring that minimal noise and interference occurs during the procedure, which may distract the patient and so cause them to move. Conversely, if the procedure is long, it may be difficult for the patient to stay still on an uncomfortable table/bed and therefore sedation may be administered or a combination of general and regional anaesthesia may also be a considered option (Avidan et al, 2003).

The Association of Anaesthetists recommends minimum standards of monitoring during anaesthesia and recovery. During induction of anaesthesia, this will include pulse oximeter, non-invasive blood pressure monitoring, electrocardiogram and capnography (measurement of CO_2 in expired air at end of respiration) (Wheeler, 2002). For those patients undergoing complex procedures, or are high risk due to co-morbidities, monitoring of urine output, body temperature and invasive monitoring such as central venous pressure and arterial pressure are essential.

During the induction of anaesthesia it is important that all personnel are calm and that noise, disruption and disturbance are minimal, as hearing is the last sense to go when the patient loses consciousness. Such ambience will aid the patient's state of mind at this time (Griffiths, 2000).

During the maintenance of anaesthesia the anaesthetic nurse will observe and monitor the patient's well-being. Eye pads may be applied over the eyes to prevent corneal abrasions and to maintain closure of the eyelids to prevent drying of the corneas due to a reduced eye reflex.

The nurse will also assist the operating team to position the patient safely, to minimize potential anaesthetic complications during transfer and the procedure itself (King, 1998).

THE PRINCIPLES OF INTRAOPERATIVE CARE

Patient and staff safety is paramount throughout the perioperative environment and a proactive clinical risk management strategy involves assessing, identifying, controlling, monitoring, reducing and evaluating

Table 2.2 Anaesthetic pharmacology

Type of drug	Names	Functions and side-effects
Induction agent	Propofol; thiopental	Administered in a rapid bolus. Patient unconscious within a few seconds. Maintained in this state until maintenance anaesthesia has taken over. May also be administered as a continuous infusion to maintain anaesthesia or sedation in intensive care. Reduces cardiovascular, respiratory and nervous system activity
Inhalation agent	Isoflurane, halothane, sevoflurane, enflurane, desflurane	Possess relaxing, sleep-inducing and minor analgesic properties. May be used for induction as well as for maintenance. Colourless liquids, but become gases when bubbled through oxygen. Affects heart rate and blood pressure. Relaxes skeletal muscle
Local anaesthetic	Lidocaine (lignocaine), bupivacaine, cocaine	Localized action around site of administration. Drug diffuses into neural sheaths and axonal membranes, then combines with nerve receptor and blocks nerve conduction. Also has a vasodilatation effect so may be combined with a vasoconstrictor. Duration of action, strength and toxicity dependent on each drug and patient's age, vascular supply and general health
Muscle relaxants: depolarizing	Suxamethonium	Drug that induces paralysis to facilitate intubation. Inhibits neuromuscular transmission by preventing muscle being polarized through chemical interference. Blood enzymes break the drug down and muscle becomes repolarized. Rapid onset time and has a short action. Reduced amount of blood enzyme leads to suxamethonium apnoea
Muscle relaxants: non-depolarizing	Atracurium, rocuronium, vecuronium, mivacurium, pancuronium	Drugs that induce paralysis to assist surgical intervention and easier ventilation. Compete at nerve receptor sites and build up as body's response continues to break down competing acetylcholine. Reversal agents such as neostigmine enable rapid build up of acetylcholine to displace muscle relaxant
Analgesics	Morphine, diamorphine, fentanyl, codeine, diclofenac, ketorolac, alfentanil, remifentanil	Basic constituent of anaesthesia. They do not induce sleep. These drugs block nerve responses to painful stimuli by action on receptors, or inhibit chemicals associated with pain. Personal perception of pain based on several factors (sociological and physiological influences) as well as own threshold. Opioids cause respiratory depression, nausea and vomiting and hypotension. Non-opioid analgesics can combine both methods of action and be more effective with reduced side-effects. Non-steroidal anti-inflammatory drugs provide anti-inflammatory action, but can cause gastrointestinal disturbances and defective coagulation

Source: from King (1998), Griffiths (2000) and Simpson and Popat (2002).

risks to improve the quality of care delivered (Wilson, 2000). Within the intraoperative phase, the patient is vulnerable and totally reliant on perioperative nurses and other members of the team to ensure that they come to no harm. Some of these risks have already been addressed with patient identification, informed consent and patient monitoring in the anaesthetic room. Intraoperatively, such clinical risks are associated with patient positioning, the risk of infection, risk of deep vein thrombosis, risk of hypothermia and the risk to both staff and patients from the use of equipment. This list is not exhaustive but identifies those potential risks to each patient undergoing surgery. For each risk, strategies are discussed to minimize the risk to patients and staff.

SURGICAL ACCESS AND POSITIONING

Positioning the patient correctly to enable easy surgical access requires coordination and cooperation from

Table 2.3   Common surgical positions

Surgical position	Description and potential risks	Procedures performed
Supine	Patient lies on their back, with their arms folded and secured across their chest, or on an arm board at less than 90° degrees to the body to prevent brachial plexus injury, or at their side. A lumbar support should be used to prevent postoperative backache. Pressure-relieving devices for the ankles should not hyperextend the knee as this may result in injury	Administration of general anaesthesia. Patient transfer to and from the operating table. Abdominal, breast and lower limb surgery
Lateral	Patient is turned on to their side and the head, rear of chest and pelvis is supported with padded table attachments. Arms are secured to allow venous access. A pillow should be placed between the knees to prevent pressure on bony contact	Hip surgery. Some kidney procedures. Thoracic surgery
Prone	Patient lies on their stomach with their head supported on a ring or turned to one side, and their arms positioned to prevent extension and abduction at the shoulder, either above their head or by their side. The chest must be supported to allow movement of the abdomen for respiration	Spinal surgery. Neurosurgery
Trendelenburg	Patient is in a supine position with a head-down tilt. Abdominal organs fall towards diaphragm due to gravity, allowing greater surgical access. Legs may be bent at the knee to add stability	Lower abdominal surgery, e.g. abdominal hysterectomy. Lower limb surgery, e.g. varicose veins
Lithotomy	Patient lies supine with their legs raised in supporting poles. These may support the calf to ankle or just the ankles are secured. The patient's arms are secured across their chest while the end of the table is removed. The legs are elevated, lowered and positioned simultaneously to prevent lower back injury, sacroiliac ligament damage and pelvic asymmetry. Nerve damage may occur from pressure applied directly from lithotomy poles, which are inadequately padded, to the medial or lateral side of the leg. A lumbar support will prevent postoperative backache	Gynaecological procedures. Urological surgery. Rectal surgery. Obstetric procedures

Source: from Taylor and Campbell (2000a) and Stoker (2002).

the whole team (Table 2.3). Manual handling regulations recommend that the team involved undertake a risk assessment for the moving and positioning of each individual patient, and that relevant aids and methods are used to reduce patient movement and potential injury to both staff and patients (Turner et al, 2000). An assessment will include the physical condition of the patient, nature of the intervention and individual patient needs (NATN, 1998). When positioning patients, consideration should be given to avoiding nerve and joint injury, avoiding mechanical trauma such as shearing, friction burns and damage to soft tissue, and ensuring that at all times the anaesthetized patient is physically well supported.

Nerve injuries are an outcome of poor positioning, with direct pressure resulting in ischaemia to that area: e.g. radial nerve injury can occur if the arm is left hanging over the edge of the operating table; ulna nerve injury due to compression by an inappropriately placed arm support; and fibular nerve injury due to compression when using the lithotomy poles. Perioperative nurses must therefore ensure that mechanical aids and supports are padded and used appropriately (Stoker, 2002).

Shearing forces can occur when moving the patient on the operating table, resulting in tissue damage, which may go undetected. The use of gel mattresses or similar pressure-relieving adjuncts can redistribute the pressure across a wider area (O'Reilly, 2001).

Common sites for skin pressure injury during surgery are the elbows, heels, buttocks and sacrum (Stoker, 2002). A study in the Netherlands identified that pressure ulcer development during surgery is a potentially serious problem and preventative measures should be in place to reduce the risk and incidence. The findings revealed that ulcers developed on the heels and sacrum (Schoonhoven et al, 2002). The risk to the patient increases as the surgery time increases but all patients undergoing surgery are at risk of intraoperative ulceration and Hartley (2003) supports the argument that pressure-reducing overlays for operating tables must be used for all patients.

PREVENTION OF DEEP VEIN THROMBOSIS

Deep vein thrombosis (DVT) is a serious postoperative complication and one where the actions of perioperative nurses can influence the outcome for the patient. DVT occurs as a result of venous haemostasis, tissue or vessel wall trauma and increased coagulant activity. DVT prophylaxis includes the use of graduated compression stockings, low molecular weight heparin and intermittent pneumatic compression (IPC) devices. However, each patient should be assessed to ensure that the appropriate prophylaxis is administered. Intermittent pneumatic compression has been shown to benefit patients undergoing surgery and to be as effective as low molecular heparin but may be limited due to a lack of resources on the ward (Arnold, 2002a; Quantrill, 2001). Risk assessments on each individual patient allow clinicians and perioperative nurses to make an informed decision about the regime for thromboembolic prophylaxis (Arnold, 2002a).

PREVENTION OF INADVERTENT HYPOTHERMIA

Inadvertent hypothermia – i.e. unintended loss in body temperature – is a potential problem for all patients undergoing a surgical procedure. The main contributory factors are:

- the ambient temperature – kept cool to suit the staff comfort
- use of fluids at room temperature – intravenously or on the skin

- unnecessary exposure of the patient before the surgical team is ready
- the patient's age (very young or very old)
- type and length of procedure
- patient's mobility
- effects of anaesthetic agents.

The detrimental effects of hypothermia include increased rates of wound infection, increased blood loss and increased length of stay in recovery and hospital (Harper et al, 2003; Turner et al, 2000). Perioperative nurses can adopt a variety of measures to control and maintain the patient's temperature throughout a surgical procedure and these include the control of the environmental temperature (21–24°C), use of forced air warming blankets, warming intravenous fluids, irrigation and skin preparation fluids and the monitoring of a patient's core temperature. Scott et al (2001) also found that warming therapy reduced the incidence of pressure ulcers intraoperatively.

INFECTION CONTROL IN THE PERIOPERATIVE ENVIRONMENT

The prevention of infection necessitates the understanding of policies and protocols, and the knowledge and skills to adapt them to the perioperative environment. A surgical intervention requires a break in skin integrity and the insertion of instruments and other foreign material into the body tissues, therefore exposing the patient to the potential to acquire an infection. Infection prevention comprises various components, all of which are aimed at reducing the risk of infection to the patient (Table 2.4).

TECHNOLOGY AND ADVANCEMENTS IN SURGICAL PRACTICE

Minimally invasive surgical procedures, drug therapy (particularly in anaesthesia) and the development of electrical equipment (lasers, microwaves) have revolutionized the patient's surgical pathway, altering the length of stay, reducing recovery time and increasing the potential for an early return to normal activity. However, as new technology is introduced, perioperative nurses must understand the principles and specifics of each new piece of equipment, drug or procedure. Turner et al (2000) recommend that every department has a protocol for the introduction of new technology, which includes risk assessments. Nurses are accountable for their own practice and should ensure that they and their colleagues do not harm the patient (NMC, 2002); therefore they should know how

Table 2.4 Infection control practices within the operating theatre department

Area	Infection control
Theatre design	• Location of operating theatre department within the hospital • Ventilation system with minimum 20 air changes per hour • Scheduled preventative maintenance • Controlled access to the department by visitors
Cleaning	• Cleaning between patients • Cleaning at the end of a list • Policies for using correct cleaning fluid depending on purpose • Correct disposal of waste and linen
Staff	• Wearing of correct clothing: i.e. scrub suits, hats and footwear • Appropriate use of personal protective equipment and adoption of standard precautions • Appropriate use of masks • Hand washing • Safe handling and disposal of sharps • Scrubbing and gowning techniques based on evidence and best practice • Maintenance of aseptic technique • Correct sterilization and disinfection procedures
Patient preparation	• Hair removal if needed in theatres immediately prior to the procedure • Use of alcohol skin preparation fluids • Identification of risk factors such as old age, obesity, malnutrition, other co-morbidities • Surgical intervention such as operative site, duration of surgery, wound contamination (such as bowel contents, pus)

Source: from NATN (1997) and Wilson (2001).

the equipment works, any potential dangers, how to avoid them and to acknowledge when they do not have the required knowledge (Turner et al, 2000).

Electrosurgical units and the use of diathermy is now commonplace in the perioperative environment. Electrosurgical units are used in most areas of surgery where coagulation or cutting of tissues is required. Electrosurgery is efficient, effective and can be used for many tasks, although it basically involves the burning of human tissue. Modern units have many safety features to reduce risk, but the use of electrosurgery units is still fraught with potential dangers for both staff and patients (Moyle, 2002; Wicker, 2000). Perioperative staff must have a basic knowledge and understanding of the principles of electrosurgery before delivering safe care to the patient.

Burns constitute the main danger to patients from the inappropriate use and lack of procedures to ensure that safety checks on all associated equipment are made prior to their use. Table 2.5 details some of the risks associated with using electrosurgery and how they may be prevented.

Lasers are used in a wide range of surgical procedures and various types of laser exist. Laser is an acronym for Light Amplification by the Stimulated Emission of Radiation (light energy), and lasers are usually distinguished by the colour of the light they produce and the medium in which they are transported, such as carbon dioxide, argon and potassium titanyl phosphate (KTP).

Potential risks to the staff and patients are:

- from fire due to the use of high temperatures
- eye injury due to laser light inadvertently striking the cornea and destroying it or the retina behind
- skin injury due to burns by the laser beam
- the biological hazards of smoke plume.

Several legislative safety standards exist in all hospital departments where lasers are used and include the requirement for a Laser Safety Officer in each area. The utilization of lasers is rigorously controlled, monitored and recorded, and each perioperative practitioner must have appropriate knowledge and skills so as to be able to participate during a surgical procedure where lasers are used (Taylor and Campbell, 1998; NATN, 1998).

Minimally invasive surgery (keyhole surgery) is now commonplace in many operating theatre departments. Laparoscopic procedures provide an excellent internal view of the abdominal organs, causing less trauma to the abdominal cavity itself, and provide access for removal of the gall bladder (cholecystectomy), appendix, repair of inguinal and hiatus hernias, and in the past few years bowel resections and renal procedures. Complications can arise on trocar and Verres needle insertion, inadvertent insufflation of gas directly into a vessel (pneumoperitoneum) and diathermy injuries, which occur outside the view of the surgeon (McCabe, 2000; Welsh and Singh, 2003). Perioperative nurses must ensure that they are skilled and trained on the equipment and are familiar with the surgical procedure so that actions can be taken to prevent and control such incidences. The use of electrosurgery during laparoscopic procedures presents added risks to those already mentioned. These are due to the proximity of other instruments in a close, confined space, lack of direct all-round vision and the

Table 2.5 Electrosurgery risks

Electrosurgery hazard	Prevention
Insulation on equipment not intact	• Ensure that all equipment, including cables, surgical instrumentation and patient plates, are fully insulated and that any faulty equipment is removed immediately and reported as per hospital policy • Always ensure that surgical electrosurgery equipment is kept within an insulated container throughout the procedure • Do not coil the return electrode cable while in use
Using alcohol-based fluids Alcohol-based fluids are commonly used to prepare the operative skin area prior to surgery. However, if the fluid is allowed to dry or remains pooled in the patient's skin or drapes, then it may be ignited by a spark from the electrosurgery, resulting in a burn	• Alcoholic skin preparations should be avoided. Ensure that if alcohol-based preparation fluid is used that it is allowed to dry or removed with a sterile swab • Ensure that surgical drapes are free from contact with alcohol • Avoid any fluid contact with the electrosurgery unit
Alternative pathways Unintended routes for the electrical pathway due to the patient being in contact with other conductors, or if the patient is wearing a pacemaker	• Patient plate should be as close to the surgical site as possible to reduce length of pathway through patient • Ensure no exposed metal, e.g. from armrests, mayo table stands or metal infusion poles, are touching the patient • For patients with a pacemaker, diathermy should be avoided, or if it cannot, then precautions should be taken to minimize the interference from the electrical current
Smoke inhalation Research has shown that surgical smoke is hazardous to the surgical team who are exposed on a daily basis. The risks are from biological and chemical hazards found in the particulate matter of the smoke (Biggins and Renfree, 2002). Patients require protection too (Rose, 2002)	• Utilization of dedicated smoke evacuators • Wearing of compliant respiratory masks • Regular changing of filters and maintenance of theatre departments
Patient preparation Incorrect preparation of the patient could mean an increase in current density to one area and result in a burn	• Ensure that the patient plate (return electrode) is clean and if single-use is never reused • Ensure good contact with the plate and the patient by placing the plate over a muscular area, away from bony prominences or scar tissue, and remove hair from directly below the plate prior to positioning • If the patient is moved during surgery, ensure that the plate remains intact or replace with another • Record the position of the plate on the patient and the skin condition before and after

Source: from Wicker (2000) and Moyle (2002).

increase in heat energy leaking through the port or entry sites (Moyle, 2002; Wicker, 2000).

SWAB AND INSTRUMENT COUNTING

Managing other risks to patients from within the perioperative environment includes the use and handling of instrumentation; care and handling of specimens; and the swab, needle and instrument count. Perioperative nurses are accountable for delivering a high standard of care that does not cause the patient harm. Negligently using defective equipment during invasive procedures and leaving foreign objects within patient cavities is against the law, as all clinical staff have a duty of care to the patient (NATN, 2003). All swabs, instruments, needles and other sharps must be accounted for at all times throughout the surgical procedure, and are recorded on a 'swab board' for all invasive procedures where swabs, instruments or needles could be retained. A count is performed by the scrub nurse and a circulating practitioner, who may be unqualified. The surgeon is informed at the end of the procedure that the count is correct and the scrub nurse documents this in the patient's care plan (NATN, 2003).

PREPARATION FOR TRANSFER OF PATIENT TO RECOVERY

At the end of the procedure, the patient's perioperative care plan (whether this is an electronic or paper record) is completed: this details the procedure; patient position; position of diathermy plate and other equipment used; skin condition due to position and site of diathermy plate; signatures confirming that the needle, swab and instrument count are correct; skin closure used; and indication of presence of any drains or catheters (NATN, 1999b). The patient is prepared for transfer to the recovery or post anaesthetic unit, which may involve moving the patient to another bed or trolley. Preservation of the patient's dignity and maintaining their safety is paramount. Once the patient has been transferred, the theatre can be cleaned and prepared for the next patient in accordance with local hospital policy.

IMMEDIATE POSTOPERATIVE CARE

For this chapter, the author will use the term 'recovery room' as the word recovery identifies that the care for each patient is being aimed at safeguarding them against the trauma and effects of surgery and anaesthesia (Hatfield and Tronson, 2001). The main objectives of recovery room care are to critically evaluate and stabilize the patient postoperatively, to anticipate and prevent potential complications and to safeguard the patient's well-being until they are able to do so themselves (Starritt, 2000a). The room itself is easily accessible and usually situated within the operating theatre department or in an adjacent area.

The recovery nurse is a skilled and knowledgeable practitioner, able to deal quickly and efficiently with any changes in the patient's condition. Within the perioperative environment, recovery nurses have the greatest autonomy, as they manage a patient's care in the recovery area from arrival through to discharge, only requesting medical assistance when needed. Postregistration courses exist specifically for recovery room nurses but others may opt for high dependency or intensive care training. Recovery room nurses must also have knowledge of both anaesthetic and operating theatre techniques.

The postoperative phase of a patient's journey starts when the patient is transferred from the theatre to the recovery room. However, preparation for each individual patient commences well before the patient arrives. All equipment such as resuscitation, oxygen and monitoring is checked and additional resources acquired if the surgery or anaesthesia indicates that this may be so: e.g. patient warming apparatus if the surgery has been long, provision of analgesic pumps, or pillows if the patient needs to be nursed sitting up due to surgery on the neck. The patient's age will also influence the size of the equipment needed, particularly for children. The transfer cannot occur until the anaesthetist is satisfied that the patient's condition is stable.

During transfer, the anaesthetist and a nurse from the perioperative team accompanies the patient to the recovery area. On arrival, the patient's care is transferred to the recovery room nurse.

The recovery nurse assesses the patient immediately on arrival, with a focus on airway, breathing and circulation (Hatfield and Tronson, 2001; Sharp, 1998; Starritt, 2000a).

AIRWAY

- The patient's airway must be patent, clear of blood or mucus.
- Adequate ventilation must be achieved and this may require assistance with the position of the head/neck or an airway adjunct; e.g. guedal or laryngeal mask airway (which may be present from theatres).
- The patient's position may also affect ventilation, and therefore the patient will need to be moved. The patient should be nursed on their side or supine, depending on the clinician's instructions.
- Oxygen therapy is commenced immediately via an oxygen mask or nasal cannulae. Usually, this is at 40%. Contraindications include chronic obstructive airways disease or where a prescribed percentage of oxygen is required.
- A pulse oximeter is attached to monitor oxygen saturation.
- Professional organizations such as the Royal College of Anaesthetists and the American Society of Post Anaesthesia Nurses recommend that until the patient is able to maintain their own airway continuous one-to-one observation is required.

BREATHING

- Observe the movements of the chest to ensure bilateral even movement and feel the air flowing in and out of the mouth.

- Noisy breathing is obstructed breathing and action must be taken to relieve the obstruction. The nurse may support the patient's airway. However, obstructed breathing is not always noisy, as complete obstruction is characterized by silence.
- Skin colour (lips, nailbeds) may indicate cyanosis.
- Respiratory rate is taken to include depth and pattern. Changes could be an early indication of future respiratory or cardiac arrest.

CIRCULATION

- Once the airway has been established, blood pressure and pulse can be monitored.
- Assessment of perfusion status includes conscious state, skin temperature and pulse and blood pressure, as an indication of perfusion to all vital organs.
- Inspection of wounds and drains for evidence of haemorrhage.

However, it must be remembered that monitors alert staff to changes in condition, but ongoing physical visual assessment and observation will allow staff to detect subtle changes in condition without relying on monitors. The patient may be hypoxic despite a 98% reading on the pulse oximeter (Hatfield and Tronson, 2001).

Once the initial assessment has been completed, the nurse can gather information through an extensive handover from the anaesthetist and theatre/anaesthetic nurse. This should include past medical history, surgical procedure, vital signs, pharmacology given (particularly analgesics), blood loss, intravenous infusions, catheters and drains. It will detail any untoward events that occurred during the surgery and highlight any potential problems for the postoperative period. The anaesthetist will outline any specific postoperative instructions for each patient: e.g. analgesics regime, oxygen therapy and any additional monitoring requirements.

The nurse can then carry out a more thorough patient assessment to include:

- checking of consciousness levels and signs of protective reflexes returning
- intravenous infusions – type, rate and patency of site
- drains – types, amount draining and rate
- urinary catheters – patency, colour of drainage and amount.

Monitoring will include:

- temperature (hypothermia remains a potential risk)

- pulses and sensation following arterial or limb surgery
- wound site
- plaster of Paris casts
- pressure areas

(Hatfield and Tronson, 2001; Starritt, 2000a).

All postoperative assessment and observations must be recorded in the patient's documentation. The immediate postoperative period is fraught with potential complications for each patient, and the recovery room nurse plays a vital role in detecting, preventing and managing dangerous life-threatening conditions by continuous, ongoing assessment of the patient visually and with the aid of monitors.

Waking up from an anaesthetic can be a frightening experience for the patient. The bright lights, uncharacteristic noises, lack of familiarity with the surroundings and pain may disorientate and confuse the patient. Constant communication with the patient during this phase and throughout their recovery is vital to reduce the patient's anxiety. The nurse should communicate any procedures being undertaken even before the patient regains consciousness, as hearing is the first sense to return.

Recovery rooms are often large areas with bays segregated by curtains or screens. Maintaining confidentiality, privacy, dignity and respect is a challenge to all recovery room nurses, as they must juggle the individual needs with those of patient safety.

MANAGING A PATIENT'S PAIN

The objective of effective pain management is to pre-empt pain before it starts. Acute pain is brief in duration, ranges from mild to severe and eases as healing occurs (Starritt, 2000b). However, pain is a subjective and highly individual experience and an accurate assessment can only be made of the severity and extent of the pain with the actual patient. In the postoperative period this can be difficult if the patient is drowsy, confused or crying. The recovery nurse can observe non-verbal clues such as restlessness, grimacing and hyperventilation (Avidan et al, 2003). Hypoxia, hypothermia, anxiety, nausea, fatigue and pain are all symptoms of the body's stress response to surgery. Pain postoperatively can magnify these responses and delay a return to normal function, as well as impair wound healing and predispose the patient to infection (Hatfield and Tronson, 2001).

Planning an analgesics regime postoperatively can start at the preoperative assessment clinic, where staff can discuss the amount of pain to be expected, how long it will last and the options available for managing this after surgery. The patient's perception of the pain can be reduced if they are prepared for and expecting it (Avidan et al, 2003; Hatfield and Tronson, 2001; Starritt, 2000b). The administration of early effective analgesics will optimize the recovery outcome. The patient in pain is anxious, distressed and agitated, yet explanations, reassurance and support can be equally as effective as pharmacological methods (Starritt, 2000b).

Analgesics can be administered through a variety of techniques and routes, i.e. intramuscular injection, intravenous bolus, intravenous patient-controlled analgesia (PCA), epidural, or rectally. Recovery nurses must have the knowledge and skills to understand and administer the different methods and analgesics available, and monitor the incidence and severity of side-effects. PCA is popular with both patients and clinicians, as it avoids the use of injections, eliminates the delay to the patient in receiving analgesia and allows the patient to feel more in control of their own pain and its management (Chumbly et al, 2002).

Assessment of the patient is ongoing, in order to monitor the efficacy of the pain relief. If the pain is controlled, then the patient should be able to move easily on the trolley/bed, take deep breaths and overall feel more comfortable and less anxious. Documentation of the assessment and actions taken must be made in the patient's care plan. (See Ch. 7 for more detailed information on pain management in the surgical patient.)

MANAGING POSTOPERATIVE NAUSEA AND VOMITING

Postoperative nausea and vomiting is a significant postoperative complication and causes the patient stress, discomfort and additional pain. Avidan et al (2003) state that postoperative nausea and vomiting occurs in up to 15% of patients postoperatively, and is the commonest complication in day surgery necessitating overnight admission.

Arnold (2002b) reviewed the factors influencing postoperative nausea and vomiting and how preoperative assessment can assist anaesthetists and perioperative nurses to improve patient care by administering the appropriate treatment promptly. Patients may become pale and experience excessive swallowing or salivation and tachycardia prior to vomiting. If a patient vomits they may be embarrassed, particularly if other patients are in the room, and preserving a patient's dignity and respect at this time is central to the delivery of a high standard of patient care.

Other postoperative complications include:

- pulmonary complications (upper airway obstruction, pneumothorax, aspiration of gastric contents)
- shock
- neurological complications (loss of sensation to affected limb)
- cardiovascular complications (hypotension, arrhythmias, myocardial ischaemia)
- postoperative bleeding
- for diabetic patients, hypo- or hyperglycaemia

(Avidan et al, 2003; Hatfield and Tronson, 2001; Sharp, 1998).

DISCHARGE OF THE PATIENT TO THE WARD

The patient's stay in the recovery room varies considerably, depending on the patient, type of anaesthetic, surgical procedure and postoperative recovery. Guidelines offer advice to staff on the minimum criteria for the safe discharge of patients back to the ward from the recovery room. It is decided by the recovery nurse based on an assessment of the patient's conscious level, respiration, circulation, pain control, haemostasis and wound care (Reed, 2003). These criteria include definitions of acceptable normal limits of postoperative observations, guidance on written information and headings to provide an accurate handover to the ward staff. The recovery room nurse must provide detailed information to a competent nurse who will take on the responsibility for that patient's care.

GENERAL POSTOPERATIVE CARE ON THE WARD

The ward nurse then escorts the patient back to the ward, monitoring the patient's condition throughout the transition. Having settled the patient on the ward, regular recording of vital signs and systemic observation can reveal early indicators of postoperative complications. Close monitoring of the patient will allow immediate action to be taken in the event of a complication. Observations should be recorded initially every 30 minutes and compared to baseline assessment by the anaesthetist and preassessment clinic, and observations in recovery, to provide an overall view of the patient's condition. Observations and their frequency can be reduced as the patient's condition improves (Table 2.6).

The aim of the care is to allow the patient to move along the patient dependence–independence continuum.

Table 2.6   General postoperative nursing care

Observation	Action and rationale	Complication
Level of consciousness	• Patient can be roused easily • Patient becomes gradually aware of surroundings • Patient can explain where they are and what has happened to them	Patient not rousable or confused: • check baseline admission nursing and medical notes • review medication in theatres or recovery • inform medical staff immediately
Respirations	• Monitor rate, depth and chest movement • Breathing should be unhindered • Skin colour is pink or based on baseline assessment of the individual patient • Alert for signs of cyanosis and poor oxygenation • Sitting patient upright as soon as possible will encourage lung expansion and oxygenation	• Reduced respiratory rate may indicate early respiratory arrest • Reduced respiratory rate may be due to analgesics or other drugs administered, and nurses should be aware of what the patient has received and its potential side-effects • Nurses must be aware of patient's medical history when administering oxygen
Pulse	• Monitor and assess against baseline recording • Monitor rate, volume and irregularities • Nurses need to be aware of drugs given in theatre and recovery as they can affect pulse rate	• Rising pulse rate may indicate reduced circulating volume due to haemorrhage • Arrhythmias may indicate cardiac problems and therefore an ECG may be required • Bradycardia may indicate reaction to drugs or cardiac arrest. Inform medical staff immediately
Blood pressure	• Monitor and assess against baseline recording • Nurses need to be aware of drugs given in theatre and recovery as they can affect blood pressure • Blood pressure should return to within patient's normal limits	• Hypotension may indicate haemorrhage or lack of fluid replacement • Hypotension may also be indicative of pain or nausea
Temperature	• Body temperature can alter significantly in surgery and should be monitored on the ward	• Continuing reduction in body temperature may indicate inadvertent hypothermia, reaction to surgical assault or drugs. Warmed blankets, increasing the room temperature and specifically designed warming blankets may be used • Increase in body temperature may indicate postoperative infection; inform medical staff so that appropriate action can be taken
Pain and nausea	• Monitoring of patient's pain and nausea by scoring or dependency • Type and rate of analgesics must reflect patient's needs • Nurses need to be aware of patient's allergies and any drugs administered in theatre and recovery	• Restlessness, agitation, confusion and non-verbal clues indicate increasing pain levels • Restlessness, hypotension and excessive salivation can indicate nausea
Fluid intake	• Encourage fluid intake as soon as possible, dependent on the surgery performed • Accurately record fluid intake if intravenous infusion sited • Monitor infusion site, rate of infusion and type of fluid being administered	• Oral intake should be gradual and halted if the patient is nauseous until more comfortable • Intravenous site becomes blocked or damaged, then it may need to be resited, depending on patient's condition and needs postoperatively • Administration of a blood transfusion requires careful observations and monitoring of the patient
Fluid output	• Every postoperative patient should have noted on their records when they pass urine • Urinary catheters must be checked for patency and flow of urine • The colour, smell and amount of urine must be recorded	• Restlessness and agitation may indicate a full bladder. The patient must be assisted and encouraged to pass urine • If catheterized, ensure patency, no blockages and if no flow a bladder washout may be performed on medical instructions

Table 2.6   (*Continued*)

Observation	Action and rationale	Complication
Neurovascular status	• Monitor colour, warmth, sensation and movement, and circulation return to the affected limb	• Report any change in condition as this may reflect constriction of blood supply or nerve damage • Dressings and plaster casts may also restrict blood supply and may need to loosened or reapplied
Wounds and drains	• Observe for excess blood loss or haemorrhage • Ensure patency of drain	• Excessive blood loss may indicate further haemorrhage. Further pressure wound dressings may be applied and the patient's overall physical status observed closely.

Source: from Torrance and Serginson (1997), Smith (2000) and Hatfied and Tronson (2001).

CONCLUSION

Entering the perioperative environment is a daunting prospect both for student nurses and the patient. Yet it is an essential part of the surgical patient's journey.

Perioperative nursing is perceived as technical, assisting the surgeon or anaesthetist – 'handmaidens' and as such not real nursing. The author hopes that through providing a rationale for nurse's actions, that those who visit the operating theatre department can gain an understanding of the high standard of nursing care that is required and delivered to the individual patient undergoing a surgical procedure. The Code of Professional Conduct clearly states that in caring for patients and clients we must:

- 'Respect the patient or client as an individual'
- 'Protect confidential information'
- 'Co-operate with others in the team'
- 'Maintain your professional knowledge and competence'
- 'Act to identify and minimize risk to patients and clients'.

(NMC, 2002: p 2).

Each perioperative nurse, no matter what their role is, is personally accountable for their practice and the author has demonstrated that the concept of perioperative nursing is centred on the well-being of the patient.

Summary of key points

This chapter has

■ provided a broad introduction to the holistic care given by practitioners within the perioperative environment during the patient's immediate preoperative, intraoperative and postoperative phases of their surgical experience

■ defined the patient's perioperative journey and the nurse's role in delivering individualized patient care

■ discussed the importance of good communication skills irrespective of the area where the nurse is working

■ explored in depth the needs of patients during these phases of their surgical experience, and how care for the individual physical and psychological needs can be adapted

■ identified potential risks for each patient in all three areas in the operating theatre department and the actions taken to prevent these occurring

■ illustrated how technology and innovation has changed perioperative patient care.

References

Arnold, A. (2002a) DVT prophylaxis in the perioperative setting. *British Journal of Perioperative Nursing* 12(9):326–331.

Arnold, A. (2002b) Postoperative nausea and vomiting. *British Journal of Perioperative Nursing* 12(11):24–30.

Avidan, M., Harvey, A., Ponte, J., et al (2003) *Perioperative Care, Anaesthesia, Pain Management and Intensive Care.* Edinburgh: Churchill Livingstone.

Biggins, J. & Renfree, S. (2002) The hazards of surgical smoke – not to be sniffed at. *British Journal of Perioperative Nursing* 12(4):136–143.

Boore, J. (1978) *Prescription for Recovery.* London: Royal College of Nursing.

Chumbly, G., Hall, G. & Salmon, P. (2002) Patient-controlled analgesia: What information does the patient want? *Journal of Advanced Nursing* 39(5):459–471.

Copp, G. (1988) Intra-operative information and pre-operative visiting. *Surgical Nurse* 1:27–29.

Dean, A., & Fawcett, T. (2002) Nurses use of evidence in pre-operative fasting. *Nursing Standard* 17(12):33–37.

Griffiths, R. (2000) Anaesthetic drugs. In: *NATN Back to Basics Perioperative Practice Principles.* Harrogate: NATN.

Harper, C.M., McNicholas, T. & Gowrie-Mohan, S. (2003) Maintaining perioperative normothermia: a simple, safe and effective way of reducing complications of surgery. *British Medical Journal* 326 (7392):721–722.

Hartley, L. (2003) Reducing pressure damage in the operating theatre. *British Journal of Perioperative Nursing* 13(6):249–254.

Hatfield, A. & Tronson, M. (2001) *The Complete Recovery Room Book,* 3rd edn. Oxford: Oxford University Press.

Hayward, J. (1975) *Information: Prescription against Pain.* London: Royal College of Nursing.

Hind, M. (2000) Accountability and the law in perioperative care. In: Hind, M. & Wicker, P. (eds) *Principles of Perioperative Practice.* Edinburgh: Churchill Livingstone.

Hughes, S. (2002) Anaesthetic nursing. *Nurse2Nurse* 2(12):37–39.

Jester, R. (1999) Pre-operative fasting: putting research into practice. *Nursing Standard* 13(39):33–35.

King, R. (1998) Anaesthetic practice. In: Clarke, P. & Jones, J. (eds) *Brigden's Operating Department Practice.* Edinburgh: Churchill Livingstone.

McCabe, J. (2000) Minimally invasive surgery. In: Pudner, R. (ed.) *Nursing the Surgical Patient,* 1st edn. Edinburgh: Baillière Tindall.

Moyle, J. (2002) Surgical diathermy. *Surgery* 20(5):112–114.

National Health Service Modernisation Agency (2002) *Step Guide to Improving Operating Theatre Performance.* London: NHS MA.

NATN (1996) *Nursing the Paediatric Patient in the Adult Perioperative Environment.* Harrogate: NATN.

NATN (1997) *Universal Precautions and Infection Control in the Perioperative Setting.* Harrogate: NATN.

NATN (1998) *Principles of Safe Practice in the Perioperative Environment.* Harrogate: NATN.

NATN (1999a) *Respecting Cultural Diversity in the Perioperative Setting.* Harrogate: NATN.

NATN (1999b) *Operating Department Records.* Harrogate: NATN.

NATN (2003) *Swab, Instrument & Needles Count: Managing the Risk.* Harrogate: NATN.

NATN, AODP, RCN et al (1998) *Safeguards for Invasive Procedures: The Management of Risks.* Harrogate: NATN.

Nursing & Midwifery Council (2002) *Code of Professional Conduct.* London: NMC.

O'Reilly, D. (2001) An analysis of perioperative care. *British Journal of Perioperative Nursing* 11(9):402–409.

Phillips, N. (2004) *Berry & Kohn's Operating Room Technique,* 10th edn. St. Louis: Mosby.

Quantrill, S. (2001) Deep vein thrombosis – incidence and physiology. *British Journal of Perioperative Nursing* 11(10): 442–451.

Reed, H. (2003) Criteria for the safe discharge of patients from the recovery room. *Nursing Times* 99(38):22–24.

Reid, J. (2003) Valid consent to surgery – dispelling the myth and establishing the evidence. *British Journal of Perioperative Nursing* 13(7):288–296.

Rose, R. (2002) The hazard of diathermy smoke plumes. *Nurse2Nurse* 2(12):40–43.

Rowe, J. (2000) Pre-operative fasting: is it time for a change? *Nursing Times* 96(17):14–15.

Schoonhoven, L., Defloor, T. & Grypdonck, M. (2002) Incidence of pressure ulcers due to surgery. *Journal of Clinical Nursing* 11(4):479–487.

Scott, E., Leaper, D., Clark, M. & Kelly, P. (2001) Effects of warming therapy on pressure ulcers – a randomised trial. *AORN* 73(5):921–938.

Sharp, J. (1998) Recovery practice. In: Clarke, P. & Jones, J. (eds) *Brigden's Operating Department Practice.* Edinburgh: Churchill Livingstone.

Simpson, P. & Popat, M. (2002) *Understanding Anaesthesia,* 4th edn. Oxford: Butterworth Heinemann.

Smith, D. (2000) Perioperative care. In: Pudner, R. (ed.) *Nursing the Surgical Patient,* 1st edn. Edinburgh: Baillière Tindall.

Starritt, T. (2000a) Patient assessment in recovery. In: *NATN Back to Basics Perioperative Practice Principles.* Harrogate: NATN.

Starritt, T. (2000b) Pain management in recovery. In: *NATN Back to Basics Perioperative Practice Principles.* Harrogate: NATN.

Stoker, M. (2002) Care and monitoring of the anesthetised patient including the prevention of injuries. *Surgery* 20(3):60–66.

Taylor, M. & Campbell, C. (1998) Surgical practice. In: Clarke, P. & Jones, J. (eds) *Brigden's Operating Department Practice.* Edinburgh: Churchill Livingstone.

Taylor, M. & Campbell, C. (2000a) Patient care in the operating department. In: *NATN Back to Basics Perioperative Practice Principles.* Harrogate: NATN.

Taylor, M. & Campbell, C. (2000b) Communication skills in the operating department. In: *NATN Back to Basics Perioperative Practice Principles.* Harrogate: NATN.

Torrance, C. & Serginson, E. (1997) *Surgical Nursing,* 12th edn. London: Baillière Tindall.

Turner, S., Wicker, P. & Hind, M. (2000) Principles of safe practice in the perioperative environment. In: Hind, M. & Wicker, P. (eds) *Principles of Safe Practice.* Edinburgh: Churchill Livingstone.

Welsh, F. & Singh, S. (2003) Abdominal access techniques, including laparoscopic access surgery. *Surgery* 21(5):125–128.

Wheeler, D. (2002) Principles of anaesthesia: perioperative plans. *Surgery* 20(3):54–58.

Wicker, P. (2000) Electrosurgery in perioperative practice. In: *NATN Back to Basics Perioperative Practice Principles.* Harrogate: NATN.

Wilson, J. (2000) Perioperative risk management. In: Hind, M. & Wicker, P. (eds) *Principles of Perioperative Practice.* Edinburgh: Churchill Livingstone.

Wilson, J. (2001) *Infection Control in Clinical Practice,* 2nd edn. Edinburgh: Churchill Livingstone.

Further reading

Bowler, G. (2002) The role of the scrub nurse. *Nurse2Nurse* 2(12):44–45.

Department of Health (2001) *Consent – What You Have a Right to Expect.* London: DOH.

Fairchild, S. (1999) *Perioperative Nursing: Principles and Practice,* 2nd edn. Boston: Jones and Bartlett.

Meeker, M. & Rothrock, J. (eds) (2002) *Alexander's Care of the Patient in Surgery,* 11th edn. St.Louis: Mosby.

NATN (2001) *Risk and Quality Management System.* Harrogate: NATN.

NATN (2001) *Future Ways of Working Unleashing the Potential of Perioperative Practice.* Harrogate: NATN.

NATN (2004) *Standards and Recommendations for Safe Perioperative Practice.* Harrogate: NATN.

Relevant website addresses

http://www.aorn.org. (accessed 27 February 2004). Association of periOperative Registered Nurses. Restricted access for non-members. American website useful for journal articles and references related to perioperative practice.

http://www.icna.org.uk (accessed 27 February 2004). Infection Control Nurses Association. Restricted access for non-members. Useful for journal articles and references related to any infection control issues in the UK. Details events and study days.

http://www.natn.org.uk (accessed 27 February 2004). National Association of Theatre Nurses. Restricted access for non-members. UK website useful for journal articles and references related to perioperative practice. Details study days and events.

http://www.aspan.org (accessed 27 February 2004). American Society of PeriAnethesia Nurses. Restricted access for non-members. American website useful for journal articles and references related to anaesthetic and recovery practice.

http://www.barna.co.uk (accessed 27 February 2004). British Anaesthetic and Recovery Nurses Association. Restricted access for non-members. UK website useful for journal articles and references related to anaesthetic and recovery practice. Details study days and events.

http://www.modernnhs.uk/theatreprogramme (accessed 27 February 2004). Details all aspects of the Operating Theatre and Preoperative Assessment Programme, including publications, national guidance, 'good news' stories, and examples from practice and diagnostic tools.

Chapter 3

Day surgery

Melanie Oakley

Key objectives of the chapter

At the end of the chapter the reader should be able to:

- give a definition of day surgery and an explanation of what it involves

- discuss the history and development of day surgery

- state the advantages and possible disadvantages of day surgery

- discuss the surgical and anaesthetic techniques employed in day surgery

- describe the recovery of the patient following surgery

- discuss the discharge criteria for the day surgery patient.

INTRODUCTION

WHAT IS DAY SURGERY?

A surgical day case is a patient who is admitted for investigations or an operation on a planned non-resident basis and who nonetheless requires facilities for recovery in a ward or unit set aside for this purpose (Royal College of Surgeons, 1992).

In 1992 the Royal College of Surgeons indicated that day surgery was the best option for 50% of all patients undergoing elective surgical procedures. Patients could receive a faster, more efficient service as day surgery patients, and hospital costs would decrease (Audit Commission, 1990). The National Health Service Management Executive (NHSME) Day Surgery Taskforce (1993) estimated that 60% of all elective surgery should be performed as day cases by 1997–98. Currently, 68% of all elective surgery is carried out as day surgery, but the NHS Plan predicts that this should increase to 75% (Department of Health, 2002).

Day surgery is a specialist area of care where patients are admitted into a designated day surgery unit for minor and intermediate surgery and discharged home the same day. Specialist training and education are recognized as important elements for the provision of high-quality patient care in this area, and guidelines have been produced to ensure that patients receive high-quality care (NHS Modernisation Agency, 2002).

HISTORY AND DEVELOPMENT OF DAY SURGERY

The history of performing operations as day cases goes back nearly a century when it was reported in the *British Medical Journal* that Professor James Nicholl, a paediatric surgeon, and his colleagues had been performing day case operations at a children's clinic in Glasgow (Nicholl, 1909, cited by Bradshaw and Davenport, 1989). Despite explaining the cost-saving implications and the benefits, the development of day surgery in the UK has been slow compared with that in North America.

During the past decade there has been a steady increase in day case treatments and operations. The results of research demonstrate the quality and acceptability of such care alongside cost advantages (Audit Commission, 1991; NHS Modernisation Agency, 2002). Day surgery has become popular, and its practice has accelerated throughout Europe.

ADVANTAGES OF DAY SURGERY

The economic benefits of day surgery can be seen as reductions in waiting lists and the increased availability of inpatient hospital beds. However, reduced costs should not be seen as the only advantage of day surgery. High-quality patient care and patient acceptability need to be achieved alongside cost savings, in order to maintain an economical, efficient and quality service. Day surgery allows for a high throughput of patients and reduces surgical waiting lists. It also has a low incidence of major morbidity, reduced cross-infection risks and lends itself to audit (NHS Modernisation Agency, 2002).

Box 3.1   The Audit Commission 'basket of 25'

- Orchidopexy
- Circumcision
- Inguinal hernia repair
- Excision of breast lump
- Anal fissure dilatation and excision
- Haemorrhoidectomy
- Laparoscopic cholecystectomy
- Varicose vein stripping and ligation
- Transurethral resection of bladder tumour
- Excision of Dupuytren's contracture
- Carpal tunnel decompression
- Excision of ganglion
- Arthroscopy
- Bunion operations
- Removal of metal ware
- Extraction of cataract with/without implant
- Correction of squint
- Myringotomy
- Tonsillectomy
- Submucous resection
- Reduction of nasal fracture
- Operation for bat ears
- Dilatation and curettage/ hysteroscopy
- Laparoscopy
- Termination of pregnancy

Box 3.2   British Association of Day Surgery 'trolley' of procedures suitable for day surgery in some cases

- Laparoscopic hernia repair
- Thoracoscopic sympathectomy
- Submandibular gland excision
- Partial thyroidectomy
- Superficial parotidectomy
- Wide excision of breast lump with axillary clearance
- Urethrotomy
- Bladder neck incision
- Laser prostatectomy
- Transcervical resection of endometrium (TCRE)
- Eyelid surgery
- Arthroscopic menisectomy
- Arthroscopic shoulder decompression
- Subcutaneous mastectomy
- Rhinoplasty
- Dentoalveolar surgery
- Tympanoplasty

Many patients prefer to have their aftercare at home rather than in hospital, and patient surveys indicate high levels of satisfaction with day case treatment (Theus et al, 1995). Patients can avoid an unnecessary hospital stay, have minimal disruption of daily routine and can return home to recover in familiar surroundings. Day surgery is not a new concept of care; it has been used throughout the century. However, now that the benefits of day case procedures are evident, it has become increasingly popular.

Most surgical specialties can utilize a day surgery unit. In 1990 the Audit Commission produced a 'basket of procedures', which numbered 20; however, this 'basket' was updated in 2001 (Audit Commission, 2001) (Box 3.1). Furthermore, the British Association of Day Surgery have put forward a further list of more major procedures that can also be performed as day surgery in 50% of cases, which is based upon the complexity, length and anaesthesia involved in the surgery (Cahill, 1999) (Box 3.2).

DISADVANTAGES OF DAY SURGERY

There are still some medical staff and managers who are unenthusiastic about the concepts of day surgery care, but training and education programmes have now been developed to increase interest and change attitudes. High standards of preoperative patient assessment and suitable anaesthetic techniques are necessary to run a successful day surgery unit, and both nurses and doctors require training in these areas, prior to accepting responsibility for day care management.

A few patients may refuse to have their operation on a day basis for fear of something unexpected happening at home after discharge, or being an extra burden on relatives. However, with good preoperative assessment, discharge planning in advance and a high input of patient education, these anxieties may be reduced, thereby enabling the patient to find day surgery care more acceptable. Patients are required to be physically fit for day surgery, have a responsible adult to care for them for at least 24 hours and a suitable home environment in which to recover. Day surgery units require good equipment and facilities; and education, audit and research into day surgery should be supported to run a successful day surgery unit.

DAY SURGERY NURSING

Day surgery nursing differs from ward or theatre nursing because of the potential for nurses to work in all areas of the day surgery unit. Most planned day surgery units have areas identified for preoperative assessment, anaesthetics, operating theatre, recovery and ward facilities. All nurses working in day surgery should ideally be trained to be multiskilled and able to work in each area, perhaps on a rotation system. Staff can expand their practice by becoming competent anaesthetic, operating theatre and recovery nurses, as well as being skilful in patient assessment before and after surgery (Hodge, 1999).

The benefits of staff rotation are greater job satisfaction, more effective and efficient staffing and good staff morale. Patients also benefit from a more knowledgeable nursing staff, and it highlights the specialized role of the day surgery nurse. The rotation system prevents work becoming too routine, and allows staff to become competent in nursing patients from a variety of specialities (Hodge, 1999).

In order to facilitate nurse rotation throughout a day surgery unit, nurses should be intensively trained so that they achieve a variety of skills. They will need theatre nursing skills, knowledge of anaesthetic techniques and the ability to deliver immediate postoperative care to patients. This is in addition to demonstrating good communication skills and a caring attitude towards patients and their relatives (Hodge, 1999).

DAY SURGERY NURSING – PATIENT CARE

Although day surgery is seen as a major vehicle in reducing long waiting lists, it must not be regarded as a panacea for waiting list problems. The shift away from conventional hospital stays towards shorter periods in hospital will herald a change not only in hospital size and layout but also in nursing practice. It is essential, therefore, that nurses take on board these changes and realize the contribution they must make to ensure that they deliver a high standard of patient care within a high-quality service. The commitment of nurses in the day surgery setting to achieve this is paramount, in order to instil in their patients the confidence to accept this shift towards shorter hospital stays and to be adequately prepared for their hospital stay and their discharge home.

The time spent by patients in the day surgery unit is short, with the pre- and postoperative periods being condensed into hours rather than days. It could be argued that the patient requires less time to recover from their treatment because of this; however, it must be recognized that, on the whole, although the hospital stay may be shorter, the period of convalescence may not alter greatly from that of an inpatient for the same procedure. The place at which the convalescence period is spent is changed, however, in that it takes place outside of the hospital environment. Whether this period takes 1 day or longer, the impact on the patient may be great. Hospitalization and subsequent recovery at home will impinge on the patient's social circumstances. It will have implications for work commitments, and the necessary help and arrangements will be needed to achieve a satisfactory and uneventful recovery. It should not be forgotten that fears and anxieties regarding treatment may be just as real in the day surgery patient (Mitchell, 1997).

PREOPERATIVE ASSESSMENT IN DAY SURGERY

The role of the preoperative assessment for surgical patients has been discussed in depth in Chapter 1. However, it is worth illustrating at this point how preoperative assessment in day surgery is integral to the whole process. Day surgery has led the way in preoperative assessment, because particularly at the inception of widespread day surgery there were very strict criteria laid down as to the patients who were suitable for day surgery and those who were not. Also, there were strict discharge criteria and initially these were very inflexible. However, as day surgery has become the 'norm' rather than a new phenomenon, these guidelines have been adjusted to suit the needs of the patient and the service. It is sensible that when the preoperative assessment was rolled out to incorporate all patients undergoing surgery, preoperative assessment in day surgery was looked at as the model upon which to base it.

ADMISSION TO THE DAY SURGERY UNIT

When patients are admitted to the day surgery unit, there is only a short amount of time available for the nursing staff to assess, plan, implement and evaluate the care required to ensure that the needs of the patient are met. However, the opportunity to practise excellent nursing care should not be dependent on the length of a patient's hospital stay, and effective communication skills should be used to establish information and understand the patient's fears and anxieties. Communicating with the patient, putting them at their ease and giving clear understandable information forms the basis of good day surgery care. The nurse in the day surgery unit should recognize that, to each patient, their operation is a major source of anxiety and will be a stressful event: however minor their surgical condition may seem, there is no such thing as a 'minor' general anaesthetic.

On admission to the day surgery unit, the nurse should explain to the patient the routine they should expect, and offer adequate preoperative instructions and information. It should be remembered that the patient will be very anxious and nervous, and the nurse should ascertain that the patient understands the information given and allow time for any questions. The patient's preoperative assessment questionnaire will be checked by the nurse to identify any change in the patient's health status since their first assessment. The patient's baseline observations will also be measured and recorded. It is important that all patients should have a responsible adult to take them home after the operation and to stay with them for the first 24 hours. This will ensure patient safety, as their coordination and memory may be impaired following general anaesthesia. Therefore, the patient's discharge arrangements should be carefully checked during the admission procedure.

ANAESTHESIA IN DAY SURGERY

As stated previously, there is no such thing as a 'minor' general anaesthetic. The anaesthetic technique for day surgery must ensure adequate anaesthesia and analgesia without compromising the recovery and subsequent discharge of the patient. Thus, the technique is tailored specifically to minimize the pain the patient will experience postoperatively, without the use of drugs that will hinder discharge from the day surgery unit. Added to this, an antiemetic anaesthetic technique will be employed to reduce the incidence of postoperative nausea and vomiting. It is obvious from this that the anaesthetic service in a day surgery unit should be consultant-led. The day unit is a good area for teaching and development, but always in a supervised capacity by the consultant anaesthetist.

The ideal anaesthetic for the day surgery patient should produce very little cardiorespiratory depression, and the induction should be smooth and rapid. The anaesthetic must facilitate the fast turnover of day surgery without pain and postoperative nausea and vomiting, and a rapid return of psychomotor state with minimal hangover effects, allowing for a prompt discharge.

Patients walk into the operating theatre to undergo induction of anaesthesia on the operating table. A nurse or operating department practitioner (ODP) will escort the patient into theatre and is, therefore, responsible for collecting the correct patient for the correct procedure. The nurse stays beside the patient until anaesthesia has been induced.

Induction of anaesthesia is facilitated by the use of an induction agent. The most commonly used agent is propofol, and indeed it is safe to say that propofol has made day surgery possible. It has a rapid onset and facilitates airway management easily, particularly the insertion of the laryngeal mask airway (LMA). Its main advantage is that patients tend to wake following its administration with very little of the 'hangover' effects seen with, for example a thiopental anaesthetic. Propofol has very few side-effects, although it can be painful on injection into the small veins of the back of the hand, so lidocaine (lignocaine) is added just before the propofol is administered. Propofol can also be used as a continuous infusion, which then negates the need for the use of maintenance agents such as isoflurane or enflurane. This method of maintaining anaesthesia is referred to as a 'total intravenous anaesthetic technique' (TIVA), and has been implicated in the reduction of postoperative nausea and vomiting (Millar, 2000). Thus, it makes it the ideal anaesthetic of choice for day surgery, as postoperative nausea and vomiting will delay the discharge of the patient.

Anaesthesia is maintained by either the use of TIVA (as mentioned above), or maintenance agents such as isoflurane, enflurane, halothane, sevoflurane or desflurane. The patient inhales these agents and, in so doing, anaesthesia is maintained. The drawback of using these agents is that they are emetic and delay the recovery of the patient when used for prolonged periods of time.

Even while asleep, the patient is not pain free, and so analgesics must be given during anaesthesia. The most commonly used analgesics in anaesthesia are fentanyl, alfentanil and remifentanil. These are synthetic opioids that are not suitable for postoperative analgesia because they are short acting and cause profound respiratory depression; however, they are ideal for anaesthesia where they are titrated to the patient's needs. Other forms of analgesics routinely used in day surgery are wound infiltration and non-steroidal anti-inflammatory drugs (NSAIDs).

If the patient is to be ventilated, a muscle relaxant will be given. Muscle relaxants fit into two categories: depolarizing and non-depolarizing. Depolarizing muscle relaxants act by mimicking the action of acetylcholine, a neurotransmitter, and are broken down naturally in the body by plasma cholinesterase. The only depolarizing muscle relaxant in clinical use in the United Kingdom is suxamethonium. It is primarily used in emergency situations where intubation has to be carried out quickly (Harper, 1995).

Non-depolarizing muscle relaxants work by blocking the receptor sites at the motor end plate at the neuromuscular junction. The action of non-depolarizing muscle relaxants has to be reversed, and this is done by the administration of an anticholinesterase such as neostigmine, which is given in conjunction with glycopyrronium bromide. Non-depolarizing muscle relaxants commonly used in clinical practice in the United Kingdom are atracurium, mivacurium, vecuronium, rocuronium and pancuronium. Of these, the first four are the most appropriate to be used in day surgery anaesthesia (Millar et al, 1997).

The airway is maintained during anaesthesia primarily with the aid of the LMA. This is a relatively new form of airway maintenance and negates the need for intubation in many instances although not all. The LMA was introduced in 1988 and has become the most popular way to manage an airway (Brimacombe, 1993). It is quick and easy to insert, and the insertion does not require muscle relaxants. It is tolerated at lighter plains of anaesthesia, so usually a bolus dose of propofol is administered and, once the patient has lost consciousness, the LMA is inserted. It allows the anaesthetist to have their 'hands free', and there is less incidence of a sore throat than with intubation, 7% as opposed to 28–47% with an endotracheal tube (Millar et al, 1997). The disadvantage of the LMA is that it cannot be used in patients who have a history of reflux or a full stomach, because it does not protect the airway from vomit and the patient is at risk of aspiration. However, this category of patients is unlikely to fit the day surgery criteria (Owens et al, 1995).

RECOVERY IN DAY SURGERY

Recovery in day surgery can be divided into two distinct phases: first stage recovery, where the patient comes to straight from theatre, and second stage recovery, which is usually where they are discharged. In first stage recovery, the care of the patient is that which is given to any post-anaesthesia patient – i.e. airway and pain management and, where necessary, management of postoperative nausea and vomiting. Where day surgery recovery is at variance from inpatient recovery is that the patient will not be allowed to 'sleep it off', as the main aim is one of discharge. That is not to say that all care will not be given to the patient and analgesics will be given as appropriate, but it will be given with a view to getting the patient into second stage recovery and discharge.

FIRST STAGE RECOVERY

The majority of patients will arrive in first stage recovery with an LMA in place and this will maintain the airway until the patient wakes up. The LMA is removed fully inflated to allow secretions to be removed with it and usually the patient is encouraged to take it out themselves.

The two most important areas in first stage recovery are the management of the patient's pain and the prevention of postoperative nausea and vomiting. Both of these are main reasons why patients cannot be discharged from the day surgery unit and have to be admitted as inpatients (Millar et al, 1997).

Pain management

The prevention of pain is managed right from pre-assessment of the patient, where patients are told what to expect and how the pain will be treated. The anaesthetic technique will incorporate strategies that will enable the patient to be pain free in the recovery period, and each unit will have protocols in place as to the analgesics the patient will take home following surgery. Obviously, the use of opioids postoperatively are avoided in favour of other forms of analgesics, but opioids should not be withheld if the patient really needs them, and the implications of this can be dealt with as they occur and the patient may have to be admitted, but rather this than the patient experiencing pain.

Management of nausea and vomiting

Postoperative nausea and vomiting is common after anaesthesia and surgery and the reasons for this are multifactorial. The incidence of postoperative nausea and vomiting in day surgery varies from 30% to 68% (Millar et al, 1997). In the general surgical population, it can range between 8 and 92% (Arnold, 2002). However, whereas it can occur in the immediate postoperative period, many patients experience nausea and vomiting post discharge. Good day surgery technique, both surgical and anaesthetic, should focus on being as antiemetic as possible. Strategies that should be used to prevent postoperative nausea and vomiting include identifying high-risk patients and operations: consider the use of prophylactic antiemetics for this group. An anaesthetic technique should be chosen which minimizes the risk of postoperative nausea and vomiting such as TIVA. All units should have protocols for the treatment of established postoperative nausea and vomiting, which recovery staff should be able to use without recourse to the anaesthetist.

There are a number of factors which predispose to postoperative nausea and vomiting. Some surgery such as laparoscopic surgery is particularly emetic. The longer the surgery, the longer the period of fasting and the increased risk of pain, which will all contribute to the patient suffering postoperative nausea and vomiting (Broomhead, 1995). In addition, there are patient characteristics which make some patients more prone than others to postoperative nausea and vomiting. These include age: postoperative nausea and vomiting is highest in children and young adults (Tate and Cook, 1996). Women are more prone than men (Beattie et al, 1991), as are patients with a body mass index of more than 30 (Thompson, 1999). Patients who have

a history of previous postoperative nausea and vomiting and those with a history of motion sickness are all more likely to suffer nausea and vomiting postoperatively (Jolley, 2001).

SECOND STAGE RECOVERY

Once the patient is conscious, pain free, not suffering from postoperative nausea and vomiting and all observations are within normal limits, they will be moved to second stage recovery. This will vary from unit to unit. Some units have their patients on beds/trolleys, whereas others have recliner chairs. At this point, the staff will start encouraging the patient to get up and start taking oral fluids and food. Once clinical staff are happy that the patient is ready to go home, the patient will be discharged.

DISCHARGE OF THE PATIENT FROM THE DAY SURGERY UNIT

In the day surgery setting, patients are usually discharged home by nurses, following protocols laid down by the medical staff. The nursing staff are responsible for assessing the patient's fitness for discharge from the day surgery unit once the anaesthetist and surgeon have seen the patient postoperatively. All patients have to fulfil a series of discharge criteria designed by the medical staff (Box 3.3). If the nurse is unhappy with the patient's condition, the anaesthetist or the surgeon should return to the unit to reassess the patient.

Failure to fulfil all these criteria will mean either a delay in the patient's discharge or their transfer to an inpatient bed. No compromises can be made, as the safety of the patient is paramount and only patients who fulfil the criteria for discharge can be discharged home. Readmission rates had been reported as high as 1.3% (Meaden and Ralphs, 1998). However, Hay et al (1999) found that over a 2-year period the readmission rate was 0.88%; furthermore, they established that only 0.59% of those were due to complications from day surgery.

Patients attending a day surgery unit require a great deal of education and support if they are to go home and care for themselves competently within a few hours of having received a general anaesthetic. Working in an area where nurses care for patients from their admission to discharge home within a compressed time span, imposes a responsibility for nurses to educate their patients prior to their discharge from the day unit.

Box 3.3   Criteria for discharge

- The patient should be alert and orientated
- The patient should have tolerated diet and fluids, i.e. not vomiting
- The patient should have voided urine, although anecdotally many units do not insist on this
- The patient should be comfortable and mobile, i.e. should be pain free
- Baseline observations must be satisfactory
- Wound checks must be satisfactory, i.e. the dressing is dry, there is no fresh bleeding
- Any follow-up appointments (if required) should be arranged
- Any mobility aids such as crutches (if required) should be supplied
- The patient must have a discharge letter for their general practitioner
- Verbal and written discharge information should be given
- Any medication to take home (if required) must be given

Box 3.4   Summary of patient advice

- How and when to take medication, if any is required
- How to manage wound care, e.g. when to remove any dressings
- When or if to bathe while any sutures/staples are in place
- When and what exercises can be taken
- When to return to work
- When to start driving following surgery
- Advice about diet and fluids, e.g. to avoid alcohol for 24 hours postoperatively
- Whether a follow-up appointment is necessary in the outpatient clinic
- When any sutures/staples will be removed
- Warnings about nausea and light headedness that may occur
- What activities may and may not be carried out in the immediate postoperative period, e.g. not to drive a car or operate machinery for 24 hours following discharge

POSTOPERATIVE INFORMATION

It is important to give clear written and verbal instructions outlining essential postoperative information, because a patient's ability to understand and remember information may be impaired following a general anaesthetic (Lock, 1999). It is therefore important for all nursing staff to develop and maintain a high standard of interpersonal and teaching skills. Many patients have unrealistic expectations and believe that, because they are only staying in hospital for a short time, they will be completely well before going home. Therefore, the importance of educating and informing patients cannot be overstressed. Prior to discharge, the nurse must check the patient understands their aftercare at home. Information should be given about whom to contact if a problem arises, how to cope in an emergency situation, and advice should be given on pain management and wound management if appropriate. Details of further appointments, suture/staple removal or specific aftercare instructions should also be given (Box 3.4).

The nurse discharging the patient should ensure that the patient fully understands the effects of the anaesthesia, and the importance of not driving or drinking alcohol for 24 hours. A responsible escort should collect the patient from the day surgery unit, as

the patient will not be allowed to travel home alone by car or on public transport. It is the nurse's responsibility to ensure the safety of the patient at all times in the unit, and this is also carried beyond the hospital stay to the post-discharge period. Adequate arrangements for patients' aftercare must be ensured, with back-up facilities arranged as necessary. Arrangements for informing the general practitioner must be adhered to. Failure to abide by strict criteria could result in unpleasant and perhaps dangerous consequences for the patient, and this is unacceptable. The day surgery nurse who strives for excellence of nursing care has the satisfaction of looking after their patient from admission until discharge, and, through the discharge process, ensures that care continues at home.

CONCLUSION

In this chapter the principles of caring for the patient as a day surgery case have been discussed. Where possible, this chapter has followed the patient journey through the day surgery unit. Day surgery is a team effort and nurses working within the unit have to be skilled in more than one area. However, this is what makes day surgery attractive to many nurses, because it means that they may be doing pre-assessment one day and recovery the next. The scope for a nurse to develop their professional portfolio is inexhaustible as new surgical techniques are developed and the role of the day surgery nurse is enhanced.

Day surgery is preferable for patients, as most patients prefer to come to hospital for one day, and in many cases half a day, and then go home to their own environment to recover. Day surgery is here to stay and will continue to push the boundaries in terms of nursing, surgical and anaesthetic development.

Summary of key points

- Day case surgery has proved to be universally popular with carefully selected patients.

- The economic benefits of day case surgery may be observed in terms of reduced waiting lists and cost savings.

- Anaesthetic and surgical technique must be tailored to patient discharge.

- Discharge planning and patient education play major roles in the duties of nurses in day surgery units.

References

Arnold, A. (2002) Postoperative nausea and vomiting in the perioperative setting. *British Journal of Perioperative Nursing* 12(1): 24–32.

Audit Commission (1990) *A Short Cut to Better Services: Day Surgery in England and Wales*. London: HMSO.

Audit Commission (1991) *Measuring Quality: The Patient's View of Day Surgery*. London: HMSO.

Audit Commission (2001) *Acute Hospital Portfolio Review of National Findings Day Surgery*. London: Audit Commission.

Beattie, W. S., Lindblad, T., Buckley, D. N. & Forrest, J. B. (1991) The incidence of post-operative nausea and vomiting in women undergoing laparoscopy is influenced by the day of menstrual cycle. *Canadian Journal of Anaesthesia* 38(3): 298–302.

Bradshaw, E. G. & Davenport, H. T. (eds) (1989) *Day Care Surgery, Anaesthesia and Management*. London: Edward Arnold.

Brimacombe, J. (1993) The Laryngeal Mask Airway: Tool for airway management. *Journal of Post-Anesthesia Nursing* 8(2): 88–95.

Broomhead, C. J. (1995) Physiology of postoperative nausea and vomiting. *British Journal of Hospital Medicine* 53(7): 327–330.

Cahill, J. (1999) Basket cases and trolleys – day surgery proposals for the millennium. *Journal of One Day Surgery* 9(1): 11–12.

Department of Health (2002) *Day Surgery: Operational Guide*. London: Department of Health.

Harper, N. J. N. (1995) Suxamethonium. In: Harper, N. J. N. & Pollard, B. J. (eds) *Muscle Relaxants in Anaesthesia*. London: Edward Arnold.

Hay, H., Lowndes, K. & King, T. A. (1999) Readmissions following day surgery. *Journal of One Day Surgery* 9: 12–14.

Hodge, D. (ed.) (1999) *Day Surgery a Nursing Approach*. Edinburgh: Churchill Livingstone.

Jolley, S. (2001) Managing post-operative nausea and vomiting. *Nursing Standard* 15(40): 47–52.

Lock, E. (1999) Preparation for procedures. In: Hodge, D. (ed.) *Day Surgery a Nursing Approach*. Edinburgh: Churchill Livingstone.

Meaden, S. & Ralphs, D. N. L. (1998) Are day surgery patients discharged too early? Abstract from the British Association of Day Surgery 9th Annual General and Scientific Meeting and Exhibition, Harrogate.

Millar, J. M. (2000) Postoperative nausea, vomiting and recovery. In: Padfield, N. L. (ed.) *Total Intravenous Anaesthesia*. Oxford: Butterworth Heinemann.

Millar, J. M., Rudkin, G. E. & Hitchcock, M. (1997) *Practical Anaesthesia and Analgesia for Day Surgery*. Oxford: Bios Scientific Publishers.

Mitchell, M. (1997) Patients' perceptions of preoperative preparation for day surgery. *Journal of Advanced Nursing* 26(2): 356–363.

National Health Service Management Executive Day Surgery Task Force (1993) *Day Surgery*. London: HMSO.

National Health Service Modernisation Agency (2002) *National Good Practice Guidance on Preoperative Assessment for Day Surgery*. London: NHS Modernisation Agency.

Nicholl, J. H. (1909) The surgery of infancy. *British Medical Journal* 2: 967–968.

Owens, T. M., Robertson, P., Twomey, C., et al (1995) The incidence of gastroesophageal reflux with the Laryngeal Mask: a comparison with the face mask using esophageal lumen pH electrodes. *Anesthesia and Analgesia* 80(5): 980–984.

Royal College of Surgeons of England (1992) *Guidelines for Day Case Surgery. Commission on the Provision of Surgical Services* (revised edition). London: RCS.

Tate, S. & Cook, H. (1996) Postoperative vomiting 1: physiology and aetiology. *British Journal of Nursing* 5(16): 962–973.

Theus, R. J., Go, P. M. N. Y. H. & van Wijmen, F. (1995) Quality assessment in a day surgery unit. *Ambulatory Surgery* 3(4): 195–198.

Thompson, H. (1999) The management of post-operative nausea and vomiting. *Journal of Advanced Nursing* 29(5): 1130–1136.

Further reading

Cahill, H. & Jackson, I. (1997) *Day Surgery – Principles and Nursing Practice*. London: Baillière Tindall.

Penn, S., Davenport, H. T., Carrington, S. & Edmondson, M. (1996) *Principles of Day Surgery Nursing*. Oxford: Blackwell Science.

Radford, M., County, B. & Oakley, M. (2004) *Advancing Perioperative Practice*. Cheltenham: Nelson Thornes.

Sutherland, E. (1996) *Day Surgery: A Handbook for Nurses*. London: Baillière Tindall.

Useful websites

http://www.aagbi.org.uk (accessed 13 April 2004). The Association of Anaesthetists of Great Britain and Ireland.

http://www.bads.co.uk (accessed 13 April 2004). British Association of Day Surgery.

http://www.barna.co.uk (accessed 13 April 2004). British Anaesthetic and Recovery Nurses Association.

http://www.natn.org.uk (accessed 13 April 2004). National Association of Theatre Nurses.

Chapter 4

Wound healing in the surgical patient

Rosie Pudner

Key objectives of the chapter

At the end of the chapter the reader should be able to:

- describe the structure and function of the skin

- discuss the different mechanisms of wound closure

- discuss the normal physiological process of wound healing and the factors which may affect healing

- state the various methods used in wound closure

- discuss the use and care of surgical wound drains

- discuss the principles of caring for a patient with a surgical wound

- discuss the complications of wound healing.

INTRODUCTION

Surgical wounds are formed from an incision in the skin and underlying structures, which is usually performed in a clean environment where asepsis is maintained at all times. The majority of surgical wounds heal by primary (first) intention, with minimal intervention from the nurse. The type of incision, manner and type of materials used in skin closure, and length of time spent in hospital have changed dramatically in recent years, which has influenced the delivery of wound management.

The main principles of surgical wound management are:

- to achieve healing of the wound
- to avoid complications, e.g. infection
- to achieve good pain control
- to ensure a cosmetically acceptable scar
- and to allow the individual to return to a normal lifestyle as soon as possible.

An holistic approach to the care of a surgical patient will assist in achieving the above. Postoperative complications of the wound can be minimized by the preoperative care given to the patient, patient education and an evaluation of healing of the wound. A sound knowledge of the structure and functions of the skin, the physiology of wound healing and factors which may interfere with this process are essential if a nurse is to deliver an optimum standard of wound care. This knowledge is fundamental to the assessment of an individual with a wound and the future management, with regard to cleansing and the application of an appropriate wound dressing.

THE STRUCTURE AND FUNCTION OF THE SKIN

The skin is one of the largest organs of the body, covering a surface area of approximately 2 square metres. The skin covers the body and gives protection to underlying structures. It varies in thickness in different parts of the body and has variations in its pigmentation too (Tortora and Grabowski, 2003). The skin performs five main functions:

1. *Protection*: the skin acts as a physical barrier, protecting underlying structures from minor mechanical trauma, chemicals and gases, bacterial invasion, dehydration, cold, heat and ultraviolet (UV) radiation.

2. *Sensation*: the skin is the largest sensory organ of the body as it contains numerous nerve endings which are sensitive to temperature, pain, touch, pressure and vibration, giving information about the external environment which can then be acted upon.

3. *Temperature regulation*: the skin plays a vital role in maintaining a constant core temperature. Homeostasis is achieved by conduction, convection or radiation of heat from the surface of the

skin. Secretion and evaporation of sweat assists in cooling the body. The circulatory mechanisms of vasodilatation and vasoconstriction also help to control the temperature of the body.

4. *Excretion*: water, salts and other organic materials are excreted through the skin.

5. *Synthesis of vitamin D*: the effect of ultraviolet rays falling on the skin brings about the synthesis within it of vitamin D from 7-dehydrocholecalciferol, which indirectly promotes the absorption of calcium from the gut.

The skin also has an absorptive capability, as it can absorb various substances, e.g. oestrogens, glyceryl trinitrate, etc. These substances can be applied as a slow-release skin patch, allowing the substance to be slowly absorbed through the skin (Hinchliff et al, 1996). Certain cells within the epidermis, i.e. Langerhans cells, also undertake a role in bolstering immunity.

The skin is a complex and multilayered structure, comprising the epidermis, dermis and subcutaneous tissue. These layers and the structures within each layer will now be discussed.

THE EPIDERMIS

The epidermis is the most superficial layer and is connected to the dermis. It is avascular, receiving nutrients from the dermis below, and is composed of keratinized stratified squamous epithelial cells. Four principal types of cells are found in this layer: keratinocytes, melanocytes, Langerhans cells and Merkel cells. The epithelial cells are produced in the basal layer and gradually migrate upwards over a period of 40–56 days.

The epidermis is made up of four to five layers of cells, depending on the location in the body. The first layer, next to the dermis, is the stratum basale. Cell division occurs here, with the cells dipping down into the dermis to surround sweat glands and hair follicles. Keratin is manufactured by the keratinocytes found in this layer. Keratin is an insoluble protein that is resistant to changes in temperature and pH, and helps waterproof and protect the skin. Also found in this layer are Merkel cells, which are in contact with the flattened end of sensory neurons, and are involved in the sensation of touch. The second layer is the stratum spinosum, which contains prickle cells and Langerhans cells (Tortora and Grabowski, 2003). The prickle cells prevent cell separation by their intercellular bridges. Langerhans cells participate in immune responses and are thought to have a role in allergic or immunological skin disorders (Bennett and Moody, 1995).

The third layer is the stratum granulosum, where the keratinocytes flatten and accumulate lamellar granules. Secretions from the lamellar granules slow the loss of body fluids and entry of foreign materials (Tortora and Grabowski, 2003). The fourth layer is the stratum lucidum, which is only found in the thick skin on the palms of hands and soles of the feet, i.e. areas of excessive wear and tear. The cells in this layer start to undergo nuclear degeneration and contain large amounts of keratin. The fifth and final layer is the stratum corneum, consisting of many layers of dead cells that are completely filled with keratin. These cells are constantly shed from the body surface, i.e. desquamation, as a result of friction and washing. They also have the ability to soak up extra moisture (Hinchliff et al, 1996).

THE DERMIS

The dermis lies beneath the epidermis and forms the main part of the skin, providing the skin with its strength and elasticity. It is formed of connective tissue containing collagen and elastic fibres, and contains blood and lymph vessels, sensory nerve endings, hair follicles, sweat and sebaceous glands. In the dermo–epidermal junction, melanin is produced by melanocytes, under the influence of sunlight. Melanin gives colour to various body structures, e.g. hair, iris and skin, but the main function of melanin is to protect the body from ultraviolet light (Tortora and Grabowski, 2003).

The upper region of the dermis is the papillary region, which consists of a series of undulations called dermal papillae. This cellular arrangement prevents the epidermis shearing off from the dermis when shearing forces are applied to the skin. The reticular layer is the remaining portion of the dermis, and consists of dense, irregularly arranged connective tissue containing interlacing bundles of collagenous, reticular and coarse elastic fibres. It is within the spaces between these fibres that hair follicles, sensory nerves and sweat glands are located (Hinchliff et al, 1996).

The dermis is constructed of ground substance or matrix, various fibres and cells. Ground substance is an amorphous matrix, resembling a gel, which provides connective tissue with its bulk. It is permeated by strands of collagen, elastin and fibronectin and other cells. The gelatinous material is composed of water, electrolytes, glycoproteins and proteoglycans, and is synthesized by fibroblasts (Hinchliff et al, 1996).

Collagen, reticular fibres and elastin fibres are all produced by mesodermal fibroblasts, situated in the dermis. Collagen is a family of connective tissue proteins with immense tensile strength, due to their rigid and durable structure. The fibres come together to form thick bundles in which numerous cross-links form, so increasing the strength of the fibres. Collagens are important as a structural support, but also control many cellular functions, including cell shape and differentiation. Ascorbic acid is necessary for the formation of collagen. There are many types of collagen which have been identified, with Types I and III being found to be important in wound healing (Fletcher, 2000). Type I is usually physically allied with Type III collagen, whereby Type III collagen synthesis is dominant in the early stage of wound healing, but with Type I synthesis being more predominant in the later stages of healing. The reticular fibres form a loose framework in the dermis and envelop the collagen bundles. The elastin fibres (elastin) are branching yellow fibres which provide elasticity and resilience to the skin (Hopkinson, 1992).

Four types of cell are found in the dermis: fibroblasts, tissue macrophages, tissue mast cells and white blood cells. The fibroblasts lie between the collagen bundles and are concerned with collagen and elastin synthesis. The tissue macrophages or histiocytes are wandering phagocytic cells. Tissue mast cells produce histamine and heparin, and are found near blood vessels and hair follicles. Neutrophils, lymphocytes and monocytes are transient cells, and are constantly moving between blood vessels (Hinchliff et al, 1996).

The cutaneous blood vessels lie entirely within the dermis and have a rich sympathetic nerve supply, so allowing vasoconstriction or vasodilatation, depending on the local environment. The lymphatic vessels are found throughout the dermis and are responsible for draining excess tissue fluid and plasma proteins which may have leaked into the tissues. The dermis contains sensory nerves which have three types of nerve ending, each responding to a specific stimulus. The hair follicles lie in the dermis, each surrounded by its own blood and nerve supply. The basal layer of the epidermis dips down to surround the hair follicle, so the process of epithelialization can occur from this area. The sweat glands – eccrine and apocrine – are formed as coiled tubular downgrowths from the epidermis. The sebaceous glands are formed as outgrowths of the developing hair follicles, producing sebum which waterproofs the skin and has some action against fungal and bacterial infections (Hinchliff et al, 1996).

SUBCUTANEOUS FAT

Adipose tissue lies beneath the dermis and is a valuable store of triglycerides, which provide a potential source of energy. The adipose tissue insulates the body, so preventing heat loss, and acts as a shock absorber, so preventing trauma to the underlying structures. It has very little ground substance, and the tissue is divided into lobes by septa which carry blood vessels and nerves. The cells which make up adipose tissue consist of a flat nucleus surrounded by a large single fat globule.

MECHANISMS OF WOUND CLOSURE

There are three mechanisms of wound closure: primary intention, secondary intention and tertiary intention or delayed primary closure.

- *Primary intention.* The skin edges are pulled together and held in apposition by a mechanical means, e.g. sutures, staples, adhesive strips or tissue adhesive. This method of closure is adopted in most surgical incisional wounds.
- *Secondary intention.* The wound is left open to allow granulation, contraction and epithelialization to occur. This method is adopted if there is extensive tissue loss, a large superficial surface area or presence of infection.
- *Tertiary intention or delayed primary closure.* The wound is initially left open to allow granulation to begin, and after approximately 3–5 days wound closure is achieved by either approximation of the skin edges or by the application of a skin graft. This method is adopted in wounds where there is a high risk of contamination and possible infection; a poor blood supply which may lead to non-viable tissue; or excessive swelling in the area, as in orthopaedic trauma. The wound is managed in this manner in order to ensure that the wound is not infected, has a good blood supply and swelling has reduced before skin closure is attempted (Westaby, 1985).

THE PROCESS OF WOUND HEALING

Wound healing is a complex systematic process comprising a complex interaction of cellular, chemical and physical events. This process is often divided into four stages or phases of wound healing (Westaby, 1985). As wound healing is a continuous process, there will be some overlap between the phases. The phases of wound healing are known as the inflammatory phase, the destructive phase, the proliferative phase and the maturation phase.

The extent and timing of these phases are controlled by a variety of mediators, e.g. growth factors. Growth factors are proteins which are secreted from a variety of cells, acting as soluble mediators in cutaneous repair. Their effects are exerted locally via specific receptors on the surface membrane of the targeted cells within the wound. They create a vital signalling network for the regulation, coordination and control of cellular interactions during wound healing (Cox, 1993).

THE INFLAMMATORY PHASE

The inflammatory phase occurs from the time of injury to approximately 3 days. The body's immediate response to wounding is to stop bleeding and prevent the entry of microorganisms. Vasoconstriction occurs in the immediate area, due to the release of serotonin and other chemical mediators from the platelets, which helps to reduce the flow of blood to the wound. Damage to the blood vessels in the wound causes the platelets to become sticky and clump together to form a platelet thrombus, so further reducing blood loss. The clotting cascade is also initiated following injury to the vascular endothelium, resulting in the formation of a fibrin thrombus in the wound (Silver, 1994).

Inflammation is a natural response to trauma. A number of mediators (chemical substances), including prostaglandins, are released into the wound, resulting in vasodilatation, increased capillary permeability and the stimulation of pain fibres. The effect of increased capillary permeability is that mediators, plasma proteins, antibodies, neutrophils and monocytes migrate into the wound and surrounding tissue. The neutrophils and macrophages phagocytose any microorganisms or dead tissue present in the wound space. The wound and surrounding area will therefore appear red, swollen, hot and painful, with possible loss of function.

THE DESTRUCTIVE PHASE

The destructive phase occurs approximately 2–5 days after injury. The polymorphonuclear leucocytes (polymorphs) and macrophages continue the process of phagocytosis, so cleaning the wound of any debris or microorganisms. The tissue macrophages also control wound healing through the production of a variety of growth factors, e.g. platelet-derived growth factor (PDGF), transforming growth factor (TGF), interleukin (IL) and tumour necrosis factor (TNF) (Steed, 1997). These growth factors stimulate the production of various cells, e.g. PDGF stimulates the growth of blood vessels (angiogenesis). This process demands substantial resources and energy, and considerable amounts of heat and fluid can be lost, especially in an open wound.

THE PROLIFERATIVE PHASE

Following the initial inflammatory response, the phase of tissue repair takes place. This occurs from approximately 4–28 days, but may be longer in some

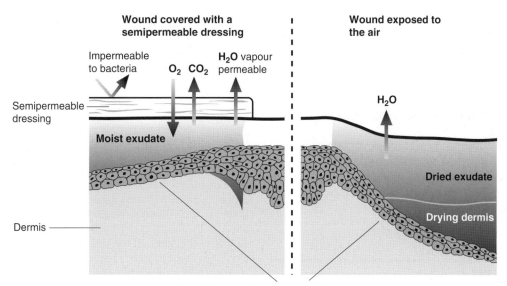

Figure 4.1   Epithelialization in wound healing in a moist and in a dry environment.

wounds. The macrophages continue phagocytosis of cell debris and microorganisms. Through monocyte-derived growth factor (MDGF), the macrophages attract fibroblasts to the area. The fibroblasts, in the presence of vitamin C, ferrous iron, nutrients, oxygen and a slightly acidic environment, produce collagen fibrils, which are laid down in a haphazard fashion. Vitamin C is vital in this phase of healing, as it is involved in the hydroxylation of proline in collagen to hydroxyproline, which aids the cross-linkage of the collagen fibres. Endothelial cells respond to the secretion of various growth factors and form new capillaries, which grow into the wound. This process is known as angiogenesis and is stimulated by the hypoxic environment (Silver, 1994). The matrix of the collagen fibres forms a scaffolding for the new capillaries, while the new capillaries provide nutrients and oxygen for continued growth. This process is often called granulation because, in a wound healing by secondary intention, the wound bed appears red and granular. As the wound defect is filled with the newly formed tissue, the numbers of macrophages and fibroblasts diminish.

Contraction of the wound can also occur in some wounds during this phase of healing, and is thought to be due to the presence of myofibroblasts within the wound. Myofibroblasts are cells containing the features of a fibroblast and a smooth muscle cell, which appear to have contractile qualities, so reducing the surface area of the wound (Butterworth, 1993).

Epithelialization is the last step in this phase of wound healing. Epithelial cells at the wound edges divide and migrate across the surface of the wound until they meet other epithelial cells. When this occurs, migration ceases, a process called contact inhibition. If the remnants of hair follicles are still present in the wound bed, epithelial cells will migrate from these areas and traverse the wound bed until they meet other epithelial cells. The rate of epithelialization is enhanced by maintaining a moist environment, as it allows the epithelial cells to migrate across the surface of the wound more easily (Winter, 1962) (Fig. 4.1). However, in surgical wounds it is important that the incisional wound is not allowed to become too wet as maceration can occur, so affecting the cosmetic result of the scar.

THE MATURATION PHASE

This is the final phase of wound healing and occurs from 15 days to 365 days approximately. The original Type III collagen laid down in the wound bed is converted to Type I collagen, which is laid down following the tension lines within the wound, and is also cross-linked so as to give strength to the scar tissue. As the remodelling process continues, cellular activity reduces and there is a gradual closure of the nutrient blood vessels in the wound. The scar should become paler and flatter in appearance.

During this final phase of healing, shortening or contracture of the scar may occur due to the reorganization of the collagen as a reaction to stretching and extension. This contracture, combined with the lack of elasticity in the scar, can cause problems of tightness or limitation of joint mobility (Silver, 1994). For some people this process may lead to hypertrophic scars, whereas keloid scarring is due to a local disturbance during the healing process (Robson, 1988).

FACTORS AFFECTING THE HEALING PROCESS

A variety of factors can affect the healing process, slowing down the rate of healing or impairing healing altogether. These factors can be divided into intrinsic and extrinsic factors (Box 4.1).

INTRINSIC FACTORS

Advanced age

The inflammatory response is reduced, so increasing the likelihood of invasion by microorganisms and infection. Increasing age reduces fibroblastic activity and migration. Collagen metabolism is reduced, with the collagen being weaker and thinner and so not able to support the blood vessels in the dermis, causing the blood vessels to be easily damaged. Angiogenesis is delayed and epithelialization is hindered (Desai, 1997). Advanced age is also often accompanied by multiple medical problems which may affect wound healing, e.g. cardiac and respiratory problems.

Dehydration

A person who is dehydrated is not able to metabolize efficiently, and subsequent electrolyte imbalance can impair cellular function. An adequate intake of 2–2.5 litres of fluid a day is required for efficient metabolism.

Disease processes

Cancer, diabetes, inflammatory diseases, jaundice and diseases affecting the immune response all have an influence on wound healing (Moncada, 1992). Patients suffering from cancer often receive chemotherapy in order to destroy the malignant cells in the body, or undergo radiotherapy. Radiotherapy has a fibrosing effect on the local blood vessels, so impairing the blood supply to that area. At the end stage of the disease the patient may suffer from cachexia, i.e. a chronic state of malnutrition produced by the absorption of toxins.

Diabetes can delay healing for a variety of reasons, due to the altered metabolism associated with diabetes (Silhi, 1998). If a diabetic person has a high blood glucose level, invading microorganisms will multiply dramatically, so causing infection. Hyperglycaemia has a deleterious effect on phagocytosis, so increasing the risk of infection. Decreased tensile strength is due to a decreased collagen synthesis and retarded capillary ingrowth (Hotter, 1990). Jaundice appears to affect the tensile strength of the wound, and is sometimes associated with abdominal wound dehiscence (Carlson, 1997). Uraemia causes a delay in the proliferative stage in healing, relating to the laying down of granulation tissue and collagen (Orgill and Demling, 1988).

Impaired blood supply to the area

Insufficient supply of nutrients and oxygen to the tissues can be caused by hypotension or arteriosclerosis. Without oxygen, ischaemia results and the newly formed tissue is compromised (Cooper, 1990). Excessive caffeine intake, through drinking large amounts of coffee or cola drinks, can lead to vasoconstriction (Bonavita, 1985), which will lead to impaired tissue perfusion.

Impaired nutritional status

Adequate supplies of protein, calories, vitamins C and K, zinc and copper are required for wound healing. If supplies are inadequate due to poor intake, abnormal absorption or greatly increased demands, this can result in poor wound healing, reduced tensile strength of the scar, increased risk of wound dehiscence, increased susceptibility to infection and poor-quality scars (McLaren, 1992). (See Ch. 5 for further information on nutrition and wound healing.)

Box 4.1   Factors affecting wound healing

Intrinsic	Extrinsic
Advanced age	Drug therapy
Dehydration	Infection
Disease processes	Inappropriate wound
Impaired blood supply	management
Poor nutritional state	Obesity
Reduced supply of	Poor surgical
oxygen	technique
	Smoking
	Stress
	Wound temperature

Social factors	Psychological factors
Poverty	Motivation of the patient
Poor housing	Concordance with treatment
Cultural/religious	Knowledge and understanding
beliefs	of patient/carer
Patient's lifestyle	Altered body image

Reduced supply of oxygen

This can be caused by prolonged hypoxia due to shock, anaemia, impaired arterial blood supply, or in patients with chronic obstructive airways disease. Inflammation is delayed, as the neutrophils are not able to reach the wound, and collagen synthesis and epithelial growth are impaired.

Smoking

Smoking has a vasoconstricting effect, inhibits epithelialization, can affect the immune response and can cause problems with scarring. Siana et al (1992) found that the width of scars was twice as wide in smokers as it was in non-smokers, and the scars of smokers tended to be lighter, so giving an overall poorer cosmetic result. Smoking can also lead to a deficiency in vitamin C, an essential factor needed for tissue repair.

EXTRINSIC FACTORS

Drug therapy

Steroids and non-steroidal anti-inflammatory drugs (NSAIDs) reduce the normal inflammatory response. Corticosteroids also suppress the synthesis of fibroblasts and collagen, with long-term usage leading to 'tissue paper' skin, which is easily damaged. Cytotoxic drugs delay the inflammatory response, suppress protein synthesis and inhibit the replication of cells. Immunosuppressive drugs reduce white blood cell activity, delaying the inflammatory response and increasing the risk of infection. Anticoagulant therapy, if not given in the correct dosage, can cause excessive bleeding and the potential formation of a haematoma.

Infection

Healing is delayed as invading bacteria compete with the macrophages and fibroblasts for oxygen and nutrients at the wound surface. Infection can lead to further local tissue destruction as a result of the ensuing inflammatory response, and can cause the formation of an abscess and breakdown of the wound. Collagen synthesis is delayed, and newly formed tissue is damaged (Orgill and Demling, 1988).

Inappropriate wound management

The inappropriate application of a dressing which causes maceration of the surrounding skin or adheres to the wound bed, inaccurate assessment of the patient and their wound or failure to evaluate care can all lead to inappropriate management of the patient's wound.

Obesity

It has been shown, especially in abdominal surgery, that obesity can lead to an increased risk of infection in clean wounds (Cruse and Foord, 1973). Obesity decreases perfusion to the wounded tissues, and, as a consequence, wound infection and wound dehiscence can occur (Jacobson, 1994). Contraction is reduced and the risk of dehiscence is also increased, because of the amount of tension exerted on the wound in an obese patient.

Poor surgical technique

If any type of tissue is handled roughly during surgery, then it can become devitalized and so provide a suitable site for infection. If haemostasis is not achieved or a drain is not inserted in a dead space, then a haematoma can form. This can cause tissue damage through the pressure exerted at the edges of the wound, and is also an ideal environment in which microrganisms can grow. The inappropriate use of diathermy can also cause problems with healing, and if sutures or staples are applied too tightly, then the result is damaged tissue and tissue death, and a poor cosmetic result (Singer et al, 2002).

Stress

Psychological problems may well affect the health of a patient, and it is known that stress has an effect on the immune system (Maier and Laudenslager, 1985) and on wound healing (Kielcolt-Glaser et al, 1995). The stress of surgery is known to stimulate the sympathetic nervous system, and continues into the postoperative period. Stress caused by hypoxia, hypothermia, pain and hypovolaemia stimulates the sympathetic nervous system, whereby excess levels of noradrenaline (norepinephrine) cause vasoconstriction and altered peripheral perfusion, so decreasing the oxygen available for healing (West, 1990). The release of glucocorticoids inhibits fibroblast activity, collagen synthesis and the formation of granulation tissue (Flanagan, 1997).

Temperature

Frequent dressing changes and the use of cleansing solutions at room temperature significantly reduce intrawound temperature. Cell division takes place at normal body temperature, and with a drop of 1°C it takes up to 3 hours for mitotic cell division to recommence (Lock, 1980), so delaying the healing process.

SOCIAL AND PSYCHOLOGICAL FACTORS

Social factors

Poverty can lead to a poor nutritional intake. It can also affect the patient's ability to afford to have sufficient heating during the cold weather, so causing peripheral vasoconstriction and a decreased blood supply to the wound. Poor housing can mean a lack of cleanliness, so increasing the risk of wound infection. Cultural and religious beliefs can have an influence on the patient's diet, hygiene and acceptance of medical interventions. The lifestyle of the patient can influence healing, especially if the person smokes, drinks excessive amounts of alcohol or abuses drugs.

Psychological factors

Poor motivation of the patient and/or carers can affect concordance with treatment, as they may lack the capability to continue with the recommended treatment of the wound. This may also be linked to a lack of knowledge or understanding of the wound and how it is to be managed. The effect of surgery on the body and the resulting scar can alter the patient's body image. (See Ch. 6 for further information on altered body image and the surgical patient.)

METHODS OF SKIN CLOSURE

The purpose of wound closure is to achieve approximation of the wound edges to produce a strong scar, with minimal disturbance of function and a good cosmetic result (Sauvage and Quinton, 1995). In wounds healing by primary intention, various types of suture material, staples, adhesive strips and tissue adhesive can be used to bring the skin edges together and hold the edges in apposition until healing has occurred. Choice of wound closure and technique depends upon the type of tissue, the position of the wound and the surgeon's preference.

SUTURES

Sutures are used to promote healing by eliminating dead space in a wound, realigning tissue planes and holding the skin edges in apposition until healing has taken place and the wound no longer needs the support of the suture material. They can be used to aid haemostasis, but if applied too tightly they can cause necrosis of the surrounding tissue. The type of suturing technique, technique of knot tying and the width of the tissue bites all affect wound strength and healing (Spotnitz et al, 1997).

Suture materials are chosen for their strength, handling characteristics and absorptive properties. Different types of suture material are required in a variety of circumstances, and for different types of tissue and parts in the body: e.g. an absorbable suture is required in the urological tract to prevent stone formation around any persistent foreign material (Leaper

and Lucarotti, 1992). Absorbable suture material is also used to prevent the collection of material build-up by the suture, which might cause an obstruction and possible leakage of contents.

The choice of suture material depends on the rate at which the tissue is likely to heal, the amount of strain or stress to which the wound site will be subjected, the likely growth of the wound and whether the suture is to give temporary or permanent support to the wound (Spotnitz et al, 1997). The surgeon will select a suture material which loses its strength relative to the gain of strength in the wound itself as it heals.

Types of suture material

Suture materials are either absorbable or non-absorbable (Table 4.1). Absorbable sutures are made out of material which is either digested by proteolytic enzymes released from the polymorphonuclear cells, or by hydrolysis whereby the action of water on the suture causes the breakdown of the material. The action of hydrolysis is increased by a rise in temperature or a change in the pH. As the suture material is absorbed, it loses its tensile strength (Capperauld, 1985). Non-absorbable sutures are made out of materials which resist enzymatic digestion, and therefore need removal when applied to the skin, e.g. silk, Prolene.

Non-absorbable skin sutures are left in place for different periods of time, depending on the site of the wound and the amount of tension the wound is under (Box 4.2). Any non-absorbable suture material that is left in place for too long can cause excessive scarring, and is a focus for infection, leading to the formation of a stitch abscess or sinus (Harding and Jones, 1996). However, it is frequently used in hernia repairs in a form of mesh, and Prolene is often used for suturing blood vessels and grafts in place.

Suture material is either monofilament or multifilament. Monofilament sutures are made from a single strand of material, and because of their smoothness, they are easy to handle and reduce tissue trauma. Multifilament sutures ensure that handling and knotting are excellent, although they may increase the risk of infection, as the braided nature of the suture can attract bacteria to it.

It is important to remember that no one suture material is suitable for all purposes, and that the choice of material depends upon the individual wound. It is also important to be aware that all suture materials within the wound stimulate their own inflammatory response, which lasts for about 7 days, but will return later, in wounds where absorbable sutures have been used, as the absorption of the suture material starts (Spotnitz et al, 1997).

Table 4.1 Types of suture material

Suture	Type	Effective wound support	Area of use
Natural absorbable			
Plain surgical	Multifilament	7–10 days	Ligation; superficial blood vessels; closure of subcutaneous fatty tissue
Chromic surgical	Multifilament	10–14 days	Most tissues except skin
Synthetic absorbable			
Coated Vicryl Rapide	Multifilament	7–10 days	Closure of skin and mucosa when of benefit to avoid patient having sutures removed, e.g. oral surgery, perineal repair, paediatric surgery, scalp wounds and wounds under a plaster cast
Monocryl	Monofilament	20 days	Subcuticular skin and soft tissue closure, e.g. biliary or gastrointestinal tract, urology, peritoneum, plastic surgery
Coated Vicryl	Multifilament	30 days	For soft tissue closure, e.g. ligation in general surgery, muscle and gynaecological surgery
PDS II	Monofilament	42 days	For slow-healing tissue and for patients where healing may be delayed, e.g. fascia, tendon, meniscus, oesophagus, rectum, colon
Natural non-absorbable			
Surgical silk	Multifilament	1 year	Ligation; skin closure
Synthetic non-absorbable			
Ethilon	Monofilament	Permanent	Fascia; skin; blood vessels
Prolene	Monofilament	Permanent	Fascia; skin; blood vessels
Ethibond	Multifilament	Permanent	Most body tissues; blood vessels
Mersilene	Multifilament	Permanent	Cornea
Nurolon	Multifilament	Permanent	Most body tissues; skin
Surgical stainless steel	Multi or monofilament	Permanent	Sternum closure and tendon repair

Source: Ethicon (2000).

Box 4.2   Suggested times for removal of sutures

- skin on head or neck, 2–5 days
- upper limbs, 7 days
- trunk or abdomen, 10 days
- lower limbs, 14 days
- retention sutures, 2–6 weeks

Source: Ethicon (2000).

Suturing techniques

The choice of suturing technique relates to the type of tissue and site and size of the wound. Westaby (1985) states that there are three vital factors in the technique of inserting sutures:

- the tightness of the suture tie
- the size of tissue bite, i.e. amount of tissue taken up
- the distance between the sutures.

If these are not addressed, then wound healing may be impaired as well as giving poor cosmetic results.

Sutures which are pulled too tight do not allow for swelling, and may induce vascular compromise at the wound edges, which will lead to necrosis, delayed healing and a poor cosmetic result. The marks left by the sutures may also be very prominent, affecting the cosmetic result. If sutures are inserted too loosely, it can cause the wound to gape, as the wound edges have not been brought together. If the wound edges are allowed to overlap, this may lead to dehiscence or cause a ridge effect, which results in a poor and obvious scar. In the event that the sutures are placed too near to the edge of the wound, this can result in the sutures pulling apart from the wound edges and causing further trauma to the wound (Castille, 1996).

Sutures can be inserted in a continuous or an interrupted manner. The continuous method of insertion is used to close an incision with one running stitch, which is tied to the skin at each end, ensuring the tension is the same along the incision, e.g. subcuticular, continuous over-and-over stitch, blanket stitch and mattress stitch (Fig. 4.2). When a Prolene subcuticular suture is inserted, it is held in position by means of a bead at each end of the incision (see Fig. 4.2). One disadvantage of using a continuous suture is that, if it breaks, the wound edges are not held together and so the suture has to be reinserted. Interrupted sutures are where a suture is knotted and cut individually along the incision, e.g. interrupted over-and-over stitch, vertical or horizontal mattress stitch (Fig. 4.3). It produces a stronger incisional line and avoids devascularization of the skin edges. Abdominal incisions are generally closed using a layered approach, where each layer is closed separately with either continuous or interrupted sutures.

Sometimes a purse string suture is inserted around a drain. This is a continuous suture which is placed around an opening, so that once the drain is removed, the edges can be pulled together, e.g. removal of a chest drain.

Retention or deep tension sutures are used when there is the risk of gross contamination of the wound, excessive tissue damage, recurrent suturing of a wound, or the patient is very obese, and is mainly used in abdominal surgery. By passing the retention sutures through all the layers of the wound and by approximating the skin edges with large non-absorbable sutures, as well as the smaller interrupted sutures, it reduces tension and holds the wound edges together until healing is complete. A bolster or plastic sleeve is placed over the retention sutures so as to prevent the sutures from cutting into the skin.

Removal of sutures

The time period for removal of sutures depends upon the position of the wound (see Box 4.2), condition of the skin and any underlying pathologies which may delay the healing process, e.g. steroid therapy. When removing sutures it is important to remember that the suture material which has been above the skin should not be pulled through under the skin edges, as microorganisms may be dragged through into the underlying tissue and so cause infection. In interrupted sutures, each suture is lifted by the knot and cut below the knot at the point where it has been withdrawn from the skin, and as near to the skin as is possible. The suture is then pulled out towards the side on which it has been cut, to avoid the risk of dragging the skin edges apart. It is important to ensure that no portion of the suture has been left behind, as it will act as a foreign body and set up a local inflammatory response.

Subcuticular

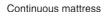
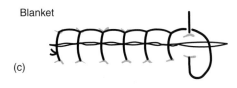

(a)

Continuous over-and-over

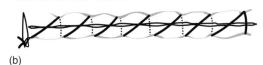

(b)

Blanket

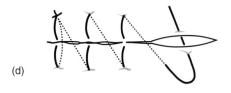

(c)

Continuous mattress

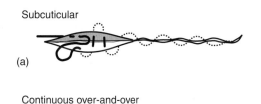

(d)

Subcuticular prolene suture and beads

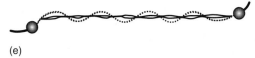

(e)

Figure 4.2   Types of continuous suturing techniques.

Interrupted over-and-over

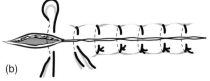

(a)

Interrupted vertical mattress

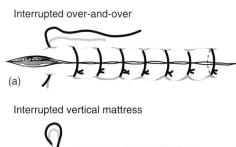

(b)

Interrupted horizontal mattress

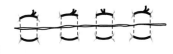

(c)

Figure 4.3   Types of interrupted suturing techniques.

In continuous subcuticular sutures, one end of the suture is cut, and the suture is then gently pulled away from the incision, ensuring the wound is supported during this procedure, as it can be very uncomfortable for the patient. In a subcuticular Prolene suture with beads, one end of the suture is cut and the bead removed, while the opposing beaded end is pulled in order to remove the suture. In other types of continuous sutures, several cuts in the suture are required to ensure that all the suture material is removed, without causing contamination to the underlying tissues.

STAPLES

The use of staples for skin closure is often preferred if the cosmetic appearance of the scar is a concern, as well as for their time-saving nature in application and painless removal. As the stapler is squeezed, the open staple is forced against an anvil located in the nose of the stapler. This action bends the staple legs, causing them to penetrate the everted skin edges, and results in the staple's final rectangular shape (Fig. 4.4). They will also allow haemostasis without causing necrosis to the tissue. In many instances the use of Michel clips has now been superseded by the use of staples, as they are easy to remove and should leave an excellent cosmetic result.

Removal of staples is achieved by inserting the lower jaw of the staple remover under the staple and closing together the two edges of the staple remover. The staple needs to be placed in the V-shaped retaining slot situated in the bottom jaw of the staple remover, in order to ensure it is removed correctly. Squeezing the handles of the staple remover reforms the staple, so that it can be lifted from the skin.

ADHESIVE SKIN TAPES

Adhesive skin tapes are used for some types of skin closure, especially if the cosmetic appearance of the scar is a concern of the patient. Westaby (1985) states that the lax skin of the face and abdomen makes them amenable sites for wound closure by tapes, whereas the skin over joints is subjected to frequent movement, and so limits the adherence of the tapes and success of wound closure. Westaby (1985) also claims that the use of adhesive skin tapes keeps inflammation at the skin edges to a minimum, and results in a good cosmetic outcome with only minimal scarring.

Adhesive skin tapes are also used in conjunction with subcuticular continuous sutures, to give extra support to the wound in some types of surgery, e.g. reconstruction of the breast. The adhesive skin tapes are usually left in place until they peel off by themselves. However, if there is leakage of exudate from the wound, the adhesive skin tapes may need to be carefully removed and then reapplied, until healing has occurred.

USE OF TISSUE ADHESIVES AND FIBRIN SEALANTS

The use of tissue adhesives as a method of wound closure has become increasingly popular in managing some minor traumatic lacerations, and especially with children, as it requires no anaesthesia. The wound edges are approximated and a small amount of glue is applied to the outside surface of the closed wound, and left for approximately 30 seconds. A study undertaken by Applebaum et al (1993) showed that the use of tissue adhesive is a quick, efficient and painless method of wound closure in some traumatic wounds, with a low overall complication rate.

Studies are being undertaken into the use of a fibrin sealant, which is a biological tissue adhesive that possesses both adhesive and haemostatic properties. It is suggested it can be used as an adjunct to sutures, or used on its own in primary wound closure where sutures are unable to control bleeding or the sutures would aggravate bleeding. Its use so far has resulted in a low rate of infection and has been found to promote healing (Spotnitz et al, 1997).

These methods of wound closure, although needing skill to achieve satisfactory results, have the added

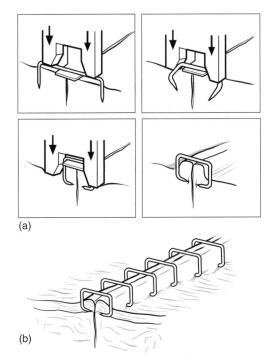

(a)

(b)

Figure 4.4   (a) Formation of skin staples. (b) Skin staples in situ. (Reproduced with permission from Ethicon Ltd.)

advantage of requiring no anaesthesia, and with nothing to remove, so reducing the need for follow-up care in the early postoperative period.

TOPICAL NEGATIVE PRESSURE

Topical negative pressure is a non-invasive technique whereby negative pressure is delivered in a uniform manner to a wound. The VAC therapy system is used to deliver topical negative pressure, and consists of a foam dressing that is cut to the shape of the wound and applied over the wound itself. Suction tubing is inserted into the foam dressing, and the foam and suction tubing is covered with an occlusive film dressing. The suction tubing is then connected to the vacuum unit, and the unit is set to the amount and type of pressure required. The negative pressure can be set at continuous or intermittent, and can be administered at between 50 mmHg and 200 mmHg, depending on patient comfort (Baxendall, 1996) and the system used. The foam dressing should be changed every 48 hours, unless the wound is infected, when it should be changed twice a day. However, if VAC therapy is used on meshed skin grafts, the foam should not be changed. The canister should be changed weekly or when half full.

The technique of using topical negative pressure creates a non-compression force to the tissues, which encourages the arterioles to dilate. This improves blood flow, promotes a moist environment and assists in the proliferation of granulation tissue. It has also been found to reduce the amount of bacterial colonization within the wound, and can remove excess fluid from the area, so reducing oedema (Banwell and Téot, 2003). The use of topical negative pressure results in progressive wound closure in wounds healing by secondary intention, e.g. following dehiscence of a wound, and following the application of a skin graft. It is contraindicated in wounds containing necrotic tissue, malignancy in the wound and the presence of any fistulae, and caution should be taken in actively bleeding wounds or in patients who are receiving anticoagulant therapy (Collier, 1997).

USE OF WOUND DRAINS

Surgical drainage is a procedure which is undertaken for the following reasons:

- where an accumulation of fluid or cellular debris is expected within the wound
- to remove air, serum or fluid from a cavity or dead tissue space.

The insertion of a surgical drain provides a channel to the body surface for fluid which might otherwise collect in the wound space. This can reduce the incidence of infection, and allows closer apposition of the tissues, so facilitating the healing process (Torrance, 1993). Drainage of fluid takes place along the surface of the drain, and the flow of fluid is affected by the size, shape and number of holes in the drainage tube. Patency of the drain is paramount, so that fluid and other materials are drawn into the lumen of the drain, or along its channels (Fay, 1987). However, there are several disadvantages of surgical drainage: surgical drains are a foreign body and so cause a local inflammatory response; they can cause pressure against vital structures, e.g. blood vessels, which can then lead to pressure necrosis; and microorganisms on the skin can gain entry to the wound and cause infection (Westaby, 1985). The risk of infection due to the presence of a drain in a clean wound increases significantly after 3–4 days, as does the risk of mechanical damage to local tissues (Dougherty and Simmons, 1992).

Surgical drainage can be said to be either therapeutic or prophylactic (Torrance, 1993; Westaby, 1985). Therapeutic drainage is undertaken to remove bacteria, dead tissue and other infected material that has collected in an area, e.g. drainage of an abscess, or to remove excess inflammatory mediators so as to reduce further damage to healing tissues. This will reduce the amount of dead tissue space, alter the fluid environment of the wound and reduce the risk of bacterial contamination. Therapeutic drainage may be undertaken by needle aspiration or by the insertion of a drain (Torrance, 1993).

Prophylactic drainage is undertaken for a variety of reasons, one being to prevent infection developing within the wound (Torrance, 1993). It is adopted whenever physiological fluid is expected to collect after a surgical procedure, or when an anastomosis or closure of a viscus may leak, e.g. leakage of bile into the peritoneal cavity after surgery on the common bile duct. This method of drainage is also used to redirect body fluids along an alternative route in order to rest an anastomosis: e.g. insertion of a T tube following exploration of the common bile duct, or insertion of a nephrostomy tube following urinary diversion. If haemostasis has been difficult to achieve, the insertion of a surgical drain allows early diagnosis of a secondary or reactive haemorrhage. It can prevent the formation of a haematoma, and is used when a seroma or haematoma may affect the healing of a skin flap, as used in mastectomy, amputations of a limb and plastic reconstructive surgery (Westaby, 1985).

TYPES OF WOUND DRAINS

There are many different types of drain available (Table 4.2), and these adopt either passive or active

Table 4.2   Types of surgical drain

Passive drainage	Active drainage
Gauze wick	Redivac
Penrose drain	Chest drain
Corrugated drain	
Yeats drain	
T tube	

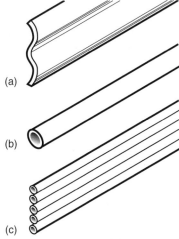

Figure 4.5   Types of passive drain: (a) Corrugated; (b) Penrose; (c) Yeats.

drainage (Torrance, 1993). Both passive and active drainage should remove fluid efficiently, avoid damage to the surrounding tissue, avoid the risk of infection and be easily removed (Dougherty and Simmons, 1992).

Passive drainage is achieved by two methods:

- a closed system drains via a tube into a bag, which is under the force of gravity or capillary action
- an open system drains into a bag or dressing, and is dependent on capillary action, gravity or changes in intra-abdominal pressure.

This type of drain must be inserted at an upward angle, in order to facilitate drainage. Examples of this type of drain are a Penrose drain, a corrugated drain or a Yeats drain (Fig. 4.5).

An active drainage system depends on a vacuum for drainage, e.g. Redivac (Fig. 4.6). These drains are usually inserted through a stab wound, which is situated near to the main incisional wound. The drainage tubing is more rigid, in order to prevent it collapsing under the pressure of the vacuum. It is often held in place by a loop suture to the skin, except in orthopaedic surgery, when removal is often required from under a plaster cast. This type of drainage system

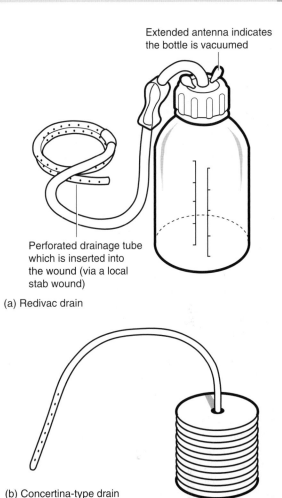

Extended antenna indicates the bottle is vacuumed

Perforated drainage tube which is inserted into the wound (via a local stab wound)

(a) Redivac drain

(b) Concertina-type drain

Figure 4.6   Types of active drain: (a) Redivac; (b) Concertina-type.

also allows an accurate record to be kept on the volume of fluid drained (Torrance, 1993).

CARE OF SURGICAL DRAINS

An aseptic technique should be used when dealing with the drainage system, which should be handled as little as possible in order to reduce the risk of infection. A sterile keyhole dressing should be placed around the drain, to absorb any leaking exudate. A passive drain should either have a sterile absorbent dressing placed over the drain, or a drainage bag should be applied over it, to collect the drained fluid (McLean and Hale, 1990). Standard precautions should be undertaken when dealing with body fluids, e.g. emptying a drainage bottle or removing a surgical drain.

Patency of the drainage system should be regularly checked to ensure free drainage of fluid from the wound site, so as to reduce the risk of infection. The amount

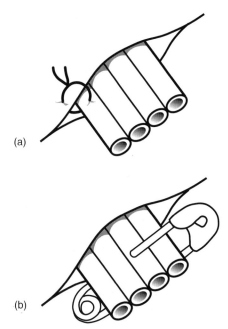

(a)

(b)

Figure 4.7   Methods of securing a passive drain in place:
(a) Yeats drain secured in place by a suture; (b) Yeats drain
secured in place by a safety pin.

and type of wound drainage should be monitored and
recorded. There is usually a high level of serous
drainage in the first 24 hours following surgery, which
reduces to approximately one-third of the previous
day's amount in the following 24 hours (Fay, 1987).
Excessive amounts of wound drainage should be
reported, as this may indicate haemorrhage which may
need investigating further, or may lead to excessive
fluid and electrolyte loss.

The drain, bag or drainage bottle should be well
secured and easily observed. The drainage tubing
should be protected from kinking, blockage or accidental removal. The area around the drain should be
inspected regularly, in order to detect signs of infection,
although the surrounding skin is often inflamed due to
local trauma caused by movement of the drain. The
patient should also be assessed in relation to the amount
of pain or discomfort the drain may be causing them.

REMOVAL OF SURGICAL DRAINS

The drain should be removed when drainage has
stopped, the abscess cavity has closed, wound repair is
complete or if there is a risk of drain-related complications, e.g. infection, tissue ingrowth or obstruction.
Prior to removal of the drain, it is important to inform
the patient of what is to happen, as this can reduce
anxiety and fear. Some patients may require analgesics, and these must be given in sufficient time

before undertaking the procedure, in order to be effective and thus minimize the pain the patient may feel
during removal of the drain. Gloves should be worn
by the nurse, in order to adhere to the policy of standard
precautions. If the drain has a retaining suture in place,
this suture will need to be cut and removed prior to the
drain's removal. In the case of an active, suction drain,
the suction or vacuum created by the bottle should
be released prior to removal of the drain, in order
to reduce trauma to the tissues during its removal
(Torrance, 1993). Once the drain has been removed, a
small absorbent dressing is required over the drain
site, and the dressing should be observed for excessive
amounts of leakage.

In the case of passive drains, some surgeons request
the drain to be shortened daily, to facilitate healing
from the base of the wound. The retaining suture
needs to be cut before the drain is shortened by 1–2 cm.
In order for the drain to stay in place and not fall out,
or be drawn back into the wound, a sterile safety pin is
inserted into the drain (Fig. 4.7). The drain is then
shortened by 1–2 cm every 24–48 hours, until it falls
out. A small absorbent dressing should be applied to
the drain site until healing has occurred, and the
amount of leakage closely monitored.

PRINCIPLES OF CARE FOR A PATIENT WITH A SURGICAL WOUND

As a surgical wound is a premeditated wound, the
main area of nursing care is to monitor the progress of
wound healing, so that any problems can be identified
early. It is well accepted that undertaking certain preventative measures in planned surgical interventions
can reduce the incidence of wound infection and lead
to an improved postoperative recovery.

RISK FACTORS FOR SURGICAL SITE INFECTION

Various epidemiological studies undertaken over the
past years have identified a number of factors which
are linked with an increased risk of postoperative
wound infection (Briggs, 1996a). The two most important factors in determining whether a patient develops
a wound infection are the number and virulence of
bacteria within the wound and the host's resistance.

A surgical classification of wounds (Box 4.3) was
proposed by the National Research Council Ad Hoc
Committee on Trauma in 1964 (cited by Briggs, 1997),
which has shown a strong association with the incidence of wound infection. In elective surgery the degree
of wound contamination relates to the type of operation,
i.e. clean, clean contaminated, contaminated or dirty.

Box 4.3   Surgical classification of wounds

- *clean surgical wound*: operation where there is no opening of the bronchi, genitourinary or gastrointestinal tracts
- *clean contaminated wound*: operation where the bronchi, genitourinary or gastrointestinal tract is opened
- *contaminated wound*: open fresh traumatic wound or incision where there is non-purulent inflammation
- *dirty wound*: old traumatic wound and wound involving abscess or perforated viscera

Source: National Research Council Ad Hoc Committee on Trauma (1964), cited by Briggs (1997)

Mishriki et al (1992) found in a study of 1242 patients that four specific factors were shown to have a significant association with the development of a wound infection. They were patient age, preoperative stay, preoperative shaving and the individual surgeon. Other factors which may increase the risk of wound infection are the duration of the surgical procedure, use of wound drains, use of prophylactic antibiotics, skin preparation of the operation site, surgical technique and method of wound closure. Reilly (2002) developed a mathematical model for identifying risk of infection in clean, elective surgical wounds. From a 3-year prospective cohort epidemiological study, it was found that smoking, a higher body mass index (BMI), malignant disease, presence of haematoma, increased numbers of people in the operating theatre, use of adherent dressings and longer times before removal of sutures increased the risk of surgical wound infection. Some of these factors will now be discussed in more detail.

Age of the patient

The incidence of wound infection increases with age (Mishriki et al, 1990), and may be due to various factors associated with ageing (see p. 50).

Length of preoperative stay

Prolonged hospital stay can allow nosocomial acquisition of resistant organisms, e.g. methicillin-resistant *Staphylococcus aureus* (Leaper, 1995); therefore, the longer the hospital stay prior to surgery, the higher the risk of the patient developing a wound infection (Cruse and Foord, 1980).

Preoperative showering and bathing

It appears to be general practice that the patient has a shower or a bath prior to surgery. There is much debate as to whether a skin disinfectant is of value in reducing postoperative wound sepsis, although few studies have been undertaken in this area.

Removal of body hair

Body hair is frequently removed as part of the patient's preoperative preparation, with the belief that it can reduce the risk of wound infection. However, Seropian and Reynolds (1971) found that wound infection was nine times higher in those patients whose body hair was removed by a razor, compared with those who had not shaved or had used depilatory creams. Cruse and Foord (1980) found an infection rate of 2.5% in those patients who had shaved preoperatively, compared with 0.9% in those who had not shaved preoperatively. These studies illustrate how shaving can have an adverse effect on wound infection rates, although removal of body hair immediately prior to surgery carries less risk of infection than shaving undertaken 24–48 hours prior to surgery. Clipping of body hair may be an alternative to shaving but it can also damage the skin and so provide an entry point for microorganisms, which can then become a focus of infection postoperatively. Depilatory creams may be less traumatic to the skin, but may cause sensitivity in some patients.

Mishriki et al (1992) found that there was a significant association between preoperative shaving and the development of wound sepsis. Despite the evidence against the routine removal of body hair, McIntyre and McCloy (1994) found that many of the surgeons and ward staff still undertook shaving, as they believed it decreased the risk of wound infection. It is clear that all medical and nursing staff need to be made aware of the adverse effects of shaving. However, removal of body hair may be required in extremely hairy patients where the hair may interfere with the suturing or stapling of the wound, prior to applying skin adhesive tapes, or where dressings may adhere, causing pain and discomfort on removal.

Duration of surgical procedure

The risk of wound infection has been shown to be proportional to the length of the surgical procedure. Cruse and Foord (1980) found that the incidence was increased with longer operations, and Garibaldi et al (1991) found that a surgical procedure longer than 2 hours was associated with an increased risk of wound sepsis.

Perioperative interventions

Perioperative hypothermia in some surgical procedures may stimulate thermoregulatory vasoconstriction, leading to a decreased subcutaneous oxygen tension. Kurz et al (1996) found that if intraoperative core temperature dropped 2°C below the normal range, the incidence of wound infection was tripled and hospital stay was extended by 20%. Greif et al (2000) identified that the administration of supplemental oxygen during and 2 hours following surgery reduced the incidence of surgical wound infection. These studies illustrate how maintaining normothermia during surgery and giving supplemental oxygen can decrease the risk of surgical site infection.

Use of surgical drains

As has been previously discussed, wound drains can assist in the removal of a dead space and in the prevention of the formation of a haematoma. However, the drain can act as a channel through which skin contaminants can gain access to deeper tissues of the wound, although this risk should be reduced if a closed system is used.

Use of prophylactic antibiotics

It is recognized that specific types of surgery, especially where a prosthesis or prosthetic material is inserted, carry an increased risk of infection, as opportunistic organisms may infect the implanted material. A broad-spectrum antibiotic is therefore prescribed (Leaper, 1992). However, Garibaldi et al (1991) found that patients who received perioperative antibiotics were likely to develop infections with resistant bacteria. They advocate that narrow-spectrum antibiotics should only be given in order to reduce the emergence of multiresistant pathogens.

Skin preparation of the operation site

The aim of cleansing the operation site with an antiseptic solution, e.g. 0.5% alcoholic chlorhexidine (Hibiscrub) or alcoholic 10% povidone-iodine (Betadine), is to remove transient and pathogenic organisms on the surface of the skin and reduce the number of resident flora. One application of either solution can reduce skin flora by 80–95% (Leaper, 1995).

Surgical technique

This relates to the manner in which the surgeon handles the tissues during surgery, excessive use of diathermy and the manner of wound closure. The use of an inappropriate suture material and poor technique of wound closure will also affect the healing of

the wound, which can lead to infection of the wound (Leaper, 1995). Mishriki et al (1992) also found that there was a strong association between the surgeon undertaking the operation and the incidence of wound infection.

POTENTIAL POSTOPERATIVE WOUND COMPLICATIONS

A variety of complications may occur following surgery: haemorrhage, haematoma, infection, wound dehiscence, sinus formation or fistula formation.

Haemorrhage

Haemmorhage can occur at the time of surgery, in the immediate postoperative period and up to 10 days postoperatively (secondary haemorrhage). Failure to control bleeding during surgery, or failure to tie blood vessels securely, often accounts for haemorrhage in the early postoperative period, whereas secondary haemorrhage is usually associated with infection. It is also thought that perioperative bleeding may affect fibroblast function, with respect to collagen production, leading to a weakened suture line (Taylor et al, 1987). Haemorrhage can be visually detected by the amount of blood loss via a drain, or into the dressing itself. The patient may need to return to theatre to have the bleeding point tied off.

Haematoma

A collection of blood in the tissues can exert internal pressure, which can restrict the blood supply and so cause tissue damage. It also appears to have a direct toxic effect on the tissues, and the haematoma can harbour microorganisms, all of which can lead to infection. Haematoma can be detected by a raised, hard area close to the incisional wound, or when it is released following removal of sutures or staples. Release of the haematoma can be achieved by gently probing the wound to allow drainage of the collection of haemoserous fluid.

Surgical site infection

The presence of a wound infection means that healing, and the patient's discharge, will be delayed, so increasing costs to the hospital, community and the patient (Reilly et al, 2001). According to Smyth and Emmerson (2000), surgical site infection (SSI) accounts for 14–16% of all nosocomial infections in hospital inpatients.

The Nosocomial Infection National Surveillance Service collected data on surgical site infections over a 4-year period and found that the incidence of surgical site infections varied between hospitals (Public Health Laboratory Service, 2002). Amputation of limbs most frequently lead to infection, and one-fifth of SSIs were due to a deep or organ/space infection. It was also identified that the incidence of SSI increases with the number of risk factors, i.e. state of the patient prior to surgery; their ASA score; type of operation; length of surgery; and wound classification (Public Health Laboratory Service, 2002).

Noel et al (1997) found that surgical wound infection was often not seen before 3–4 days postoperatively when the patient may have returned home, and many patients are not seen on follow-up. This prospective study found an SSI rate of 9%, and identified the costs to the patient, i.e. a delay in returning to work, and possible loss of income for a period of time.

The diagnosis of wound infection is often based on clinical criteria, i.e. signs of inflammation, pyrexia, discharge of pus, pain in the area and possible breakdown of the wound. However, it is possible that the early inflammatory stage of wound healing may be mistaken for the beginning of a wound infection. Surgical wounds which are healing by secondary intention may present with different clinical features (Box 4.4) (Cutting and Harding, 1994; Cutting and White, 2003).

Wound infection is often confirmed by the clinical symptoms and a positive result from a wound swab, which should be taken prior to antibiotic therapy. However, it must be remembered that the swab may also pick up contaminants as well as the pathogenic microorganisms that are causing the infection. There is great debate as to whether a wound should be cleaned prior to swabbing, in order to remove the contaminants and so gain a clearer picture of the organisms responsible for the infection. Lawrence (1993) and Wilson (1995) suggest that the wound should be swabbed prior to cleaning, as the maximum number of bacteria are present, whereas Kerstein (1996) suggests that the wound should be cleaned prior to swabbing in order to remove the contaminants within the wound. It is important that nurses adopt whichever method is advocated by their microbiology department, and that as much patient-related information as possible is given to the laboratory in order for them to detect the infecting organism. Microscopy, culture and sensitivity of wound exudate will identify the pathogenic organism, and will allow the appropriate antibiotic to be prescribed; if left untreated, infection can lead to lymphadenitis, bacteraemia, septicaemia and even death (Lawrence, 1993).

Several scoring systems devised to quantify the major signs of wound infection may be of value when assessing the patient with a suspected wound infection. Wells et al (1983) developed a grading system for classifying

---

Box 4.4   Criteria for identifying wound infection in surgical wounds

Surgical wounds healing by primary intention
- abscess
- cellulitis
- discharge
- delayed healing
- discoloration
- unexpected pain or tenderness
- bridging of epithelium or soft tissue
- malodour
- wound breakdown

Surgical wounds healing by secondary intention
Additional criteria to the above:

- abscess/pus
- erythema
- heat
- oedema
- friable granulation tissue
- pocketing at the base of the wound

Source: Cutting and White (2003).

---

the external incisional wounds of patients undergoing cardiothoracic surgery in order to distinguish between a normal incisional wound and one that was infected. Wilson et al (1990) designed the ASEPSIS wound scoring method, which makes assessment of wound infection more objective, by allocating points for both the appearance of the wound in the first week and the clinical consequences of infection. This wound scoring method was found to be more sensitive than other methods in identifying wound infection and wound breakdown, and may be of value in clinical trials or as a method of surveillance, although it may be regarded as time consuming as it takes 3 hours a day to process the data (Wilson et al, 1990). Bailey et al (1992) devised the Southampton Wound Assessment Scale to audit surgical wound infection in patients following hernia surgery in the community setting. The wounds were graded before discharge and 10–14 days postoperatively into one of four categories: normal healing; minor complication; wound infection; and major haematoma.

Another scoring method for wound infection was developed by the Centers for Disease Control following their study on the effect of nosocomial infection control (SENIC), whereby a simple predictive index is calculated based on a score of 0 or 1 for each of the following four patient factors: an abdominal operation; an operation lasting 2 hours or more; an operation which is contaminated; and a patient who has three or more diagnoses at discharge, exclusive of wound infection (Hunt and Hopf, 1997). The risk of infection increased as the numerical score increased, and was consistent with other studies.

The prevalence and incidence of surgical site infection is often used as an outcome indicator (Reilly et al, 2001). However, this information is difficult to obtain due to the variation in definitions of surgical wound infection (Bruce et al, 2001; Mishriki et al, 1993), and difficulty in following up patients in the community. Wilson et al (1998) identified that many of the tools used in audit are labour intensive; however, Reilly et al (2001) was able to demonstrate the potential cost savings by auditing surgical wound infection.

Dehiscence

Dehiscence is the term used when there is partial or complete separation of a surgically closed wound. It is often seen in abdominal wounds and may result in a 'burst abdomen'. It is also a potential problem following sternotomy, episiotomy and caesarean section (Perkins, 1992). According to Perkins (1992), wound dehiscence may be classified as 'early' or 'late'. Early wound dehiscence occurs during the early stages of healing and is related to the sutures and/or suturing technique. Late wound dehiscence is most likely attributed to wound infection, although there are a number of local and systemic factors which may also cause late wound dehiscence (Box 4.5).

A lack of development of a ridge of skin along either side of the incision line, and a discharge of serosanguinous fluid from the wound, are signs that wound dehiscence may occur. Complete wound dehiscence is often said by the patient to be that 'something has given way' and may be associated with a warm, wet sensation.

The degree of dehiscence will determine the management of the wound. Total dehiscence will require surgical intervention to explore the wound, remove any devitalized tissue and closure of the wound. Gauze packs soaked in sterile normal saline 0.9% should be placed over the wound until the patient returns to the operating theatre. If there is partial dehiscence, the wound cavity can be lightly filled with an appropriate dressing, e.g. alginate or hydrofiber rope.

Sinus formation

A sinus is a blind-ending track which opens onto the body surface (Fig. 4.8(a)). It is caused by the presence of an abscess, or foreign material which is an irritant and has become a focus for infection, e.g. suture material. It is often recognized as a point on the incisional wound which will not heal, or repeatedly breaks down. The extent of the problem and possible cause of the sinus can be established by a sinogram. The most effective way of managing a sinus is surgical excision and removal of the foreign material, or laying open of the sinus to facilitate growth of healthy granulation tissue from the base of the wound.

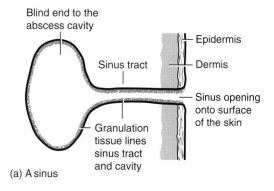

(a) A sinus

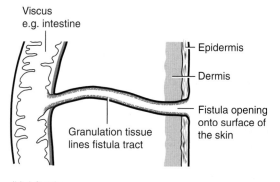

(b) A fistula

Figure 4.8   The difference between a sinus and a fistula: (a) a sinus; (b) a fistula.

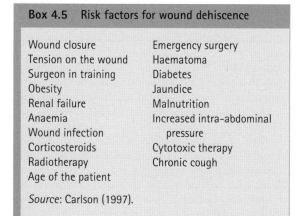

Box 4.5 Risk factors for wound dehiscence	
Wound closure	Emergency surgery
Tension on the wound	Haematoma
Surgeon in training	Diabetes
Obesity	Jaundice
Renal failure	Malnutrition
Anaemia	Increased intra-abdominal
Wound infection	pressure
Corticosteroids	Cytotoxic therapy
Radiotherapy	Chronic cough
Age of the patient	

Source: Carlson (1997).

Fistula formation

A fistula is an abnormal track connecting two viscera (Fig. 4.8(b)), e.g. rectum and vagina, or between a viscera and the body surface, e.g. gastric fistula, and can occur following surgery where an anastomosis of the gastrointestinal tract has taken place, e.g. sigmoid colectomy. The wound will ooze large amounts of fluid, and examination of the fluid will determine the source of the fistula. Most fistulae will close spontaneously, and are therefore managed conservatively. The aims of management are to:

- maintain the integrity of the skin around the fistula
- maintain fluid and electrolyte balance
- give nutritional support
- use an appropriate ostomy or wound drainage device.

ASSESSMENT OF PATIENT AND THE WOUND

Assessment of the patient's general condition should be undertaken, and factors which may influence the healing process should be identified. Assessment of the wound should identify the method of closure, the presence of any drains, and indicate any complications of wound healing. If the wound is healing by primary intention, it should be observed for the normal signs of inflammation, which is seen in the first few days following surgery. However, if the wound appears inflamed and clinical infection is suspected, the patient should be treated accordingly. A surgical wound that is healing by secondary intention should be observed in relation to the appearance of the wound bed; the size, shape and depth of the wound; the amount and type of exudate; and the presence of any complications, e.g. necrotic/sloughy tissue, or infection.

The assessment should be conducted in a structured manner, as it provides baseline information and enables the progress of wound healing to be monitored. The information gained from this assessment should be clearly documented to facilitate communication between the nurse, patient and carer/relative. A variety of tools and charts have been utilized for the purpose of assessing a wound, many of which are designed for patients with wounds healing by secondary intention (Pudner, 1997a). The use of a wound assessment chart should be considered, as it can assist the nurse by providing a suitable framework to structure the process of assessment and documentation.

WOUND MANAGEMENT

It is important that the optimum environment for healing is maintained at all times, both with patients and their wounds. Factors such as the nutritional state of patients and their general health status should be taken into consideration, and if deficiencies exist they should be corrected. This means that the patient should be in an optimum physical condition if possible, and an optimum environment should be maintained at the wound interface. The wound should be kept warm and moist, and measures should be taken to avoid causing any kind of trauma to the wound during the changing of the dressing.

A large number of wound dressing products are now produced, with most available in the community on the Drug Tariff (i.e. FP10), a sample of which are highlighted in Box 4.6. When considering which dressing product is most suitable, the nurse should take into account the patient; their occupation; the position and type of wound; and the amount of exudate being produced, especially in those surgical wounds healing by secondary intention.

Surgical wounds healing by primary intention

These wounds will initially have a light dry dressing applied, to protect the wound and absorb any excessive amounts of exudate, which is then removed after 24–48 hours. The wound may then be left exposed if there is no leakage of exudate (Chrintz et al, 1989), although many patients prefer a small dressing over the wound for cosmetic reasons and comfort. The dressing should only be changed if there is leakage of exudate or clinical infection is suspected.

If haemostasis has been achieved and minimal exudate is expected postoperatively, a vapour-permeable film dressing may be applied over the incisional wound, and left in place until removal of the sutures or staples. This has the advantage of allowing the wound to be monitored without having to remove the dressing, as well as allowing the patient to bathe. Briggs (1996b) found that those patients who had a vapour-permeable film dressing applied postoperatively had less pain than those patients who had their wound exposed after 24 hours. Hultén (1994) and Holm et al (1998) also found that hydrocolloid dressings were of value in surgical wounds healing by primary intention.

These incisional wounds rarely need cleansing, except when excessive leakage has occurred. If this is the case, the wound should be gently cleaned with warm normal saline 0.9% or tap water (Gilmour, 2000), in order to remove any excess wound exudate, prior to the new dressing being applied.

Surgical wounds healing by secondary intention

The wound deficit will be lightly filled with an absorbent dressing material to assist in haemostasis;

Box 4.6   Classification of wound dressing products

- **Absorbent dressings:** e.g. *Mepore, Mepore Ultra, OpSite-Plus, Medipore, Tegaderm + Pad*. These will absorb exudate from the wound, and should only be used on clean incisional wounds, or as a secondary dressing. If applied to a granulating wound, they will cause trauma on removal. *Mepore* should not be stretched on application, as it can cause shearing forces to the skin, resulting in blistering of the skin underneath the dressing.

- **Alginate dressings:** e.g. *Algosteril, Algisite M, Kaltostat, Melgisorb, SeaSorb Soft, Sorbalgon, Sorbsan, Tegagen, Urgosorb*. These are dry absorbent dressings made from seaweed. They contain calcium and sodium salts of alginic acid, a polymer composed of mannuronic acid and guluronic acid residues. On contact with exudate, they form a hydrophilic gel, so providing a moist, warm and particulate-free dressing. They all have haemostatic properties and are of value in exuding wounds healing by secondary intention. An appropriate secondary dressing is required to maintain a moist environment. The dressing should be removed without causing trauma to the wound bed. However, if it has dried out, irrigation with normal saline 0.9% will cause the dressing to gel, and so allow an atraumatic removal of the dressing.

- **Foam dressings:** e.g. *Allevyn range, Allevyn Cavity, Cavi-Care, Lyofoam range, 3M Foam, Transorbent*. These are hydrophilic, semiocclusive dressings which provide a warm and moist environment, and are suitable for healthy, exuding, granulating wounds. They can all be left in situ for periods of up to 7 days, depending on the amount of exudate from the wound. The non-adhesive foams can be cut to size, as long as there is a clear margin of 1.5–2 cm from the edge of the wound. For granulating cavity wounds, *Allevyn Cavity* or *Cavi-Care* can be used. *Allevyn Cavity* conforms easily to fill the cavity. It requires a secondary dressing to keep it in place, and can be left in situ for up to 5 days. *Cavi-Care* needs to be mixed prior to being poured into the wound. *Cavi-Care* will form a stent, which takes up the shape of the wound, and is suitable for clean cavities of a regular shape. A secondary dressing is needed to hold the stent in place. The stent will need to be removed and cleaned every 24–48 hours in order to prevent colonization of the stent.

- **Hydrofiber dressings:** e.g. *Aquacel, Aquacel Ag*. This a soft, non-woven pad or ribbon dressing composed of hydrocolloid fibres, which converts from a soft conformable dressing into a cohesive gel when exudate is absorbed into the dressing. The dressing can absorb high amounts of exudate, which is held within the fibres, so reducing the risk of maceration and excoriation. It should be changed when saturated or after 7 days, and requires a secondary dressing. *Aquacel Ag* contains silver and is of value in controlling bacterial burden in colonized wounds.

- **Hydrocolloid dressings:** e.g. *Comfeel* range, *CombiDERM, DuoDERM Extra Thin, Granuflex* range, *Hydrocoll, Tegasorb, Versiva*. These are occlusive dressings which provide an ideal moist environment. They are 'interactive' in contact with wound exudate. Fluid is absorbed into the dressing, leading to a change in the physical state of the dressing, which forms a gel. *CombiDERM* and *Versiva* have the ability to absorb moderate to large amounts of exudate and lock it away within their unique structure, so avoiding maceration of the wound and skin edges, but maintaining a moist wound environment

  Pain can often be relieved after application of these dressings, as the lack of macrophages, resulting from the lack of surface oxygen, prevents the stimulation of prostaglandins which cause pain. The occlusive environment also encourages angiogenesis, but can cause overgranulation in wounds healing by secondary intention. These dressings can be left in situ for up to 7 days, depending on the amount of exudate. They should be used with caution in diabetic patients, and can only be used in clinically infected wounds if the patient is receiving systemic antibiotic therapy.

- **Hydrogel dressings:** e.g. *Aquaform, GranuGel, Intrasite, Nu-Gel, Purilon*. These consist of insoluble polymers with hydrophilic sites, which interact with aqueous solutions, absorbing and retaining significant volumes of water. They aid rehydration of slough and necrotic tissue to ease debridement. A secondary dressing is required. They are contraindicated where an anaerobic infection is suspected. *Aquaform, GranuGel, Intrasite* and *Nu-Gel* can be inserted into cavity wounds, or sinuses. *Nu-Gel* and *Purilon* contain alginate properties, which aid the absorption of exudate.

- **Hydropolymer dressings:** e.g. *Biatain* range, *Tielle* range. These dressings consist of a mixture of polymers which are hydrophilic and interact with aqueous fluids. They provide a moist environment, while removing excess exudate away from the wound and into their absorbent layer.

- **Paraffin gauze dressings:** e.g. *Jelonet, Unitulle*. These are gauze dressings impregnated with various amounts of paraffin. They are designed for granulating wounds but can adhere to the wound bed and so cause trauma on removal. A secondary absorbent dressing is required.

- **Non/low adherent dressings:** e.g. *Mepitel, Mepilex, N-A Ultra, Release, Tegapore, Tricotex, Urgotul.* These dressings provide protection to surgical incisional wounds and granulation tissue from harmful external influences but allow gaseous exchange and evaporation of water vapour. They provide a moist environment, and are free from particulate contamination. They all require a secondary dressing, except *Release* and *Mepilex*, which have some absorbency, and can be left in place for several days.

   Mepitel and *Tegapore* are dressings which are designed to be placed on the wound bed and left in place for 7–10 days, with a secondary dressing being changed as required. As the wound bed is not disturbed, these dressings reduce pain at dressing change.

- **Vapour–permeable film dressings:** e.g. *Bioclusive, C-View, Mefilm, OpSite Flexigrid, Tegaderm.* These are thin, sterile, vapour-permeable, hypoallergenic, adhesive-coated film dressings. They are permeable to both water vapour and oxygen but impermeable to microorganisms, and provide a moist environment by reducing water vapour loss from the exposed tissue. In these conditions, scab formation is prevented and epidermal regeneration takes place at an enhanced rate. They are only suitable for surgical incisional wounds or shallow, low-exuding wounds but can be used in conjunction with other products in order to maintain a moist environment.

- **Polysaccharide dressings:** e.g. *Iodoflex, Iodosorb.* These products consist of hydrophilic polysaccharide beads containing cadexomer iodine, which is released into the wound as the exudate is absorbed into the dressing. They are of benefit in surgical wounds which have become infected and dehisced to form a small cavity wound. A secondary dressing is required. The dressing should be changed once the product has become saturated. The gel can be removed with gentle irrigation of the wound.

Source: Morgan (2003).

---

absorb exudate, as large amounts of exudate can be produced in surgically created cavities; and facilitate the development of granulation tissue from the base of the wound.

The traditional dressing for this purpose has been ribbon gauze soaked in an antiseptic solution. However, this dressing will dry out, causing adherence of the dressing to the wound bed, which when removed causes the wound to bleed and much discomfort and pain for the patient (Bethell, 2003). Various dressing materials can be used, e.g. alginate or hydrofiber rope, foam cavity filler, or foam stent (see Box 4.6). They are more suitable than ribbon gauze, as they should not adhere to the wound bed and should be able to be removed without causing pain and discomfort for the patient (Briggs and Torra I Bou, 2002; Pudner, 2001a,b). It is also important that the dressing material is laid lightly in the wound bed, as tightly packing the wound can lead to excessive local pressure on the capillary loops, which will result in ischaemia and tissue death as well as causing pain and discomfort for the patient. Topical negative pressure may also be used to promote wound closure (see p. 56).

Wounds healing by secondary intention may need cleansing, in order to remove excessive amounts of exudate from the wound edges. This may be achieved by the patient having a shower and irrigating the wound with warm water, as opposed to using an aseptic technique or using antiseptic solutions which may have a detrimental effect on healing (Gilmour, 2000; Pudner, 1997b).

The wound will need to be redressed according to whichever dressing material is used. An alginate or hydrofiber dressing will need to be replaced once it is fully saturated, which may be daily in the initial days postoperatively, and then every 3–5 days as the amount of exudate diminishes. If a cavity filler is used, it can stay in place until it is fully saturated, and then be replaced with another cavity filler. If a foam stent is used, it will need to be removed and cleaned every 24–48 hours, and can be used until the stent does not fit the shape of the wound, indicating that another stent will need to be made. The use of this type of dressing may also mean that patients can manage the wound themselves, instead of having to visit the clinic or surgery for daily wound dressings.

As healing of the wound progresses, the amount of exudate will be reduced and the shape of the cavity will change, becoming much shallower and eventually showing signs of epithelialization. The wound dressing will need to be changed accordingly, and a non-adherent dressing used, so as to protect the new epithelial tissue.

Infected wounds

If the wound has become infected, the most important intervention is the prompt removal of pus, devitalized tissue, or accumulated fluid, as well as giving the appropriate antibiotic therapy. The edges of the wound may need to be gently pressed to release any discharge that has collected within it, and the wound irrigated to remove any purulent material. A drainage bag may be needed if there is a large amount of drainage, ensuring observation of the amount and type of discharge, as well as keeping the patient clean and dry and protecting the surrounding skin from excoriation. Once the amount of discharge has reduced, an appropriate dressing should be applied, depending on the size and shape of the wound (Galvani, 1995).

DISCHARGE ADVICE

Prior to the patient's discharge, they will need advice as to how their wound should be managed at home. This may also include the patient's carer and/or relative. If the patient is discharged home prior to having their sutures or staples removed, they will need to return to the hospital or visit their general practitioner, to arrange for the nurse to remove the sutures/staples. The patient should be given information regarding the signs to look out for that will indicate a wound infection, and what to do if this happens. If a dressing is still needed, the patient will need to be given information as to when, where and by whom it will be changed. This may often need to fit in with his family and work commitments.

Many patients want to know if they have to continue wearing a dressing once the wound has healed and whether they can bathe or shower. Once the wound has healed, the patient does not require a dressing, although if the scar is irritated by clothing, a light dressing may be required to protect the scar from any friction or rubbing. Some patients may also find that the scar feels very sensitive to touch, and again will prefer to wear a light dressing over the scar to avoid any unpleasant sensations. The patient will be able to bathe or shower normally, although they may need to pat the scar dry in order to avoid any discomfort. If the wound is still exuding, they can still bathe or shower, and will need to apply an appropriate dressing afterwards. Patients should always be given a contact number in case of any concerns or problems that they may have with their wound.

CONCLUSION

Surgical wounds are premeditated wounds, and so the surgeon will endeavour to reduce any risks of complication to a minimum. It is well recognized that a number of factors can increase the risk of the patient's wound becoming infected, and strategies should be adopted by all healthcare practitioners to reduce these risks to a bare minimum. In the USA the Centers for Disease Control and Prevention has produced guidelines to reduce the incidence of surgical wound infection (Mangram et al, 1999). Postoperative complications can be minimized by the preoperative care the patient receives, the amount of information and education given to the patient, as well as evaluation of the healing process.

Summary of key points

- Surgical wounds can heal by primary, secondary or tertiary intention.

- There are many factors that can influence the healing process and increase the risk of wound infection.

- Choice of wound closure depends upon the type of tissue and position of the wound.

- Surgical drainage can reduce the incidence of wound infection, and allows closer apposition of the tissues.

- Postoperative wound complications are usually related to infection.

- The patient and their wound should be assessed in order to plan appropriate interventions.

- Wound cleansing is not required unless there is excessive exudate or presence of purulent material.

- Wound dressings should maintain an optimum environment for healing, and not cause pain or trauma on removal.

- Advice on how to manage the wound should be given to the patient and/or carer prior to discharge.

References

Applebaum, J., Zalut, T. & Applebaum, A. (1993) The use of tissue adhesion for traumatic laceration repair in the emergency department. *Annals of Emergency Medicine* 22(7): 1190–1192.

Bailey, I. S., Karran, S. E., Toyn, K., et al (1992) Community surveillance of complications after hernia surgery. *British Medical Journal* 304(6825): 469–471.

Banwell, P. E. & Téot, L. (2003) Topical negative pressure (TNP): the evolution of a novel wound therapy. *Journal of Wound Care* 12(1): 22–28.

Baxendall, T. (1996) Healing cavity wounds with negative pressure. *Nursing Standard* 11(6): 49, 51.

Bennett, G. & Moody, M. (1995) *Wound Care for Health Professionals*. London: Chapman & Hall.

Bethell, E. (2003) Why gauze dressings should not be the first choice to manage most acute surgical cavity wounds. *Journal of Wound Care* 12(6): 237–239.

Bonavita, L. (1985) Free tissue transfer. *American Journal of Nursing* 85(4): 384–387.

Briggs, M. (1996a) Epidemiological methods in the study of surgical wound infection. *Journal of Wound Care* 5(4): 186–191.

Briggs, M. (1996b) Surgical wound pain: a trial of two treatments. *Journal of Wound Care* 5(10): 456–460.

Briggs, M. (1997) Principles of closed surgical wound care. *Journal of Wound Care* 6(6): 288–292.

Briggs, M. & Torra I Bou, J. E. (2002) Pain at wound dressing changes: a guide to management. In: Calne, S. (ed.) *Pain at Wound Dressing Changes*. EWMA Position Document. Available at http://www.tendra.com/files/Tendra/safetac/ENGLISH.pdf (accessed 11 December 2003).

Bruce, J., Russell, E. M., Mollison, J. & Krukowski, Z. H. (2001) The quality of measurement of surgical wound infection as the basis for monitoring: a systematic review. *Journal of Hospital Infection* 49(2): 99–108.

Butterworth, R. (1993) Wound contraction: a review. *Journal of Wound Care* 2(3): 172–175.

Capperauld, I. (1985) Sutures in wound repair. In: Westaby, S. (ed.) *Wound Care*. London: Heinemann Medical Books.

Carlson, M. (1997) Acute wound failure. *Surgical Clinics of North America* 77(3): 607–636.

Castille, K. (1996) Suturing. *Nursing Standard* 10(51): 49–54.

Chrintz, H., Vibits, H., Cordtz, T., et al (1989) Need for surgical wound dressing. *British Journal of Surgery* 76(2): 204–205.

Collier, M. (1997) Know how: vacuum-assisted closure (VAC). *Nursing Times* 93(5): 32–33.

Cooper, D. (1990) Optimizing wound healing. *Nursing Clinics of North America* 25(1): 165–180.

Cox, D. (1993) Growth factors in wound healing. *Journal of Wound Care* 2(6): 339–342.

Cruse, P. & Foord, R. (1973) A five-year prospective study of 23,649 surgical wounds. *Archives of Surgery* 107(2): 206–210.

Cruse, P. & Foord, R. (1980) The epidemiology of wound infection – a 10 year study of 62,939 wounds. *Surgical Clinics of North America* 60(1): 27–40.

Cutting, K. F. & Harding, K. G. (1994) Criteria for identifying wound infection. *Journal of Wound Care* 3(4): 198–201.

Cutting, K. F. & White, R. J. (2003) Criteria for identifying wound infection – revisited. Poster presentation at Wounds UK 2003, November 2003, Harrogate International Conference Centre; Harrogate.

Desai, H. (1997) Ageing and wounds. Part 2: healing in old age. *Journal of Wound Care* 6(5): 237–239.

Dougherty, S. H. & Simmons, R. L. (1992) The biology and practice of surgical drains: Part 1. *Current Problems in Surgery* 29(8): 561–623.

Ethicon (2000) *Wound Closure Manual*. Edinburgh: Ethicon.

Fay, M. (1987) Drainage systems. *AORN Journal* 46(3): 442–443, 445, 447, 449–452, 454–455.

Flanagan, M. (1997) *Wound Management*. Edinburgh: Churchill Livingstone.

Fletcher, J. (2000) The role of collagen in wound healing. *Professional Nurse* 15(8): 527–530.

Galvani, J. (1995) Nursing care of a superficial surgical site infection. *British Journal of Nursing* 4(18): 1084–1086.

Garibaldi, R. A., Cushing, D. & Lerer, T. (1991) Predictors of intraoperative-acquired surgical wound infections. *Journal of Hospital Infection* 18(Suppl. A): 289–298.

Gilmour, D. (2000) Is aseptic technique always necessary? *Journal of Community Nursing* 14(4): 32, 35

Greif, R., Horn, E-P., Kurz, A. & Sessler, D. I. (2000) Supplemental perioperative oxygen to reduce the incidence of surgical wound infection. *The New England Journal of Medicine* 342(3): 161–167.

Harding, K. & Jones, V. (1996) *Wound Management: Good Practice Guidance*. London: Macmillan.

Hinchliff, S., Montague, S. & Watson, R. (eds) (1996) *Physiology for Nursing Practice*, 2nd edn. London: Baillière Tindall.

Holm, C., Petersen, J. S., Grønbœk, F. & Gottrup, F. (1998) Effects of occlusive and conventional gauze dressings on incisional healing after abdominal operations. *European Journal of Surgery* 164(3): 179–183.

Hopkinson, I. (1992) Molecular components of the extracellular matrix. *Journal of Wound Care* 1(1): 52–54.

Hotter, A. (1990) Wound healing and immunocompromise. *Nursing Clinics of North America* 25(1): 193–203.

Hultén, L. (1994) Dressings for surgical wounds. *The American Journal of Surgery* 167(1A Suppl): 42S–45S.

Hunt, T. & Hopf, H. (1997) Wound healing and wound infection. *Surgical Clinics of North America* 77(3): 587–606.

Jacobson, T. (1994) Obesity and the surgical patient: nursing alert. *Ostomy/Wound Management* 40(2): 56–58, 60–63.

Kerstein, M. (1996) Wound infection: assessment and management. *Wounds: A Compendium of Clinical Research and Practice* 8(4): 141–144.

Kielcolt-Glaser, J. K., Marucha, P. T., Malarkey, W. B., et al (1995) Slowing of wound healing by psychological stress. *The Lancet* 346(8984): 1194–1196.

Kurz, A., Sessler, D. I. & Lenhardt, R. (1996) Perioperative normothermia to reduce the incidence of surgical wound infection and shorten hospitalization. *The New England Journal of Medicine* 334(19): 1209–1215.

Lawrence, J. (1993) Wound infection. *Journal of Wound Care* 2(5): 277–280.

Leaper, D. (1992) Surgical management of wounds. In: Harding, K., Leaper, D. & Turner, T. (eds) *Proceedings of the 1st European Conference on Advances in Wound Management.* London: Macmillan Magazines.

Leaper, D. J. (1995) Risk factors for surgical infection. *Journal of Hospital Infection* 30(Suppl.): 127–139.

Leaper, D. J. & Lucarotti, M. (1992) Sutures and staples. *Journal of Wound Care* 1(4): 27–30.

Lock, P. M. (1980) The effects of temperature on mitotic activity at the edge of experimental wounds. In: Sundell, B. (ed.) *Symposium on Wound Healing. Plastic Surgical and Dermatological Aspects.* Sweden: Mölndal.

McIntyre, F. J. & McCloy, R. (1994) Shaving patients before operation: a dangerous myth? *Annals of the Royal College of Surgeons of England* 76(1): 3–4.

McLaren, S. (1992) Nutrition and wound healing. *Journal of Wound Care* 1(3): 45–54.

McLean, F. & Hale, C. (1990) Comparing drainage bags. *Nursing Times* 86(15): 66, 69.

Maier, S. F. & Laudenslager, M. (1985) Stress and health: exploring the links. *Psychology Today* 19(8): 44–49.

Mangram, A. J., Horan, T. C., Pearson, M. L., et al, the Hospital Infection Control Practices Advisory Committee (1999) Guideline for prevention of surgical site infection, 1999. *American Journal of Infection Control* 27(2): 97–132.

Mishriki, S. F., Law, D. & Jeffery, P. (1990) Factors affecting the incidence of postoperative wound infection. *Journal of Hospital Infection* 16(3): 223–230.

Mishriki, S. F., Jeffery, P. & Law, D. (1992) Wound infection: the surgeon's responsibility. *Journal of Wound Care* 1(2): 32–36.

Mishriki, S. F., Law, D. & Jeffery, P. (1993) Surgical audit: variations in wound infection rates according to definition. *Journal of Wound Care* 2(5): 286–288.

Moncada, G. (1992) The healing wound: clinical management. *Plastic Surgical Nursing* 12(2): 56–60.

Morgan, D. (2003) *Formulary of Wound Management Products.* Available at http://www.euromed.uk.com/formulary10update.htm (accessed 30 October 2003)

Noel, I., Hollyoak, V. & Galloway, A. (1997) A survey of the incidence and care of postoperative wound infections in the community. *Journal of Hospital Infection* 36(4): 267–273.

Orgill, D. & Demling, R. (1988) Current concepts and approaches to wound healing. *Critical Care Medicine* 16(9): 899–908.

Perkins, P. (1992) Wound dehiscence: causes and care. *Nursing Standard* 6(34) (Tissue Viability Suppl.): 12, 14.

Public Health Laboratory Service (2002) *Surveillance of Surgical Site Infection in English Hospitals 1997–2001.* Available at http://www.hpa.org.uk/infections/publications/ninns/NINSS-SSI2000.pdf (accessed 11 December 2003)

Pudner, R. (1997a) Assessing a patient with a wound. *Journal of Community Nursing* 11(5): 28, 30, 32, 34.

Pudner, R. (1997b) Wound cleansing. *Journal of Community Nursing* 11(7): 30, 32, 34, 36.

Pudner, R. (2001a) Alginate and hydrofibre dressings in wound management. *Journal of Community Nursing* 15(5): 38, 41–42.

Pudner, R. (2001b) Foam, hydrocellular and hydropolymer dressings in wound management. *Journal of Community Nursing* 15(11): 26, 28, 31–32, 34.

Reilly, J. (2002) Evidence-based surgical wound care on surgical wound infection. *British Journal of Nursing* (Tissue viability supplement) 11(16): S4–S12.

Reilly, J., Twaddle, S., McIntosh, J. & Kean, L. (2001) An economic analysis of surgical wound infection. *Journal of Hospital Infection* 49(4): 245–249.

Robson, M. C. (1988) Disturbances of wound healing. *Annals of Emergency Medicine* 17(12): 1274–1278.

Sauvage, A. & Quinton, D. (1995) Procedure for closure of traumatic wounds. *Update* 50(8): 531–532, 534–536.

Seropian, R. & Reynolds, B. (1971) Wound infections after preoperative depilatory versus razor preparation. *The American Journal of Surgery* 121(3): 251–254.

Siana, J., Frankild, S. & Gottrup, F. (1992) The effect of smoking on tissue function. *Journal of Wound Care* 1(2): 37–39.

Silhi, N. (1998) Diabetes and wound healing. *Journal of Wound Care* 7(1): 47–51.

Silver, I. (1994) The physiology of wound healing. *Journal of Wound Care* 3(2): 106–109.

Singer, A. J., Quinn, J. V., Thode, H. C. & Hollander, J. E. (2002) Determinants of poor outcome after laceration and surgical incision repair. *Plastic and Reconstructive Surgery* 110(2): 429–435.

Smyth, E. T. M. & Emmerson, A. M. (2000) Surgical site surveillance. *Journal of Hospital Infection* 45(3): 173–184

Spotnitz, W., Falstrom, J. & Rodeheaver, G. (1997) The role of sutures and fibrin sealant in wound healing. *Surgical Clinics of North America* 77(3): 651–669.

Steed, D. (1997) The role of growth factors in wound healing. *Surgical Clinics of North America* 77(3): 575–586.

Taylor, D. E., Whamond, J. S. & Penhallow, J. E. (1987) Effects of haemorrhage on wound strength and fibroblast function. *British Journal of Surgery* 74(4): 316–319.

Torrance, C. (1993) Introduction to surgical drainage. *Surgical Nurse* 6(2): 19–23.

Tortora, G. & Grabowski, S. R. (2003) *The Principles of Anatomy and Physiology*, 10th edn. New York: John Wiley and Sons.

Wells, F., Newsom, S. & Rowlands, C. (1983) Wound infection in cardiothoracic surgery. *Lancet* (May 28): 1209–1210.

West, J. (1990) Wound healing in the surgical patient: influence of the perioperative stress response on perfusion. *AACN Clinical Issues in Critical Care Nursing* 1(3): 595–600.

Westaby, S. (1985) Wound closure and drainage. In: Westaby, S. (ed.) *Wound Care.* London. Heinemann Medical Books.

Wilson, J. (1995) *Infection Control in Clinical Practice.* London: Baillière Tindall.

Wilson, A. P., Weavill, C., Burridge, J. & Kelsy, M. C. (1990) The use of the wound scoring method 'ASEPSIS' in postoperative wound surveillance. *Journal of Hospital Infection* 16(4): 297–309.

Wilson, A. P., Helder, N., Theminimulle, S. K. & Scott, G. M. (1998) Comparison of wound scoring methods for use in audit. *Journal of Hospital Infection* 39(2): 119–126.

Winter, G. D. (1962) Formation of the scab and rate of epithelialisation in the skin of the young domestic pig. *Nature* 193: 293–295.

Further reading

Bale, S. & Jones, V. (1997) *Wound Care Nursing*. London: Baillière Tindall.

Briggs, M. (1997) Principles of closed surgical wound care. *Journal of Wound Care* 6(6): 288–292.

Dealey, C. (1999) *The Care of Wounds,* 2nd edn. Oxford: Blackwell.

Flanagan, M. (1997) *Wound Management*. Edinburgh: Churchill Livingstone.

Hampton, S. & Collins, F. (2004) *Tissue Viability.* London. Whurr.

Hinchliff, S., Watson, R. (eds) (1996) Innate defences. In: Hinchliff, S., Montague, S. & Public Health Laboratory Service (2002) *Physiology for Nursing Practice*, 2nd edn. London: Baillière Tindall. *Surveillance of Surgical Site Infection in English Hospitals 1997–2001.* Available at http://www.hpa.org.uk/infections/publications/ninns/NINSS-SSI2000.pdf (accessed 11 December 2003).

Morgan, D. (2003) *Formulary of Wound Management Products.* Available at http://www.euromed.uk.com/formulary10update.htm (accessed 30 October 2003).

NICE (2001) *Guidance on the Use of Debriding Agents and Specialist Wound Care Clinics for Difficult to Heal Surgical Wounds.* Available at http://www.nice.org.uk/pdf/woundcareguidance.pdf (accessed 30 January 2004).

http://www.worldwidewounds.com Resource for dressing materials and practical wound management (accessed 30 January 2004).

Chapter 5

Nutrition and the surgical patient

Susanne Wood

Key objectives of the chapter

The nurse will be able to promote recovery and well-being and reduce the harmful effects of undernutrition following surgery through understanding:

- the relationship between surgery, metabolism and nutrition

- the causes of undernutrition and their assessment in the surgical patient

- methods of preventing and treating undernutrition.

INTRODUCTION

The relationship between poor nutritional status and postoperative complications has been recognized for over 50 years (Mulholland et al, 1943; Studley, 1936). Malnutrition increases the risk of complications arising from physical weakness and impaired immunity such as chest and wound infections (Haydock and Hill, 1986; Meijerink et al, 1995). It also contributes to pressure ulcer formation and delays wound healing (Thomas, 1994). In addition, the undernourished patient is often apathetic, with little desire to eat and drink or engage in other therapeutic activities.

Weight loss around the time of surgery is common. Food and drink intake is often inadequate to meet nutritional needs, needs which may be increased by the metabolic response to the stress of surgery, infection or cancer. In addition, nutrients may also be required to replace those lost through drainage of body fluids.

Of all healthcare professionals, nurses have the most constant, intimate contact with patients and play a pivotal role in identifying potential and actual nutritional problems, and ensuring the delivery of adequate nourishment. Nurses should never assume that other professionals are aware of factors evident only during the delivery of nursing care. Communicating nursing observations and evaluations of care to doctors, dietitians, pharmacists and other professionals is of equal importance as direct nursing interaction with patients, in ensuring good nutrition.

This chapter aims to provide background information on the metabolic and nutritional alterations which occur after surgery and to highlight the importance of nutritional status in the surgical patient. It will describe ways in which nurses can take a proactive role in the planning, delivery and evaluation of nutritional care.

NUTRITIONAL REQUIREMENTS

The body requires an adequate balanced intake of nutrients and fluid to maintain body weight, body composition and to function optimally. Daily requirements for protein, energy, fluid, sodium and potassium can be estimated using Table 5.1.

ENERGY

Sufficient energy from food is required for growth, maintenance of body functions such as the beating of the heart, maintenance of body temperature and for physical activity. Energy may also be expended in response to drugs, metabolic changes which may occur in injury or trauma, including surgery, wound healing and after the ingestion of food (thermogenic response to food intake).

Energy in food is measured in kilocalories or kilojoules. An adequate intake of energy is also required to allow the use of protein for production of body tissues, rather than its breakdown to provide energy. Energy in the diet is provided primarily by fat and carbohydrate.

PROTEIN

Dietary proteins are made up of long chains of amino acids. Protein makes up the main structural and functional components of all cells in the body and is therefore essential for the structure and function of body cells and tissues. All amino acids contain nitrogen, and often protein intake and requirements may be discussed in terms of 'nitrogen balance'. Proteins within the body are continuously being broken down and resynthesized, with the result that some nitrogen is excreted from the body each day in urine, faeces and via the skin. Additional losses may occur through loss of blood, heavily exuding wounds, or via the gastrointestinal tract such as via a stoma or fistula. This balance of protein breakdown and synthesis may be altered by trauma or surgery.

ELECTROLYTES

The electrolytes sodium, potassium and chloride are essential to maintain the correct composition of body fluids. Sodium and chloride are present mainly in the extracellular fluid. Both these electrolytes are conserved by the body by an efficient reabsorption mechanism in the kidneys and by reabsorption of intestinal fluids in the large bowel. Sodium depletion may occur in a number of circumstances, such as:

- excessive sweating (due to pyrexia for example)
- if there are losses from the small bowel, such as in the case of a small bowel fistula or ileostomy
- in cases of profuse diarrhoea
- or if there are excessive sodium losses from the kidney.

Table 5.1   Nutritional requirements per kg actual body weight – adults

Patient group	Protein (g/kg)	Energy (kcal/kg) [kJ/kg]	Fluid (mL/kg)	Sodium (mmol/kg)	Potassium (mmol/g protein)
Normal and mildly stressed	1.0	30 [125]	30–35	1.0 minimum 50 mmol/day	5.0
Moderately stressed	1.3–1.9	35–40 [150–170]	30–35	1.0	5.0
Severely stressed	2.0–3.0	40–60 [170–250]	30–35	1.0	7.0

Source: Elwyn (1980).
Adapted and printed with permission from the Parenteral and Enteral Group of the British Dietetic Association (1989).
For each 1°C rise in temperature, the patient requires an additional: 500–700 mL fluid; 30 mmol sodium; 10% energy requirements.

Often depletion of body sodium occurs in conjunction with water loss, and restoration of the body's fluid balance requires the oral administration of water and sodium salts, usually sodium chloride or intravenous saline 0.9% solution.

Potassium occurs mainly within the cells, with only 2% of the total body stores existing in the extracellular fluids. Increases in plasma potassium levels may occur when tissues are destroyed and potassium is released from the cells. A fall in plasma potassium usually occurs when losses from the body are increased, e.g. in diarrhoea or increased losses from the kidney.

VITAMINS AND MINERALS

Adequate quantities of vitamins and minerals are essential for optimal functioning of the body. Daily requirements for healthy individuals are discussed in detail in the Department of Health publication *Dietary Reference Values for Food Energy and Nutrients for the United Kingdom* (Department of Health, 1991).

Requirements for some vitamins and minerals may be increased in surgical patients because of an increase in metabolic rate. In the surgical patient, absorption of vitamins and minerals may be reduced by malabsorption, poor gastrointestinal motility or loss of intestinal mucosa. Losses of vitamins from the body, particularly water-soluble vitamins, may be increased due to diarrhoea, fluids from fistulae or drainage of gastric contents via a nasogastric tube (Shenkin, 1995).

Some vitamins and minerals are of particular importance to the surgical patient and may need to be given in doses higher than those recommended for healthy individuals.

Vitamin C (ascorbic acid) is essential for the formation of collagen and therefore for wound healing. Deficiency of vitamin C, known as scurvy, impairs the formation of collagen and may result in delayed wound healing or in wound breakdown. Vitamin C has been shown to have beneficial effects in the healing of pressure ulcers. In a group of surgical patients with pressure ulcers, a daily supplement of 500 mg of ascorbic acid twice daily was demonstrated to significantly improve the rate of healing of the pressure ulcers (Taylor et al, 1974).

Vitamin A (retinol) is necessary for the formation of collagen and enhances granulation and epithelialization of healing wounds. Vitamin A deficiency is rare in Western countries, and care must be taken to avoid exceeding reference nutrient intakes, because of the toxicity of fat-soluble retinol (Department of Health, 1991).

Vitamin K is necessary for clotting of the blood. Although requirements are not known to be increased in the surgical patient, the action of vitamin K may be altered by drugs. Anticoagulant drugs such as warfarin block the recycling of vitamin K, and broad-spectrum antibiotics destroy the bacteria responsible for producing menaquinones, which have vitamin K activity (British Medical Association and Royal Pharmaceutical Society of Great Britain, 2004).

Zinc is necessary for division of cells within the body. Rapid loss of lean body mass – i.e. muscle – encourages loss of zinc from the body (Pichard and Jeejeebhoy, 1994). In patients who are depleted of zinc, zinc supplementation may help wound healing. Wound healing was enhanced in patients with low serum zinc when they were given oral supplementation with 200 mg zinc sulphate three times daily (Hallbook and Lanner, 1972).

Requirements for iron may be raised in the patient who experiences blood loss during or after surgery. Blood transfusions provide the body with a non-dietary source of iron.

Whenever possible, vitamin and mineral requirements should be met by intake of food and fluids. Where dietary intake is inadequate or requirements are raised, a multivitamin and mineral preparation may be necessary to ensure an adequate intake. For patients with particularly poor wound healing, supplements of vitamin C and zinc, as described above, may be of benefit. There is no benefit to be gained from excess or 'mega-doses' of vitamins or minerals. Intakes in excess of requirements may not be absorbed, may be excreted by the body as in the case of water-soluble vitamins such as vitamin C, or stored within the body and potentially produce toxic side-effects as in the case of vitamin A and selenium (Department of Health, 1991).

FLUID

Water is an essential component of body tissues, constituting approximately 50–70% of the total body weight. About two-thirds of the water exists within cells and one-third in the extracellular fluid. Water is ingested as fluid drunk and in food eaten, and is excreted in urine, faeces, sweat from the skin and is exhaled from the lungs. Requirements for fluid may be increased with increases in body temperature, diarrhoea and vomiting.

NUTRITIONAL CHANGES DURING STARVATION

When food intake is reduced, metabolic adaptations occur to delay the loss of tissues and therefore prolong survival. A reduction in energy intake results in the body mobilizing adipose tissue fat to be used to meet energy requirements. Carbohydrates stored within the liver as glycogen are released to provide glucose for the brain. As starvation proceeds, there is a breakdown of the body's protein, initially skeletal muscle, to provide amino acids. The amino acids are processed by the liver and kidneys and converted to glucose. Nitrogen contained within the amino acids is excreted in the urine as urea and ammonia.

All these changes are consistent with the body's breaking down its own tissues to provide the necessary energy for body functions, and maintenance of body temperature. As starvation proceeds, there is a reduction in nitrogen loss from the body, and the metabolic rate falls as the body tries to conserve depleted tissues. Without food, death would occur within 40–60 days, as irreversible damage to vital organs would occur (Pichard and Jeejeebhoy, 1994).

METABOLIC AND NUTRITIONAL CHANGES AFTER SURGERY

Surgery or trauma can cause metabolic changes which influence the patient's nutritional status. In starvation, the body adapts to a reducing food intake, conserving protein stores within the body and reducing metabolic rate. After trauma or surgery, hormonal changes cause a prolonged increase in metabolic rate, which can cause rapid depletion of body tissues (Broom, 1994).

There are two main phases in the response to trauma: the ebb or shock phase and the flow phase.

THE EBB OR SHOCK PHASE

The initial response of the body to injury is caused by hormonal changes. Adrenaline (epinephrine), cortisol and antidiuretic hormone are released into the bloodstream. Blood vessels become dilated, cardiac output falls and the patient goes into 'shock'. The most important factors in treatment during this phase are that blood volume is maintained with intravenous fluids, to help maintain cardiac output and tissue perfusion, and that pain is relieved. Nutritional support during this phase, which may last up to 24 hours, is of little value or importance.

THE FLOW PHASE

The flow phase occurs after the ebb or shock phase and can be divided into two parts: the catabolic and the recovery phase.

During the catabolic phase, oxygen consumption, body temperature and energy expenditure increase dramatically to above normal levels. There is a rapid increase in protein breakdown and loss of lean body mass. The duration of the catabolic phase varies depending on the severity of the injury and measures taken to counteract the shock. It may be from 24 hours for a minor procedure or up to 5 days or longer for major surgery. Patients who return to theatre for any reason will go through the ebb and flow phases again, thereby having prolonged periods of time when metabolic rate is raised. Increase in energy expenditure may vary from 10% above resting energy expenditure in minor surgery, to up to 50–60% above resting energy expenditure in major surgery and sepsis (Elwyn, 1980). Sepsis may further increase energy expenditure and can cause metabolic alterations which encourage more rapid loss of lean body mass.

Although the metabolic alterations which occur during the catabolic phase cannot be prevented, the effects on the body can be reduced if nutritional support is given through this period. Many patients at this stage are unable to eat and drink enough to meet their needs, and benefit from oral nutritional supplements or enteral tube feeding. Intravenous (parenteral) feeding is required by those unable to absorb nutrients or in whom rest of the gastrointestinal tract is prescribed (Broom, 1994).

During nutritional support, some nitrogen continues to be lost from the body as a result of protein breakdown, although feeding the patient stimulates protein synthesis. Excessive feeding, however, in an attempt to restore lean body mass, is not advisable, as it may provide an additional stress to the body. Changes in metabolism as a result of the stress hormones adrenaline (epinephrine) and cortisol may prevent the efficient use of glucose. The recovery phase occurs after the catabolic phase when the body is no longer hypermetabolic, and intakes of energy and nitrogen can be given safely in quantities to restore lean body mass (Elwyn, 1980).

THE EVIDENCE FOR NUTRITIONAL SUPPORT IN THE SURGICAL PATIENT

PREOPERATIVE NUTRITIONAL SUPPORT

Preoperatively, patients may become malnourished due to a poor appetite, dysphagia, malabsorption, malignant disease, inflammatory bowel disease or periods of not eating due to hospitalization. Sepsis may also increase nutritional requirements. The length of time the patient is kept nil by mouth for investigations is a further contributory factor. Nutritional support is more likely to replete body stores when given preoperatively, because of the absence of the catabolic changes which occur following surgery. Studies on the value of preoperative nutritional support have often failed to demonstrate a clear clinical benefit (Allison, 1995). This has been attributed to poor study design, too few patients and insufficient focus on patients who were most nutritionally depleted.

POSTOPERATIVE NUTRITIONAL SUPPORT

Studies on postoperative nutritional support have shown clinical benefit in patients who were initially malnourished as identified by a significant degree of weight loss (Allison, 1995). Supplementary feeding in malnourished patients has been demonstrated to reduce rehabilitation time, improve muscle strength, reduce the rate of serious infections and improve the rate of wound healing (Lennard-Jones, 1992; Robinson et al, 1987). This may represent huge financial savings in terms of reduced patient days in hospital and a reduced cost per day compared with the malnourished patient or patients who do not receive appropriate nutritional support (Lennard-Jones, 1992). This has been demonstrated in elderly women after surgical repair of a femoral neck fracture (Bastow et al, 1983). Women who received additional enteral nutrition had a shorter recovery and were discharged from hospital sooner. The evidence of this study is of particular importance when considering the increasing elderly population in the United Kingdom and their health-care needs.

There is evidence of improved clinical outcome resulting from immediate postoperative enteral feeding, including an early positive nitrogen balance, reduction in days of stay and improved sepsis resistance (Mainous and Deitch, 1994). Poor tolerance to early feeding is usually a result of poor gastric motility, which may occur in ventilated patients, multiple trauma, postabdominal surgery and abdominal sepsis (Silk, 1995). However, recent studies indicate that early enteral feeding, by tube, directly into the duodenum or jejunum, following major abdominal surgery, can be safe and effective (Beier-Holgersen, 2001).

PRESSURE ULCERS AND WOUND HEALING

Malnutrition may predispose the surgical patient to the development of pressure ulcers and contribute to impaired healing of pressure ulcers for a number of reasons (Olde Damink and Soeters, 1997). Loss of body fat and muscle results in a loss of the cushioning effect between the bones and skin. Protein depletion, as occurs in the catabolic phase of trauma or injury, may hamper the healing of pressure ulcers and surgical wounds (Mulholland et al, 1943). Improved nutritional intake, either by oral liquid supplements or by enteral

tube feeding, has been shown to promote healing of pressure ulcers (Breslow et al, 1991).

The following factors will increase the chances of the surgical patient becoming malnourished:

- existing preoperative malnutrition
- oral intake withheld or refused for more than 5–7 days, e.g. in oral or gastrointestinal surgery
- postoperative complications, e.g. sepsis, wound breakdown, intestinal ileus.

(Thomas, 1994).

PLANNING AND DELIVERING NUTRITIONAL CARE TO THE SURGICAL PATIENT

NUTRITION SCREENING

The purpose of screening is to grade an individual patient's level of risk of malnutrition and formulate an action plan. All patients are at risk; therefore, all patients should be screened. To be of value, screening needs to occur on first contact with the patient and at regular intervals thereafter. Changes in the underlying condition will influence risk: e.g. in one study, 34% of patients experienced significant weight loss following gastrointestinal surgery (Fettes et al, 2002). Patients requiring elective surgery should ideally be screened prior to admission, allowing time for the benefits of nutritional support, for those who are malnourished, to be effective. This may involve advice regarding an increased food intake, the use of oral nutritional supplementation or even nasogastric feeding for patients unable to take sufficient food and drink orally.

A wide range of screening instruments are available. The British Association for Parenteral and Enteral Nutrition Maladvisory Group recommends the *Malnutrition Universal Screening Tool (MUST)* (BAPEN, 2003). The scores for body mass index (BMI), unplanned weight loss and the presence of acute disease activity and current nutritional intake are added to provide a low-, medium- or high-risk grading for malnutrition, from which specific management guidelines can be instituted.

For patients for whom both height and weight are known, BMI can be calculated from the following equation:

$$\text{Body mass index} = \frac{\text{weight (kg)}}{\text{height (m}^2)}$$

Ideal BMI falls in the range 20–25 kg/m^2. The determination of BMI enables comparison of the individual's

Table 5.2 Severity of nutritional complications for varying degrees of weight loss

% Weight loss from normal in 6-month period	Severity of nutritional complication
0–10	Minor
10–35	Major – seriously impairs host defence mechanism and ability to withstand surgery
Over 35	Life threatening

Source: Elwyn (1980).

body weight and height in relation to the ideal. However, it gives no indication of recent weight loss. An accurate weight history helps to identify an increased risk of nutritional problems.

$$\% \text{ loss of body weight} = \frac{\text{normal weight} - \text{current weight}}{\text{normal weight}} \times 100$$

Oedema, which may arise due to disease or drugs, may distort measurements of weight (i.e. $1\,kg = 1\,L$).

The severity of nutritional complications for varying degrees of weight loss are shown in Table 5.2.

Patients who are obese may still experience nutritional depletion and the postoperative risks associated with malnutrition. Calculation of the percentage change in body weight allows the obese but malnourished patient to be recognized.

NUTRITIONAL ASSESSMENT

This is a more detailed evaluation of those patients, identified through screening, to be at high risk of malnutrition and is usually performed by a dietitian. Some elements – e.g. observation of the ability to eat and functional impairment – are, however, best performed by the nurse during the delivery of nursing care. Close working practices and communication between the nurse and dietitian are therefore beneficial.

There is no one single objective test that can accurately define whether a patient is malnourished. It is now thought that the most practical way to assess malnutrition is to undertake a bedside 'subjective global assessment' (Pichard and Jeejeebhoy, 1994). All of the following factors contribute information which indicates the possible causes and consequences of malnutrition in an individual patient. With this information, nutrient requirements can be calculated and the most effective method of achieving good nutritional intake determined.

ELEMENTS OF SUBJECTIVE GLOBAL ASSESSMENT

Ability to eat and functional impairment

Physical factors
- Age: energy intakes are often reduced in the elderly.
- Poor dentition: may make eating some foods difficult or impossible.
- Obstruction of the gastrointestinal tract: e.g. cancer of the mouth, throat or oesophagus.
- Gastrointestinal symptoms: e.g. nausea, vomiting or diarrhoea.
- Breathlessness (dyspnoea): e.g. in chronic obstructive airways disease.
- Neurological impairment: unconscious, or inability to feed.
- Anorexia: due to sepsis or severe systemic illness; may also be caused by excessive consumption of alcohol.
- Poor mobility: e.g. due to pain, osteoarthritis.
- Poor manual dexterity: e.g. in rheumatoid arthritis; may make food preparation and feeding difficult.

Emotional factors
- Anxiety.
- Apathy.

Social and environmental factors
- Social circumstances
  - low income
  - poor cooking facilities
  - poor access to shops.
- Iatrogenic starvation – repeatedly kept nil by mouth for tests.

Disease stress

The patient may have increased nutritional requirements because of the disease state, e.g. cancer, burns or sepsis.

Clinical wasting

This can be assessed by a physical examination, looking for loss of subcutaneous fat, muscle wasting and dry skin. Ankle and sacral oedema may be present. Other indicators of recent weight loss are loose clothing, rings and dentures. The presence of unhealed wounds is another indicator of poor nutritional status. Physical examination is particularly valuable when the patient cannot be weighed or give information about recent weight changes.

Assessing recent food intake

As patients may be unable to recall even the previous meal, calculating the recent intake of nutrients requires skilled questioning. Nurses can assist the patient and dietitian by recording intake of food and drink on a food monitoring chart. Direct observation of intake is crucial for accuracy as patients with little appetite often report having eaten well following very small meals, due to early feelings of fullness.

Special considerations

Bowel preparation

For patients undergoing elective gastrointestinal surgery, bowel preparation may be necessary to ensure that the contents of the bowel are cleared as much as possible prior to surgery. A regimen of a low-fibre diet, avoiding fruit, vegetables and wholegrain cereals, may be started 3–4 days preoperatively. At 24–48 hours prior to surgery, the patient may be allowed clear fluids only, such as water, black tea, black coffee, consommé, meat extracts, fruit squash or glucose drinks. Laxatives, such as Klean-Prep or Picolax, are used the day before surgery to clear the bowel of faecal matter. A few days of reduced nutritional intake is unlikely to be significant for the well-nourished patient, although for the already malnourished patient it may further exacerbate their depleted nutritional state.

Insulin-dependent diabetes mellitus

Diabetic patients must be given a 5% dextrose saline infusion in conjunction with a sliding-scale insulin administration when required to be nil by mouth prior to surgery, to avoid hypoglycaemia. Patients taking oral hypoglycaemic agents must be advised on taking such drugs. It is usual to stop the drugs when the patient is unable to eat, to avoid hypoglycaemia.

Intravenous hydration

Intravenous hydration is usually provided by sodium chloride 0.9% or 5% dextrose. It is important to remember that this provides fluid replacement only, and even dextrose is of little nutritional value in the quantities given.

Ethics

Ethical considerations underpin every aspect of nutritional care. For example, nutritional screening is an ethical action, because failure to identify and treat malnourished patients has been shown to increase the risk of complications. When planning care, the wishes of the patient are paramount and health professionals must carefully explain, in an unbiased and clear way, the rationale for any proposed nutritional therapy. A competent patient may refuse any intervention, and sensitivity is needed to determine the reason why. In current English law, feeding through a tube is viewed as medical therapy. As with any other medical intervention, the benefit must be balanced against the risk or burden it imposes. Complex situations, such as artificial feeding when patients are approaching the end of life, are often helped by establishing a goal for nutritional management, assisted by an ethical framework (Planas and Camilo, 2002).

POSTOPERATIVE NUTRITIONAL SUPPORT

Opinion as to the speed of introduction of food and fluids to the gut varies (Keohane et al, 1984). Although recent evidence supports the use of early duodenal or jejunal tube feeding following major abdominal surgery, oral fluids and food are commonly started postoperatively when the surgeon is satisfied that gastric emptying and gut function have resumed. This may take several days. Small amounts of water, 30–60 mL/h may then be allowed initially before the patient proceeds to taking free fluids and a light diet. Intravenous hydration must be maintained until the patient is drinking sufficient fluids orally. There is no universal definition of a light diet, although it is often considered to be based on foods which have a moderate fat and low-fibre content such as soup, eggs, fish, potatoes, yoghurt and ice cream. As oral intake increases, intravenous fluids may be decreased. Patients undergoing surgery not involving the gastrointestinal tract may usually start eating and drinking as soon as they wish postoperatively.

In the case of emergency surgery, there may be little or no information on the patient's preoperative nutritional status. Nutritional assessment should be performed at the earliest opportunity and a plan of care developed and commenced, to prevent a deterioration in nutritional status.

Intake of fluid and foods is often poor in the initial postoperative period. This may be due to anorexia induced by stress, poor gastric motility, pain or nausea. Patients need guidance and encouragement to achieve a nutritional intake to meet their requirements (see section on nutritional requirements). Any concern regarding nutritional intake should prompt referral to the dietitian.

Methods of nutritional support

- Oral: food and drink, oral liquid supplements.
- Enteral tube feeding: nasogastric, gastrostomy or jejunostomy.
- Parenteral feeding: via a central or peripheral vein.

IMPROVING DIETARY INTAKE

Food availability and presentation

It is essential that the foods available suit the patient's personal preferences, ethnic and cultural needs. In the hospital setting it is important to liaise with the catering and dietetic departments, to facilitate patients receiving food which they would like to eat and which is of a suitable consistency: e.g. soft foods for the dysphagic patient.

Timing of meals

Encouraging patients to eat when they can, may help dietary intake. Mealtimes are often at set times within the hospital setting, although it may be possible for snacks or nourishing drinks to be taken between meals.

Appetite stimulants

For the severely anorexic patient an appetite stimulant may be useful, such as alcohol, a low dose of steroids if appropriate, or medroxyprogesterone acetate or megestrol acetate (Bruera et al, 1990).

Nutritional supplements

Various nutritional supplements are available which may help improve intake.

Meal supplements or nutritionally complete liquid supplements

Examples are Build-Up (Nestlé), Complan (Glaxo), Ensure and Ensure Plus (Ross Laboratories). Additional fruit-flavoured drinks are available, such as Enlive (Ross) or Fortijuce (Nutricia Clinical). These may be used to replace meals completely or, more often, are given to supplement a poor food intake. Semisolid supplements are available for patients who are unable to swallow liquids, such as Formance (Ross Laboratories) and Fortipudding (Nutricia Clinical).

Energy supplements

Powdered glucose polymers can be used in drinks, soup, yoghurts, desserts and cereals. Examples are Maxijul (Scientific Hospital Supplies) and Polycose (Ross Laboratories). Liquid glucose in a concentrated form can be mixed with water, fruit squash, fruit juice and fizzy drinks. Examples are Hycal (SmithKline Beecham) and Polycal Liquid (Nutricia Clinical).

Combined glucose and fat powders or liquids are available to use in drinks and in cooking, e.g. Duocal (Scientific Hospital Supplies).

Protein supplements

Powdered protein supplements are available, such as Casilan 90 (Heinz) and Maxipro (Scientific Hospital Supplies). They can be added to drinks, soups and desserts but are rarely used in isolation, since protein alone is ineffective in restoring positive nitrogen balance. An adequate energy intake is essential to improve nutritional status. Studies have demonstrated that high energy drinks taken between meals do not alter the overall solid food intake and may even contribute to an improvement in main meal intake (Hessov, 1995).

ENTERAL TUBE FEEDING

Enteral feeding through nasogastric, gastrostomy (into the stomach) or jejunostomy (into the small intestine) tubes may be necessary in patients who have a functional gastrointestinal tract and are:

1. unable to eat, e.g. due to oral surgery, upper gastrointestinal surgery or dysphagia
2. able to eat but not in sufficient amounts to achieve an adequate nutritional intake, e.g. severely anorexic patients or those who have undergone gastrointestinal surgery and have a limited capacity to eat.

Nasogastric feeding

A nasogastric tube is often used when tube feeding is required for a period of less than 3–4 weeks. A fine-bore tube, usually made of polyurethane, is preferable to a wider-bore PVC Ryles tube, for patient comfort (Payne-James, 1995). Tubes may also be introduced through the nose and advanced through the pylorus for nasoduodenal or nasojejunal feeding. In addition, double lumen tubes are available which allow duodenal/jejunal feeding in conjunction with gastric aspiration. This method is indicated when gastric emptying is slow, or there is a risk of feed being regurgitated into the oesophagus due to poor function of the lower oesophageal sphincter.

During placement, tubes may coil in the pharynx or pass into the respiratory system; therefore, the position must be confirmed prior to commencing the feed and at regular intervals (usually every 24 hours) thereafter. The following techniques are used for nasogastric tubes:

- measuring the pH of gastric aspirate, which should be less than 4
- auscultation of the epigastrium while injecting air through the tube
- chest and/or abdominal X-ray.

(Methany, 1993).

X-ray is the 'gold standard' but delays the start of feeding, exposes the patient to ionizing radiation and is costly. It should, however, always be performed if gastric aspirate cannot be obtained or the pH is above 5. Auscultation is not reliable and must never be used as the sole method of confirming tube position (Methany et al, 1990).

Gastrostomy feeding

When longer-term feeding is anticipated, a gastrostomy tube may be placed directly into the stomach, during surgery or under radiological or endoscopic control. The latter tube is known as a percutaneous endoscopic gastrostomy or PEG. The tube is held in the stomach by an internal flange or balloon. An external retention device prevents internal migration of the tube. Haemorrhage and infection are risks associated with PEG placement. Percutaneous endoscopic gastrostomy tubes may remain in place for a number of years (Grant, 1993).

Jejunostomy feeding

For patients who have undergone surgery to the stomach or have pyloric obstruction, a feeding jejunostomy provides an alternative route. A fine-bore catheter is inserted into the jejunum and brought out through the anterior abdominal wall.

Feeding regimens

There are many commercial enteral feeds available which can be divided into the following categories.

1. *Polymeric feeds* require digestion before they can be absorbed and are used in patients with a normally functioning gastrointestinal tract. Examples include Ensure, Ensure Plus, Osmolite, Jevity (Ross Laboratories), Nutrison, Nutrison Energy Plus (Nutricia Clinical).

2. *Predigested chemically defined elemental feeds* require little or no digestion prior to being absorbed. They may be used in patients with an impaired gastrointestinal tract such as in short bowel syndrome or Crohn's disease. Examples include Elemental 028 (Scientific Hospital Supplies) and Peptamen (Nestlé Clinical).

3. *Disease-specific formulations* are designed for particular diseases. For example, high fat-to-carbohydrate ratio for cardiopulmonary failure; altered protein or amino acid composition for renal or liver failure, e.g. Nepro and Pulmocare (Ross Laboratories).

4. *Opportunistic feeds* are designed to improve various aspects of organ function, such as that of the gastrointestinal tract and the immune system. Various additions to the feed include arginine, glutamine and *n*-3 fatty acids. Examples include Alitraq (Ross Laboratories).

5. *Modular feeds* are composed of protein, fat, carbohydrate, vitamins and minerals from separate sources. They allow adaptation of food to meet the patient's specific requirements.

Administration of enteral feeding

The following regimens may be used to administer an enteral feed.

1. *Continuous, controlled feeding via an enteral pump.* This method is commonly used for patients starting enteral tube feeding, for patients in intensive care or for patients with poor tolerance. It avoids the administration of a large volume of feed into the gastrointestinal tract, which may cause rapid intestinal transit. This increases absorption of the feed (Payne-James, 1995). A short break in feeding of 4–6 hours allows the gastric pH to fall and helps to prevent bacterial overgrowth (Lee et al, 1990).

2. *Intermittently via an enteral feeding pump.* Generally used for patients with a good tolerance to enteral tube feeding and for those also taking food and fluids orally. Overnight feeding may be used to allow patients to eat and drink during the day.

3. *Bolus feeding.* The administration of 200–400 mL of feed over 15 minutes to 1 hour. This is only occasionally used, as it may increase the risk of side-effects such as diarrhoea and bloating (Payne-James, 1995).

Initially, full-strength feed is given at a slow rate, e.g. 30 mL/h. There is evidence to suggest that it is unnecessary to dilute the feed, and that the incidence of side-effects is unchanged when a full-strength feed is used to commence feeding (Keohane et al, 1984). When gut function is impaired due to starvation, drugs, disease or surgery, a slow introduction of feed may be required. Gastric emptying is assessed by aspirating every 2–3 hours. Residual gastric volume of greater than 200 mL from a nasogastric tube or 100 mL from a gastrostomy tube may indicate intolerance to the feed (Payne-James, 1995). The patient will require intravenous hydration until intake of the full volume of feed is achieved. The quantity of feed required can be assessed by using the figures in Table 5.1 and the known composition of the feed.

Problems of administration and complications of enteral tube feeding

Pulmonary aspiration

Aspiration may occur after vomiting or in patients who are unconscious. The latter should be nursed with a minimum of 45° elevation of thorax, head and neck. Postpyloric feeding, as in jejunostomy feeding, reduces the risk of aspiration.

Tube blockage

Feeding tubes should be flushed with water before and after periods of feeding and the administration of medications. The tube should also be flushed between each individual medication. Water, bicarbonate of soda in water and pancreatic enzymes may be used to facilitate unblocking of tube (Taylor, 1989).

Displacement of tube

Patients should be advised to avoid excessive tension on the feeding tube, as it may become dislodged accidentally. The tube should be securely fixed to the nose and face and administration sets attached to night attire. The tube should be examined for retrograde migration at least twice daily. A partially displaced tube must be re-inserted and the position checked in accordance with hospital policy.

Diarrhoea

Diarrhoea associated with enteral tube feeding may be due to:

- the administration of high osmolarity feeds, e.g. elemental feeds
- fast and irregular feeding
- infusion of cold feeds
- bacterial contamination or infection
- hypoalbuminaemia
- drugs such as those used in chemotherapy, and antibiotics
- or impaired gut motility.

Treatment of this complication must always be directed to the cause of the diarrhoea. Drugs such as codeine phosphate or loperamide may be useful in helping relieve the symptoms. When handling a tube or any part of the enteral feeding system, bacterial contamination from the hands must be avoided (Beattie and Anderton, 1999).

Constipation

Constipation may occur as a result of drugs which slow the action of the bowel, such as codeine-containing drugs or morphine, and when fluid requirements are underestimated (Heberer and Marx, 1995). Additional fluid, laxatives and enemas may be required. Patients on long-term enteral feeding may benefit from the use of fibre-containing feeds.

PARENTERAL FEEDING

Parenteral feeding is the provision of nutrients directly into the bloodstream, bypassing ingestion, digestion and absorption. It is indicated when the small intestine is unable to absorb sufficient fluid and nutrients, or when there is a therapeutic need to eliminate nutrients from the gastrointestinal tract. Although it is an effective method of nutritional support, it should only be used when enteral feeding is impossible, as it is associated with life-threatening septic, metabolic and thrombotic complications. In addition, it is now recognized that the presence of nutrients in the gastrointestinal tract may reduce the risk of bacterial translocation across the gut mucosa and therefore reduce the risk of infection (Silk, 1995).

Surgical patients who may require parenteral feeding include those who:

- are nil by mouth for longer than 5 days
- are intolerant to enteral feeding, e.g. uncontrolled vomiting or diarrhoea
- have an intestinal fistula necessitating bowel rest
- have pre- or postoperative bowel obstruction
- have a paralytic ileus.

Nutrients are provided in a form which can be used directly by the body: amino acids as the protein source, long-chain triglycerides as the fat source, glucose, electrolytes, vitamins, minerals and trace elements. Often the daily requirements are mixed in pharmacy and provided to the ward as an 'all-in-one' bag, which is administered over 24 hours. The high strength (hypertonicity) of some parenteral nutrition fluids necessitates their administration into the superior vena cava, where rapid dilution occurs due to the high blood flow of this large vein, so reducing the thrombotic effects. Other less hypertonic mixtures may be administered into a peripheral vein for short-term feeding when peripheral veins are satisfactory.

The aims of nursing care are:

- to deliver the parenteral feed at the correct rate over the correct time period
- to prevent septic, metabolic, thrombotic and other intravenous catheter-related complications
- to help the patient cope emotionally.

As formulations are quite complex, prescription forms specific to parenteral nutrition are an aid to safe checking and administration. The nutrient solutions are a rich culture media for bacteria, which may enter the circulation from the fluid in the container, connections in the administration system or from the skin at the catheter entry site. Clear protocols for infection control must be available and strictly adhered to at all times.

Concentrated glucose solutions are incorporated into all parenteral nutrition formulations; therefore, the blood glucose level should be monitored carefully. A volumetric infusion pump must be used to control the infusion rate, to prevent fluctuations in glucose administration.

Fluid balance should also be monitored through records and, when possible, measuring the body weight daily (1 litre is equivalent to 1 kilogram) . When serum albumin levels are low, fluid may be retained as oedema, which has the potential to interfere with physiological functions such as respiration.

Abnormal liver function and cholestasis may also occur, the cause of which has yet to be fully determined. The presence of the intravenous catheter or the administration of hypertonic fluids into a small vein can cause thrombosis, and the insertion of the intravenous catheter into the subclavian vein may result in a pneumothorax.

Patients needing parenteral nutrition are often very ill, with multiple clinical problems. Emotional support for the patient, family and, if the illness is protracted, the healthcare team is vital, as poor morale can be a major problem. Patients requiring long-term parenteral nutrition at home may wish to contact a patient support group such as Patients on Intravenous and Nasogastric Nutrition Therapy (PINNT).

Care from clinical nutrition teams composed of specialist nurses, doctors, pharmacists and dietitians who are familiar with this specialized area of nutritional support has been shown to reduce complications (Trujillo et al, 1999).

MONITORING NUTRITIONAL SUPPORT

1. *Body weight*: should be measured weekly or with a frequency appropriate to the nutritional therapy and the patient's clinical condition. Rapid changes in weight are usually due to alterations in fluid balance.
2. *Nutritional intake and fluid balance records*: a record of the patient's intake of fluid, food, sip feeds, enteral tube feed and parenteral nutrition should be documented to monitor the actual, rather than perceived intake.
3. *Physical examination*: obvious changes in physical appearance, the amount of subcutaneous fat, muscle power and mental state may give an indication of improving or deteriorating nutritional status (Lennard-Jones, 1992).

The dietitian or nutritional support team may use additional measures such as BMI, skinfold thickness, hand grip dynamometry, or biochemistry of blood or urine, to contribute to the monitoring of nutritional status (Thomas, 1994).

TERMINATION OF NUTRITIONAL SUPPORT

Enteral tube feeding must not be terminated until an adequate intake of nutrients is achieved orally. In the case of parenteral feeding, oral or enteral tube feeding must be adequate. Abrupt cessation of nutritional support usually causes the patient to have an insufficient nutritional intake.

THE MULTIDISCIPLINARY TEAM

Nutritional support of the surgical patient is the joint responsibility of a number of professions and departments within the hospital setting. Nurses, doctors, dietitians, pharmacists and the catering department all have responsibilities regarding the adequate screening, assessment, provision and monitoring of nutritional care. A team approach with good communication between disciplines has been shown to be a cost-effective way of providing advice on the support of individual patients, in addition to developing protocols, guidelines and standards (Silk, 1994).

Summary of key points

- Good nutritional status is essential to reduce complications, promote wound healing and reduce length of hospital stay.

- The nurse caring for the surgical patient needs to consider the following as part of the overall care of the patient:
  1. Screening. All surgical patients should undergo a nutritional screening prior to and after surgery. Patients who are malnourished or at risk of becoming malnourished must be referred to the dietitian or hospital nutrition team.
  2. Provision of nutritional support. The following methods may be used:
     - oral: diet and nutritional supplements
     - enteral tube feeding
     - parenteral feeding.

- The most appropriate form of support must be selected and monitored for efficacy and safety.

References

Allison, S. (1995) Malnutrition in hospitalised patients and assessment of nutrition support. In: Payne-James, J., Grimble, G. & Silk, D. (eds) *Artificial Nutrition Support in Clinical Practice*. London: Edward Arnold.

Bastow, M. D., Rawlings, J. & Allison, S. (1983) Benefits of supplementary tube feeding after fractured neck of femur: a randomised controlled trial. *British Medical Journal* 287(6405): 1589–1592.

Beattie, T. K. & Anderton, A. (1999) Microbiological evaluation of four enteral feeding systems which have been deliberately subjected to faulty handling procedures. *Journal of Hospital Infection* 42(1): 11–20.

Beier-Holgersen, R. (2001) The importance of early post operative enteral feeding. *Clinical Nutrition* 20(Suppl. 1): 123–127.

Breslow, R. A., Hallfrisch, J. & Goldberg, A. P. (1991) Malnutrition in tubefed nursing home patients with pressure sores. *Journal of Parenteral and Enteral Nutrition* 15(6): 663–668.

British Association for Parenteral and Enteral Nutrition (2003) *Malnutrition Universal Screening Tool ('MUST')* [online]. Available at http://www.bapen.org.uk/pdfs/Must/MUST-Complete.pdf (accessed 19 April 2004).

British Medical Association and Royal Pharmaceutical Society of Great Britain (2004) *British National Formulary No 47*. London: British Medical Association.

Broom, J. (1994) Sepsis and trauma. In: Garrow, J. S. & James, W. P. T. (eds) *Human Nutrition and Dietetics*, 9th edn. Edinburgh: Churchill Livingstone.

Bruera, E., Macmillan, K., Kuehn, N., et al (1990) A controlled trial of megestrol acetate on appetite, caloric intake, nutritional status and other symptoms in patients with advanced cancer. *Cancer* 66(6): 1279–1282.

Department of Health (1991) *Panel on Dietary Reference Values for Food Energy and Nutrients for the United Kingdom*. London: HMSO.

Elwyn, D. H. (1980) Nutritional requirements of adult surgical patients. *Critical Care Medicine* 8(1): 9–20.

Fettes, B. S., Davidson, I. M., Richardson, R. A. & Pennington, C. R. (2002) Nutritional status of elective gastrointestinal surgery patients pre and post operatively. *Clinical Nutrition* 21(3): 249–254.

Grant, J. P. (1993) Percutaneous endoscopic gastrostomy: initial placement by single endoscopic technique and long-term follow-up. *Annals of Surgery* 217(2): 168–174.

Hallbook, T. & Lanner, E. (1972) Serum zinc and healing of venous leg ulcers. *The Lancet* (Oct 14): 780–782.

Haydock, D. A. & Hill, G. L. (1986) Impaired wound healing in surgical patients with varying degrees of malnutrition. *Journal of Enteral and Parenteral Nutrition* 10(6): 550–554.

Heberer, M. & Marx, A. (1995) Complications of enteral nutrition. In: Payne-James, J., Grimbley, G. & Silk, D. (eds) *Artificial Nutrition Support in Clinical Practice*. London: Edward Arnold.

Hessov, I. (1995) Oral diet administration and supplementation. In: Payne-James, J., Grimble, G. & Silk, D. (eds) *Artificial Nutrition Support in Clinical Practice*. London: Edward Arnold.

Keohane, P. P., Attrill, H., et al (1984) Relation between osmolarity of diet and gastrointestinal side effects in enteral nutrition. *British Medical Journal* 288(6418): 678–680.

Lee, B., Chang, W. R. S. & Jacobs, S. (1990) Intermittent nasogastric feeding: a simple and effective method to reduce pneumonia among ventilated ICU patients. *Clinics in Intensive Care* 1: 100–102.

Lennard-Jones, J. E. (1992) *A Positive Approach to Nutrition as Treatment*. London: King's Fund Centre.

Mainous, M. R. & Deitch, E. A. (1994) Nutrition and infection. *Surgical Clinics of North America* 74(3): 659–676.

Meijerink, W. J. H. J., von Meyenfeldt, M. F. & Soeters, P. B. (1995) Nutrition support for the surgical patient. In: Payne-James, J., Grimble, G. & Silk, D. (eds) *Artificial Nutrition Support in Clinical Practice*. London: Edward Arnold.

Methany, N. (1993) Minimizing respiratory complications of nasogastric tube feedings: state of the science. *Heart and Lung* 22(3) 213–223.

Methany, M., McSweeney, M., Wehrle, M. A. & Wiersema, L. (1990) Effectiveness of the auscultatory method in predicting feeding tube location. *Nursing Research* 39(5): 262–267.

Mulholland, J. H., Co Tui, Wright, A. M., et al (1943) Protein metabolism and pressure sores. *Annals of Surgery* 118(6): 1015–1023.

Olde Damink, S. W. M. & Soeters, P. B. (1997) Nutrition in practice: nutrition and wound healing. *Nursing Times* 93(30) (Suppl. 4): 1–6.

Payne-James, J. (1995) Enteral nutrition: tubes and techniques of delivery. In: Payne-James, J., Grimble, G. & Silk, D. (eds) *Artificial Nutrition Support in Clinical Practice*. London: Edward Arnold.

Pichard, C. & Jeejeebhoy, K. N. (1994) Nutritional management of clinical undernutrition. In: Garrow, J. S. & James, W. P. T. (eds) *Human Nutrition and Dietetics*, 9th edn. Edinburgh: Churchill Livingstone.

Planas, M. & Camilo, M. E. (2002) Artificial nutrition: dilemmas in decision-making. *Clinical Nutrition* 21(4): 355–361.

Robinson, G., Goldstein, M. & Levine, G. M. (1987) Impact of nutritional status on DRG length of stay. *Journal of Parenteral and Enteral Nutrition* 11(1): 49–51.

Shenkin, A. (1995) Adult micronutrient requirements. In: Payne-James, J., Grimble, G. & Silk, D. (eds) *Artificial Nutrition Support in Clinical Practice*. London: Edward Arnold.

Silk, D. B. A. (1994) *Organisation of Nutritional Support in Hospital* – a report by a working party for the British Association for Parenteral and Enteral Nutrition (BAPEN), Secure Hold Business Centre, Studley Road, Redditch, Worcs B98 7LG.

Silk, D. B. A. (1995) Enteral diet choices and formations. In: Payne-James, J., Grimble, G. & Silk, D. (eds) *Artificial Nutrition Support in Clinical Practice*. London: Edward Arnold.

Studley, H. O. (1936) Percentage of weight loss, a basic indicator of surgical risk in patients with chronic peptic ulcer. *Journal of the American Medical Association* 106: 458–460.

Taylor, S. (1989) Preventing complications in enteral feeding. *The Professional Nurse* 4(5): 247–249.

Taylor, T. V., Rimmer, S., Day, B., et al (1974) Ascorbic acid supplementation in the treatment of pressure sores. *The Lancet* (Sept 7): 544–546.

Thomas, B. (ed.) (1994) Surgery (Chapter 5.5). In: *Manual of Dietetic Practice*, 2nd edn. Oxford: Blackwell Scientific.

Trujillo, E. B., Young, L. S., Chertow, G. M., et al (1999) Metabolic and monetary costs of avoidable parenteral nutrition use. *Journal of Parenteral and Enteral Nutrition* 23(2): 109–113.

Further reading

Lennard-Jones, J. E. (1992) *A Positive Approach to Nutrition as Treatment.* London: King's Fund Centre.

McLaren, S. (1992) Nutrition and wound healing. *Journal of Wound Care* 1(3): 45–54.

Useful address

PINNT : PO Box 3126, Christchurch, Dorset BH23 2XS.
Email: PINNT@dial.pipex.com

Chapter **6**

Altered body image and the surgical patient

Adèle Atkinson and Rosie Pudner

Key objectives of the chapter

At the end of the chapter the reader should be able to:

- discuss the meaning of body image and altered body image

- discuss perceptions of body image

- discuss the effects of surgery on body image

- identify the effects of altered body image on body reality, body presentation and body ideal

- discuss coping mechanisms and strategies

- highlight the role of the surgical nurse in supporting the patient with an altered body image.

INTRODUCTION

The importance of physical appearance as an aspect of identity is very closely allied with the notion of who we are as people. Body image carries significant meaning, and is consistent with self-concept, self-esteem and identity. The very nature of surgery is a traumatic invasion upon the body and the self, and will invariably cause temporary or permanent changes. Some of these changes may not be anticipated or only emerge after the patient has been discharged. The issue of altered body image, and the degree to which it might affect patients' quality of life and self-concept, has become an increasingly important factor to consider when caring for patients undergoing surgery. This chapter will predominately discuss issues related to patients undergoing planned/elective surgery, but will highlight issues related to patients undergoing emergency surgical procedures where appropriate.

WHAT IS MEANT BY BODY IMAGE?

Body image is a widely used but poorly defined term. The concept of body image is generally taken to include the psychological and social aspects of behaviour. At the simplest level, body image has been described as how we think and feel about our bodies (Schilder, 1935 cited in Price, 1990a). It is also believed to be the perception and evaluation of one's physical functioning and appearance (Fisher and Cleveland, 1958). Other authors have emphasized the dynamic and ever-changing nature of body image and the external changes that can alter perceptions of body image (Janelli, 1986; Norris, 1970; Price, 1990b; Salter, 1997; Schontz, 1969).

Physical appearance and behaviour are influenced by society, and the predominant sociocultural values of youth, physical attractiveness, health and wholeness are constantly reinforced through the media and by social contact. A wealth of evidence from studies of the psychology of person perception indicates that, regardless of other variables such as sex, age, intelligence and class, the physically attractive are favoured over others across a wide range of situations (Clifford and Walster, 1973; Dermer and Thiel, 1975; Dion et al, 1972; Morse et al, 1974).

Further evidence has shown that perceptions and feelings about body size, function and appearance are also included in body image and have an impact on levels of self-esteem (Price, 1990a). This means that body image is a psychological experience focusing on conscious and unconscious attitudes and feelings. There is no single static image of the body, as it is always in the process of revision, being shaped according to the current situation of the individual.

Price (1990b) identified three major aspects of body image which, when in balance, constitute a healthy body image and a sense of well-being (Fig. 6.1). These three components are described as:

- *body reality*, i.e. the physical body as it is
- *body ideal*, i.e. the individual's desired body image
- *body presentation*, i.e. the body as it is presented to the world.

Most people will have experienced dissatisfaction in all areas at one time or another due to the natural

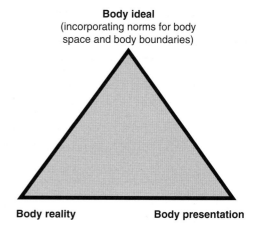

Body ideal
(incorporating norms for body
space and body boundaries)

Body reality   **Body presentation**

Figure 6.1   A body image model.

consequences of their genetic make-up, or the processes of physical maturation, ageing or other environmental events which cause changes in body image and subsequently in self-concept. It is also suggested that body image is the root of our identity, self-esteem and self-worth, and thus the basis from which man functions (Wassner, 1982).

The influence of body image on personal self-image is an easier concept to comprehend, as it suggests that self-image is built upon valuing the opinions and respect of others and that body image is used in society to negotiate and develop a sense of self-worth. Views on what constitutes the 'self' are the subject of endless debate, but perhaps it is fair to say that self-image is our own assessment of our social worth and is important for our self-confidence, motivation and sense of achievement (Price, 1990a).

PERCEPTIONS OF ALTERED BODY IMAGE

Body image perceptions adapt to the naturally changing events in life such as puberty, pregnancy and ageing. However, unpredictable or unavoidable changes to body image, such as those that can occur due to the trauma of surgery, sometimes precipitate long-term consequences. These may alter perceptions of body presentation and consequently self-image.

Body image is a very personal matter and depends upon the experiences and the adaptability of the individual. Mind and body are closely linked together, so that what happens to the body can have an effect on emotional health and vice versa. It can also determine a person's behaviour, as a result of the effect on self-concept. If people are not feeling well, they may not take as much care with their personal appearance, e.g. not washing hair, not wearing make-up or not shaving. This has the effect that when people look at themselves in the mirror their physical appearance reinforces how they feel. Since body image disturbance is the state in which an individual experiences a disruption in the way in which the body is perceived, it could be assumed that the consequences of surgery might have an effect on that individual's quality of life. At the same time, the individual may have to come to terms with the fact that the surgery is not a question of choice and that the treatment can be as bad as the disease, e.g. formation of a stoma following removal of a bowel tumour.

Certain operations can arouse specific fears in addition to the fear of pain and even the threat to life – e.g. mastectomy, formation of an ileostomy, colostomy or urostomy, amputation and certain types of plastic surgery – where fears of mutilation can be highly stressful. These fears can be related to the consequences of the change in daily life, and thus the perceived alteration of a concept of self.

Both the concept and the psychological effects of altered body image have been well studied, particularly in relation to the more obvious states of illness or injury, such as from the perspectives of oncology, burns, stomas, mastectomy and skin diseases (Elcoat, 1986; Goin, 1982; Kelly, 1987; Raab, 1986; Salter, 1997).

Changes that occur as a result of the surgical procedure, such as the insertion of a wound drain or intravenous infusion, may cause a disruption in body image; thus, a holistic approach to care should always consider the issue of altered body image as an integral part of a person's well-being. The nurse is in a unique position to engage the patient in conversation while caring for them, seeking in these dialogues to re-examine the meaning, if any, of altered body image and its impact on the patient. Perceptions of damaged or altered body image, and thus self-image, may significantly affect the patient's rehabilitation. This presupposes that health professionals are fully aware of the many meanings that changes in body image could have for the patient, the burdens that are carried by the individual and the factors that affect those burdens.

The individual interpretations of a person's experiences are concerned with perceptions and behaviours. Nurses need to help patients to cope with their reactions to the effects of surgery, and, since nurses are involved in determining patient needs, it is important that they have an insight not only into the obvious but also into the less obvious aspects of psychological perceptions. For example, in some situations a small scar may cause a patient more anxiety than a larger scar. Altered body image is therefore defined by the patient and not by health professionals.

Assessment of the perceived effects of altered body image is also complex because of the subjective nature of the phenomenon of body image. The nurse may have had some experience in reviewing her own body image, as well as the nature of body image in general, as she will have been exposed to caring for others who have suffered physical trauma or who are dying. These experiences usually give a greater insight and empathy with the patient.

REACTIONS TO ALTERED BODY IMAGE

Being a patient in hospital and requiring assistance with any acts of daily living has been identified as a threat to body image, because of the changes in body presentation and the body ideal (Webb, 1985). How a person responds when faced with changes in body image depends on many factors. These are mainly bound up with their personality and the way in which that person perceives and values their own body, and their ability to adapt to stress. It also depends on the nature of the change to their body image, how it was brought about, and whether the change is visible, prominent or hidden, as in the case of a woman having a hysterectomy. This may involve making adjustments for the future or it could be life threatening. The significance of this change in body image may impact on the person's work, social or sex life and be perceived to have a negative effect on their future lifestyle. However, there are some patients who do not perceive a change in body image as a threatening disability or a problem, and this should be recognized by the nurse. It should therefore not be an assumption that the surgical patient will interpret a change in body image in a negative fashion.

Cultural issues are also associated with body image, and need to be taken into consideration when caring for patients from different cultures. Dewing (1989) identified the sexual connotations related to the breast in Western society, and that women undergoing a mastectomy may no longer feel attractive to their partner and alter the clothes they would normally wear. Smith (1997) highlights the fact that a change in body image can affect patients as to how they are seen by their family members and the community they live/work in. The ethnic background of the patient may also create anxieties with body image: e.g. risk of keloid scarring in the Afro-Caribbean population. Religious faith can also impact on body image, as for those patients who follow the Sikh faith it is paramount for the body to remain intact. This could therefore create a problem if a man had to undergo an emergency circumcision for paraphimosis. Patients who practise the islamic faith may experience difficulties if they have a stoma, as they are not permitted to perform ablutions during prayer times (Smith, 1997). This may cause problems for the patient if his stoma works within the confines of the mosque, and the potential risk of this occurring may prevent the patient from attending the mosque.

Surgery on specific parts of the body also impacts on body image. Wounds resulting from surgery on the breast, uterus or genitalia can have significant meaning for women, as it is connected to their reproductive functions, while surgery on the male genitalia links to reproduction and sexual prowess. Women may see the surgery as a loss of their feminity and a loss of body ideal, while men undergoing prostatic surgery or an orchidectomy may fear impotence and loss of their manhood, also affecting their body ideal.

Breast surgery, either a lumpectomy or mastectomy, changes the shape of the breast and so affects body reality (Keeton and McAloon, 2002), and may impact on the woman's role in society. For Chinese or Vietnamese women, especially if they are of child-bearing age where in traditional Chinese medicine the breast is important in breast feeding, a damaged breast means an outward sign of inner turmoil. There may also be an associated feeling of shame and the woman may withdraw from an intimate relationship with her partner/husband (Smith, 1997). In Western society, much emphasis is put on the shape and size of the perfect breast, so a change in shape or size following breast surgery can cause psychological trauma in some women.

If patients have a stoma formed – either temporary or permanent – it is a violation of body integrity (Borwell, 1997) and can threaten the patient's self-esteem. It may alter their position in their social/cultural community and may lead to a life of isolation; separation from their family in relation to cooking, eating and caring; and preclusion from their place of worship. In some instances, they may be seen as permanently unclean and untouchable. A Chinese woman with a stoma may even withdraw from public life, as the stoma is seen as unhealthiness in the person (Smith, 1997).

The face is also extremely important. This is because the face equates with attractiveness, so surgery to the face may alter the patient's perception of their attractiveness (Berscheid and Gangstad, 1982). If surgery to the face interferes with eating or talking, then this may further reinforce feelings of unattractiveness and helplessness.

Amputation of a limb not only alters body image but also extends it, as a prosthesis has to be worn and crutches, a walking stick or wheelchair may be used to get around. The manner in which patients construct meaning out of the experience will affect their attitude

---

Box 6.1   Psychological reactions to altered body image which resemble the grief response

- Shock
- Denial
- Anger
- Depression
- Bargaining
- Acceptance

Source: Kubler-Ross (1969)

---

and concordance to wearing the prosthesis (Desmond and MacLachlan, 2002).

Hidden body image changes should not be forgotten, as these may also impact on the patient. This may include gynaecological surgery, or loss of fertility following hysterectomy. Also, areas of skin normally covered by clothing are more likely to be exposed in the summer months and when undertaking certain sporting activities such as swimming. A patient with a scar on the top of the arm may not want to expose it and prefer to wear short-sleeved tops rather than sleeveless tops, or a scar on the top of the leg may mean that a man will not wear shorts.

However, if there is conflict, and anxiety exists as a result of an altered body image, the nurse is well placed to recognize reactions which are often manifested in the form of a grief response (Kubler-Ross, 1969; Parkes, 1972). Some surgical procedures may make a person look or feel 'different', presenting a major challenge. Patients who are able to come to terms with a 'new body image' appear to follow the grief response, such as those described by Kubler-Ross (1969) (Box 6.1). It is important to note that the phases of the grief response can overlap and may take years to complete. The individual may also shift backwards and forwards between the various phases.

Patients may grieve for the loss of their 'old' body image and this is particularly exacerbated for the patient with a stoma, amputation or any mutilating surgery. However, this is not just limited to individuals with a visibly altered body image, as many patients may grieve for less-obvious losses, such as changes in relationships, lifestyle and loss of personal freedom. A woman may have a sense of loss following a hysterectomy, as she may feel that she has lost her feminity. Likewise, a man may have a sense of loss following an orchidectomy, as he may feel that his masculinity and sexual prowess have been affected by the surgery.

Loss of body image causes a grief reaction which will release in the afflicted person feelings of insecurity, particularly if the person perceives the change as a crisis. Tension and depression are typical reactions, and their recognition is the key to understanding the person's stress, sometimes perceived by the health team as being out of proportion to the magnitude of the actual surgical event. Yet, grief, loss and mourning are all terms which have been associated with changes in body image, regardless of the cause, and can continue long after the patient has been discharged.

Bereavement may also be encountered by patients with an altered body image, and Dewing (1989) identified the following four stages of bereavement:

1. *Impact* – the initial shock and anger which can precipitate depression and pessimism regarding recovery. This reaction is exacerbated by those patients who have experienced sudden traumatic changes in body image and have had little or no time to receive information about, or prepare themselves for, the implications of the surgery, e.g. patients undergoing emergency surgery.

2. *Retreat* – a phase of mourning for the affected part and a desire to return to the previous self. There is often denial, avoidance and emotional withdrawal.

3. *Acknowledgement* – confrontation of the problem, reliving events, searching for a cause and seeking information to aid coping mechanisms.

4. *Reconstruction* – recognition of implications, accepting the use of aids and planning for the future.

Coping mechanisms are often employed unconsciously and are a normal human reaction to control fear and anxiety. A crisis associated with body image might be revealed by certain types of behavioural defence mechanisms which have been observed by Wright (1986) (Box 6.2). Adjustment can be enhanced by the nurse with the appropriate skills to care for patients with an altered body image.

Regardless of the cause of altered body image, it is argued that patients who have had a sudden traumatic change, e.g. following emergency surgery, may experience greater difficulty in coming to terms with the perception of loss, and will need more time to accept the event and their feelings regarding it (O'Brien, 1980). If a person can discuss, and more importantly, be allowed to discuss, the fears and anxieties of forthcoming surgical procedures, it can promote healthier coping mechanisms and better reintegration of body image. The introduction of preadmission and preassessment clinics is a place where this can be facilitated. It has also been identified by Price (1990a) and Salter (1997) that support networks are also important in helping patients to adapt to a change in body image.

Box 6.2   Types of behavioural defence mechanisms

- *Passivity.* A change of mood or affect which can lead to sadness or withdrawal. The patient does not wish to be involved with their own care and may feel they are unacceptable. Motivation is poor and there is a loss of purpose and initiative.

- *Denial.* The patient refuses to look at or touch the altered part and may even deny its absence, trying to carry on as before. This dissociation from changes in body image demonstrates a distortion of reality which is a clear sign of psychological disequilibrium. The therapeutic relationship may be threatened by this resistance.

- *Reassurance.* The patient persistently seeks attention to check that they are still acceptable, sometimes making self-denigrating remarks to initiate a compliment. This can be a powerful affirmation that a person's attraction does not depend on a wholesome body reality.

- *Isolation.* This may be self-imposed because the patient feels unacceptable and fears risking rejection.

- *Hostility.* This may be due to a strong protest about what has been perpetrated on that person. It can also be a manifestation of anger against the medical profession and is often associated with grief and loss.

Source: Wright (1986).

The physiological response to stress is well documented (Carola et al, 1992; Clancy and McVicar, 1995), and the surgical nurse needs to be familiar with the signs and symptoms of arousal of the sympathetic nervous and endocrine systems causing what is commonly known as the 'fight-or-flight' response, a homeostatic response of adaptation. Selye (1956, 1976, 1985) carried out much research in this area, particularly examining what happens to the body when stress is prolonged. He identified a series of physiological reactions which he named the 'general adaptation syndrome' (GAS):

1. *Alarm reaction* – in which the body is mobilized to defend itself against the perceived stressor. Preoperatively, patients become aware that surgery is necessary, which creates anxiety, e.g. removal of a sebaceous cyst or appendectomy.

2. *Stage of resistance* – in which the body attempts to adapt to the stress. The physiological arousal

remains higher than normal but shows few outward signs of stress. However, the ability to resist new stressors is impaired, and there is an increased vulnerability to health problems. Preoperatively, the patient is trying to come to terms with impending surgery and reduce anxiety levels. This also relates to the period of time prior to surgery (e.g. waiting time) which can increase the level of anxiety. Hence, the role of preadmission and preassessment clinics, where the patient can openly discuss any fears or concerns regarding their forthcoming surgery with a healthcare professional. Wilson-Barnett (1978) found that well-informed patients had lower levels of stress postoperatively.

3. *Stage of exhaustion* – in which the body's reserves are depleted and the ability to resist may collapse, leading to further serious physiological damage if severe stress continues or is repeated. This implies that there is a state of altered body image.

THE PREOPERATIVE PHASE

The prospect of imminent surgery and its hidden consequences naturally causes a considerable amount of fear for the patient. The preoperative phase is a time when the nurse can discuss the patients' fears and anxieties and the likely events during their hospital stay, and patients are able to express any concerns regarding a change in their body image. An important piece of research which had an impact on nursing practice focused on giving information about the physical experiences which may be expected following surgery, with the result that postoperative pain was generally found to be reduced (Hayward, 1975). Boore (1978) also found that giving patients information preoperatively about their future care and treatment reduced stress in patients postoperatively. As this will reduce the amount of circulating adrenaline (epinephrine), pain should therefore be reduced. However, if a patient is admitted for emergency surgery, there is limited time for this to occur.

Four main stressors can be identified which can be seen during various stages in the preoperative period:

1. loss of control over the events
2. fear of the unknown
3. loss of dignity
4. lack of privacy.

Loss of control over the events

The reaction to life in a hospital surgical ward and the adjustment to patient status can manifest itself in an initial hostility (Kelly, 1985), and the ward routine can undermine confidence. The loss of independence and a familiar environment poses a threat to the patient, which is often not appreciated by the ward staff to whom the ward is a familiar and non-threatening environment, and this can therefore affect body ideal. In order to fit into the ward environment, patients will often take the line of least resistance and become passive recipients of care.

Sometimes the surgical procedure may be quite minor, such as the removal of a small cyst, or it may be a more substantial operation such as bowel surgery. Whatever the circumstances of the surgery, the surgical nurse needs to demonstrate that nursing care includes sensitivity to patient perceptions of possible changes in body image, no matter how small, and that facilitating patient control over events as much as possible can do much to sustain body ideal and self-esteem, e.g. giving patients information so that they are aware of the potential appearance of the scar.

Effective preoperative assessment of patients undertaken in a holistic manner can ascertain valuable information on perceptions of their present body image, and can also elicit from their own experiences something of the nature of their coping mechanisms in times of stress. Stress is sometimes difficult to identify, and it appears that nurses are often unable to accurately recognize anxiety and stress in their patients (Biley, 1989).

The patient and their family may also meet with the specialist nurses who can give them more detailed information about the surgical procedure; discuss their expectations following the surgery; and give details of relevant support groups if appropriate.

Giving the patient information on the forthcoming procedure helps the patient to feel involved and thus able to maintain a sense of control (Wilson-Barnett, 1978). Using photographs to illustrate how the patient may look after the surgery can help to reassure the patient. A well-informed patient feels more independent and less reliant on the hospital staff, and may also exhibit a better postoperative adjustment to surgery (Johnston, 1980). The admission procedure should ensure consultation with patients to encourage a sense of control over events and help patients make informed choices about the nursing care or therapy they will be receiving. This also helps to maintain their individuality within the hospital experience.

There will be times when the patient is unable to be in control, such as when they are anaesthetized or recovering from the anaesthetic, in which case the nurse is of necessity caring for the patient. It is important for patients to anticipate this and to feel confident that their needs will be dealt with respectfully. The surgical nurse should therefore be aware that this lack of control makes the patient feel very vulnerable in this preoperative phase.

Fear of the unknown

On admission, nurses need to recognize that patients may adopt defensive behaviours, due to their anxieties about forthcoming surgery which may affect their body image. Nurses appear to underestimate the impact of surgery on body image, due to the familiarity of routine operations and their after-effects (Kelly, 1985). They may know the temporary nature of the ensuing scars, as they have seen it all before, but the patient does not know this and has very real fears about their own body and the potential expected changes affecting it.

Patients typically have many concerns, and real anxieties, about what the operated part will look like and how other people might react to it, e.g. the partial or total loss of a breast, or formation of a stoma. These fears might be unfounded; therefore, it is important to make time to discuss any concerns and listen to the patient's feelings. The nurse should be honest about the anticipated altered body image and allow the patient to talk through the reality of the forthcoming changes of body form and function, e.g. use of photographs to show before and after images. Patients also worry about how other people will react, fearing rejection, and it may be appropriate to discuss potential coping strategies with them at this point.

The transfer of the patient to the operating theatre can be the time of greatest stress for the patient, and the time during which the surgical nurse needs to be very conscious of the support that may be needed by the patient. Many patients are more concerned about the anaesthetic than they are about the surgery, as anaesthesia evokes fears due to loss of consciousness, which in some instances is equated with death.

Loss of dignity

One of the fears of surgical patients is the loss of bodily awareness while anaesthetized and of not being in control of their body. This fear can be exacerbated by previous bad experiences. It is important that the patient's dignity should be respected at all times by all healthcare professionals during the surgical experience.

Some of the more practical issues affecting body image arise from the need for physical preparation of the patient prior to surgery, which may affect body reality (Price, 1990a). This may involve procedures such as preoperative shaving of the affected part, marking of the skin of planned operation sites and the removal of false teeth, contact lenses and make-up. Some of these alterations to body reality are the subject of controversy, and subsequent results of research have changed some of these rituals of practice, e.g. preoperative shaving (Seropian and Reynolds, 1971).

Other preparations for surgery which might impinge adversely upon a patient's perceptions of body image are the need to remove personal adornments such as make-up, jewellery and nail polish. These things can be an important aspect of a person's body presentation and are closely associated with self-worth.

The necessary removal of dentures can embarrass the patient and make them feel particularly vulnerable, as this is often only done in private and significantly alters body presentation. Another area that may make the patient feel vulnerable is the removal of their contact lenses. If contact lenses are removed too soon, the patient may feel anxious that they cannot see what is going on around them. The removal of dentures and contact lenses should therefore be undertaken just before the patient leaves the ward/day surgery unit.

Lack of privacy

Marking of the patient's skin to identify the operation site(s) is an important patient safety measure. Health professionals should have an understanding of how it might affect the patient's privacy and body image in relation to body reality, and inform the patient as to why it is undertaken.

THE PATIENT IN THEATRE

One of the patient's identified fears, as stated previously, is the loss of bodily control under anaesthesia, coupled with the loss of dignity and privacy. Although it is vital for the surgeon to have optimal exposure in order to operate, it is the responsibility of the theatre nurse to act as the patient's advocate and ensure that the dignity of the patient is preserved as far as it is possible.

Increasing numbers of operations are being carried out in day surgery units, and many are performed under a local anaesthetic. It is therefore essential that the patient's dignity is maintained during their surgical procedure, and that patients have been fully informed in the preoperative phase as to the events that will occur during surgery.

POSTOPERATIVE PHASE

Many of the factors discussed below will influence the patient's body reality, as surgery directly alters this. Body presentation may also be altered, especially if it is difficult for the patient to hide drains, wound dressings, etc. This may have a direct influence on patients' body ideal, as they may find it harder to achieve their body ideal by the manner in which they present themselves to friends and the rest of society.

Following surgery, the assessment of the patient is primarily geared to the patient's physiological condition by the observation and monitoring of vital signs, level of consciousness, etc., together with the relevant specific care, as described in other appropriate chapters concerned with specialist surgery.

Patient comfort and related perceptions in body image may not become apparent or be an issue until the patient has become alert enough to be aware of them. This may relate to gaining consciousness and becoming aware of an intravenous infusion in situ, or the long-term realization of the appearance of the scar, and this will alter the patient's body reality.

Following surgery, the patient may find his body image has extended or been breached, due to the necessity for tubes such as nasogastric tubes, urinary catheters, wound drains and intravenous infusions, so affecting his body presentation. As soon as possible, the nurse should reinforce the reasons behind why they are necessary, as well as whether they are of a temporary or permanent nature. The temporary nature of drains, etc., may result in minor threats to body image (Price, 1990b). This is probably because there is no need for long-term adjustment. Even so, it is important to realize that the patient may still grieve until the drains, etc., have been removed. If the changes are of a more permanent nature, then the patient will have to come to terms with their 'new' body image.

Nasogastric tubes are particularly distressing to the patient, as they occupy a facial position, make the face asymmetrical and cannot be hidden. The angle of the tube should be as comfortable as possible, not pulling or distorting the nostril, and attention should be paid to nasal toilet, since it is not possible for the patient to blow their nose. This may alter the patient's body reality, as the patient becomes more dependent on the nurse, albeit for a short period of time. A minimal amount of tape to hold the tube in position should be used in order to keep the tube secure, and prevent pulling of the skin, which could cause distortion of the face. The nurse should also always check that the patient's view is not compromised by a loop of the tubing in front of the eyes.

For many patients the presence of a urinary catheter can be distressing, since it is invasive and is placed in a normally private part of the body. It is essential that the urinary catheter is appropriately secured, so as to reduce urethral trauma and possible pain or discomfort. If there is a drainage bag attached to the catheter, it can be supported in a wire holder attached to the side of the bed. Once the patient is mobile, the presence of a urinary drainage bag to be carried around in a wire cradle can affect body presentation, and something more discreet, such as a support belt or leg bag, should be used.

Wound drains can also be a problem, particularly if attached to a drainage bottle, although their presence is often short term. If the patient is mobile and still has a wound drain in situ, the same discreet principle for carrying it around can be used as for the urinary catheter, thus helping to preserve the patient's body presentation.

Intravenous infusions should be positioned with some thought to the patient's comfort and abilities: for example, the non-dominant arm is the best choice unless there is some medical reason to do otherwise. This leaves the patient with the ability to use the dominant arm and also preserves some independence, an important factor in maintaining some personal control.

Removing the operation gown and allowing the patient to wear their own nightdress/pyjamas as soon as possible represents a limited return of control for the patient. A return to normality is also achieved when the patient is allowed to wear their own dentures/glasses/hearing aid, etc., again.

The majority of surgical procedures will leave a wound. This may be an incisional wound or it may be a larger wound which will heal by secondary intention. If wounds are not hidden, then patients may go to great lengths to ensure that they are covered so that others do not see them (Neil, 2000). If patients do not want to draw attention to their wound, then the colour of the wound dressing is important, as few dressings actually blend into the skin. Some dressing products are bulky and may prevent patients from wearing the clothes or shoes that they wish to (Atkinson, 2002).

All wounds will heal, leaving a scar. A survey by the Scar Information Service (1999) found that the majority of patients who were concerned about their scars had small scars, and most respondents dressed differently in order to hide their scar. The survey also found that patients perceived healthcare professionals to be less sympathetic to those with small scars, giving more sympathy to those with larger and more obvious scars. The importance of listening to patients' worries cannot be overstated as an important aspect in the nursing care of a surgical patient. Using pictures from previous patients may help them appreciate the amount of scarring that they will have.

It must also be remembered that it may take years to adjust to a new body image (Atkinson, 1997), especially if the body part that is affected has particular significance for the patient. Mock (1993) found that women were still adjusting to their altered body image 1 year following mastectomy.

Pain following an operation is often one of the patient's greatest anxieties, and the fear of it should be discussed as part of the preoperative assessment, although this may not be able to be undertaken in patients undergoing emergency surgery. Pain can be a challenge to body image because it is a body experience – sometimes unpredictable and always unpleasant. Price (1990a) believes that pain affects body image, as the person can no longer trust their body, as they do not know when the pain will return. The surgical nurse must reassure the patient that, while pain is sometimes inevitable following the surgical procedure, it can be controlled, and no patient should be in pain or discomfort postoperatively. Assessment of, and nursing interventions for, the patient with postoperative pain are dealt with in more detail in Chapter 7.

All pain produces anxiety and reduces pain tolerance; therefore, increased pain is experienced by the anxious patient (Wall and Melzack, 1984). It is imperative to ensure that patients continue to be kept informed and are able to discuss any fears or anxieties they may have. Early and prompt relief of postoperative pain usually results in decreased anxiety, less sensitivity to pain, earlier postoperative activity and a reduction in the total need for analgesics.

SOCIAL SUPPORT AND COPING STRATEGIES

The desire to maintain body integrity is a profound need, which is usually internalized until such time as it is threatened. People look for social approval of their appearance, especially when faced with illness, trauma or surgery. Alterations to the way the body image is perceived can sometimes be so threatening that a crisis is precipitated. Stress appraisals carried out on ill adults typically include concerns for the future, such as disfigurement, disablement or even death (Sarafino, 2002).

Many people have difficulty in coping with physical changes resulting from surgery, despite psychological support in the form of information giving and listening to patients' anxieties. Helping patients to adjust psychologically through rehabilitation and to achieve a satisfactory body image will contribute to a more positive self-concept and feelings of self-worth.

People vary considerably in the way they cope psychologically with stress: sometimes confronting a problem directly and rationally, and sometimes not facing up to the reality of the situation. The complex interplay of psychological and physiological reactions to stress are determined in part by genetic predisposition and the early environmental experiences that an individual brings to a stressful situation. These determine a person's psychological vulnerability and ability to deal with conflict (Dubovsky, 1985). The emotional and physical strain that accompanies stress is uncomfortable, upsetting the psychological equilibrium, and the response is to try to reduce that stress.

Social support can help to modify the impact of stress on the individual, and is referred to as 'the perceived comfort, caring, esteem or help a person receives from other people or groups' (Sarafino, 2002:98). This can be through family or friends, work colleagues, or local support groups.

Social support can be classified as five main types (Sarafino, 2002):

- *Emotional support*: expression of empathy, caring and concern towards the individual, e.g. companionship; giving a shoulder to cry on.
- *Esteem support*: expression of positive regard for the individual; positive comparison of the individual with others. This encourages the individual's feelings of self-worth.
- *Tangible support*: direct assistance from someone in relation to finances or help in the home.
- *Information support*: giving advice/suggestions or feedback as to how the individual is doing.
- *Network support*: provides a feeling of membership in a group of individuals who share similar interests/ activities.

Patients who are able to discuss their anxieties with someone who has experienced similar treatment can help develop a more positive outlook. Partners, immediate family and close friends should also be included in counselling, in order to promote understanding of the loss and the patient's need for time to work through to acceptance. Both the patient and their partner and/or family frequently look to nurses for the opportunity to talk about their concerns; thus, the ability to build a good interpersonal relationship with both the patient and their immediate family can promote the adaptation and mature coping of all parties. The type of support the patient needs or receives will depend on the situation, although not all patients get the social support they need, e.g. elderly patients living alone; patients who are not sociable with others; or those patients who do not ask for help. However, social support can reduce the stress directly, e.g. changing how a person looks at a situation (a patient accepting a scar as body reality), or by giving a patient information which allows them to calm down and be less anxious.

What each individual actually does to manage the perceived stress is known as 'coping'. Benner and Wrubel (1989) emphasize the individuality of this process, suggesting that a person's history and individual personality will determine what is perceived to be a stressor and what possible coping mechanisms are employed by the individual.

Several different definitions of coping exist (Lazarus and Folkman, 1984; Lazarus, 1987) but, generally, coping is seen to be the process by which people try to manage a perceived discrepancy between the demands of the stressor and the resources available. Managing the stressful situation does not necessarily lead to a solution, but the coping efforts can help to alter the patient's perception of a discrepancy; to tolerate or accept the harm or threat; and to avoid or escape the situation. Coping is not a single event but is a dynamic series of 'continuous appraisals and reappraisals of the shifting person–environment relationships' (Lazarus and Folkman, 1984:142). Thus the re-evaluation of what is happening can influence subsequent coping efforts of adjustment and adaptation to perceived changes in body integrity.

The Lazarus model divides coping into two types:

- Problem-focused coping – in which a patient actively attempts to tackle the problem and tries to view the problem as manageable, e.g. purchasing and using a silicone gel sheet to reduce hypertrophic scar tissue following surgery.

- Emotional-focused coping – whereby the patient attempts to deal with the feelings associated with the problem. This can be through behavioural approaches such as drinking alcohol or talking to friends; or by using cognitive approaches such as rationalization; or by denying unpleasant facts, e.g. denying that a breast lump is malignant and that it is only a cyst.

Problem-focused coping strategies appear to be more beneficial and more positive than emotional-focused coping strategies (Drageset and Lindstrøm, 2003). The coping ability of the individual depends on two psychological factors: namely, the degree of perceived threat and the person's ego strength, i.e. how someone uses their mental defence mechanisms.

Anxiety and uncertainty of outcome can also lead to the use of defence mechanisms (Drageset and Lindstrøm, 2003), such as:

- passivity – where the patient does not appear to want to be involved in their care and leaves decisions to the healthcare staff
- reassurance – where the patient uses attention-seeking strategies to ensure that things will turn out alright
- isolation – where the patient believes they 'look' unacceptable and withdraws
- denial – where the patient appears to deny the 'altered body part' and attempts to carry on as before.

Erikson and Ursin (1999) (cited in Drageset and Lindstrøm, 2003) found that people who use more emotional-focused coping strategies tend to take longer to come to terms with the problem, in this case an alteration in body image.

The nurse's caring role in helping patients and families cope with perceived changes in body image is very important, and yet it is something that some nurses find difficult to address, preferring to deal with more concrete and familiar patient needs. Patients need to be able to express their feelings in an atmosphere of trust and confidence, and the nurse can help the facilitation of such expression, which in itself is therapeutic.

Assessing a patient's body image is complex, as there are many facets to it. On first meeting, the patient may not tell you all, as information is usually disclosed over a period of time. Nurses can observe patients for their reactions and how they dress, and listen to the words that they use, e.g. patients may not maintain eye contact, or they may wear dark clothes to divert attention. Assessment will also take account of any potential threats to body image, e.g. anxiety due to surgery. It is also helpful for the nurse to reflect over what has caused problems in other patients and bear these in mind (Price, 1995).

It is important that the nurse responds to the patient with 'positive-regard', to help build up a trusting relationship. When a patient starts to trust the nurse, then it is possible to start to explore their body image with them. Price (1995) noticed that patients talked about how they felt about their bodies in terms of how they would perform in the future, rather than focusing on the now. Neil and Barrell (1998) found that one person in their study brought in photographs to show how she had looked before and after having a wound to show how she felt her whole body had changed, even though the photographs were not of the area where the wound was.

In reality, it may be impractical, in a busy surgical ward, to use a lengthy assessment tool for assessing body image. Price (1990b) suggests that the need for extensive and formal assessment tools is much reduced where the nurse is able to develop a patient profile through observation, reflection and effective communication, and can then formulate a tailored care plan which outlines the patient's concerns and perceptions.

Awareness of people's various coping strategies, and the different social resources that a patient can draw upon, will help the nurse to anticipate and understand the patient's reactions. The ability to communicate and actively listen will lead to trust. The knowledge and skills required by surgical nurses to comprehend why people react as they do, and the ability to help a patient overcome the problems of altered body image, are all concerned with good interpersonal skills, trust, empathy and touch.

CONCLUSION

It is essential for surgical nurses to be aware of the invasive effects of surgery, however minor they may seem, and to have a clear understanding of the personal meaning of body image. This includes knowledge of the effects of the stress response, and the psychosocial adjustments needed for a patient to be able to cope in a positive manner when faced with perceived altered body image. Using strategies that will build up a trust with the patient, such as active-listening skills and 'positive-regard', will hopefully assist patients in coming to terms with their altered body image.

Summary of key points

- Appearance is an important aspect of identity.

- Body image is related to self-esteem and self-worth.

- Perceptions of disruption, damage or changes in body image due to surgery differ from one individual to another, and so do responses to an altered body image following surgery.

- Assessment of the surgical patient's concerns, anxieties and fears related to body image should be considered during the assessment process.

- Surgical nurses should be aware of potential pre-, peri- and postoperative situations that can cause an alteration in the patient's body image.

- Pain following surgery can also be a challenge to a patient's body image.

- An individual patient's reaction to a perceived altered body image can be linked with reactions to grief.

- The surgical nurse has an important role in incorporating sensitive awareness and support strategies into the care of a surgical patient.

References

Atkinson, A. (1997) Body image disturbance in burns. In: Salter, M. (ed.) *Altered Body Image – The Nurse's Role*, 2nd edn. London: Baillière Tindall.

Atkinson, A. (2002) Body image considerations in patients with wounds. *Journal of Community Nursing*, 16(10): 32–38.

Benner, P. & Wrubel, J. (1989) *The Primacy of Caring*. Reading, Mass.: Addison-Wesley.

Berscheid, E. & Gangstad, S. (1982) The social psychological implications of facial physical attractiveness. *Symposium on Social and Psychological Considerations in Plastic Surgery* 9(3): 289–295.

Biley, F. C. (1989) Nurses' perception of stress in pre-operative surgical patients. *Journal of Advanced Nursing* 14(7): 575–581.

Boore, J. R. P. (1978) *Prescription for Recovery*. London: RCN.

Borwell, B. (1997) Psychological considerations of stoma care nursing. *Nursing Standard* 11(48): 49–55.

Carola, R., Harley, J. P. & Noback, C. R. (1992) *Human Anatomy and Physiology*, 2nd edn. New York: McGraw-Hill.

Clancy, J. & McVicar, A. J. (1995) *Physiology and Anatomy—A Homeostatic Approach*. London: Edward Arnold.

Clifford, M. & Walster, E. (1973) The effect of physical attractiveness on teacher expectations. *Sociology of Education*. 46(2): 248–258.

Dermer, M. & Thiel, D. (1975) When beauty may fail. *Journal of Personality and Social Psychology* 31(6): 1168–1176.

Desmond, D. & MacLachlan, M. (2002) Psychological issues in the field of prosthetics and orthotics. *American Academy of Orthotists and Prosthetists* 14(1): 19–22 [online] Available at: http://gateway2.uk.ovid.com/ovidweb.cgi (accessed on 19 May 2004).

Dewing, J. (1989) Altered body image. *Surgical Nurse* 2(4): 17–20.

Dion, K., Berscheid, E. & Walster, E. (1972) What is beautiful is good. *Journal of Personality and Social Psychology* 24(3): 285–290.

Drageset, S. & Lindstrøm, T. C. (2003) The mental health of women with suspected breast cancer: the relationship between social support, anxiety, coping and defence in maintaining health. *Journal of Psychiatric and Mental Health Nursing* 10(4): 401–409.

Dubovsky, S. L. (1985) The psychophysiology of health, illness and stress. In: Simons, R. C. (ed.) *Understanding Human Behaviour in Health and Illness*, 3rd edn. Baltimore: Williams & Wilkins.

Elcoat, C. (1986) *Stoma Care Nursing*. London: Baillière Tindall.

Erikson, H. & Ursin, H. (1999) Subjective health complaints: is coping more important than control? *Work Stress* 13: 238–252.

Fisher, S. & Cleveland, S. E. (1958) *Body Image and Personality*. Princeton, N.J.: Van Nostrand.

Goin, M. K. (1982) Psychological reactions to surgery of the breast. *Clinics in Plastic Surgery* 9(3): 347–354.

Hayward, J. (1975) *Information: A Prescription Against Pain*. London: Royal College of Nursing.

Janelli, L. (1986) Body image in older adults: a review of the literature. *Rehabilitation Nursing* 11(4): 6–8.

Johnston, M. (1980) Anxiety in surgical patients. *Psychological Medicine* 10(1): 145–152.

Keeton, S. & McAloon, L. (2002) The supply and fitting of a temporary breast prosthesis. *Nursing Standard* 16(41): 43–46.

Kelly, M. P. (1985) Loss and grief reactions as responses to surgery. *Journal of Advanced Nursing* 10(6): 517–525.

Kelly, M. P. (1987) Adjusting to ileostomy. *Nursing Times* 83(33): 29–31.

Kubler-Ross, E. (1969) *On Death and Dying*. London: Tavistock.

Lazarus, R.S. (1987) Coping. In: Corsini, R. J. (ed.) *Concise Encyclopaedia of Psychology*. New York: Wiley.

Lazarus, R. S. & Folkman, S. (1984) Coping and adaptation. In: Gentry, W. D. (ed.) *Handbook on Behavioural Medicine*. New York: Guilford.

Mock, V. (1993) Body image in women treated for breast cancer. *Nursing Research* 42(3): 153–157.

Morse, S. J., Reis, H. T., Gruzen, J. & Wolff, E. (1974) The eye of the beholder: determinants of physical attractiveness judgements in the U.S. and South Africa. *Journal of Personality* 42(4): 528–542.

Neil, J. A. (2000) The stigma scale: measuring body image and the skin. *Dermatology Nursing* 12(1): 32–36.

Neil, J. A. & Barrell, L. M. (1998) Transition theory and its relevance to patients with chronic wounds. *Rehabilitation Nursing* 23(6): 295–299.

Norris, C. M. (1970) The professional nurse and body image. In: Carson, C. E. (ed.) *Behavioural Concepts and Nursing Interventions*. Philadelphia: Lippincott.

O'Brien, J. (1980) Mirror, mirror, why me? *Nursing Mirror* 150(17): 36–37.

Parkes, C. (1972) *Bereavement: Studies of Grief in Adult Life*. London: Tavistock.

Price, B. (1990a) *Body Image—Nursing Concepts and Care*. London: Prentice Hall.

Price, B. (1990b) A model for body image care. *Journal of Advanced Nursing* 15(5): 585–593.

Price, B. (1995) Assessing altered body image. *Journal of Psychiatric and Mental Health Nursing* 2(3): 169–175.

Raab, D. M. (1986) Helping patients develop a positive postoperative image. *Health Care* (February): 16–18.

Salter, M. (ed.) (1997) *Altered Body Image—The Nurse's Role*, 2nd edn. London: Baillière Tindall.

Sarafino, E. P. (2002) *Health Psychology—Biopsychosocial Interactions*, 4th edn. New York: John Wiley and Sons.

Scar Information Service (1999) *Scarring: A Research Report into Keloid and Hypertrophic Scarring*. London: Smith and Nephew.

Schilder, P. (1935) *The Image and Appearance of the Human Body*. London: Kegan Paul.

Schontz, F. C. (1969) *Perceptual and Cognitive Aspects of Body Experience*. New York: Academic Press.

Selye, H. (1956) *The Stress of Life*. New York: McGraw-Hill.

Selye, H. (1976) *Stress in Health and Disease*. Sevenoaks, Kent: Butterworths.

Selye, H. (1985) History and present status of the stress status. In: Monat, A. & Lazarus, R. S. (eds) *Stress and Coping*, 2nd edn. New York: Columbia University Press.

Seropian, R. & Reynolds, B. (1971) Wound infections after pre-operative depilatory versus razor preparation. *American Journal of Surgery* 121(3): 251–254.

Smith, J. (1997) Cultural issues associated with altered body image. In: Salter, M. (ed.) *Altered Body Image – The Nurse's Role*, 2nd edn. London: Baillière Tindall.

Wall, P. D. & Melzack, R. (1984). *Textbook of Pain*. New York: Churchill Livingstone.

Wassner, A. (1982) The impact of mutilating surgery or trauma on body image. *International Nursing Review* 29(3): 86–90.

Webb, C. (1985) *Sexuality, Nursing, and Health*. London: Heinemann.

Wilson-Barnett, J. (1978) Patients' emotional responses to barium X-rays. *Journal of Advanced Nursing* 3(1): 37–46.

Wright, B. (1986) *Caring in Crisis*. Edinburgh: Churchill Livingstone.

Further reading

Bailey, R. & Clarke, M. (1993) *Stress and Coping in Nursing*. London: Chapman & Hall.

Hyland, M. E. & Donaldson, M. L. (1989) *Psychological Care in Nursing Practice*. London: Scutari Press.

MacGinley, K. J. (1993) Nursing care of the patient with altered body image. *British Journal of Nursing* 2(22): 1098–1102.

Price, B. (1993) Dignity that must be respected; body image and the surgical patient. *Professional Nurse* 8(10): 670–672.

Chapter **7**

Concepts of pain and the surgical patient

Sharon Kitcatt

Key objectives of the chapter

At the end of the chapter the reader should be able to discuss the following:

■ the classification of pain

■ the gate control theory of pain

■ general principles in the management of acute pain

■ factors that can affect the experience of acute pain

■ pain assessment

■ the physiological response to pain and the dangers of poorly managed acute pain

■ methods of administering postoperative analgesia

■ pharmacology in acute postoperative pain management

■ the role of the nurse and the acute pain team.

INTRODUCTION

Pain is a complex, multidimentional experience and it is unique to the person experiencing it. Pain is often seen as a warning sign that something is wrong and is a common reason for people to consult their general practitioner. The International Association for the Study of Pain (1992:2) describes pain as 'an unpleasant sensory and emotional experience associated with actual or potential tissue damage or described in terms of such damage'.

The management of postoperative pain has received much attention in the past few years, particularly since the publication of the Joint Report of the Royal Colleges of Surgeons and Anaesthetists 'Pain after Surgery' (Royal College of Surgeons of England, 1990). This report highlighted the continuing failings in postoperative pain management and made several recommendations for the improvement of the situation. The development of acute pain services in general hospitals undertaking surgery was one of those recommendations.

Postoperative pain should not be expected or seen as being an inevitable part of recovery and it can be assumed that patients should not suffer unnecessarily. Health professionals have an ethical duty to provide pain relief, and this is reinforced in Article 3 of the Human Rights Act (1998), which states: 'No one shall be subjected to torture or to inhuman or degrading treatment or punishment'.

In addition, poorly managed postoperative pain can activate several physiological responses which can be harmful, and may delay recovery from surgery and ultimately the patient's discharge from hospital. It is difficult to state that good pain relief alone will reduce length of stay, as this is only one part of the patient's journey, but it is reasonable to expect that a patient who experiences a manageable level of pain is less likely to experience postoperative complications and hence is likely to recover more quickly.

Unfortunately, it is likely that many patients are still being failed in this area of care due to many factors. An extensive review of postoperative pain management by Dolin et al (2002) suggested that one in five patients still report severe pain postoperatively. Similarly, a survey of over 44 000 NHS inpatients (Picker Institute Europe, 2002) found that two-thirds of those surveyed had experienced pain at some point during their hospital stay. Although the methodology of the study is unclear and those surveyed had not necessarily had surgery, the results are disturbing. Additionally, a study by Scott and Hodson (1997) suggested that many patients have a poor understanding of the nature of postoperative pain and how it is managed and will maintain a passive role in this part of care, preferring to leave decisions about pain to be made by health professionals who they may regard as being the experts.

CLASSIFICATION OF PAIN

Acute pain is pain of recent onset and limited duration. It usually has an identifiable cause and an identifiable beginning and end. Acute postoperative pain is nociceptive pain. Nociception is the term used to describe the processing of noxious or damaging stimuli, and nociceptive information is transmitted by specific pain fibres called nociceptors. Tissue injury starts the process of inflammation by stimulating the release of inflammatory mediators such as bradykinin, histamine and prostaglandins from the damaged tissue cells (Kidd and Urban, 2001). This process will cause nociceptors to become further sensitized to pain. Acute pain is also associated with the stimulation of the sympathetic nervous system, which can lead to the activation of several potentially harmful physiological responses. Nociceptive pain can be visceral or somatic. Visceral pain arises from internal organs and may be difficult to localize. Somatic pain relates to skin, muscle or joints and tends to be localized.

Chronic pain may be defined as that pain which has persisted, either continuously or intermittently, for 3 months or more and does not respond to traditional medical or surgical treatment. Bonica (1990:19) defined chronic pain as 'pain that persists a month beyond the usual course of an acute disease or a reasonable time for an injury to heal, or that is associated with a chronic pathological process that causes continuous pain or the pain recurs at intervals for months or years'. Chronic pain is unlikely to stimulate the sympathetic nervous system. However, it can totally disrupt normal life by taking over the life of the sufferer and of those close to them. Chronic pain can be complex and multidimensional in nature, which can lead to the sufferer seeking many different treatments. It is important to note that inadequately controlled acute pain can lead to chronic pain.

Chronic pain after surgery was described by Macrae (2001) as a common problem which seemed to be neglected despite causing disability and distress. Common operations causing chronic pain after surgery were cited as breast surgery, hernia repair, cholycystectomy and thoracotomy.

Neuropathic pain can be described as pain initiated or caused by a primary lesion or dysfunction in the nervous system. This is a very distressing pain and early diagnosis and treatment is crucial, as it may become more difficult to treat over time. Patients will often describe neuropathic pain as burning, shooting or stabbing in nature and the pain may also be associated with abnormal sensations such as numbness and hyperalgesia. Neuropathic pain can occur following a viral infection such as shingles; following surgery such as amputation; or it may be linked to a medical condition such as diabetes (diabetic neuropathy). An important part of postoperative pain management is the recognition of neuropathic pain. Staff should be alerted to signs of an increase in pain, perhaps of a shooting or stabbing nature, particularly when the level had started to diminish. If the pain is requiring increasing amounts of opioids with little or no effect, this may be a sign of neuropathic pain, as generally this pain does not tend to respond well to opioids (Bridges et al, 2001; NHMRC, 1999).

PAIN THEORIES: A BRIEF HISTORY

In primitive times, it was believed that pain was caused by an external force. Pain from internal disease caused great mystification (Bonica, 1985). The ancient Egyptians believed that pain, other than that from obvious wounds, entered the body through an orifice and that it was caused by demons or spirits of the dead. They learned that pain could be affected by rubbing, heat and cold, although they did not know why, and they believed that pain would leave the body by sneezing or within waste fluids. Aristotle believed that pain was experienced in the heart as an emotion, opposite to pleasure. The ancient Romans were the first to link pain to the phenomenon of inflammation, with the associated redness, swelling and heat, although it was hundreds of years before the concept of pain was linked to the brain and spinal cord and a network of sensory and motor nerves.

The 'specificity' theory was the traditional pain theory, described by Descartes in 1644 (cited by Fordham and Dunn, 1994). This proposed that a specific pain system carried pain messages directly to a pain centre in the brain, producing a uniform and invariable response, which helped form the belief that the intensity of the pain experience was directly linked to the severity of an injury. The 'pattern' theory was based on the belief that there were nerve pathways exclusively conducting pain information and that every sensory stimulus was capable of producing pain if the stimulus reached sufficient intensity.

In 1965, Melzack and Wall suggested a new theory for pain, the 'gate control' theory, which assumes that pain perception is controlled by a gate mechanism in the spinal cord, as well as being influenced by input from other areas of the central nervous system. The gate control theory provides the basis for much of our current understanding of the physiology of pain.

THE GATE CONTROL THEORY OF PAIN

The gate control theory suggests that pain perception can be influenced by a gating mechanism in a specific area of the spinal cord called the substantia gelatinosa. The substantia gelatinosa is located within the dorsal horn of the cord. The dorsal horn is constructed in layers called laminae, numbered from I to IX, and laminae II and III form the substantia gelatinosa. Pain information reaches the brain from the dorsal horn via a pathway called the spinothalamic tract. This tract relays sensory information to the thalamus and also carries information to another tract called the spinoreticular tract. The spinoreticular tract relays information linked to the emotional aspects of pain perception to the limbic system.

Three types of nerve fibres are described in relation to the gate control theory, although only two of these fibre types, called A delta and C fibres, carry actual pain impulses. The A delta fibres are small, myelinated fibres. Myelin is a fatty sheath that envelops the nerve, helping the rapid transmission between synapses. Hence, the myelinated A delta fibres respond to fast, sharp pain such as the initial pain following a surgical incision or a pinprick. The small, unmyelinated C fibres respond to chemical, mechanical and thermal stimuli. They transmit information linked to slow, dull pain such as the residual pain due to inflammation. Chemical mediators from damaged tissues and some of those produced at the dorsal horn will have an excitatory effect on C fibres, thus increasing the pain.

A third type of fibre, called A beta fibres, have a role in external pain modulation. A beta fibres are myelinated and have a lower stimulation threshold than A delta and C fibres. They are stimulated by temperature change, pressure or vibration. If the impulses transmitted by the low-threshold A beta fibres exceed those transmitted by the small nociceptive A delta and C fibres, then inhibitory neurotransmitters will be released within the substantia gelatinosa, inhibiting the release of excitatory substances, thereby closing the gate. Modulation can also occur due to descending inhibitory mechanisms from the brain, including descending chemical inhibition, information from the autonomic nervous system and the release of endogenous opioids at the dorsal horn.

However, if the firing of the nociceptive A delta and C fibres is greater than that of the A beta fibres, then there will be no inhibitory influence and the gate will be open. An important chemical transmitter involved in this excitatory response is substance P, which is secreted by some nerve endings.

GENERAL PRINCIPLES IN THE MANAGEMENT OF ACUTE PAIN

The desired outcome for postoperative pain management is for the patient to report that they are comfortable, or that their pain is at a level which is acceptable to them, with minimal side-effects such as nausea and vomiting or oversedation. Pain must be assessed and recorded, and the assessment acted upon. The assessment must involve the patient where possible and should be a dynamic pain assessment, measured on moving or coughing, or during procedures which might cause pain. Pain should be considered as the fifth vital sign, to ensure that it is considered routinely along with other observations such as temperature and pulse recordings (Campbell, 1995). The effects of analgesics given must be evaluated and reviewed regularly, according to the response indicated by the patient.

The strongest available analgesic should be used, and opioid analgesics are the mainstay in the management of moderate to severe pain (NHMRC, 1999). However, analgesics must be given using the most appropriate route at that time. For example, it is appropriate to administer intravenous opioids in a postoperative recovery area, but local policies will dictate routes of opioid administration on general surgical wards in respect of continuous infusions or intravenous bolusing by ward staff.

In addition, the use of different types of analgesics as multimodal analgesia will improve the effectiveness of the analgesia (NHMRC, 1999). For example, simple oral analgesics should be prescribed and administered 'by the clock' rather than according to the pain level in addition to 'as required' opioids.

Epidural analgesia and patient-controlled analgesia (PCA) are commonly used to provide postoperative analgesia. McQuay and Moore (2002) recommend the use of high-tech analgesia in the postoperative setting, reducing the amount and technique from high to low as the pain reduces or goes away over time. The patient must be nursed in the most appropriate environment for the method of analgesia that they are receiving, and consideration for this must be made in relation to the whole 24-hour period.

WHAT CAN AFFECT THE EXPERIENCE OF ACUTE PAIN?

Pain is a complex interaction of both mind and body, and the outcome of postoperative pain management is subject to many contributing factors. For example, staff and patient attitudes, particularly in relation to fears of addiction from the use of opioids, may prevent a patient from receiving adequate analgesics. Education of all staff involved in the management of patients postoperatively is essential, to ensure that such attitudes are challenged.

It is important to undertake a full assessment of the patient's pain history, so as to ascertain whether he has had any surgery before, whether he is currently taking analgesics or if analgesics have been taken before. Any

fears or misunderstandings about analgesics such as worries about addiction or side-effects can also be discussed. Other factors are important, such as the age of the patient, which can affect the quantity and type of analgesics given. Many elderly patients can be stoic about pain and may not feel that they should report it. Equally, the elderly may have other ongoing pain problems due to conditions such as arthritis, and they may already take other analgesics.

A patient's personality can strongly influence the way in which pain is expressed. A patient who appears quiet and comfortable may not necessarily be so. It has been suggested that people with extroverted personality types are more likely to complain and to express their pain than introverted personality types. If this is so, then it could be argued that extroverts will probably receive more analgesics (Bond, 1984). A person's culture can also strongly influence perception of pain and how pain is expressed, which will affect the outcome of treatment. In addition, the nurse's own culture can influence how they assess pain and it is important for nurses to recognize how a cultural bias on their part can affect this (Davitz and Davitz, 1985).

Past experience may be reflected in the response of an individual to pain. Many of these responses are learnt during childhood and carried through into adult life, with associated personal beliefs and coping mechanisms.

It has been suggested that comparable stimuli in different people do not necessarily produce the same pain, either in duration or intensity (Melzack and Wall, 1991). This highlights the misconception that a particular operation or injury will produce a predictable level of pain. Interestingly, most people have a fairly uniform pain sensation threshold, which is the lowest intensity at which pain is felt, but pain perception and tolerance are not static. Pain perception and tolerance can be influenced by feelings of exhaustion, boredom, anxiety and isolation.

Wall (1999) anecdotally describes several reports illustrating how the meaning of the pain can influence the experience of the individual. It is also important to consider what the pain means to the patient and how this links in with the meaning of the surgery. For example, a patient undergoing a joint replacement will know that this is likely to improve their quality of life, whereas a patient who has had surgery related to cancer will have many anxieties.

PAIN ASSESSMENT

Assessment of pain is crucial if effective pain management is to be delivered and evaluated. The patient must be involved in pain assessment where possible (Royal College of Surgeons of England, 1990), as it is the patient who knows how severe the pain is. A study by Seers (1987) found that nurses frequently recorded the patient's pain to be less severe than the patient's own assessment, and it is probable that this still remains an issue.

Pain assessment should be carried out regularly, like other routine observations, and not seen as an extra task used in isolation to other routine postoperative observations. Pain assessment is not just about using a chart, and other aspects must be considered. For example, health professionals may use the term 'pain', which the patient may consider to mean only severe or excruciating pain rather than soreness or aching which can also prevent them from carrying out their daily activities. It is therefore important to ascertain what words patients use to describe their pain. It is also important to find out whether the patient usually takes any medication which may affect postoperative analgesic use, including analgesics, homeopathic medicines, alcohol and nicotine.

Pain assessment in the acute or postoperative setting tends to focus on pain intensity. This is because a quick assessment is required in order for treatment to be given as soon as possible. Although a dedicated pain assessment chart can be used, it may be more acceptable to staff if pain assessment is incorporated into a general observation chart. The most common measure in the acute pain setting is the categorical scale (Fig. 7.1). This uses words such as 'no pain', 'mild pain', 'moderate pain' and 'severe pain' to describe the severity of the pain. Numbers can be added alongside this verbal description to help the patient to use the tool and also to assist with analysis of data for audit purposes.

Pain assessment using the categorical scale may be difficult for some patients, such as the elderly or cognitively impaired. Pain assessment in the elderly must also consider other coexisting pain problems, which must be distinguished from the acute postoperative pain (Moddeman, 2002). Victor (2001) suggested that the use of standard pain tools should not be automatically excluded for elderly patients who may be cognitively impaired, and that additional simple, specific questioning can be helpful. The same author recommended the use of other measurements such as facial expression, sweating, increased heart rate, agitation and guarding. These observations can be used for any patient who is unable to verbalize pain.

Pain assessment tools are often standardized within individual hospitals, to avoid uncertainty when staff move between areas. If possible, patients should be introduced to a pain assessment tool preoperatively and written information given about how to use the

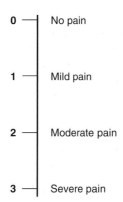

Figure 7.1   Categorical pain scale.

tool and what to do if their pain is not controlled. The preoperative assessment clinic is an ideal environment for the dissemination of this preoperative information, although it is likely that the patient will be given a great deal of information at that time and this may need revisiting on admission.

THE PHYSIOLOGICAL RESPONSE TO PAIN AND THE DANGERS OF POORLY MANAGED PAIN

Severe acute pain can be physiologically harmful due to the stimulation of the sympathetic nervous system. The role of the sympathetic nervous system is to protect the body in times of stress, and stimulation causes several physiological responses known as the 'surgical stress response'. These include the release of hormones such as cortisol and growth hormone; increased levels of blood glucose; and fluid and electrolyte imbalances. Increased metabolism will lead to an increased catabolism, requiring higher levels of oxygen. It has been suggested that the provision of adequate pain relief may reduce this automatic response (Kehlet and Holte, 2001). The use of continuous epidural analgesia with the inclusion of a local anaesthetic agent is the choice for providing this level of analgesia because the local anaesthetic will block the sympathetic nerves.

Poorly managed acute pain may be particularly harmful to the elderly or those with pre-existing cardiac morbidity because of the resulting increased workload on the heart. Pain may also prevent the elderly person from breathing adequately, thus reducing oxygenation. More oxygen will be required if the heart is forced to work harder and this could be compounded further if the patient is unable to breath properly due to pain. In addition, the elderly patient will have an altered response to analgesics due to physiological changes such as less circulating blood volume, less muscle mass and reduced hepatic and renal clearance of drugs (Cooper, 2002) within their bodies which may affect the metabolism of drugs. The elderly are also more susceptible to adverse drug reactions (NHMRC, 1999), probably due in part to polypharmacy.

METHODS OF ADMINISTERING POSTOPERATIVE ANALGESIA

The administration of strong opioids is the first-line treatment for pain following surgery. The actual route of administration will depend on the type of surgery and the expected level of pain. The route of analgesic administration will also be dependent on where the patient is being cared for: i.e. patients with continuous epidural analgesia may need to be nursed in a high-dependency setting and staff will need to be trained in the management of this.

ORAL ADMINISTRATION

Oral administration of analgesics is the most acceptable route for patients, and it should be the first choice if at all possible. However, this route is seldom appropriate in the immediate postoperative phase, as gut motility is often reduced or the type of surgery may make the route impossible. If the oral route is used inappropriately, then there can be delayed absorption at an unpredictable time. In addition, if the patient is nauseated or is vomiting, there will be very little absorption of the drug.

RECTAL ADMINISTRATION

Some analgesics such as paracetamol and non-steroidal anti-inflammatory drugs (NSAIDs) can be administered rectally. The drug is systemically absorbed through the rectal mucosa. This method may not be acceptable to patients, and it is essential that verbal consent is obtained and recorded prior to administering drugs in this way. If the patient consents to this method, then it allows early implementation of balanced analgesia even if the patient is 'nil by mouth'.

TRANSDERMAL ADMINISTRATION

This is a useful route for the administration of lipophilic drugs such as fentanyl, as the route avoids first-pass metabolism. Patients who cannot take oral medications may have analgesics by this route. However, the transdermal route is not usually used in the postoperative period, because the absorption is unpredictable and it may take up to 24 hours for effective plasma levels to be reached. Analgesics such as fentanyl and buprenorphine can be given in this way but neither are currently licensed for use in postoperative acute pain.

THE INTRAVENOUS ROUTE

The intravenous route is a rapid way of administering analgesics, including some NSAIDs and opioids. The administration of opioids by this route is often limited to areas where there are high staff to patient ratios. The intravenous route is fast acting and easy to titrate to pain levels, but it requires the nurse to stay with the patient during administration and for some time afterwards, which may not be possible in a busy general ward. Hence, this method is frequently reserved for use in more specialist areas or by the acute pain service in general wards. Goodman and Gilman (1996) suggested that respiratory depression following the administration of intravenous opioids was most likely to occur within 7–10 minutes of administration; hence, it could be argued that the nurse would need to stay with the patient for at least 10 minutes following the last injection. Best practice would also suggest that naloxone should be immediately available during administration, and that the nurse administering the opioid would remain responsible for the safekeeping of any unused portion of the drug until no more was required and any remainder could be discarded.

The use of a continuous intravenous infusion is another method of administering opioids. However, this may lead to accumulation of the analgesic and patients should be nursed in an area where they can be closely observed for the whole time that they are receiving opioids by this route (Dodds and Hutton, 2002).

THE INTRAMUSCULAR ROUTE

The intramuscular route is frequently used for the intermittent 'as required' dosing of opioids and remains the traditional method of administering analgesics postoperatively, although it commonly fails for several reasons. First, most patients do not like injections, because they are painful. Also, the nurse has control of the analgesia instead of the patient, and many patients worry about bothering the nurses if they are in pain, especially if the nurses look busy.

Seymour (1996) highlighted that, when using another method of analgesia such as PCA, patients felt that they were not being a bother to the nurses. Additionally, both the prescribing and administration of intramuscular opioids tends to be inadequate and the pharmacokinetics are unpredictable, therefore it is difficult to achieve a constant level of analgesia. This may lead to intermittent analgesia and sedation, identified by Lovett et al (1994) as a bolus comfort sedation cycle, due to the wide fluctuation in plasma concentrations that can occur with intramuscular injections (Koh and Thomas, 1994).

However, the intramuscular route of administering opioids may be the most appropriate route of administration for a particular clinical setting (e.g. if that area has no staff trained in the management of epidurals); hence, there should be some effort made to make this a more reliable and effective method of analgesia. One recommendation of the Joint Report of the Royal Colleges of Surgeons and Anaesthetists 'Pain after Surgery' (1990) was to utilize existing methods of analgesia more effectively and challenge traditional beliefs and attitudes. Harmer and Davies (1998) demonstrated that by introducing simple changes on the method of giving intramuscular analgesics, the patient experience could be improved. They did this by recommending the introduction of an algorithm which would allow the hourly administration of opioids using an indwelling intramuscular cannula. This enabled staff to work within a much more flexible but safe system. Hourly administration of intramuscular opioids was also recommended by Dodds and Hutton (2002), who felt that this would be advantageous not only because patients would be less likely to experience peaks and troughs of analgesia but also because the dose could be more easily titrated and patients would have their pain assessed more frequently along with other vital signs. However, it was also recognized that such a change in practice may increase the workload for nursing staff if two nurses were required to check the analgesics.

THE SUBCUTANEOUS ROUTE

The subcutaneous route requires no alterations to dosage or frequency of dosing as the absorption of the drug is similar to when given intramuscularly (Macintyre and Ready, 1997) and an indwelling cannula can also be used, as described above.

PATIENT-CONTROLLED ANALGESIA (PCA)

PCA is a common method of administering postoperative analgesia and many patients have benefited from using it. The patient can choose when they have analgesics without having to bother staff, and the dose can provide analgesia quickly, as well as providing a sense of control and empowerment for the patient. PCA allows the patient to self-administer analgesics within set parameters. The concept lies in the aim to keep plasma levels of opioid at a consistent, effective level without causing side-effects, and without causing peaks and troughs of analgesia, which could happen with the administration of intramuscular analgesics.

PCA is frequently used for both adults and children postoperatively. The most obvious criteria for its use are that the patient is physically able to use the chosen device and that they have the ability to understand the concept. Some patients may not feel that PCA is appropriate for them, as they may not wish to take on this part of their care or they may associate the use of an opioid with drug addiction.

To help ensure best practice in the use of PCA, every step must be taken to reduce risk, such as the standardization of equipment and the use of prescribing guidelines or protocols. Any changes made within these to allow for individual patient need must be made absolutely clear by the prescriber. Administration lines used must be designed for PCA use, incorporating a one-way valve port for the safe attachment of intravenous infusions plus an anti-siphon valve to prevent gravity-induced siphoning if the pump is placed too high or if there is a crack in the syringe. All staff using PCA equipment must be trained in its use, and this training must be provided as an ongoing programme.

It is important that all staff caring for patients using PCA are able to manage the equipment. This must include being able to monitor the amount of drug given in milligrams or micrograms (depending on the drug used) plus the equivalent volume in millilitres (mL). This information should be recorded with each set of observations, and it is also advisable to record this information each time a different nurse takes over the care of the patient. Most PCA pumps enable the patient and staff to obtain a history of the total number of demands made and how many of those demands resulted in successful delivery of analgesics. Staff must also be able to troubleshoot potential problems with the equipment and replace PCA syringes or infusion bags as needed, so as to ensure that the patient does not have a break in analgesia.

Description of terms used in patient-controlled analgesia

The *bolus dose* is the amount of analgesic drug that the patient will self-administer on a successful demand with PCA. The bolus should be enough to provide good analgesia with minimal side-effects. Morphine is frequently used for PCA and a 1 mg dose every 5 minutes, if required, appears to be a fairly standard dose for most adult patients. This would appear to go against the argument that we should be providing analgesia which is tailored to the individual, but consistency in prescribing will reduce risk in relation to prescribing or administration errors.

The *lockout time* is the time during which the PCA pump will not deliver any dose of analgesic. The patient must be reassured that the PCA will not give a dose of analgesic during this time, no matter how many times the demand is pressed. The time is set to allow for the opioid to have full effect. Lockout times of between 5 and 10 minutes are commonly used, although it is accepted that this may not be long enough for the full effect of some drugs to be seen (Macintyre, 2001).

It is good practice to provide initial analgesia in the form of an intravenous *loading dose* for the patient, so that the patient can maintain this with PCA. Due to the small amount of drug used with each patient bolus, PCA is unlikely to provide adequate initial analgesia to a patient who is in severe pain. The loading dose is given by a doctor or a nurse who has received the appropriate training. The amount of analgesic given as a loading dose will depend on the individual analgesic requirement for each patient. The loading dose can be given as a separate injection or by using the loading dose facility on an electronic PCA pump.

Patient education

Patients must have a clear understanding of how to use the PCA equipment prior to using it. This may be difficult if the patient is undergoing emergency surgery or if they are given information too far in advance and their understanding of how to use the PCA is not checked. A study of patients using PCA showed that structured teaching may make a difference as to how patients managed their pain with this method, although it was not clear when the teaching should be undertaken in order to be most effective (Timmons and Bower, 1993). The use of an information leaflet may be helpful. Chumbley et al (2002) undertook a study involving patient focus groups in the design of a patient information leaflet for PCA. This led to the production of a more informative leaflet that was more acceptable to patients.

Common problems with patient–controlled analgesia

If the patient is not receiving adequate analgesics, the nurse should check that the patient is using the PCA equipment correctly. The pump history must be checked, as the patient may not be using the pump enough due to a lack of understanding. If the patient is not using the PCA appropriately, then further advice

and support can be given to help the patient to get the greatest benefit.

One of the main principles of acute pain management is to provide multimodal analgesia with simple analgesics given regularly rather than waiting until the pain becomes problematic. It is therefore important for the nurse to ensure that the patient has other analgesics prescribed alongside the PCA and to ensure that these are given. If no regular analgesic is prescribed, then it is the responsibility of the nurse to get the analgesic prescription reviewed. If the patient has used the PCA to the maximum and has received other analgesics, but the level of pain remains unacceptable to them, then their drug regime must be reviewed. Extra analgesics in the form of an intravenous rescue dose may be required to reinstate analgesia. It is not appropriate to give an opioid intramuscularly as an addition to PCA, as the effect of this may be unpredictable and could lead to oversedation and respiratory depression.

It is also common for patients using PCA to have pain on waking from sleep. This is a common problem which can only be addressed by advising the patient to press the button as soon as they awake. It could be argued that a solution to this problem is to give the patient a continuous background infusion of opioid in addition to PCA, but this may simply lead to a higher incidence of side-effects such as respiratory depression rather than an improvement in analgesia (Macintyre, 2001).

During early use of PCA, many patients who were known or suspected to be drug users were often denied it, as it was believed that this would encourage a drug habit. It should now be accepted that PCA is an appropriate method of administering postoperative pain relief to this specific client group. Postoperative care of this client group should encompass effective pain management while preventing physical withdrawal symptoms (Jage and Bey, 2000). Maintenance of their usual opioid requirement will need to be maintained, in addition to postoperative analgesics. This can be achieved with a background infusion plus PCA. This approach may also be appropriate for other patients who take regular opioid-based analgesics, including patients with cancer or chronic non-malignant pain problems.

Morphine is the most common drug used, although diamorphine or fentanyl can also be used for PCA. Pethidine is not recommended for PCA use, as the potentially high dose that could be used may lead to the accumulation of the toxic metabolite norpethidine, particularly during the first 24 hours of use (Macintyre, 2001). More recently, analgesics such as tramadol have been used and the opioid oxycodone is now licensed for use in PCA. The most common route of PCA administration is intravenous, but the subcutaneous route is also used in some places. This requires a different lockout time, and dose duration may be over a few minutes to allow more comfortable administration for the patient.

All opioids administered by any route have the potential to cause oversedation and respiratory depression (see p. 109). Whenever PCA is prescribed and used, the staff caring for the patient must be able to recognize these problems early on, and follow clear guidelines for subsequent management of the patient. Patients using PCA must only be nursed throughout the 24-hour period in clinical areas where staff have received the appropriate training. This must be understood by and strictly adhered to by all staff, including the prescribing doctor. It is considered good practice to prescribe oxygen therapy for all patients who are receiving PCA for the duration of PCA use (Dodds and Hutton, 2002).

It could be argued that if the patient is using the PCA unaided, then the natural control would be that they would stop using it if oversedation occurred. However, oversedation is a possibility, particularly if another person is pressing the demand button on behalf of the patient. The basic principle of PCA requires only the patient to press the button and if they became too drowsy to press the demand button then they would not do so. However, if another person such as a family member or a healthcare professional presses the button, this would override the natural control loop and the patient could easily become overdosed. Visitors are to be actively discouraged from pressing the PCA demand for a patient and must be informed of the potential dangers of doing so. If the patient is unable to understand how to use the PCA or is unable to press the demand for themselves without prompting, then the PCA must be discontinued and an alternative method of analgesia prescribed.

Over sedation may be a more accurate early indicator of opioid-induced respiratory depression (NHMRC, 1999). If a patient becomes sedated at a level that they are difficult to rouse or they are unrousable, then the PCA handset must be removed from the patient and the patient closely observed until they become less sedated. Close observation means direct observation by a trained nurse who is also constantly monitoring sedation, respiratory rate and oxygen saturations, because a reduced level of sedation such as this is likely to be accompanied by a reduction in respiratory function. If a patient has oxygen saturations of less than 95% on oxygen accompanied by a respiratory rate of less than 8 breaths per minute and is sedated, then the nurse should communicate this to medical staff immediately and ensure that naloxone is available and ready for rapid use if required to reverse the action of the opioid. Local policies will dictate at which point naloxone should be used and whether nursing staff are able to administer it.

The patient may show other signs of opioid overdose such as constricted pupils and cyanosis. Other potential side-effects of opioids such as pruritus, nausea and vomiting, hypotension and constipation are discussed in the pharmacology section of this chapter.

EPIDURAL ANALGESIA

The use of epidural analgesia for postoperative pain has the potential to provide a level of analgesia that is superior to other methods such as intramuscular opioids. Epidural analgesia involves the injection of drugs into the epidural space. *Epi* means above therefore, this means that the injection is administered into the space above the dura and not directly into the cerebrospinal fluid, which is contained below the dura. Drugs injected through the dura into the cerebrospinal fluid would be intraspinal or intrathecal.

Many patients receive epidural analgesia following major surgery and most centres use a mixture of opioids and local anaesthetics in a continuous infusion to deliver balanced analgesia. A continuous epidural infusion containing both an opioid and a local anaesthetic has the potential to provide excellent analgesia, while blocking the potentially harmful stimulation of the sympathetic nervous system (sympathetic blockade). It has been hypothesized that using an epidural containing local anaesthetic is the only way to reduce the body's stress response to surgery (Kehlet and Holte, 2001) (see p. 101).

Common opioids used epidurally are fentanyl and diamorphine. These are most commonly administered in addition to a local anaesthetic agent such as bupivacaine. The local anaesthetic component acts by blocking the action potential in the spinal nerves, hence preventing pain messages from reaching the brain. Other drugs such as clonidine and adrenaline (epinephrine) can be added to the epidural mixture. These drugs act as 'adjuvants', meaning that they enhance the effect of analgesics while not having a direct analgesic action. Patients receiving a continuous epidural infusion containing an opioid must not receive opioids by any other route for the duration that they have the epidural, so as to prevent accidental opioid overdose.

Opioid analgesics administered epidurally will be partly absorbed through the epidural veins and fat, but the majority will diffuse across the dura into the cerebrospinal fluid. They ascend rostrally in an upward spiral to the brain but also act upon opioid receptors in the dorsal horn of the spinal cord, mimicking the action of endogenous opioids.

An epidural will not be appropriate for all patients. The anaesthetist responsible for the patient will assess whether it is safe to undertake the procedure. The absolute contraindication to an epidural is if the patient does not consent to the procedure. The patient should give verbal consent prior to the insertion of an epidural and must receive an explanation about the procedure and the possible complications. Harmer (2002) suggested that formal written consent of postoperative pain procedures may become a requirement in the future but, in the meantime, patients should be given the opportunity to fully discuss the pain management procedure, including alternatives, if a particular method of analgesia is not available.

Caution should be exercised in the following situations, although these are not necessarily absolute contraindications:

- The presence of a clotting disorder or if the patient is being anticoagulated may increase the risk of bleeding into the epidural space.
- Any abnormal spinal anatomy can narrow the vertebral canal or the epidural space, and may make it difficult to site the epidural catheter.
- The presence of aortic valve stenosis may reduce the ability of the body to compensate in situations of hypotension. Equally, any untreated hypovolaemia can compound the hypotension caused by epidural local anaesthetic agents.
- Patients with any head injury may not be suitable for epidural placement in case of damage to the dura.
- Any local or generalized infection may put the patient at risk of meningitis or an epidural abscess.

A key role of an acute pain service is the management of a ward-based epidural service. Key tasks for the acute pain nurse are to minimize risk by educating staff in the management of epidurals, standardizing equipment, auditing problems and ensuring that appropriate observation of the patient is carried out in accordance with local policy. All nurses caring for patients with epidurals must be aware of the potential effects of local anaesthetics and opioids and how to manage potential problems, including the management of the epidural equipment. Potential problems associated with the administration of opioids are discussed in the pharmacology section (see p. 109).

Local policy will dictate the type and frequency of observations carried out for patients with continuous epidural analgesia. It would be realistic to suggest that blood pressure, heart rate, respiratory rate and oxygen saturations, pain levels, sedation and any nausea and vomiting are measured and recorded at least 2 hourly during the first 24 hours and 4 hourly for the remainder of the time that the epidural infusion is in progress. In addition, monitoring of sensory and motor block must be carried out at least 4 hourly, plus observation of the epidural site whenever a different nurse takes over the care of the patient or if the patient reports an increase in pain.

Patients with an epidural must be able to move and be able to take a deep breath and cough with minimal, if any, pain. If a patient has pain, staff should follow their local guidelines to manage the situation before calling for assistance from anaesthetic staff or from the acute pain service. Patients will rarely report a sudden increase in pain unless the epidural catheter has fallen out or the infusion has been interrupted for any other reason. An increase in pain is likely to be accompanied by increased blood pressure, heart rate and a sensory block that is below the level of the surgery. If the patient reports pain, then the nurse must check the sensory level, the epidural site and general observations and also whether any other analgesics have been given, e.g. regular paracetamol. If an increase in the rate of the epidural infusion fails to improve the level of pain within 30 minutes, then advice should be sought, as it is likely that the patient will require a 'top up' administered by the acute pain service or an anaesthetist, depending on local guidelines.

A 'top up' involves the administration of a further dose of analgesics via the epidural to reinstate analgesia. If a strong solution of local anaesthetic is used, then the patient must be advised that there may be increased numbness around the wound site and a fall in blood pressure following the 'top up'. If the patient has a lumbar epidural, then it is possible that they will experience a motor block for a few hours post 'top up' and that their feet will feel warm due to the vasodilatation effect. During the 'top up', it is essential to monitor and record the patient's blood pressure, heart rate, sedation and pain level at 3–5-minute intervals plus monitoring of sensory and motor function. If a 'top up' fails to help the patient's pain levels, then an alternative method of analgesia will be required as any more time spent trying to rectify the pain may result in the patient losing confidence in the epidural.

Hypotension can occur due to vasodilatation that results from sympathetic blockade. Hypotension can lead to cerebral hypoxia and poor perfusion to other organs such as the kidneys, heart and the gut. It can also contribute to the breakdown of surgical anastamoses. A sudden drop in systolic blood pressure may occur following a 'top up' during which a bolus of local anaesthetic is given. In the absence of a 'top up', a sudden drop in systolic blood pressure could indicate migration of the epidural catheter below the dura. However, hypotension is rarely due to the epidural alone and is more commonly linked with hypovolaemia. If the patient with an epidural becomes hypotensive, then a full assessment must be carried out, including fluid management, rather than simply discontinuing the epidural. Accurate monitoring and management of fluid balance in addition to considering the possible effects of the epidural on blood pressure are essential to ensure that the patient continues to receive effective pain management.

If patients becomes hypotensive in relation to their normal systolic blood pressure, accompanied by a reduced urinary output, then a review of their fluid balance may be all that is required, particularly if they feel well otherwise. If the patient becomes symptomatic, then, in addition to the above, the patient should be laid down with legs elevated to aid venous return, and medical advice sought. It would also be appropriate to check the sensory level of the epidural to ensure that this had not risen above the dermatomal level supplied by the fourth thoracic nerve (T4). This could occur if the epidural had been topped up or if the epidural catheter had migrated. An epidural sensory level of above T4 could block the cardioaccelerator nerves, causing bradycardia in addition to hypotension. If hypotension is not responsive to an increase in fluid administration, then it may be necessary to give ephedrine. Ephedrine stimulates alpha and beta adrenergic receptors, causing vasoconstriction, and it must be available for intravenous use in all areas where patients with epidurals are nursed, and all staff must be familiar with its preparation and administration.

Testing the level of sensory block

An important measurement that is recorded for patients with continuous epidural analgesia is the sensory level, although local policy will dictate how much emphasis is placed on this. The method for carrying out this test will also vary in different hospitals. Ideally, the height of the sensory block should be at least to the top of the surgical wound. The anaesthetist will site an epidural to enable this, and it is expected that the epidural block will spread approximately two to three dermatomes above and below the level of insertion. For example, an epidural sited between the eighth and ninth thoracic vertebrae would be expected to block the area supplied between the sixth and twelfth thoracic vertebrae.

The sensory level can be tested using ice or a neurological testing pin. If ice is used, this should be placed into a plastic bag or non-sterile glove or, alternatively, a frozen sachet of 0.9% sodium chloride can be used. The cold sensation must be initially tested on the

patient's arm so that cold is clearly distinguished from touch. The ice is placed on the skin well below the anticipated area of sensory block and moved gradually upwards while asking the patient to indicate when they no longer feel the cold sensation or when it changes to a different sensation. The sensory level is measured as being the dermatome at which cold sensation returns at the same intensity as when tested on the arm.

Epidural analgesics should provide analgesia by blocking sensory nerves with minimal effect on motor nerves. The presence of a persistent motor block must be investigated without delay, as it could be an indication of a complication such as an epidural haematoma or migration of the epidural. If the catheter has migrated, the motor block will be accompanied by a sudden drop in systolic blood pressure. It may be necessary to temporarily stop the epidural infusion to ensure that normal motor function is present and the epidural infusion can then be tailored to prevent this recurring.

Some degree of motor block may be inevitable if a patient has a lumbar epidural. A motor block can impede recovery by delaying mobilization and may lead to the development of pressure ulcers due to reduced sensation. Regular checking of pressure areas must be an integral part of care for the patient with a lumbar epidural. The motor block must be tested by asking patients to move their feet, flex their knees and, if possible, lift their legs. If an epidural haematoma is suspected, then this demands immediate investigation. Patients may complain of severe pain in their back, at the site of the epidural, and this would be accompanied by a change in sensation and movement in the legs. If left untreated, an epidural haematoma can lead to permanent paralysis. An epidural haematoma is most likely to form following the siting or removal of the epidural cannula, therefore, the administration of any anticoagulants must be timed to ensure that the epidural procedure can be carried out safely (Skilton and Justice, 1998). Local policies relating to epidurals and the use of anticoagulants, including the administration of subcutaneous heparin, should be in place to help reduce this risk.

Similarly, the formation of an epidural abscess is also potentially catastrophic for the patient. Patients with an epidural in situ must have their temperature recorded 4 hourly, and the epidural site checked at the same time for redness, swelling, pain and oozing. If an abscess is suspected, then this requires immediate investigation as the outcome if untreated would be similar to that of an untreated epidural haematoma.

If a patient with an epidural feels nauseated or is actually vomiting, this could be due to the opioid in the epidural, particularly if it is accompanied by a feeling of lightheadedness or dizziness. However, nausea and vomiting may also be due to hypotension and the patient's blood pressure should always be checked if vomiting occurs. Urinary retention can occur as a side-effect of opioids, which can cause increased tone in the bladder and inhibition of the voiding reflex (Rowbotham, 2002).

Headache

The presence of a headache in the patient who has an epidural may be due to several causes. It is important to be aware of any problems encountered during the insertion of the epidural: i.e. whether there was a dural puncture or several attempts to site the epidural, or whether a combined spinal epidural injection was used, as this procedure will also pierce the dura. The anaesthetic record should be part of the handover from theatre to recovery and from recovery to the ward to ensure that staff are aware of the patient's intraoperative treatment. In the absence of any of the above, a headache may be one sign that the epidural catheter has migrated intraspinally and other symptoms should be excluded, such as a drop in systolic blood pressure or a motor block.

Nursing staff caring for patients receiving epidural analgesia must also be able to recognize signs of local anaesthetic toxicity. This may occur due to overdose or due to accidental intravenous administration. The initial signs of toxicity may be a feeling of numbness and tingling around the mouth and the tongue. This can be accompanied by visual disturbances and lightheadedness. If not detected at this stage, the patient may develop convulsions and respiratory arrest, which could lead on to a cardiac arrest (Bromley, 2002). If a patient reports any of the early symptoms, then the epidural must be stopped and medical help sought immediately.

Care of the patient who has had a spinal injection

Drugs injected below the dura are called 'spinal' or 'intraspinal/intrathecal' injections. Injection of a local anaesthetic is called 'spinal anaesthesia', whereas injection of an opioid is called 'spinal analgesia'. Some patients will have their surgery carried out under spinal anaesthesia (instead of or in addition to a general anaesthetic) and the effect of the drugs may last for several hours. Some patients may have a spinal injection followed by an epidural injection by using the same catheter; this is known as a combined spinal epidural (CSE) and is often used in orthopaedic surgery.

Spinal anaesthesia is usually performed at the lumbar level, and the administration of a local anaesthetic will provide a dense motor block which can last for several hours. Staff may be concerned about sitting patients up or allowing them to mobilize following this procedure. Patients can sit up as their general condition allows, but they should not mobilize until they have full motor power in their legs and, even then, initial mobilization must be under the supervision of two members of the clinical staff. Motor power is tested by asking patients to bend their knees and to perform a straight leg raise, which will demonstrate quadriceps strength. Patients may also experience urinary retention due to blocking of the sacral autonomic fibres and it may be necessary for a urinary catheter to be inserted to allow the bladder to empty.

Patients who have received a spinal opioid are likely to have analgesia for several hours; unless a local anaesthetic has also been given, they should not have any problems with motor power.

Potential complications following a spinal injection

A potential complication is the development of a spinal headache. The risk of a spinal headache occurring can be reduced by the use of small-bore needles. The headache is due to leakage of cerebrospinal fluid through the hole punctured in the dura by the spinal needle. This causes cerebrospinal fluid to leak out through the dura, leading to a drop in the pressure of the cerebrospinal fluid. The headache is severe and is classically worse on sitting up, as this causes a further drop in the pressure of the cerebrospinal fluid. The patient may also feel nauseated, be photophobic and have pain when flexing the neck. Patients are encouraged to rest lying down and to gradually sit up as they feel able, as well as being reassured that the condition is not life threatening. Administration of simple analgesics such as paracetamol may help, and the patient should also be encouraged to drink plenty of fluids to help increase the levels of cerebrospinal fluid. If the patient is unable to drink, then an intravenous infusion will be necessary to maintain hydration. If the headache does not resolve, then administration of a 'blood patch' may be required. During this procedure, an anaesthetist takes a blood sample from the patient and injects it into the epidural space, thus blocking the hole in the dura. Some patients will get instantaneous relief from this procedure.

PHARMACOLOGY IN ACUTE PAIN MANAGEMENT

This section will look at the types of drug commonly used in the management of acute postoperative pain, and their possible side-effects. The aim of postoperative pain management is to provide effective analgesia while causing minimal side-effects. A patient is unlikely to want to continue receiving an analgesic if they feel that it is causing nausea or other unwanted effects.

OPIOIDS

Opioids are strong analgesics used for moderate to severe pain. Opioids exert their action by mimicking the actions of endogenous opioids through activation of opioid receptors in the central nervous system. The receptors can be classified into three main types. Most opioids bind with varying degrees of affinity to μ-receptors – hence, this receptor type is associated with pain, respiratory depression and euphoria; δ-receptors are associated with pain at higher levels; and κ-receptors are linked with dysphoric effects. The degree of affinity to a receptor determines whether an opioid is classed as an agonist (has the maximum effect), partial agonist (has less effect), antagonist (has a blocking effect) or agonist/antagonist (has an effect at one receptor but blocks another).

Wherever possible, opioid dosages should be tailored to the individual patient. For adult patients, age rather than weight is the best predictor of opioid requirements (Macintyre and Jarvis, 1995). Due to the effect on the central nervous system, opioids will also have the potential to cause several side-effects, including respiratory depression, sedation, nausea and vomiting, pruritus and constipation. Respiratory depression can occur due to depression of the respiratory centre in the medulla. This effect can also lead to a reduction in tidal volumes and respiratory rate. As already discussed, measurement of respiratory rate can be a late indicator of respiratory function and the sedation level of the patient should be considered first.

Opioids given by any route can cause nausea and vomiting, as they stimulate the chemotrigger receptor zone in the medulla. The nausea related to postoperative opioid use tends to be worse on movement and it can be difficult to balance effective analgesia with the control of nausea and vomiting (Dodds and Hutton, 2002). Opioids can also delay gastric emptying and slow down the gut, causing constipation, due to the presence of μ-receptors in the gastrointestinal tract.

Pruritus can occur due to histamine release, although this can often be treated with an antihistamine drug. If this is not effective, then administration of low-dose naloxone should be considered to help reverse this effect. However, this must be carefully titrated to avoid reversing the analgesic effect of the opioid.

Some patients may experience a degree of urinary retention following the use of parenteral opioids. This is due to the action of the opioid on the voiding reflex and increased detrusor muscle tone in the bladder (Rowbotham, 2002).

The action of opioids is reversed by the opioid antagonist naloxone. The half-life of naloxone is approximately 1 hour, which is shorter than most opioids (Galbraith et al, 1999; Sasada and Smith, 1998) therefore the patient's level of sedation must be closely monitored during this time as further doses may be required.

Common opioids used in postoperative pain management are morphine, diamorphine, pethidine and fentanyl. Morphine remains the main choice for postoperative pain management and the effects of other parenteral analgesics are measured against it. Morphine is a pure μ-receptor agonist and it can be given parenterally and orally. A systematic review of the use of intramuscular morphine by McQuay et al (1999) found that 10 mg of morphine provided effective postoperative analgesia in adult patients.

Fentanyl is also commonly used in the postoperative setting. It is a synthetic, lipid-soluble opioid. Fentanyl cannot be administered orally, as it is subjected to high first-pass metabolism, but it can be administered epidurally, intraspinally or intravenously. The transmucosal and transdermal routes are not licensed for use in the postoperative setting.

Pethidine is a synthetic opioid that is shorter acting than morphine. Pethidine does not appear to have any clinical benefit over other opioids such as morphine, but the accumulation of the toxic active metabolite norpethidine, leading to central nervous system toxicity, can occur even in patients who are not felt to be at risk (Waitman et al, 2001). For this reason, pethidine is not recommended for routine use.

Once a patient is able to take oral analgesics, this should be encouraged. However, it should not be assumed that the patient will no longer need strong analgesics and there are several strong oral opioids available that are commonly used in the postoperative setting.

Morphine can be administered orally as a tablet or as an elixir. The potential side-effects are the same as with other routes of administration. The most common concentration of oral morphine elixir used for postoperative pain contains 10 mg per 5 mL. This concentration is classed as a 'prescription only' medicine, so it does not need to be stored or administered as a controlled drug (British Medical Association and Royal Pharmaceutical Society of Great Britain, 2004). However, local hospital policies may vary in this practice.

Oxycodone is an alternative oral opioid preparation that has recently been licensed for use in the postoperative setting. Oxycodone is a semi-synthetic opioid, structurally related to morphine, and is a full opioid agonist with an affinity for μ- and κ-receptors. It can be given orally or parenterally. When given orally, it is less subject to first-pass metabolism than other oral opioids and is twice as potent as oral morphine (Curtis et al, 1999). Oxycodone can be given orally as a modified release formula and it has two stages of release and absorption. The first phase is rapid and accounts for about 40% of the dose; this phase occurs by dissolution from the tablet surface and may provide analgesia within 1 hour. The second phase is a sustained release of the remainder of the dose, which may provide analgesia for up to 12 hours (Curtis et al, 1999).

Tramadol is a centrally acting analgesic which acts on μ-receptors while also inhibiting serotonin and noradrenaline (norepinephrine) reuptake (Webb et al, 2002). Both of these substances are involved in pain modulation in the central nervous system. Serotonin release is also increased. Tramadol can be administered orally or parenterally. It is an effective analgesic for moderate to severe pain and is useful in the management of neuropathic pain. It has advantages over morphine in the postoperative setting, as it has less affinity to the μ-receptor and therefore is likely to cause less respiratory depression, and less slowing of the gut. Also, although it has μ-receptor activity, it is not a controlled drug; hence, it is more convenient for staff to administer.

Codeine is an opioid analgesic that is less potent than morphine. It can be given orally or intramuscularly. Following administration, approximately 10% of the drug is metabolized to morphine by the CYP2D6 enzyme. A small percentage of the Caucasian population do not have this enzyme and will not get effective analgesia from codeine (Rowbotham, 2002). Codeine is frequently combined with paracetamol to form a compound oral analgesic.

NON–STEROIDAL ANTI–INFLAMMATORY DRUGS (NSAIDs)

NSAIDs alone are unlikely to be adequate for postoperative analgesia but the quality of opioid analgesia can be enhanced by their concomitant use (Royal College of Anaesthetists, 1998). NSAIDs have analgesic, antipyretic and anti-inflammatory actions and they work by blocking the action of cyclo-oxygenase (COX), which in turn inhibits synthesis of prostaglandins, prostacyclins and thromboxanes. There are two isoforms of COX: COX-1 and COX-2. COX-1 is a normal constituent with a protective role and is always active, synthesizing prostaglandins for homeostasis; therefore, blocking of COX-1 will lead to a reduction in protective prostaglandins. However, COX-2 is only active during inflammation. Traditional NSAIDs will block both COX-1 and COX-2; hence there is an increased likelihood of side-effects. More recently, new NSAID agents such as rofecoxib and celecoxib have been introduced which are COX-2 selective. This means that they will have more influence in blocking COX-2 rather than disturbing the balance of COX-1. The newer COX-2 inhibitors are more expensive and most patients will be prescribed traditional NSAIDs. Guidelines for the use of COX-2 drugs (National Institute for Clinical Excellence, 2001) recommend that the use of COX-2 selective inhibitors is considered for patients at high risk of developing gastrointestinal problems. Recent evidence has suggested that there may be an increased risk of cardiovascular events related to the use of COX-2 inhibitors and this remains the subject of much debate. However, the likelihood of side-effects from the traditional NSAIDs can be reduced by taking a careful history from the patient, prescribing the lowest effective dose for as short a time as possible and by giving clear, concise patient information.

The analgesic action of NSAIDs is directly related to the anti-inflammatory action and is mainly peripheral at the site of injury, although there is some central action. The anti-inflammatory action does not completely block the process, as prostaglandins are only a part of this. So, although inhibition of prostaglandin synthesis reduces the inflammatory response, other mediators such as bradykinin and histamine are unaffected. The antipyretic effect is achieved by blocking prostaglandins in the hypothalamus, which regulates normal body temperature. The role of prostaglandins and the actions of NSAIDs in blocking prostaglandins are illustrated more fully in Table 7.1. The full prostaglandin blocking effect may not occur for several days; therefore the incidence of side-effects may be reduced if NSAIDs are prescribed for a limited number of days. Side-effects will be more likely with longer-term use and higher doses.

There is often some debate regarding the use of NSAIDs for patients undergoing orthopaedic surgery or patients who have bone fractures, due to the possibility that NSAIDs may inhibit bone healing. However, there appears to be very little evidence from human studies to support this (Moore et al, 2003).

PARACETAMOL

Paracetamol is a simple analgesic which is used for the management of mild to moderate pain. It is a drug that is likely to be familiar to most patients and the majority will report taking it at some time in their lives. Paracetamol is frequently administered regularly as part of multimodal analgesia in acute pain management, as it may have an opioid-sparing effect (NHMRC, 1999).

Table 7.1   Side-effects of non-steroidal anti-inflammatory drugs (NSAIDs)

Area in which prostaglandins are present	Protective prostaglandin function	NSAID effect	Additional information and cautions in NSAID prescribing
Gastrointestinal tract	Decrease acid production, inhibit pepsinogen release, stimulate mucus and bicarbonate secretion and mucosal blood flow	Will inhibit the protective gastric functions which may lead to gastric erosions, gastritis, bleeding	• Patients may require gastric protection agents or it may be appropriate to switch to a COX-2 inhibitor. • Some NSAIDs contain a prostaglandin analogue to help decrease gastric irritant effects • Check whether patient has a history of dyspepsia or gastric ulcers. Advise to take with or after food. • Advise to stop taking the drug if any stomach pains, nausea or vomiting, vomiting of blood or development of black stools
Renal system	Prostaglandins are synthesized in the kidney and are responsible for vasodilatation and maintenance of renal blood flow. Also helps to regulate water and sodium balance	Inhibition by NSAIDs may decrease renal blood flow, causing sodium and water imbalance. Water retention may lead to hypertension. In vulnerable patients, a reduction in renal blood flow can lead to renal failure	• Side-effects are less likely to be harmful in patients with healthy kidneys. • Particular caution required if patient is hypovolaemic, dehydrated, or is taking ACE inhibitors. • Do not give to patients who have deranged serum urea and electrolyte levels
Blood	Role in the regulation and aggregation of platelets and in vasoconstriction. Production of thromboxanes when there is tissue damage	Inhibition may lead to prolonged bleeding times and inhibition of platelet formation, although this is reversible. Also, reduction in platelet adhesiveness	• Should not be given to patients with coagulation problems or those taking warfarin. • Ibuprofen must not be given concurrently with cardiac dose of aspirin, as it can inhibit the antiplatelet effect of the aspirin. Advise the patient to report any unexplained bruising or bleeding
Respiratory system	Protective mechanism is not clear	Inhibition may lead to severe bronchospasm in some asthmatics	Approximately 10% of patients with asthma will react to aspirin. It is likely that they will have the same reaction to NSAIDs. Advise the patient to stop taking the drug if there is any shortness of breath, wheezing, pruritus or facial swelling

Paracetamol can be administered orally, rectally and intravenously as the prodrug propacetamol. Oral paracetamol can be combined with a weak opioid to form a compound oral analgesic preparation. Examples of a compound drug are co-codamol, which is paracetamol with codeine, and co-dydramol, which contains paracetamol and dihydrocodeine.

Paracetamol has both antipyretic and analgesic actions and although it inhibits prostaglandin synthesis in the central nervous system, it does not actually have any anti-inflammatory properties (Lewis, 2000). It is well absorbed orally and has a high bioavailability (Lewis, 2000). Absorption is improved if taken on an empty stomach (Galbraith et al, 1999). Paracetamol is very dangerous in overdose and as little as 20 tablets can cause liver necrosis (British Medical Association and Royal Pharmaceutical Society of Great Britain, 2004). Paracetamol is not contraindicated in patients with liver disease or those who have a heavy alcohol intake but these patients should have reduced doses.

LOCAL ANAESTHETIC AGENTS

Some patients may have local nerve blocks performed as part of the anaesthetic to provide part of balanced postoperative analgesia. Local anaesthetics work by blocking membrane depolarization. The flow of ions across the nerve membrane is reduced, inhibiting the conduction of impulses and consequent sensory input into the central nervous system. Adrenaline (epinephrine) can be added to a local anaesthetic if vasoconstriction is required. Constriction of blood vessels will prolong the action of the block, by reducing absorption into the general circulation, and also reducing the risk of system toxicity. Adrenaline (epinephrine) should not be used in the extremities, as the resulting vasoconstriction of small blood vessels could result in tissue hypoxia (British Medical Association and Royal Pharmaceutical Society of Great Britain, 2004).

Potential risks of local anaesthetic use include toxicity, which is most likely if inadvertent intravenous injection occurs. A new local anaesthetic agent called levobupivacaine is available, and this has been shown to be as effective as bupivacaine for local and central blockade in terms of analgesia but has an enhanced safety profile, particularly relating to cardiac toxicity (McLeod and Burke, 2001). Nerve damage is also possible if nerve blocks are carried out. Local anaesthetic agents can also be used for wound infiltration at the end of surgery and this can provide several hours of analgesia at the wound site.

THE ROLE OF THE NURSE AND THE ACUTE PAIN TEAM

Since the publication of the Royal College of Surgeons Report (1990), a lot of work has been done to improve the management of postoperative pain. The report provided a much needed framework for the ongoing development of acute pain services, and the roles that should be undertaken within these services. Mackrodt (2001:493) suggested that acute pain services should be setting a standard to ensure that patients receive 'safe, effective, optimal pain relief without increasing side-effects.' It could be argued that the only way to achieve this is to ensure that education of staff is a major part of the work of the team. The emphasis should be on the education and support of clinical staff, particularly nurses in the general ward areas to ensure that practice is enhanced at ward level, rather than staff becoming deskilled by the acute pain team. Education can be delivered in the clinical setting, including during ward rounds as well as in formal study days, but whatever format is used, education must always include the relevant practical skills, including management of the equipment. This can be supported by the use of a skills competency framework. Critical incidents involving pain management must be managed in a supportive way, using reflection to ensure that the incident is used as a learning experience.

The nurse in the clinical area is likely to spend the most time with patients postoperatively compared to other team members. It could be proposed that it is the nurse who is best placed to enable the patient to get optimal pain relief: hence the importance of the teaching role of the acute pain service.

Many acute pain teams are nurse-led on a day-to-day basis, and roles are developing to include areas such as nurse prescribing, epidural 'top ups' and intravenous cannulation for PCA. However, nurses working within this setting also require peer support, as the role can be isolating. Membership of professional groups such as the UK Pain Network can provide nurses with up-to-date information and opportunities for networking with other nurses involved in different areas of pain management.

All acute pain services should be continually auditing their activity, and ensuring that practice is based on current evidence as much as possible. However, it is also important to question more traditional methods, as some of these can be reviewed to enhance them. This is highlighted by McQuay et al (1997:10), who said that 'the key to successful management of pain is education not new drugs or high tech delivery systems'. The acute pain team has a responsibility not only to challenge the 'old' ways of doing things but also to find the solutions to do them more effectively while maintaining safety at all times. Only then should the ongoing development of the service, such as the introduction of new drugs and of new techniques such as patient-controlled epidural analgesia, be considered. All postoperative analgesic practices should be supported by written guidelines, including guidelines for prescribing analgesics.

Finally, the acute pain team does not work in isolation. The team may work closely with other teams involved in pain, such as the chronic pain team and the palliative care team. The team is also part of the wider hospital team, and good communication by team members is essential to ensure safety and consistency in practice. Until recently, the acute pain team was almost unique in its set up, but this has changed with the introduction of critical care outreach teams. There has been some debate about whether the two should work as one team. Counsell (2001) suggested that there was common ground between the two specialties, because acute pain teams had been finding sick patients on wards for some time, and that their role has moved beyond that of simply providing analgesia. This issue remains topical and much debate continues.

Summary of key points

- Pain is a subjective and complex experience: an interaction of both mind and body. Past experiences, culture and background will affect the pain response.

- Pain must be assessed, involving the patient where possible, and this must be a dynamic pain assessment.

- Nurses often record pain to be less severe than the patient says.

- The physiological response to acute pain can be harmful.

- Poorly managed acute pain can lead to the development of chronic pain.

- The use of epidural analgesia containing a local anaesthetic agent can help to reduce the stress response to surgery.

- Multimodal analgesia forms the basis of good postoperative analgesia. Strong opioid analgesics should be used with the addition of regularly prescribed simple analgesics.

- Preoperative information and teaching may help to reduce anxiety in relation to postoperative pain.

- The patient should be involved in the choice of postoperative analgesics wherever possible.

- Addiction to opioids is unlikely to occur in the postoperative setting.

References

Bond, M. R. (1984) *Pain: Its Nature, Analysis and Treatment,* 2nd edn. London: Churchill Livingstone.

Bonica, J. (1985) History of pain concepts and pain therapy. *Seminars in Anaesthesia* IV(3): 189–207.

Bonica, J. J. (1990) *The Management of Pain,* Vol. I, 2nd edn. Pennsylvania: Lea & Febiger.

Bridges, D., Thompson, S. W. N. & Rice, A. S. C. (2001) Mechanisms of neuropathic pain. *British Journal of Anaesthesia* 87(1): 12–26.

British Medical Association and Royal Pharmaceutical Society of Great Britain (2004) *British National Formulary 47.* London: British Medical Association.

Bromley, L. (2002) Local anaesthetics. In: Hutton, P., Cooper, G. M., James, F. M. & Butterworth, J. F. (eds) *Fundamental Principles and Practice of Anaesthesia.* London: Martin Dunitz.

Campbell, J. (1995) Presidential Address to the American Pain Society [n.p.]. American Pain Society.

Chumbley, G. M., Hall, G. M. & Salmon, P. (2002) Patient-controlled analgesia: what information does the patient want? *Journal of Advanced Nursing* 39(5): 459–471.

Cooper, G. M. (2002) The elderly patient. In: Hutton, P., Cooper, G. M., James, F. M. & Butterworth, J. F. (eds) *Fundamental Principles and Practice of Anaesthesia.* London: Martin Dunitz.

Counsell, D. J. (2001) The acute pain service: a model for outreach critical care. *Anaesthesia* 56(10): 925–926.

Curtis, G. B., Johnson, G. H., Clark, P., et al (1999) Relative potency of controlled-release oxycodone and controlled-release morphine in a postoperative pain model. *European Journal of Clinical Pharmacology* 55(6): 425–429.

Davitz, L. L. & Davitz, J. R. (1985) Culture and nurses' inferences of suffering. In: Copp, L. A. (ed.) *Perspectives on Pain*. Edinburgh: Churchill Livingstone.

Descartes, R. (1644) *L'Homme. Lectures on the History of Physiology during the 16th, 17th and 18th Century* (translated by Foster, M.). Cambridge University Press. In: Fordham, M. & Dunn, V. (1994) *Alongside the Person in Pain*. London: Baillière Tindall.

Dodds, C. & Hutton, P. (2002) Postoperative care. In: Hutton, P., Cooper, G. M., James, F. M. & Butterworth, J. F. (eds) *Fundamental Principles and Practice of Anaesthesia*. London: Martin Dunitz.

Dolin, S., Cashman, J. N. & Bland, J. M. (2002) Effectiveness of acute postoperative pain management: I. Evidence from published data. *British Journal of Anaesthesia* 89(3): 409–423.

Galbraith, A., Bullock, S., Manias, E., et al (1999) *Fundamentals of Pharmacology*. Harlow: Addison Wesley Longman.

Goodman, L. S. & Gilman, A. (1996) *The Pharmaceutical Basis of Therapeutics*, 9th edn. New York: Macmillan.

Harmer, M. (2002) Consent and ethics in postoperative pain management. *Anaesthesia* 57(12): 1153–1154.

Harmer, M. & Davies, K. A. (1998) The effect of education, assessment and a standardised prescription on post-operative pain management: the value of clinical audit in the establishment of acute pain services. *Anaesthesia* 53(5): 424–430.

Human Rights Act (1998) *Article 3 Prohibition of Torture*. London: HMSO.

International Association for the Study of Pain (1992) *Management of Acute Pain: A Practical Guide*. Seattle: IASP Press.

Jage, J. & Bey, T. (2000) Postoperative analgesia in patients with substance abuse disorder: Part 1. *Acute Pain* 3(3): 140–155.

Kehlet, H. & Holte, K. (2001) Effect of postoperative analgesia on surgical outcome. *British Journal of Anaesthesia* 87(1): 62–72.

Kidd, B. L. & Urban, L. A. (2001) Mechanisms of inflammatory pain. *British Journal of Anaesthesia* 87(1): 3–11.

Koh, P. & Thomas, V. J. (1994) Patient-controlled analgesia (PCA): does time saved by PCA improve patient satisfaction with nursing care? *Journal of Advanced Nursing* 20(1): 61–70.

Lewis, K. E. (2000) Analgesic drugs. In: Pinnock, C., Lin, T. & Smith, T. (eds) *Fundamentals of Anaesthesia*. London: Greenwich Medical Media.

Lovett, P. E., Stanton, S. L., Hennessy, D. & Cashman, J. N. (1994) Pain relief after major gynaecological surgery. *British Journal of Nursing* 3(4): 159–162.

Macintyre, P.E. (2001) Safety and efficacy of patient-controlled analgesia. *British Journal of Anaesthesia* 87(1): 36–46.

Macintyre, P. E. & Jarvis, D. A. (1995) Age is the best predictor of postoperative morphine requirements. *Pain* 64(2): 357–364.

Macintyre, P. E. & Ready, L. B. (1997) *Acute Pain Management – A Practical Approach*. London: W. B. Saunders.

Mackrodt, K. (2001) The role of an acute pain service *British Journal of Perioperative Nursing* 11(11): 492–497.

Macrae, W.A. (2001) Chronic pain after surgery. *British Journal of Anaesthesia* 87(1): 88–98.

McLeod, G. A. & Burke, D. (2001) Levobupivacaine. *Anaesthesia* 56(4): 331–341.

McQuay, H., Moore, A. & Justins, D. (1997) Treating acute pain in hospital. *British Medical Journal* 314(7093): 1531–1535.

McQuay, H. J., Carroll, D. & Moore, R. A. (1999) Injected morphine in postoperative pain: a quantative systematic review. In: Moore, A., Edwards, J., Barden, J. & McQuay, H. (eds) (2003) *Bandolier's Little Book of Pain*. Oxford: Oxford University Press.

McQuay, H. & Moore, A. (2002) *An Evidence-Based Resource for Pain Relief*. Oxford: Oxford University Press.

Melzack, R. & Wall, P. D. (1965) Pain mechanisms: a new theory. *Science* 150: 971–979.

Melzack, R. & Wall, P. D. (1991) *The Challenge of Pain*. London: Penguin.

Moddeman, G (2002) Considerations for postoperative pain management in older adults. *Clinical Nurse Specialist* 16(1): 35–37.

Moore, A., Edwards, J., Barden, J. & McQuay, H. (2003) Do NSAIDs inhibit bone healing? In: Moore, A., Edwards, J., Barden, J., & McQuay, H. (eds) *Bandolier's Little Book of Pain*. Oxford: Oxford University Press.

National Health and Medical Research Council (NHMRC). (1999) *Acute Pain Management: The Scientific Evidence*. Canberra: NHMRC.

National Institute for Clinical Excellence (2001) *The Use of Cyclo-oxygenase (COX) 2 Selective Inhibitors, Celecoxib, Rofecoxib, Meloxicam and Etodolac in the Treatment of Osteoarthritis and Rheumatoid Arthritis*. London: NICE.

Picker Institute Europe (2002) Improving patients' experience (Newsletter). Picker Institute Europe [online] Available at http://www.pickereurope.org/news (accessed 22 March 2003).

Rowbotham, D. J. (2002) Opioids, NSAIDs and other analgesics. In: Hutton, P., Cooper, G. M., James, F. M. & Butterworth, J. F. (eds) *Fundamental Principles and Practice of Anaesthesia*. London: Martin Dunitz.

Royal College of Anaesthetists (1998) *Guidelines for the Use of NSAIDs in the Perioperative Period*. London: Royal College of Anaesthetists.

Royal College of Surgeons of England (1990) *Commission on the Provision of Surgical Services: Report of the Working Party on Pain after Surgery*. London: Royal College of Surgeons.

Sasada, M. & Smith, S. (1998) *Drugs in Anaesthesia & Intensive Care*, 2nd edn. Oxford: Oxford Medical Publications.

Scott, N. B. & Hodson, M. (1997) Public perceptions of postoperative pain and it's relief. *Anaesthesia* 52(5): 438–442.

Seers, K. (1987) Perceptions of pain. *Nursing Times* 33(48): 37–39.

Seymour, J. (1996) Analgesia: under patient control. *Nursing Times* 92(1): 42, 44.

Skilton, R. W. H. & Justice, W. (1998) Epidural haematoma following anticoagulant treatment in a patient with an indwelling epidural catheter. *Anaesthesia* 53(7): 691–701.

Timmons, M. E. & Bower, F. L. (1993) The effect of structured preoperative teaching on patients' use of patient-controlled analgesia [PCA] and their management of pain. *Orthopaedic Nursing* 12(1): 23–31.

Victor, K. (2001) Properly assessing pain in the elderly. *Registered Nurse* 64(5): 45–49.

Waitman, J., McCaffery, M. & Pasero, C. (2001) Meperidine – a liability. *American Journal of Nursing* 101(1): 57–58.

Wall, P. (1999) Private pain and public display. In: Wall, P. (ed.) *Pain the Science of Suffering*. London: Weidenfeld & Nicolson.

Webb, A. R., Leong, S., Myles, P. S. & Burn, S.J. (2002) The addition of a tramadol infusion to morphine patient-controlled analgesia after abdominal surgery: a double-blinded, placebo-controlled randomised trial. *Anesthesia and Analgesia* 95(6):1713–1718.

Further reading and relevant websites

http://www.jr2.ox.ac.uk/bandolier/index.html Bandolier Evidence based medicine (accessed 28 April 2004).

Horn, S. & Munafo, M. (1997) *Pain Theory, Research and Intervention*. Buckingham: Open University Press.

http://www.youranaesthetic.com Guide to postoperative pain and anaesthesia for patients (accessed 28 April 2004).

Melzack, R. (1975) The McGill Pain Questionnaire: major properties and scoring methods. *Pain* (1): 277–299.

Moore, A., Edwards, J., Barden, J. & McQuay, H. (2003) *Bandolier's Little Book of Pain*. Oxford: Oxford University Press.

http://www.health.gov.au/nhmrc/publications National Health and Medical Research Council (Australia). Acute Pain Management (accessed 28 April 2004).

http://www.nurseprescriber.co.uk Nurse prescribing on line (accessed 28 April 2004).

http://www.jr2.ox.ac.uk/bandolier/booth/painpag/ Oxford Pain Internet Site (accessed 28 April 2004).

Royal College of Surgeons of England (1990) *Commission on the Provision of Surgical Services: Report of the Working Party on Pain after Surgery*. London: Royal College of Surgeons.

Shipton, E. A. (1999) *Pain Acute and Chronic*, 2nd edn. London: Arnold.

http://www.painsociety.org The Pain Society (Great Britain) (accessed 28 April 2004).

http://www.painnetwork.co.uk/ The UK Pain Network for Nurses (accessed 28 April 2004).

http://www.mhra.gov.uk (accessed 14 March 2005)

Chapter 8

Discharge planning following surgery

Rosie Castle and Teresa Rooney-Kaymakci

Key objectives of the chapter

At the end of the chapter the reader will be able to:

- define and describe the process of discharge planning and the multidisciplinary approach

- set discharge planning within the context of Government policy and Department of Health (DoH) recommendations

- give a description of different models of discharge planning.

This chapter describes the general themes, principles and goals of patient discharge planning. The aim is to establish 'best practice' in discharge planning following all types of surgery.

INTRODUCTION

'Best practice' in discharge planning is described through reference to policy documents, research findings and the use of clinical scenarios. Age alone is a poor predictor of postoperative recovery and rehabilitation to prehospitalization lifestyle. However, elderly people are more likely than other groups of patients to live alone, suffer from chronic illness or be cared for by others who are themselves advanced in years. They are, therefore, particularly vulnerable within the discharge planning process (DoH, 1989; 2001a) and their particular needs are emphasized in this chapter.

The importance of effective discharge planning is recognized within Government policy documents, e.g. *National Service Framework For Older People* (DoH, 2001b), *Your Guide to the NHS – Getting the Most from Your NHS* (DoH, 2001c) and *Discharge from Hospital: Pathway, Process and Practice* (DoH, 2003a). These documents highlight the need for collaborative interprofessional working, using the single assessment process and patient-centred care concept.

The Government introduced a system of reimbursement for hospital discharge in April 2004. Implementing this system required best practice home discharge and interprofessional partnerships. The *Hospital Discharge Workbook* (DoH, 2003b) contains detailed and definitive guidance, and examples of good practice in all facets of hospital discharge.

Research spanning some 30 years (Skeet, 1970; Victor and Vetter, 1984; Nazarko, 1997, 1998; Munshi et al, 2002) has suggested that patients discharged from hospital often fail to receive the care they need, and that this can result in readmission, which is costly for the patient, the family and the National Health Service (Townsend et al, 1988).

Failure in discharge planning has been attributed to:

- poor communication between patients and professionals (Klop et al, 1991)
- communication breakdown between professionals themselves, particularly between those working in the hospital and those in the community (Skeet, 1970; Meara et al, 1992; Tierney et al, 1994)
- lack of appropriate patient assessment (Skeet, 1970; Harding and Modell, 1989; Wills and Ford, 2000/2001)
- over-reliance on informal care and lack of (or slow) statutory provision (Waters, 1987; Victor and Vetter, 1988)
- inattention to the special needs of the most vulnerable (Harding and Modell, 1989; Mamon et al, 1992).

The impetus to improve discharge planning has never been greater. Through advances in technology, potentially life-enhancing surgery is possible for an increasingly older population. Simultaneously, pressure on acute hospital beds, and Government policy emphasizing care delivery within a community setting (DoH, 1990, 1997, 1998, 2001a, 2003a) have encouraged rapid patient discharge. The DoH (2003a) claims that about 60% of all people that are in acute hospitals as inpatients are over 65 years of age. It warns that the acute setting is not conducive to adequate rehabilitation, leading to patient institutionalization and increased susceptibility to hospital-acquired infections such as MRSA, while waiting for care arrangements to be organized. Severing important links with the older person's care networks may occur if the process is too drawn out. *The Community Care (Delayed Discharges etc.) Act* (DoH, 2003c) enables trusts to be penalized for such delays. Paradoxically, just as the need for thorough and efficient discharge planning is heightened by surgical interventions on increasingly vulnerable individuals, the available time in which to achieve this is reduced.

DEFINING AND DESCRIBING MULTIDISCIPLINARY DISCHARGE PLANNING

Discharge planning has been described as:

A systematic, multi-disciplinary process by which the needs and resources of in-patients and their carers are assessed in order to enable comprehensive discharge preparation and the arrangements of appropriate community support and services on discharge from hospital.

(Tierney, 1993:30)

Discharge planning is an actively managed process which begins at the point of admission (Hurst, 1996; Rudd and Smith, 2002) with agreed pathways of care (DoH, 2003a). The process should identify patients who are likely to need actively managed transfers and ongoing health and social care services at the point of their admission, or as near to admission as possible.

Communication among the members of the multidisciplinary team – general practitioner (GP), hospital nurse, district nurse, discharge coordinator, occupational therapist, social worker, etc. – along with the patient/carers when community plans are being set up is vital (Salter, 2002). Nurses in the acute hospital setting and in the community should act as the receivers and completers of discharge checklists, and ensure that a number of different services are in place prior to patients' discharge (Audit Commission, 1992; DoH, 1994, 2003a). Occupational therapists assess patients' ability to cope within their home environment after treatment for the most common trauma conditions such as humeral and hip fractures (Rudd and Smith, 2002). Dietitians can offer advice and information on dietary modification, which may improve the quality of life and quicken postoperative recovery, such as diet following cholecystectomy. Provision of 'social care' within the community following discharge may fall within the remit of social services; hence, the social worker's involvement in discharge planning. Assessing social needs may be of greater importance for older patients, as some authors have claimed that this group are likely to require a higher level of care prior to admission (Nixon et al, 1998). The GP's early involvement in discharge planning can reduce the likelihood of readmission and shows better outcomes for the frail older person (McInnes et al, 1999 cited in Munshi et al, 2002).

The process of discharge planning, therefore, has a number of different phases (Mamon et al, 1992; King and MacMillan, 1993). These phases are:

- patient assessment
- development of a discharge plan
- the provision of services, including patient/family education and service provision
- follow-up and evaluation.

Victor and Vetter (1988) state that adequate notice of discharge, discussion of arrangements for aftercare with patient and family, arrangements for aftercare and liaison with primary care services are the key elements of discharge planning. The BGSADSSRCN (1988) recommended that, at discharge, a patient should have the following:

- a written discharge checklist (DoH, 2003a)
- a record of predischarge education, and competence in self-medication
- recorded current assessment of physical and mental functioning
- a speedy home assessment visit if functional capacity is an issue
- a record of formal and informal support arrangements
- a written discharge summary sent to the GP
- a care transfer plan
- reliable transport, including welcome at home
- follow-up arrangements.

The same document recommends that an identified discharge coordinator should lead and record communication with all relevant agencies, and that the goals of discharge planning should be patient-oriented and set by the patient in association with the multidisciplinary team.

DISCHARGE PLANNING WITHIN THE CONTEXT OF PAST AND PRESENT GOVERNMENT POLICY

Discharge planning takes place within the context of Government policy. This emphasizes the centrality of 'primary care' (DoH, 1998) and the growing importance of care delivery within a community setting. Certain key legislation has directly influenced patient discharge planning in recent years. The National Health Service and Community Care Act (DoH, 1990), which was enacted in 1993, divided the responsibility for provision of statutory health services between three main agencies: local authorities, health authorities and the Family Health Services Authority. Henceforth, local authorities were given responsibility for making annual agreement with their related health authorities, on the purchasing of residential and nursing home care and on arrangements for discharging patients from hospital into the community. Statutory recognition was given to the division between 'health' and 'social' care, with responsibility for provision of the latter falling to local authorities.

The split between health and social needs and between purchasers and providers of care, which was created by The National Health Service and Community Care Act (DoH, 1990), has been accused of increasing fragmentation of care (Benton, 1995) rather than enhancing the 'seamless' garment envisaged by Griffiths (DHSS, 1988). If patients are assessed, at their discharge from hospital, as having a 'social' rather than a health need, then it is the direct responsibility of the social services department of the local authority to meet that need. However, differences of opinion may exist between professional groups as to what constitutes a 'health' need or a 'social' need, respectively. A social worker, for example, may consider the hygiene needs of a postsurgical patient discharged into the community for palliative care to be a 'health' need. For the community nurse, on the other hand, that patient's need for pain relief is a health need, but his bed-bath is 'social'. Finite resources within social services departments can mean that needs are assessed according to the availability of care provision rather than as dictated by patients and their professional and nonprofessional carers. Tierney (1993) described the legislation as creating 'artificial boundaries' between hitherto closely related agencies. Within this scenario, patients, particularly those with complex needs, are likely to be transferred between agencies (Klop et al, 1991) or to disappear into the dividing void.

In 1989, the Department of Health issued guidelines on planning for discharge of patients from hospital, which recognized this potential for fragmentation. Financial penalties were threatened for those trusts lacking appropriate mechanisms by which to provide 'shared care' between health and social services, and a *Hospital Discharge Planning Workbook* (DoH, 1994) was devised as a guide to practice. Although nurses were to have a central role in the assessment of health needs, no one profession was allocated the key role of 'discharge coordinator'. Victor and Vetter (1988) saw this as an omission and recommended the appointment of a key professional to coordinate discharge planning. Exemplars of good practice (Bradbury, 1997) certainly suggest that a coordinator improves the efficiency of discharge planning for all concerned.

Delays in discharge are commonly blamed on insufficient capacity within local residential and nursing homes. The Government now advises that more intermediary care resourcing is required to allow rehabilitation and promote independence, such as community hospital beds (DoH, 2003a).

Communication problems are a recurrent theme within descriptions of poor discharge planning. Tierney (1993) found that even within one type of institution (hospitals) there were examples of communication breakdown. Professionals were unsure as to whether or not decisions should be made by the multidisciplinary team, or if they were the responsibility of individuals. Communication between hospital and community is even more problematic. Victor (1991) found that contributions from community staff to discharge planning were limited and that, while some health professionals were recognized as having a legitimate role within the discharge planning process and were therefore invited to participate in this, others were not given this recognition and remained outside the process. Staff from nursing homes may well fall within this second category and, although they will inevitably provide postdischarge care, find themselves excluded from planning arrangements.

The DoH's revised and updated version of the discharge workbook (DoH, 2003b) includes the need for a named discharge coordinator and to have interdisciplinary teamwork in the decision-making process. This is to ensure that:

- Interagency policies and agreements deliver effective and flexible discharge care pathways.
- A named person at ward/similar level coordinates the patient (and carer) journey. The ward-based care coordinator is a person who can be responsible for the holistic discharge management for those patients identified as requiring additional support. This role is widely expected to be undertaken by an experienced nurse; however, it may be appropriate in transitional or rehabilitation services for a therapist or social worker to undertake this role.

Nursing staff perceptions of current discharge planning procedures are not well documented (Nixon et al, 1998). They cite Tierney's study (1993), which found

practical issues such as ambulance/transport problems and prescription/pharmacy issues, as well as the already noted communication problems among health and social care professionals. These included the discharge notice being too short, failed provision of services, delay in discharge letters and poor communication with social work and occupational therapy departments. The updated workbook (DoH, 2003a) may help to create a more effective system.

The Audit Commission (1992, 2000) found that perspectives of patient need varied between nurses within the acute sector and those in the community. Whereas hospital-based nurses had difficulty in predicting patient needs within the home environment, community nurses found difficulty in understanding the concept of the 'named nurse'.

The advent of primary care groups and primary care trusts, which promised a new culture of collaboration and multidisciplinary working, may prove an important step in the provision of discharge planning and care. Audits to measure the effectiveness of discharge management and planning can help staff reflect on the issues involved in the process and increase staff cooperation (Rudd and Smith, 2002).

To examine recommendations for best practice in discharge planning, each phase will now be discussed in more detail.

PATIENT ASSESSMENT

In her early work, Roberts (1975) rightly claimed that discharge planning, by its very nature, implied some deficit in an individual's self-caring ability. Assessment of health need is the first step in estimating the extent of, and ultimately making good, that self-care deficit. Assessment is the foundation of all good discharge planning.

The National Health Service and Community Care Act (DoH, 1990) emphasized the position of the nurse as the lead assessor of patient-vulnerable groups, which the DoH circular on discharge planning indicated were likely to be elderly people, those living alone, those with chronic illness and those with elderly or infirm carers (DoH, 1989).

Assessment, like the entire discharge planning process, should start early. If possible, assessment should begin before admission (DoH, 2002) and certainly before the point of discharge (Waters, 1987). Guidelines on preadmission discharge assessment have been issued by the Health and Social Services Department in conjunction with the Health Boards in Scotland (Scottish Office Home and Health Department

(SOHHD), 1993), and the success of preadmission clinics throughout the United Kingdom has been well documented (Hurst, 1996). Evidence suggests that such clinics offer patients the opportunity to discuss worries and fears related to surgery, and offer professionals the opportunity to assess patients in their own environment before the trauma of surgical intervention.

The patient perspective, and that of their family, should be at the very core of assessment (DoH, 1992; SOHHD, 1993), with the professional helping the patient to overcome any initial reluctance to become involved (Waterworth and Luker, 1990; Wiffin, 1995). The benefits of patient participation in discharge planning have been well documented. These include both improved clinical outcomes (Titler and Petite, 1994) and increased patient efficacy in postdischarge self-care (Hall and Carty, 1993). Social, environmental and emotional needs must be included within the discharge assessment; an assessment of physical needs alone will not suffice. What Cass (1978) called a 'social diagnosis' is an inherent part of any discharge plan, and this can only be achieved if adequate information is documented on living conditions and support at home. However, evidence suggests that information of this type is rarely recorded within the acute setting (King and MacMillan, 1993).

The single assessment process currently being introduced in the care of older people (DoH, 2003a) contained within the edicts of the *National Standards Framework for Older People* (DoH, 2001b), provides guidance as to the depth and scale of assessment according to individual needs of the patient and carer, including a risk assessment.

Older people, in particular, often find certain tasks they managed easily before surgery more difficult following a period of hospitalization (Bowling and Betts, 1984; Waters, 1987; Victor and Vetter, 1988) and, to account for this, assessment must be dynamic and responsive to individual circumstances and needs. Moreover, although patients may cope well within the controlled hospital environment, they may find coping at home more difficult. Tierney et al (1994, cited in Nixon et al, 1998) found that for both GPs and community nursing staff, post-discharge assessment was more common. Occupational therapists have a key role in assessing patient-coping potential within a number of different environments and informing the decisions of the multidisciplinary team.

Current nursing practice promotes the importance of the partnership between nurses and older people, using a biographical person-centred assessment of an individual's potential and aspirations (Kings Fund, 1997). Therefore, using so-called objective standardized

tools provides the healthcare professional with a dilemma. Furthermore, although multidisciplinary assessment is essential to good discharge planning, problems arise when different disciplines assess the patient from professional perspectives and/or use different assessment 'tools' or instruments (Banks, 1995; Seedhouse, 1998). Frankum et al (1995) found that even when professionals use the same assessment tools, they often use them differently according to their individual professional backgrounds, training and education. A variety of formal tools certainly exist, and it has been recommended that diverse tools are used in a variety of combinations to ensure a comprehensive and meaningful patient assessment (Royal College of Physicians and the British Geriatrics Society, 1992).

Recommended assessment tools include the *Barthel Activities of Daily Living Index* (the Barthel Index) (Mahoney and Barthel, 1965). The Barthel Index covers areas such as feeding, mobility from bed to chair, personal toilet, getting on and off the toilet, bathing, walking on a level surface, going up and down stairs, dressing and incontinence. Designed originally for use with long-term hospital patients, the Barthel Index needs modification to include social activities such as shopping and cooking and to accommodate more environmental influences on individual well-being (Ross and Bower, 1995).

Other popular assessment tools focusing on physical functioning include Katz et al's (1963) *Index of Activities of Daily Living*, the *Townsend Disability Scale* (Sainsbury, 1973) and the *Clifton Assessment Procedures for the Elderly* (Pattie and Gilleard, 1979). These assessment tools all focus upon physical functioning but recognize that this will be influenced by a variety of factors such as mental state and financial situation.

Similar tools exist with which to assess mental functioning. These include the *Abbreviated Mental Test* (Hodkinson, 1972), which aims to assess orientation to time and place through a 10-item schedule of questions, and *The Geriatric Depression Scale* (Yesavage et al, 1983), which assesses mood through a 30-item scale. *The Health of the Nation Outcome Scales* (Wing et al, 1995) rate an individual's health and social functioning across 12 areas related to mental illness. More recent nursing assessment tools such as the *Minimum Data/Resident Assessment Instrument* (MDS/RAI) (1997, cited in Wills and Ford, 2000/2001) and the Royal College of Nursing Assessment Tool (1997) for nursing older people are available. These tools were designed to quantify care requirements across a broad range of need assessments. Both tools are cited as good practice examples in the National Service Framework documents for older people (DoH, 2001b). However, these tools need to be used in conjunction with other health professional tools. The one-stop assessment process (National Service Framework – standard 2) (DoH, 2001b), which will include rehabilitation potential, should dovetail into this process along with an emphasis on increasing intermediary care to avoid admission to hospital or enable early discharge (National Service Framework – standard 3) (DoH, 2001b).

In addition to assessment of physical and mental functioning, the Royal College of Physicians and the British Geriatrics Society (1992) recommend that a checklist of major social indicators, including support, housing and financial needs, be used to assess patient need. However, no one scale has been found to measure social status accurately (Ross and Bower, 1995). Although the choice of assessment tools is important, what is more important in ensuring effective discharge planning is that the chosen tool is used in a standardized manner by all members of the multidisciplinary team and that its use is documented.

DEVELOPMENT OF A DISCHARGE PLAN

In the UK, until recently, many hospitals have lacked a formal process or policy for the development of discharge plans. Jewell (1993) identified a distinctive discharge process which began at patient admission and ended with the patient leaving hospital: the discharge plan was identified as part of this process. Models of formal discharge planning are more fully described within the American literature. Tuazon (1993), for example, described a model for discharge planning with the acronym SMART: specific treatment instructions (dressing changes, etc.), medications, activity (allowed and to be avoided), referrals, and therapeutic diet and instructions.

Rothrock (1996) has described a 'Generic Care Plan' for use within the discharge planning process. The Generic Care Plan aims to aid rehabilitation following surgery through patient participation and documentation of assessment, goals and achievements. It incorporates a number of documented categories such as 'key assessment points' – e.g. age, functional abilities and learning needs – and explicitly states desired patient outcomes such as 'awareness of different referral sources'. Space within the care plan is allocated to recording of completed nursing actions. The Generic Care Plan illustrates the component parts of a good discharge plan: i.e. clear documentation, partnership with patient and family in its development, accessibility of the plan to the patient and their family, development of goals for patient and healthcare staff, and indication of the extent to which these goals have been achieved.

THE PROVISION OF SERVICES

Provision of post-discharge patient services can be provided for in two mutually complementary ways. Discharge planners can, themselves, undertake steps which lead to service provision and they can also educate patients and their families as to how best to assess their own health needs, and how to access appropriate services to meet those needs. Evidence suggests (Tierney, 1993) that it is in service provision that the discharge planning process fails most profoundly.

Once again, communication, or failures of communication, particularly between hospital and community services can be the central problem. In one study, less than half the hospital discharge notices reached the appropriate GPs within 1 week of the patient's discharge from hospital (Williams et al, 1992). Meara et al (1992) found that, although GPs were notified within 5 days of the patient's discharge, they were, on the whole, dissatisfied with the information provided. New models of discharge planning and service provision which are initiated within the community may offer some resolution to these difficulties.

Education of the patient and his family is an important part of providing services within the discharge plan. All healthcare professionals have a responsibility for patient education, but, here too, many deficits have been identified (Wiffin, 1995). Patient education includes teaching about specific postoperative measures and requirements, medication and its possible side-effects and health promotion relevant to the patient's needs.

It involves building on family resources and local networks to foster feelings of support, particularly in the first 2 weeks after surgery. The extent to which patients can participate in programmes of education will vary according to where they are positioned in the pre- and post-surgical continuum (Biley, 1992). Written information is an effective means of providing education which the patient and his family can draw upon at their respective discretion. However, problems have been identified, as Robinson and Miller (1996) found, that written instructions were often jargonized and therefore unhelpful to patients and their carers. The lesson for discharge planning is that all patient-oriented literature must be jargon-free and clearly written, with information at an appropriate level. The healthcare professional should also check the patient's understanding prior to his discharge.

Some patients will suffer more than others from failures in the provision of services. Harding and Modell (1989) found that patients who lived alone were most likely to return to an unheated home without basic food. Of those discharged patients who lived alone, 33% were found not to have been visited by family, friends or professionals within 3 days of their discharge from hospital. This failure was attributed to an over-reliance on the part of hospital staff, on supposed informal support networks and to slow initiation of statutory service provision. More recently, in an analysis of readmissions to a London teaching hospital, Munshi et al (2002) found that individuals discharged on a Friday accounted for all readmissions, i.e. a risk of readmission 3 times that of other weekdays.

EVALUATION OF DISCHARGE PLANNING

Only by thorough evaluation of the discharge planning process can progress towards improvements in care be made; evaluation must include the patient's perspective. Research presents some contradictory findings in this respect. Patients within McHale's study (1995) were generally satisfied with the arrangements for their discharge, with only 3% stating that they had encountered problems. However, other studies contrast with this, e.g. Bruster et al (1994), with over 50% of participants expressing worries about their discharge and saying that they received inadequate information. The challenge for health professionals is to devise meaningful methods of evaluation for discharge planning. Evaluation should give patients a chance to influence service provision and be part of the wider picture of total quality monitoring and clinical governance.

There have been various studies reporting on audits carried out on discharge planning/implementation for particular areas (Nixon et al, 1998; Salter, 2002; Rudd and Smith, 2002) which highlight good practice, i.e. patient-centred care, but also reinforce the need for discharge preparation on admission.

MODELS OF DISCHARGE PLANNING

Although the USA, rather than the UK, has hitherto taken the lead in developing models of discharge planning, e.g. McClelland et al's (1985) typology of five discharge planning models, some new initiatives within the UK are worthy of mention. These include the use of liaison nurses to improve the continuity of care for discharged patients in Wales (Armitage, 1990) and community-based discharge schemes (Townsend et al, 1988). The Black Country GP Practice, for example, has developed and favourably evaluated a model of case management. This involves preadmission assessment by a discharge coordinator who is also a community nurse, and support and follow-up from different members of the primary healthcare team (Bradbury, 1997). The emphasis within this and similar models is less upon merely 'discharging' the patient from hospital and more upon transferring care of the individual successfully through surgery, with rehabilitation as the ultimate goal. Primary Care Act pilot studies developed models of care delivery, which included community management of hospital admissions and discharges (Agnew, 1998).

The development of discharge planning models serves to illustrate the essential elements of good discharge planning. These include the following:

- multidisciplinary assessment and planning
- a key person to work as a discharge coordinator
- adequate notification of discharge date and identified patient need to all agencies involved
- standardized documentation for use by all agencies
- a formal, recognized and explicitly stated structure for discharge planning which effectively links the acute sector, the community, social services, the patient and his family.

The NHS, local authorities and social services departments are working hard to have systems in place now that the *Community Care (Delayed Discharges etc.) Act* (DoH, 2003c) is in place. The Government intends to introduce a system of reimbursement for hospital discharge. Part of the implementation of this strategy was the publishing of the revised and updated version of the *Hospital Discharge Book* (DoH, 1994, 2003b), which contains dated and definitive guidance of good practice in all aspects of hospital discharge. Staff training materials based on the publication *Discharge from Hospital: Pathway, Process and Practice* (DoH, 2003b) and a 'good practice checklist' for discharge from hospital are now available.

TWO CASE STUDIES

To illustrate the points made within this chapter, two different post-discharge scenarios are presented. All names and places are fictitious.

Case study no. 1: exemplar of poor discharge planning

Mr Y is a 76-year-old man with chronic hypertension and mild left ventricular failure. He is admitted to Cleaver Ward on Monday for planned surgery – transurethral resection of prostate. Ms Y, his 74-year-old sister, accompanies him and tells the ward staff that they live together in a large house on the other side of town. Neither Mr Y nor his sister have any 'real' health problems – or so they say. Ms Y does have 'brittle bones', however, but generally they are well and enjoy their lives. Surgery takes place as planned, and Mr Y is discharged on Friday with an indwelling urethral catheter. Ms Y is a little shocked at the speed of her brother's return home and is nervous about the catheter but she doesn't like to appear difficult, and after one teaching session on attachment of a night-time catheter bag the couple leave the ward.

When they arrive home Mr Y remembers that he took his antihypertensive medication into hospital with him and that it has not been returned to him at discharge. Ms Y telephones the ward, but the staff nurse on duty says that the tablets have been returned to pharmacy, which is now closed, and there is no access to replacement medication. Ms Y starts to panic, but the staff nurse tells her not to worry, as the district nurses have been told about Mr Y's discharge home and they will surely contact the couple later in the evening.

As they wait for the district nurse, Ms Y notices that her brother is much more feeble than he was either

before his operation or, indeed, on the hospital ward. She hopes that the district nurse arrives soon because she is unsure whether or not she will be able to help her brother into bed and she is unhappy about changing the catheter bag.

The notification of Mr Y's discharge reaches the community nursing office at 4.40 p.m., and the district nurse on duty assesses the information given. As the discharge notice was given to the community office before Ms Y realized her brother lacked his medication, this was not mentioned in the discharge summary. Mr Y was presented, therefore, as an elderly gentleman, generally fit, cared for by his sister, fully mobile with an indwelling urethral catheter but self-caring at 4 days after a successful transurethral resection of prostate. Friday was a particularly busy night for the district nursing team, and a visit was allocated for Monday morning.

Mr Y sleeps in his armchair on Friday night; his sister is too weak to help him upstairs. On Saturday morning, now very anxious about her brother's lack of medication and feeling guilty because she did not change the catheter bag, Ms Y climbs on a table to search for some tablets. She falls and suffers a fractured neck of femur. Mr Y hears the noise and calls an ambulance. Both Mr and Ms Y are readmitted to Cleaver Ward – Ms Y for a total hip replacement and her brother for social care.

Case study no. 2: exemplar of good discharge planning

Mr Y is booked for a transurethral resection of prostate and is assessed in his own home by the admission/discharge coordinator, who is also a district nurse from his local primary healthcare team. The coordinator assesses both Mr Y's and his sister's health needs, and they all discuss the coming surgery. Assessment of physical health and functioning (using the Barthel Activities of Daily Living Index), mental, emotional and social well-being takes place. Ms Y is anxious that her brother should come home as soon as possible after his operation, but is afraid she may be unable to meet all his needs. An occupational therapy assessment leads to the installation of bathroom aids, and a temporary bed is made in the downstairs living area – just in case Mr Y finds stairs difficult after the operation. Neither Mr nor Ms Y like undue interference in their lives, but they would like the reassurance that help is at hand should they need it. The coordinator gives them a contact

number for the 24-hour nursing service, and this is placed in a safe but accessible place.

Following surgery, Mr Y is given written discharge instructions and a leaflet on health after transurethral resection of prostate (incorporating care of an indwelling catheter). A second assessment of Mr Y's physical, emotional, mental and social state is completed by the ward staff in conjunction with the discharge coordinator, who visits Mr Y in hospital. This is documented on the care plan, which was initiated on Mr Y's preoperative assessment and maintained during his period of hospitalization. The hospital nurse and the discharge coordinator complete the checklist of discharge services needed by Mr Y – medication, transport, notification of the GP. The community nursing team telephone Mr Y on the evening of his discharge to reinforce the availability of the 24-hour nursing service and to arrange a home visit for Monday morning.

CONCLUSION

In looking to the future, goals such as appropriate and standardized documentation and improved interprofessional communication may be enhanced by the use of user-friendly information technology. New forms of data storage and transfer may facilitate a proactive management of individual patient needs, beginning before admission to hospital and certainly before discharge planning is completed. The role of the ward-based care coordinator, to include nurse-led discharge and discharge planning teams, are all exciting developments with greater use of intermediary care.

This chapter has discussed the various themes, principles and goals of discharge planning which must be addressed when professionals are considering 'best practice' methods of discharge planning, and especially of older patients following surgery. The chapter has looked at the various roles of the multidisciplinary team when assessing patients within the context of present NHS legislation and guidelines.

Summary of key points

- Discharge planning is a complex process which must involve all members of the multidisciplinary team.

- Poor discharge planning can lead to readmission to hospital at considerable cost, both emotional and financial, to the patients, relatives of the patients and the National Health Service.

- Discharge planning is important for all patients leaving hospital, but certain groups of patients, e.g. the elderly, those living alone and those whose carers are elderly, are particularly vulnerable.

- Discharge planning must start early, possibly even before admission to hospital, and must address physical, mental, emotional and social health needs.

- Key individuals may work as coordinators of discharge planning to good effect.

References

Agnew, T. (1998) A life of their own. *Health Service Journal* 108(5620): 10–11.

Armitage, S. (1990) *Liaison and Continuity of Care – Executive Summary*. Cardiff: Welsh Office.

Audit Commission (1992) *Lying in Wait: The Use of Medical Beds in Acute Hospitals*. London: HMSO.

Audit Commission (2000) *Impatient Admissions and Bed Management in NHS Acute Hospitals*. London: HMSO.

Banks, S. (1995) *Ethics and Values in Social Work*. Basingstoke: Macmillan.

Benton, D. (1995) The role of managed care in overcoming fragmentation. *Nursing Times* 91(25): 25–27.

Biley, F. (1992) Some determinants that affect patient participation in decision making about nursing care. *Journal of Advanced Nursing* 17: 414–421.

Bowling, A. & Betts, G. (1984) Communication on discharge. *Nursing Times* 80(32): 31–33.

Bradbury, P. (1997) Admission and discharge co-ordination from primary care. *Primary Health Care* 7: 41–43.

British Geriatrics Society, Association of Directors of Social Services, and Royal College of Nursing (1988) *The Discharge of Elderly Persons from Hospital for Community Care. A Joint Policy Statement by the British Geriatrics Society, the Association of Directors of Social Services and the Royal College of Nursing*. London: BGS/ADSS.

Bruster, S., Jarman, B., Bosanquet, N., et al (1994) National Survey of Hospital Patients. *British Medical Journal* 309: 1542–1545.

Cass, S. (1978) The effects of the referral process on hospital in-patients. *Journal of Advanced Nursing* 3: 563–569.

Department of Health (1989) *Discharge of Patients from Hospital. Health Circular HC(89)5*. London: HMSO.

Department of Health (1990) *The National Health Service and Community Care Act*. London: HMSO.

Department of Health (1992) *The Patient's Charter*. London: HMSO.

Department of Health (1994) *Hospital Discharge Planning Workbook. A Manual on Hospital Discharge Practice*. London. The Health Publication Unit.

Department of Health (1997) *Primary Care Act*. London: HMSO.

Department of Health (1998) *The New NHS: Modern, Dependable*. London: HMSO.

Department of Health (2001a) *House of Commons Health Committee Delayed Discharges (2001–2)*, Vol. 1, Ch. 5. London: Stationery Office.

Department of Health (2001b) *The National Service Framework for Older People*. Short summary, March. London: Stationery Office.

Department of Health (2001c) *Your Guide to the NHS – Getting the Most from Your NHS*. Available at http://www.dh.gov.uk/PublicationsAndStatistics/Press Releases/PressReleasesNotices (accessed 6 April 2004).

Department of Health (2002) *Fair Access to Care Services*. London: Stationery Office.

Department of Health (2003a) *Discharge from Hospital: Pathway, Process and Practice* (autumn 2003). *Change Agent Team – Changing Places: Report on Work of Health and Social Care*. Health and Social Care Unit. London: Stationery Office.

Department of Health (2003b) *Discharge from Hospital: Pathway, Process and Practice.* Chapter 5, Co-ordinating the patient journey. Available at http://www.doh.gov.uk/jointunit/delayed discharge/discharge-get-ri-ch5.pdf (accessed 18 September 2003).

Department of Health (2003c) *Community Care (Delayed Discharges etc.) Act.* Chapter 5. Available at http://www.uk-legislation.hmso.gov.uk/acts/acts2003/20030005.htm (accessed 18 September 2003).

Department of Health and Social Security (1988) *Community Care: Agenda for Action. A report to the Secretary of State for Social Services*. London: HMSO.

Frankum, J. L., Bray, J., Ell, M. S. & Philip, I. (1995) Predicting post-discharge outcome. *British Journal of Occupational Therapy* 58(9): 370–372.

Hall, W. A. & Carty, E. M. (1993) Managing the early discharge experience: taking control. *Journal of Advanced Nursing* 18(4): 574–582.

Harding, J. & Modell, M. (1989) Elderly people's experiences of discharge from hospital. *Journal of the Royal College of General Practitioners* 39(1): 17–20.

Hodkinson, H. M. (1972) Evaluation of a mental test score for the assessment of mental impairment in the elderly. *Age and Ageing* 1(4): 233–238.

Hurst, S. (1996) Multidisciplinary discharge planning. *Professional Nurse* 12(2): 113–116.

Jewell, S. E. (1993) Discovery of the discharge process: a study of patient discharge from a care unit for elderly people. *Journal of Advanced Nursing* 18(8): 1288–1296.

Katz, S., Ford, A. B., Moskowitz, R. W., et al (1963) Studies of illness in the aged: the index of ADL – a standardized measure of biological and psychosocial function. *Journal of the American Medical Association* 185: 914–919.

King, C. & MacMillan, M. (1993) Documentation and discharge planning for elderly patients. *Nursing Times* 90(20): 31–33.

Kings Fund (1997) *Effective Practice in Rehabilitation – The Evidence of Systematic Reviews*. London: Kings Fund Publishing.

Klop, R., van Wijmen, F. C. B. & Philipsen, H. (1991) Patients' rights and the admission and discharge process. *Journal of Advanced Nursing* 16(4): 408–412.

McClelland, E., Kelly, K. & Buckwater, K. (1985) *Continuity of Care: Advancing the Concepts of Discharge*. Orlando: Grune and Stratton.

McHale, S.A. (1995) Implementation of a patient discharge policy. *Professional Nurse* 10(9): 590–592.

McInnes, E., Mira, M., Atkin, N., et al (1999) Can GP input into discharge planning result in better outcomes for the frail aged? *Family Practice* 16(3): 289–293.

Mahoney, F. & Barthel, D. (1965) Functional evaluation: the Barthel index. *Maryland State Medical Journal* 14: 61–65.

Mamon, J., Steinwachs, D. M., Fahey, M., et al (1992) Impact of hospital discharge planning on meeting patient needs after returning home. *Health Service Research* 27(2): 155–175.

Meara, J. R., Wood, J. L., Wilson, M.A. & Hart, M.C. (1992) Home from hospital: a survey of hospital discharge arrangements in Northamptonshire. *Journal of Public Health Medicine* 14(2): 145–150.

Munshi, S., Lakhani, D., Ageed, A., et al (2002) Readmissions of older people to acute medical units. *Nursing Older People* 14(1): 14–16.

Nazarko, L. (1997) Improving hospital discharge arrangements for older people. *Nursing Standard* 11(40): 44–47.

Nazarko, L. (1998) Improving discharge: the role of the discharge coordinator. *Nursing Standard* 12(49): 35–37.

Nixon, A., Whitter, M. & Stitt, P. (1998) Audit in practice: planning for discharge from hospital. *Nursing Standard* 12(26): 35–38.

Pattie, A. H. & Gilleard, C. J. (1979) *Manual of the Clifton Assessment Procedures for the Elderly*. Sevenoaks, Kent: Hodder and Stoughton.

Roberts, I. (1975) *Discharged from Hospital*. London: RCN.

Robinson, A. & Miller, M. (1996) Making information accessible: developing plain English discharge instructions. *Journal of Advanced Nursing* 24(3): 528–535.

Ross, F. M. & Bower, P. (1995) Standardised assessment of elderly people (SAFE) – feasibility study in district nursing. *Journal of Clinical Nursing* 4(5): 303–310.

Rothrock, J. C. (1996) *Peri-operative Nursing Care Planning*, 2nd edn. New York: Mosby.

Royal College of Nursing (1997) *RCN Assessment Tool for Nursing Older People*. London. RCN.

Royal College of Physicians and British Geriatrics Society (1992) *Standardised Assessment Scales for Elderly People. A Report of the Joint Workshops. Research Unit of the Royal College of Physicians and the British Geriatric Society*. London: RCP/BGS.

Rudd, C. & Smith, J. (2002) Discharge planning. *Nursing Standard* 17(5): 33–37.

Sainsbury, S. (1973) *Measuring Disability*. London: Bell.

Salter, M. (2002) Discharge planning: patient and carer satisfaction. *Primary Health Care* 12(8): 43–46.

Scottish Office Home and Health Department (1993) *A Guide to Good Practice on Discharge from Hospital*. Edinburgh: The Scottish Office.

Seedhouse, D.F. (1998) *Ethics: The Heart of Health Care*. Chichester: Wiley.

Skeet, M. (1970) *Home from Hospital: The Result of a Survey Conducted among Recently Discharged Hospital Patients*. London: Macmillan.

Tierney, A. (1993) Discharge planning for elderly patients. *Nursing Standard* 7(52): 30–33.

Tierney, A., Macmillan, M., Worth, A. & King, C. (1994) Discharge of patients from hospital – current practice and perceptions of hospital and community staff in Scotland. *Health Bulletin* 52(6): 479–491.

Titler, M. G. & Petite, D. M. (1994) Discharge readiness assessment. *Journal of Cardiovascular Nursing* 9(4): 64–74.

Townsend, J., Piper, M., Frank, A. O., et al (1988) Reduction in hospital readmission stay of elderly patients by a community-based hospital discharge scheme: a randomised controlled trial. *British Medical Journal* 297(6647): 544–547.

Tuazon, N. C. (1993) Designing a SMART discharge plan. *Nursing Spectrum* 2: 16.

Victor, C. R. (1991) *Health and Health Care in Later Life*. Milton Keynes: Open University Press.

Victor, C. R. & Vetter, N. J. (1984) District nurses and the elderly after hospital discharge. *Nursing Times* 80(15): 61–62.

Victor, C. R. & Vetter, N. J. (1988) Preparing the elderly for discharge from hospital: a neglected aspect of patient care. *Age and Ageing* 17(3): 155–163.

Waters, K.R. (1987) Discharge planning: an exploratory study of the process of discharge planning and geriatric wards. *Journal of Advanced Nursing* 12(1): 17–83.

Waterworth, S. & Luker, K. A. (1990) Reluctant collaborators: do patients really want to be involved in decisions concerning care? *Journal of Advanced Nursing* 15(8): 971–976.

Wiffin, A. (1995) An assessment of procedures: discharge procedures and their efficiency at maintaining continuing care. *Nursing Times* 91(28): 31–32.

Williams, E. I., Greenwell, J. & Groom, L. M. (1992) The care of people over 75 years old after discharge from hospital: an evaluation of timetabled visiting by health visitor assistants. *Journal of Public Health Medicine* 14(2): 138–144.

Wills, T. & Ford, P. (2000/2001) Assessing older people, contemporary issues for nursing. *Nursing Older People* 12(9): 16–20.

Wing, J., Curtis, R. D. & Beevor, A. (1995) *HoNOS Health of the Nation Outcome Scales: Version 4*. London: Royal College of Psychiatrists Research Unit.

Yesavage, J., Brink, T., Lum, O., et al (1983) Development of a geriatric depression scale: a preliminary report. *Journal of Psychiatric Research* 17(1): 37–49.

SECTION II

Nursing care for specific surgical procedures

Chapter **9**

Patients requiring neurosurgery

Christine Eberhardie

Key objectives of the chapter

At the end of the chapter the reader should be
able to:

- give a brief overview of the anatomy and
  physiology of the central nervous system

- discuss the specialist investigations the patient
  may undergo

- describe the reasons for carrying out neurosurgery

- discuss the mechanisms and consequences of
  raised intracranial pressure and its treatment

- discuss the need to undertake a detailed neurological assessment of patients

- describe in detail the holistic nursing care of a
  patient undergoing a craniotomy

- develop an increased awareness of the
  long-term consequences of neurosurgery and
  the need for the patient, carer and society to be
  well informed.

INTRODUCTION

The specialty of neurosurgery involves surgery to the
brain and spinal cord. There is, however, an overlap
between all the head and neck disciplines. For example,
in severe traumatic brain injury, neurosurgeons, ophthalmic, maxillofacial and dental surgeons frequently

work together to reconstruct damaged tissues; vascular surgeons have also developed a technique for removing atheromatous tissue from the carotid arteries supplying the brain, called carotid endarterectomy; and spinal surgery is carried out by orthopaedic surgeons too.

Surgery to the brain and spinal cord can be life saving but it can leave the patient with serious disability. Part of the initial care is carried out in intensive care/high dependency units, and some patients will be treated in specialist neurosurgical units and then transferred back to a general hospital.

OVERVIEW OF THE ANATOMY AND PHYSIOLOGY OF THE NERVOUS SYSTEM

THE SKULL

The brain is protected by the rigid bony structure of the skull or cranium. The brain, its blood supply and a regulated amount of cerebrospinal fluid fill the cranium and are usually referred to as the intracranial contents (see Box 9.1 and section on raised intracranial pressure, p. 136).

THE BRAIN

The brain consists of the cerebrum and the cerebellum, which are separated by a double fold of dura mater known as the tentorium. The area above the tentorium is known as the supratentorial space, and the area below it is the infratentorial space.

The cerebrum is further divided into two cerebral hemispheres by the falx cerebri, which is a double fold of dura mater with a venous sinus, the superior sagittal sinus, in between the two layers of dura mater. The two hemispheres are joined by the corpus callosum. The cerebral cortex, which makes up the outer layer of the brain, comprises of neural cell bodies (grey matter). This layer of grey matter plays a most important role in the higher functions of the brain. The cerebral cortex of each hemisphere has four lobes which are not separated physically and are named after the bones that lie above them: i.e. frontal, parietal, temporal and occipital.

Box 9.1	Intracranial contents (% volume)
Brain	80%
Blood	10%
Cerebrospinal fluid	10%

The nerve fibres carrying sensory and motor information to and from the cortex and other islands of grey matter, such as the basal ganglia, are known as white matter. The white appearance is caused by the presence of myelin surrounding the neural axons making up the fibres. The myelin provides a protective insulating sheath around the axon.

THE MENINGES AND CEREBROSPINAL PATHWAYS

The brain and spinal cord are covered by the meninges, which are made up of an outer tough layer called the dura mater; a middle layer, the arachnoid mater; and a layer which lies next to the brain and spinal cord called the pia mater. The arachnoid mater is so-called because its cells have a spider-like appearance. Between the arachnoid mater and pia mater lies the subarachnoid space. The arteries of the brain, known as the circle of Willis, lie in the subarachnoid space of the brain, and cerebrospinal fluid circulates around the brain in the subarachnoid space. It is formed in the choroid plexus in all four ventricles. From the lateral ventricles it flows through the interventricular foramina (foramina of Monro) to the third ventricle. From there it flows through the central aquaduct to the fourth ventricle. The cerebrospinal fluid flows from the fourth ventricle into the subarachnoid space via the foramen of Magendie and the foramina of Luschka. There are also large collections of cerebrospinal fluid to be found in the cisterna magna at the base of the brain.

CEREBROSPINAL FLUID

Cerebrospinal fluid consists of water, glucose, protein and electrolytes. It protects and nourishes the brain, by absorbing a certain amount of shock, bringing nutrients such as glucose to the cells and providing some immunity to infection.

BASAL GANGLIA AND THALAMUS

The basal ganglia are masses of grey matter deep in the brain and contain the putamen, caudate nucleus, globus pallidus, subthalamic nucleus and substantia nigra. They are interconnected with the thalamus. The function of the basal ganglia is to coordinate voluntary muscle movement and to maintain the tone of the muscles. Disorders of the basal ganglia result in movement disorders such as chorea, athetosis, hemiballismus and the increased tone and tremor seen in Parkinson's disease.

THE HYPOTHALAMUS

The hypothalamus lies above the pituitary gland and is connected by the pituitary stalk. This area of the brain controls the autonomic nervous system and has links with the limbic system and the pituitary gland. The limbic system is a network of interlinking pathways which are responsible for the emotions, motivation and behaviour. This activity results in the monitoring and control of temperature, appetite and satiety; water regulation and thirst; physical experiences of emotion such as fear, pain, pleasure and rage; and the control of the neuroendocrine system by the production of releasing factors.

THE PITUITARY GLAND

The pituitary gland consists of two parts. One is the neurohypophysis (posterior pituitary gland), which receives hormones secreted by the hypothalamus and releases them into the capillary blood supply. The two hormones secreted by the neurohypophysis are antidiuretic hormone and oxytocin by way of the hypothalamo-hypophyseal tract. The other part of the pituitary gland is the adenohypophysis (anterior pituitary gland), which synthesizes and releases hormones into the blood when stimulated by the hypothalamic releasing factors.

THE CEREBELLUM

The cerebellum lies in the posterior fossa. It is made up of two hemispheres separated from the cerebrum above by the tentorium, i.e. a tent-shaped fold of dura mater. Each hemisphere is separated by the vermis. The function of the cerebellum is to coordinate muscle movement and to maintain posture and balance.

THE BRAINSTEM

The brainstem consists of the midbrain, pons varolii and medulla oblongata. The midbrain is the part of the brainstem nearest to the hypothalamus. The pons varolii lies between the midbrain above and the medulla oblongata below. The medulla oblongata has an oblong shape and extends to form the spinal cord.

One function of the brainstem is to control sleeping and waking. It monitors the environment during sleep in order to arouse the sleeper when necessary. Essential motor and sensory fibres pass through the brainstem, to and from the cerebral cortex. Without such information the body cannot become aware of its surroundings. It contains many of the body's vital centres such as the cardiac, respiratory and vomiting centres, and is also the source of most of the cranial nerves which play a role in specialized sensory input such as hearing, balance and taste, as well as motor functions such as chewing, swallowing and shrugging the shoulders.

THE BLOOD SUPPLY TO THE BRAIN

The arterial supply to the brain is known as the circle of Willis, which is supplied by the carotid arteries. The circle provides a collateral supply to the whole brain. If any one of the arteries is compromised, the others can take over the supply.

SPECIALIST INVESTIGATIONS

A number of specific investigations may be undertaken as part of the clinical investigations of a patient (Box 9.2).

COMPUTERIZED AXIAL TOMOGRAPHY

Computerized axial tomography (CT) is an X-ray technique which enables the brain to be X-rayed in the coronal or sagittal planes in a series of slices 2–10 mm wide. The computer then processes the information, and the end result is a series of films showing the structure of the brain or spine at various levels. It depicts the structures of the brain and spinal cord at the time the scan was taken, but it cannot demonstrate physiological activity over a period of time.

MAGNETIC RESONANCE IMAGING

Magnetic resonance imaging (MRI) scanning was developed after CT scanning and relies on the physical

---

Box 9.2   Specialist investigations

Magnetic resonance imaging	Positron emission tomography
Angiography	Digital subtraction angiography
Electroencephalogram	Cortical mapping
Video telemetry	Sensory evoked potentials
Lumbar puncture	Myelography
Skull X-rays	Transcranial Doppler
Computerized axial tomography	

properties which occur when the patient is placed in a magnetic field and a radiofrequency pulse is applied. It is particularly useful in highlighting soft structures and can show some pathological states more clearly than the CT scan. Other advantages are that the patient is not exposed to radiation and the image of the brain can be made in any plane. It has been particularly helpful in the diagnosis of multiple sclerosis. It is not capable of demonstrating physiological function over a period of time.

POSITRON EMISSION TOMOGRAPHY

Positron emission tomography or PET scan is a relatively new technique which has been developed in order to demonstrate the functional activity of the brain over a period of time (anything from 20 minutes to 2 hours depending on the substance used). It involves the production of isotopes that emit positrons, which are then used to label substances which the target organ needs. In the case of the brain, oxygen and glucose are labelled. The resulting scan shows areas of increased local uptake and activity (McCulloch, 1986). It has been used in the study of dementia, schizophrenia and many other neurological and psychiatric disorders; however, it is not used in routine clinical investigations.

ANGIOGRAPHY

Cerebral angiography is useful when it is necessary to demonstrate the state of cerebral arteries and diagnose abnormalities of the blood vessels, such as atheroma, aneurysms and arteriovenous malformations. It is also helpful in the diagnosis of brain tumours, and it is used in the newly developing techniques of embolization of vessels in the treatment of aneurysms.

DIGITAL SUBTRACTION ANGIOGRAPHY

Digital subtraction angiography is a combination of angiography and computer technology in which the computer can subtract information from the image and expose the vessels of interest more clearly.

ELECTROENCEPHALOGRAM

An electroencephalogram (EEG) is a recording of the electrical activity of the brain and is used in the diagnosis of various neurological conditions, especially epilepsy. It is also useful in the investigation of sleep disorders.

CORTICAL MAPPING

Cortical mapping is carried out during awake craniotomies for patients suffering from lesions which are near vital areas such as the speech and language areas. In this way patients can tell the surgeon what they are experiencing and enable the surgeon to be more precise and selective in the amount of tissue that is removed (Reinhardt et al, 1996).

VIDEO TELEMETRY

Video telemetry is a form of electroencephalogram which is linked to a video camera. Patients suffering from seizures and non-epileptic seizures have video telemetry to enable the medical staff to see clearly the clinical manifestations of the seizure and have the EEG recording during it.

SENSORY EVOKED POTENTIALS

Some diagnoses can be made by stimulating specific sensory pathways and recording the electrical activity of the appropriate area of cerebral cortex and/or brainstem. Visual evoked potentials are useful in the diagnosis of multiple sclerosis. Auditory evoked potentials are useful in the diagnosis of acoustic neuroma and brainstem death.

LUMBAR PUNCTURE

Lumbar puncture is a procedure carried out by a doctor, during which a spinal needle is inserted into the subarachnoid space between the third and fourth lumbar vertebrae. Cerebrospinal fluid is withdrawn for the following reasons:

- to confirm a diagnosis, e.g. subarachnoid haemorrhage or meningitis
- to instil dyes, e.g. as in myelography, or drugs, e.g. intrathecal antibiotics.

It should not be used in patients with raised intracranial pressure, as it can provoke tentorial herniation (see raised intracranial pressure, p. 136).

MYELOGRAPHY

A myelogram is a specialized X-ray of the spine. A water-soluble dye is inserted into the subarachnoid space through a lumbar puncture, and lesions of the spine are highlighted if the cerebrospinal fluid pathway around the spinal cord is impeded in any way by a disc protrusion, tumour or arteriovenous malformation.

SKULL X-RAY

Anterior–posterior and lateral radiographs of the skull are usually taken in order to diagnose skull fractures, meningiomas and other bony injuries of the skull. In cases of head injury, the radiograph should include the neck down to and including the seventh and eighth cervical vertebrae, to exclude cervical fracture/dislocation.

TRANSCRANIAL DOPPLER

Transcranial Doppler studies rely on ultrasound technology. A very low frequency ultrasound wave is passed through the skull and is useful in assessing cerebral blood flow and vasospasm in disorders such as carotid stenosis.

NEUROSURGERY

REASONS FOR NEUROSURGERY

Neurosurgery is performed for two reasons:

- the removal or repair of brain tissue in order to prevent further harm
- to give palliative relief of distressing symptoms when the cause cannot be removed.

Box 9.3 gives a brief resumé of the reasons for neurosurgery.

THE APPROACHES USED BY THE SURGEON

Burr holes

Burr holes are holes drilled into the skull with an air drill and are used for the following reasons:

- insertion of brain needles to remove tissue for biopsy, or removal of a subdural haematoma
- to insert Gigli's saw to create a bone flap in a craniotomy.

Craniotomy

A craniotomy is an opening of the cranium, as shown in Figure 9.1. It is performed when a surgeon requires direct access to a cerebral hemisphere. At the end of the operation, the bone flap is usually replaced. Pioneering surgery is being carried out in the treatment of brain tumours. The patient is woken after the skull is opened, so that by assessing the patient while mapping the cortex and dissecting the tumour the surgeon can remove more of the tumour than ever before. The patient is anaesthetized again during the closure of the

---

Box 9.3 Reasons for neurosurgery

- Trauma: e.g. fractured skull, spinal injuries, traumatic brain injury.
- Infections: e.g. cerebral and spinal abscesses.
- Vascular disorders: e.g. cerebral aneurysm, haematoma, arteriovenous malformation.
- Spinal disorders: e.g. tumours of the spine, prolapsed intervertebral disc.
- Congenital abnormalities: e.g. hydrocephalus, craniostenosis
- Cerebral and spinal tumours: e.g. glioma, meningioma
- Degenerative disorders: e.g. carpal tunnel syndrome, arthritic changes in the spine.

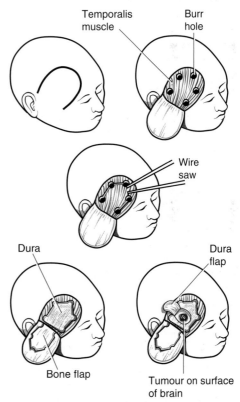

Figure 9.1 Stages of a craniotomy. (From *Neuromedical and Neurosurgical Nursing*, Baillière Tindall, 1977.)

---

skull. This procedure is also used in some forms of epilepsy surgery.

Craniectomy

A craniectomy is also an opening into the cranium, but it is smaller and the bone is usually chipped away and not replaced. This is commonly used in posterior fossa surgery.

Gamma knife surgery

Gamma knife surgery was developed in Sweden in 1968 by Professor Lars Leksell. Surgery in this case is radiosurgery, which involves precision targeting of a tumour or arteriovenous malformation with a high dose of gamma radiation.

Hypophysectomy

Hypophysectomy is the name of the operation for the removal of pituitary (hypophysis) tumours. This surgery can be done by a transsphenoidal approach through the nose, or transoral approach through the mouth, or through a craniotomy (see Fig. 9.1).

Laminectomy

Laminectomy is the term used for surgery of the spine in which the laminae have been opened to gain access to more than one level of the spinal cord.

Microdiscectomy

Microdiscectomy is a technique used increasingly by neurosurgeons to remove prolapsed intervertebral discs with the minimum of surgery. There is no bony involvement, and patients can be mobilized within 48 hours.

THE LONG-TERM CONSEQUENCES OF NEUROSURGERY

The rehabilitative process begins with the nurse's preoperative assessment and care planning. The prevention of common perioperative and postoperative complications is shared with the other disciplines discussed in this book, e.g. wound infection, deep vein thrombosis, haemorrhage and anaesthetic complications. The consequences of raised intracranial pressure (RICP) or ischaemia need to be considered, as outlined later in this chapter.

In addition, however, the results of focal damage to a particular area of the brain must be considered. As we will see with John, who underwent partial removal of a frontoparietal glioma, there were focal problems which resulted from removal of part of the frontal and parietal lobes.

PREOPERATIVE ASSESSMENT OF THE PATIENT UNDERGOING CEREBRAL SURGERY

A detailed history, functional and neurological assessment/observations can assist the nurse and other members of the critical care team to plan and monitor care. In neurosurgery, a patient's condition can deteriorate very quickly, with fatal consequences. One of the important skills of the neuroscience nurse is the ability to make detailed observations and act upon them promptly. The main cause of rapid deterioration in neurosurgery is raised intracranial pressure.

RAISED INTRACRANIAL PRESSURE

The adult brain is protected by a closed skull. The only openings in the skull are the foramen magnum, the small foramina by which the cranial nerves enter or leave the skull, e.g. optic or auditory nerves and the sinuses. The contents of the skull are such that there is little room for anything that takes up extra space. The normal intracranial pressure (ICP) is 0–10 mmHg. However, a higher upper limit of 15 mmHg is the more usual level recognized in neurosurgical practice (North and Reilly, 1990). This margin of 0–15 mmHg enables such activities as coughing, straining and bending to take place without the individual being harmed. If there is a space-occupying lesion in the brain, such as a haematoma, hydrocephalus or a tumour, the brain will compensate until it reaches a point where it cannot do so any longer. This period of autoregulation is known as Cushing's response, and during this phase the autonomic nervous system responds by slowing the pulse rate and widening the systolic and diastolic blood pressure. This is nature's attempt to overcome the pressure on the cerebral arteries and ensure cerebral blood flow. If the lesion is supratentorial, the pressure above the tentorium will be greater than that below.

In this way the pressure is funnelled toward the weakest point in the tentorium, causing tentorial herniation of the uncus of the temporal lobe. This funnel-shaped pressure wave is like an ice cream cone and gives rise to the term 'coning'. At this point there is pressure on the brainstem and the third cranial nerve (oculomotor nerve) on the affected side. This results in a change in the size and reaction of the pupil to light on the same side as the lesion.

If left untreated, the third cranial nerve on the other side becomes compromised and both pupils will become dilated and eventually cease to react to light. A Cheyne–Stokes respiratory pattern will follow, and the continuing pressure on the brainstem will disrupt the stability of the blood pressure and pulse rate, and death will follow. Neurological assessment and observations are essential to detect early signs of rising intracranial pressure and to treat them. The first sign of rising intracranial pressure may be headaches, lethargy or increased drowsiness, depending on the speed at which the intracranial pressure is increasing.

Nursing measures to treat raised intracranial pressure will be discussed in the section on postoperative care.

THE NEUROLOGICAL ASSESSMENT AND OBSERVATIONS

The major difference between neurological assessment and neurological observations is that a neurological assessment is more holistic and covers all the nervous system activity, including cognition, perception and behaviour, when it is possible to assess these aspects of the patient. It also includes neurological observations.

A full neurological assessment is taken on admission to the neurosurgical ward and will provide a baseline for planning care. A further full assessment needs to be carried out at regular intervals during the patient's stay in the unit in order to fully evaluate care and to plan for the patient's discharge or transfer to a general hospital.

The nurse should look closely at the findings made by the doctor in their history and clinical examination at the time of admission, in order to compare the patient's perception of their problems with the nurse's own findings. Sometimes patients and their carers give information to nurses because they believe the information to be of little importance to the doctor, or because they forgot to mention it, or may have been too embarrassed or frightened to talk about it.

An assessment of neurological function should include the following:

- conscious level, by using the Glasgow Coma Scale (Teasdale and Jennett, 1974)

- vital signs – temperature, pulse, respirations and blood pressure
- posture and gait (if able to walk)
- nutritional status (BAPEN, 2003a,b)
- signs of infection
- pressure ulcer risk assessment (Waterlow, 1985)
- behaviour
- perceptual problems
- pain
- vision
- sensory pathways
- cognitive function
- communication
- use of drugs, e.g. alcohol, over-the-counter drugs, prescribed and illegal drugs
- urinary continence (Woodward, 1995).

Conscious level by using the Glasgow Coma Scale

Teasdale and Jennett (1974) developed the Glasgow Coma Scale, which is a simple scale for measuring the patient's level of arousal and awareness and, by so doing, enabling clinicians to determine the patient's progress by means of a reliable and valid tool. It has since been brought into use by most neurosurgical units throughout the world, although it has been modified. There are three parts to the Glasgow Coma Scale: eye opening, best motor function in the arms and best verbal response. Each of the items on the scale is given a score. The sum of all the scores gives a maximum of 15 and the lowest possible score is 3. Figure 9.2 shows a chart for recording scores on the scale.

A coma scale observation chart

					Date
Name					
Record No.					
					Time
	Eyes open	Spontaneously			Eyes closed by swelling = C
		To speech			
		To pain			
		None			
Coma scale	Best verbal response	Orientated			Endotracheal tube or tracheostomy = T
		Confused			
		Inappropriate words			
		Incomprehensible sounds			
		None			
	Best motor response	Obeys commands			Usually record the best arm response
		Localize pain			
		Flexion to pain			
		Extension to pain			
		None			

Figure 9.2   A coma scale observation chart. (From Hinchliff et al, 1996:126.)

Many neurosurgeons do not use the total score as a reliable guide to the patient's state but tend to note the scores for each of the three modalities separately. The advantage of the Glasgow Coma Scale over any other is that it has been shown to have good interobserver reliability (Juarez and Lyons, 1995) among trained, experienced staff (Ellis and Cavanagh, 1992). The Glasgow Coma Scale cannot be used in isolation. When used with the other observations such as vital signs, speech and language, cognitive and perceptual behaviours, the nurse obtains a more complete assessment of the patient's neurological state. The frequency of these recordings will depend on the severity of the patient's condition and the likelihood of sudden deterioration, e.g. following a craniotomy when the patient may suffer from a haemorrhage or cerebral oedema.

Vital signs: temperature, pulse, respirations and blood pressure

The patient's temperature, pulse, respirations and blood pressure should be recorded regularly. In raised intracranial pressure the patient's temperature is likely to rise as pressure on the hypothalamus and brainstem increase. Having excluded infection, the patient should be kept cool by modifying the temperature of the room and by removing all but enough clothing to preserve the patient's dignity. Drugs such as paracetamol may be required to keep the temperature under control. Fans are no longer used, particularly since the possibility

of methicillin-resistant *Staphylococcus aureus* (MRSA) has become a serious threat in surgical wards. Fanning is also thought to induce shivering, which increases the metabolic rate, and this is undesirable in the hypermetabolic postoperative patient (Holtzclaw, 1990).

The nurse should observe not only the rate and quality of the pulse but also its rhythm. In raised intracranial pressure, the pulse will be strong and bounding. After subarachnoid haemorrhage, the pulse is often irregular because of disturbances of the catecholamines (Kocan, 1988).

Respiration needs to be monitored very closely, neurosurgical patients being more likely to undergo a respiratory rather than a cardiac arrest. In raised intracranial pressure, respiratory function is compromised when the pressure is so great that tentorial herniation occurs, causing torsion and pressure on the brainstem, which in turn causes pressure on the respiratory centre. The problem is not only mechanical but also biochemical. The increased pressure inside the skull causes the cerebral perfusion pressure to fall. This results in tissue hypoxia, and the level of carbon dioxide rises, which in turn leads to vasodilatation and a further increase in intracranial pressure (Fig. 9.3).

It is therefore important to monitor the patient's oxygen saturation levels. In intensive care units this is done by frequent arterial blood gas analysis to observe more accurately the patient's arterial oxygen, carbon dioxide and sodium bicarbonate levels, as well as monitoring any acidosis or alkalosis that may be

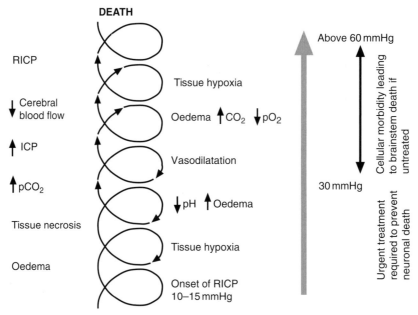

Figure 9.3   Untreated raised intracranial pressure (RICP) and its consequences.

developing (Brenner and Welliver, 1990). In other wards and departments, extra vigilance is required to ensure that the patient's mucous membranes are pink and well perfused. Pulse oximetry can be used to measure oxygen saturation if arterial blood gas monitoring is not possible (Tremper and Barker, 1989).

Blood pressure monitoring provides another good indicator of raised intracranial pressure because, as the Cushing's response takes effect, the gap between the systolic and diastolic pressure widens and the systolic pressure rises significantly, as shown in Figure 9.4. In subarachnoid haemorrhage, the blood pressure should be maintained at a constant high level, since rapid rises or falls can provoke rebleeding or vasospasm (Rusy, 1996; Segatore, 1992).

Mobility, posture and gait

The patient's ability to walk should be examined unless their condition precludes it. Among the group of patients on whom one would not be able to carry this out are those who have had a severe traumatic brain injury, a brain haemorrhage or where the level of consciousness is impaired. It is necessary to establish how far the patient can walk and whether walking aids or assistance is required. The patient should walk down the ward, with help if needed, and their posture and gait observed. Patients with ataxia tend to fall backwards or to one side. Those with lower motor neuron lesions may walk with a drop foot and have signs of increased wear on the toes of their shoes on the affected side. If there are perceptual problems, the patient may appear clumsy and knock into objects, and may also be labelled confused. When proprioception is lost, the patient may walk with a high-stepping gait and will tend to fall if he is in a darkened room.

Nutritional status

It is important to assess the nutritional status of the patient on admission. Height, weight and body mass index should be recorded, along with brief details of appetite, eating habits and food preferences, intolerance or allergies. A physical examination will identify any problems with dentition, mobility, chewing and swallowing. A social history will help to identify problems such as distance from the shops for those who have mobility problems, as well as issues related to safety and competence to prepare and cook food.

Nutritional assessment is a team activity and the nurse's role is to ensure that the appropriate members of the nutrition team – e.g. dietitian, speech and language

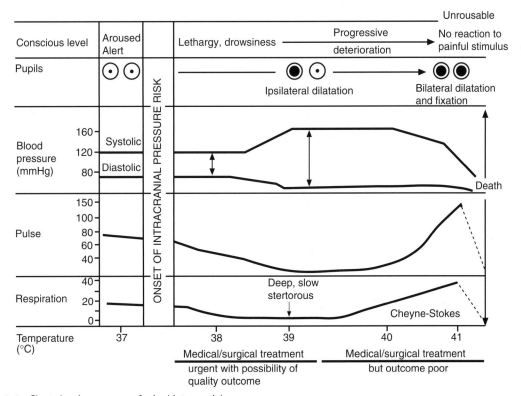

Figure 9.4   Chart showing progress of raised intracranial pressure.

therapist, occupational therapist, social worker, pharmacist and doctor – are informed of any problems.

Neurosurgery causes a massive stress response, which results in hypermetabolism, hypercatabolism and glucose intolerance. Cortisol levels rise and the patient will start to break down muscle, develop ketosis and lose weight rapidly (Ott and Young, 1991). To try to prevent this from happening, the patient should be fed a well-balanced diet high in protein as soon as possible after admission, and starved preoperatively for as short a time as is compatible with safe anaesthesia. There are commercially prepared feeds on the market which can be prescribed. They contain all the essential amino acids required to enable neurotransmitters to be formed and to prevent the breakdown of muscle. They usually contain 1–1.5 kcal/mL of feed, which enables the nurse to feed the patient adequately even when there is raised intracranial pressure, and some surgeons restrict fluid intake to 1.5 L in 24 hours by all routes, but this is currently being challenged.

To prevent overloading the patient with glucose at a time when they are liable to be intolerant, neurosurgeons usually restrict the patient to normal saline intravenously without any added dextrose.

Enquiries into the patient's preoperative diet will enable the nurse to prevent some immediate postoperative problems and give advice about a healthy diet. One of the most common problems in the postoperative phase in any patient is the sudden cessation of caffeine intake in those who drink large quantities of coffee, cola drinks and to a certain extent tea. Sudden caffeine withdrawal frequently causes headache and restlessness. The patient's ability to cough and swallow needs to be checked before they are given an oral diet.

Signs of infection

If the patient has an infection, the source should be found as soon as possible. The temperature-controlling mechanism in the hypothalamus should only be considered as the reason for the pyrexia when all other possibilities have been excluded.

Pressure ulcer risk assessment

The Waterlow risk assessment scale should be used to assess the patient's risk of acquiring a pressure ulcer (Waterlow, 1985). If the patient is paralysed, unconscious or incontinent, the risk is much higher.

Behaviour

Neurosurgical patients often seem to have 'inappropriate' or 'confused' behaviour. These two labels are often misleading, as they mask real inquiry into the nature of the behaviour. Is the patient restless, aggressive,

euphoric, depressed, dehydrated, apathetic, slow in giving responses or disinhibited? Damage to the brain can provoke any of these behaviours.

Temporal lobe disorders can cause the strange behaviour associated with partial seizures of this area, such as violent outbursts and some altered sensory perception such as strange tastes, smells and auditory hallucinations. They are simple partial seizures if consciousness is not affected and complex partial seizures if it is (Taylor, 1996).

Perceptual problems

Some of the other reasons for confused behaviour can be agnosia, dyspraxia and sensory inattention. Many of these problems cannot be fully assessed in an acute setting, but a good understanding of the underlying anatomy and physiology of the central nervous system will enable the nurse to infer the true nature of the confusion in many cases. Visual disturbances can also account for clumsy behaviour in some cases, and this will be addressed in the section on vision.

Pain

Headache, neck stiffness, back and nerve root pain are all common to neurosurgical patients. In assessing the patient's pain, its site, intensity and description should be recorded, as well as noting any self-help therapies the patient may be using to ease the pain.

With headache the nurse should note whether the pain is:

- worse in the morning
- like a tight band around the head
- localized to one area, e.g. pain behind the eye.

The type and quality of the headache can provide important information to help in the diagnosis of its cause as well as providing a baseline for the effectiveness of therapy.

With back pain, the nurse should ascertain whether it:

- is central back pain
- radiates to one side, e.g. into shoulders or hips
- radiates to one or more limbs
- is accompanied by loss of or altered sensation, e.g. hypersensitivity, tingling or numbness.

Vision

Patients with parietal lobe lesions can experience a visual pathway disorder known as homonymous hemianopia. The patient experiences blindness in the left or right field of vision in each eye. Patients with trauma or other lesions of the occipital cortex may suffer from cortical blindness. In pituitary gland tumours, many patients suffer from bitemporal hemianopia, which shows itself as tunnel vision. Although it is the doctor's role to assess the patient's visual fields and acuity, the nurse should assess the impact of partial loss of vision on the patient's safety and behaviour. The latter often requires explanation to bewildered relatives.

Sensory and motor pathways

The sensory and motor pathways will be tested by the medical staff in order to establish whether there is any loss of the sense of touch, deep pressure, tendon reflexes, paraesthesia or joint position sense. Joint position sense is so-called because stretch receptors in the joints provide the brain with information about the position of the body. Nurses should assess the motor power in each limb and, if there are any sensory changes, report them to the medical staff.

Psychological state

The patient's mental state should be assessed from the point of view of mood and affect as well as cognitive and perceptual processing. There is a need to understand the patient's comprehension of and feelings towards the injury or disability, and to give them the time to express them in a variety of ways. Sometimes the disability is such that the nurse needs to find innovative alternative strategies such as art or music therapy. For example, patients with dysphonia cannot shout or even raise their voice. How will you know when they are indignant, or enraged? Patients with dysphasia cannot express themselves in words but may be able to write or use music to express their feelings. An alternative has to be found for the paralysed individual who cannot stamp their feet or walk away.

In addition, the hopes and fears of the patient's family and principal carers should be assessed and they should be given time to express their fears and worries.

Cognitive function

The clinical examination of the patient will show any major cognitive problems such as their ability to solve simple problems, slowness of thinking, numeracy and literacy. The neuropsychologist may be asked to carry out pre- and postoperative assessments of the patient's cognitive function. However, there is evidence in the literature that there is an instrument which can be used by nurses to give a broad assessment of the patient's mental state, i.e. the Neurobehavioural Cognitive Status Examination (NCSE). Reimer et al (1990) looked at its validity in relation to head injury, and Cammermeyer and Prendergast (1997) have used it to create profiles of cognitive function in other neurological problems. Such a test will detect such problems as an inability to

calculate (dyscalculia) or write (dysgraphia), loss of memory (amnesia) and slowness to process information.

Communication

Damage to the speech and language centre of the brain can leave the patient with disorders such as dyslexia, dysphasia, dysgraphia and dysarthria. Communication difficulties of this kind need the help of a speech and language therapist who will assess the patient at an appropriate time. In the meantime, the nurse should assess the patient's ability to understand the spoken word, to exclude receptive dysphasia. If the patient can understand the nurse clearly but has an expressive dysphasia, a system of communication should be established with the patient. These patients require great patience and understanding, and the use of slang, long sentences and fast speech should be avoided.

Use of drugs: alcohol, over-the-counter, prescribed and illegal drugs

Does the patient drink large quantities of alcohol? This needs to be recorded, as some seizures after surgery may be due to alcohol withdrawal and not epilepsy. The use of alcohol and other drugs can seriously affect the assessment of patients and eventual outcome of both the neurological disorder and its treatment.

The use of eye drops to alter the pupil reaction (e.g. atropine or pilocarpine), sedatives or some analgesics can also give a misleading assessment.

If the patient has had any alcohol, this should be discounted when assessing them, in the sense that drowsiness or behavioural changes cannot automatically be put down to the alcohol. Patients should be woken at regular intervals to ensure that they are still rousable.

The patient's drug history should be recorded not only to ensure that they are not on any drugs that will cloud the accuracy of neurological assessment but also to inform the medical staff whether the patient is at risk from sudden withdrawal, e.g. from steroids or drugs of addiction.

Urinary continence

There are many reasons why patients become incontinent of urine, but there are among them some important neurological causes and these require careful assessment. Woodward (1995) has developed a continence assessment tool which is of use to nurses in a neurological setting. Damage or impaired function of the nerve supply to the bladder through cerebral or spinal pathology can result in retention or incontinence of urine.

In a short chapter on neurosurgical nursing it is not possible to describe in detail the care of patients undergoing every kind of neurosurgery. For cerebral and spinal surgery, there are some common denominators following a craniotomy. For the subtle changes which accompany certain pathologies or surgical approaches, the reader should refer to specialist neurosurgical nursing texts (see Further reading).

PLANNING CARE FOR THE NEUROSURGICAL PATIENT

The nursing care plans which follow illustrate the pre- and postoperative care of a patient who has undergone neurosurgery for partial removal of a glioma (Tables 9.1 and 9.2). The nursing care plan for any patient undergoing craniotomy has similarities to that described below. The potential complications of raised intracranial pressure, haemorrhage and infection are common to all. What makes each patient unique is the cause, the focal neurological signs, the patient's reaction to the diagnosis and surgery, and other medical, nursing, socioeconomic, cultural and spiritual considerations.

THE PATIENT

This is a fictitious patient, and the case history is a synthesis of several actual cases. All the details have been altered to preserve the patient's anonymity.

- name: John Jones (he likes to be called John)
- age: 39 years
- marital status: married to Alison (same age)
- dependants: a daughter, Claire, aged 18 years; a son, Paul, aged 16 years
- occupation: draughtsman
- home situation: a house in a London suburb. It is on a bus route and near a station. It has four bedrooms. The bathroom and toilet are upstairs
- previous medical history:
  - appendicectomy in 1965
  - no other surgery
  - otherwise healthy; no known allergies; does not smoke; drinks beer and wine occasionally.

HISTORY OF PRESENT ILLNESS

John has complained of severe headaches, lethargy and nausea for about 6 weeks. He took paracetamol regularly, but the headaches were unrelieved by it and were unbearable in the early morning. They were affecting his work and he consulted his general practitioner, who referred him to a neurologist for further investigations and opinion.

One week before his appointment was due, John collapsed at work and had a tonic–clonic seizure. He was taken to the local accident and emergency department, from which he was referred to the regional neuroscience unit.

NEUROLOGICAL ASSESSMENT ON ADMISSION

- Glasgow Coma Scale:
  - eye opening 3
  - verbal response 4
  - motor response 6
- Conscious, drowsy, opens eyes to speech; obeys commands slowly. He is fully orientated in time, place and person. His left arm is weaker than the right. Both legs move spontaneously and to command with equal power. No other apparent neurological deficits.
- Unable to fully test cognitive and perceptual function at this stage but appears to have sensory loss in left arm when moved.
- No glycosuria on urine testing. Specific gravity normal. No abnormalities discovered.
- Temperature 37.4°C; pulse 82 bpm; respirations 16 rpm, regular; colour good; blood pressure 150/80 mmHg.

INVESTIGATIONS

Investigations were carried out as follows:

- clinical examination
- blood: full blood count: Hb, WBC, RBC, lymphocytes
- radiography:
  - skull X-rays, anterior–posterior views
  - CT scan
- MRI scan
- EEG.

The scans showed that John had a large frontoparietal tumour which had the appearance of a cystic glioma. The neurosurgeons decided that surgery would be advisable to help John's headaches. He was prescribed anticonvulsants, analgesics and antiemetics. He was also prescribed dexamethasone to reduce the oedema around the tumour.

THE PRINCIPLES OF POSTOPERATIVE CARE OF A PATIENT FOLLOWING A CRANIOTOMY

The principles of care following a craniotomy are to:

- ensure a safe recovery from anaesthesia
- monitor the patient's condition for signs of raised intracranial pressure and its clinical management
- implement a nursing care plan which ensures that care is given according to the patient's degree of dependency
- promote rehabilitation.

Table 9.1 Preoperative care plan for a patient undergoing a craniotomy

Actual/potential problem	Nursing goals	Nursing action	Rationale	Outcome and evaluation
Actual deterioration in conscious level during 12 hours prior to admission due to raised intracranial pressure (RICP)	(a) To ensure that deterioration in conscious level is detected and treated as a matter of urgency (b) To monitor the effectiveness of the clinical management of raised intracranial pressure	(1) 1 hourly neurological observations using the modified Glasgow Observation Chart (2) 1 hourly pulse, respirations and blood pressure (3) 2 hourly temperature (4) Full neurological assessment (5) Report any change in patient's condition to medical staff immediately	(1) The Glasgow Coma Scale and modified Glasgow Observation Chart have been tested as valid and reliable measures of the patient's level of arousability and awareness (Teasdale and Jennett, 1974) (2) Neurological observations detect early signs of raised intracranial pressure, which if not treated can continue to rise with fatal consequences (3) As intracranial pressure rises, pressure on the brainstem and the activation of the Cushing's response cause an alteration in temperature, pulse, respiration and blood pressure (Hickey, 2001) (4) See explanation of rationale for neurological assessment in this chapter (p. 137) (5) The change can be deterioration or amelioration following the administration of dexamethasone	Neurological observations were reduced to 1 hourly after examination by neurosurgical senior registrar. John's neurological state improved after the administration of dexamethasone
John is suffering from raised intracranial pressure and is at risk of changes in respiratory pattern and respiratory arrest	(a) To monitor respiratory rate, depth and pattern (b) To be aware of the respiratory arrest procedure (c) To develop listening skills which, when away from the patient's bedside, will detect changes in a patient's respiratory pattern	(1) Record respiratory rate, depth and pattern at least 1 hourly (2) Listen carefully for changes in respiratory pattern when away from John's bed but within earshot (3) Ensure that all nursing members of the team are vigilant and able to react to a respiratory arrest	Increasing supratentorial pressure can cause sufficient pressure on the respiratory centre in the medulla oblongata to cause respiratory distress and possibly a respiratory arrest	John's respiratory rate remained within normal limits preoperatively
John has already had one tonic–clinic generalized seizure	(a) Ensure John's safety during and after the seizure (b) Monitor the seizure and record the following: (i) time of start and end of seizure	(1) Ensure John cannot fall from his bed (2) Record the data listed in (b) i–v on a seizure chart (3) Inform medical staff of seizures (4) Administer drugs prescribed	(1) Patients can harm themselves during falls associated with generalized seizures (2) Recording the patient's seizures accurately can assist in the diagnosis of the cause	John had 3 further seizures preoperatively and his anti-convulsant therapy was changed to sodium valproate *(Continued)*

Table 9.1 (Continued)

Actual/potential problem	Nursing goals	Nursing action	Rationale	Outcome and evaluation
	(ii) description of seizure (iii) presence of incontinence of urine or faeces (iv) duration of recovery period (v) oxygen saturation levels (c) Maintain a calm, efficient approach to the seizures and discuss with John and Alison their reactions to them	for John's epilepsy (5) Support John and Alison during the seizure if it takes place in Alison's presence (6) If the seizures persist, long-term drug therapy and counselling should be provided	(3) Patients can also harm themselves by not being fully aware of their surroundings as they come round from a seizure (4) Patients and onlookers are often frightened by a generalized seizure. This can lead to social isolation	
Lack of information concerning diagnosis and treatment options	(a) Ensure that John makes an informed decision about surgery based on adequate information and an opportunity to discuss it with staff and family (b) Ensure that the patient and doctor have signed the consent form before the premedication is given (c) Ensure that the patient and his immediate family are given sufficient privacy in which to discuss the diagnosis, treatment and possible outcomes	(1) Offer John and Alison an opportunity to speak to the surgeon together and separately (2) Provide a suitable environment for the interview to take place (3) Check that the consent form has been signed by John and a member of the neurosurgical team (4) Listen to John and Alison's queries and anxieties as they arise (5) If appropriate, introduce them to the local Tumour Support Group	(1) It is illegal to operate on a patient without his consent, except in an extreme emergency when this is not possible (2) The patient who is well informed is less anxious than a patient whose fear is imaginary (Cheetham, 1993; Leino-Kilpi et al, 1993) (3) Some patients are particularly frightened of diseases or damage to the brain. Some of those fears are reasonable but some can be irrational	John and Alison were devastated by the news that John had a brain tumour. John's main anxieties about surgery were: • Will it make him feel worse? • How likely is he to survive surgery? • Will he go mad? • Will he lose control of himself? • Will he be able to put his affairs in order legally before surgery? Alison's main anxieties were: • Will John die? • Will John suffer more after surgery than he does now? • What will she tell the children and how? • How will she cope?

Problem	Goal	Nursing action	Rationale	Evaluation
John is at risk of inadequate personal hygiene due to deterioration in conscious level and left arm weakness	(a) To assist John in the maintenance of his personal hygiene (b) To encourage John to be independent whenever possible	(1) Give John an assisted bath (2) Offer mouth care regularly and at least twice daily. (3) Ensure that John is lying in a clean, tidy bed (4) Assist John to change his pyjamas when necessary (5) Wash John's hair preoperatively (6) Ensure that John's nails are cut regularly	(1) Personal hygiene reduces the risk of infection and promotes the patient's sense of well-being. It also encourages a good self-image (2) A clean mouth prevents dental caries and gum infection. It also improves taste and encourages a healthy appetite	• John and Alison seen by medical social worker and John's manager John's neurological condition improved sufficiently for him to be given assisted washes. On the eve of his operation, John asked to be taken to the bathroom for a shower under supervision. His hair was washed. His skin is in good condition. His nails are well manicured and he can shave himself with an electric razor. John has all his own teeth, no crowns, caps, bridges or plates. His teeth and gums are healthy. He last visited the dentist 6 months ago
Poor nutritional status and fluid balance due to nausea and vomiting worsened by preoperative starvation	(a) To ensure that John's nutritional state is maintained/improved preoperatively	(1) Administer antiemetics if John is nauseated (2) Record John's height, weight and calculate his body mass index (BMI). Record outline details of his usual pre-morbid diet (3) Refer to dietitian if necessary (4) Offer John small but nutritionally well-balanced meals high in protein and energy (5) Encourage John to drink but not more than a total 1.5 L per 24 hours	(1) Patients undergoing neurosurgery become hypermetabolic and hyperglycaemic. (2) Long periods of starvation before investigations or surgery add to the problem, as weight loss and muscle breakdown ensue (Chapman, 1996). (3) Gut motility is stimulated by the presence of food in the stomach	John did not regain much appetite preoperatively. His nausea was controlled by antiemetics but John was too drowsy to eat much. He ate small meals but the news of his diagnosis and fear of both seizures and surgery affected his appetite. BMI: 21
John suffers from raised intracranial	(a) Prevent pressure ulcers (b) Prevent deep vein thrombosis	(1) Turn or encourage John to turn himself 2 hourly	(1) Poor ergonomics and prolonged length of time in one position causes the	John was repositioned 2 hourly on a *(Continued)*

Table 9.1 (Continued)

Actual/potential problem	Nursing goals	Nursing action	Rationale	Outcome and evaluation
pressure and is at risk of reduced mobility and its complications	(c) Prevent hypostatic pneumonia (d) Prevent muscle contractures	(2) Use a pressure-relieving mattress (3) Encourage John to move his feet and contract his leg muscles frequently to prevent deep vein thrombosis (4) Sit John up in bed at an angle of 30–40° to assist his respiratory function and reduce raised intracranial pressure (5) Assist John out of bed as soon as his raised intracranial pressure is lowered and his condition improves (6) Assess John's risk from pressure ulcers using the Waterlow scale. (7) Put John's joints through a full range of movements twice daily and position them in a neutral position in between	formation of pressure ulcers (2) Prevention of pressure ulcers is promoted by frequent change of position and pressure-relieving ergonomic mattresses and cushions (Waterlow, 1988) (3) Muscle activity increases blood flow in deep veins and discourages the formation of deep vein thrombosis	pressure-relieving mattress until his conscious level improved and he could turn himself. John was seen by a physiotherapist once a day and his limbs were put through a full range of movements. Waterlow score: 9
John has raised intracranial pressure and is at risk of urinary and faecal incontinence	(a) To prevent formation of pressure ulcers (b) To maintain John's dignity (c) To monitor John's urinary output and bowel movements	(1) Change John's bed linen if wet and/or soiled (2) Use incontinence aids to prevent soiling the bed linen and protect the skin (3) Maintain John's dignity and privacy (4) Ensure sufficient intake of fluid and diet to prevent kidney failure and constipation	Patients are more anxious about the possibility of incontinence than any other aspect of care. The patient has the right to privacy and dignity. Failure to maintain an adequate diet or fluid intake causes constipation and renal problems, including renal calculi and renal failure	John received 1.5 L of fluid per 24 hours and ate segments of orange during the day in addition to his small meals. Waterlow score: 9
Fear of anaesthesia and postoperative side-effects of anaesthesia	To listen to John's fears and allay them	(1) Liaise with anaesthetist and ensure time and privacy for them to discuss John's anxieties (2) Liaise with intensive care unit and operating theatre nursing staff	Fear of anaesthetic complications and loss of control is common before a general anaesthetic. In neurosurgery, this is compounded by a fear of mental disturbance, disability and/or death	John was seen by the anaesthetist. He remained anxious but many of his fears were allayed. John was seen by the nurses who will receive him in the anaesthetic room and

			intensive care unit. They discussed what he could expect to find when he recovered from the anaesthetic.
			Premedication given at 7.30 am. on day of surgery. John slept until time to go to operating theatre
Possible dangers of inadequate pre- and perioperative safety procedures	To carry out an established pre- and perioperative safety check	To carry out the checks listed on the preoperative check list before leaving the ward and when handing the patient over to the operating theatre staff	Preoperative checks reduce the risk of operating on the wrong patient or on the wrong part of the patient. They also reduce the risk of complications from aspiration of gastric contents, damaged teeth and deep vein thrombosis (see Ch. 2)	John was starved from 4 am prior to surgery at 8.30 am. Pre-operative check carried out and premedication given at 7.30 am.

Table 9.2 Postoperative care plan following a craniotomy

Actual/potential problem	Nursing goals	Nursing action	Rationale	Outcome and evaluation
Actual deterioration in conscious level during 12 hours prior to admission due to raised intracranial pressure and at risk of cerebral oedema and haemorrhage for at least 24 hours postoperatively. John showed signs of a rise in intracranial pressure while in intensive care unit	(a) To ensure that deterioration in conscious level is detected and treated as a matter of urgency (b) To monitor the effectiveness of the clinical management of raised intracranial pressure	(1) 1 hourly neurological observations using the modified Glasgow Observation Chart (2) 1 hourly pulse, respirations and blood pressure (3) 2 hourly temperature (4) Full neurological assessment (5) Report any change in patient's condition to medical staff immediately (6) Administer prescribed drugs for the reduction of raised intracranial pressure (7) Position head of bed at an angle of 30–40°	(1) The Glasgow Coma Scale and modified Glasgow Observation Chart have been tested as valid and reliable measures of the patient's level of arousability and awareness (Teasdale and Jennett, 1974) (2) Neurological observations detect early signs of raised intracranial pressure which, if not treated, can continue to rise with fatal consequences (3) As intracranial pressure rises, pressure on the brainstem and the activation of the Cushing's response cause an alteration in temperature, pulse, respiration and blood pressure (Hickey, 2001) (4) See explanation of rationale for neurological assessment in this chapter (p. 137) (5) The change can be deterioration or amelioration following the administration of dexamethasone and partial removal of the glioma	(1) Neurological observations were reduced to 1 hourly after examination by neurosurgical senior registrar 6 hours after surgery (2) Mannitol 20% given in intensive care unit with good diuretic effect
John has experienced raised intracranial pressure and is at risk of respiratory distress and respiratory arrest	(a) To monitor respiratory rate, depth and pattern at least 1 hourly (b) To be aware of the respiratory arrest procedure (c) To develop listening skills which, when away from the patient's bedside, will detect changes in a patient's respiratory pattern	(1) Record respiratory rate, depth and pattern at least 1 hourly (2) Listen carefully for changes in respiratory pattern when away from John's bed but within earshot (3) Ensure that all nursing members of the team are vigilant and able to react to a respiratory arrest	Increasing supratentorial pressure can cause sufficient pressure on the respiratory centre in the medulla oblongata to cause respiratory distress and possibly a respiratory arrest	John's respiratory rate remained within normal limits postoperatively
Risk of wound breakdown and infection	Prevent wound infection and ensure wound has healed	(1) Ensure that the craniotomy dressing is kept clean and the staples are removed when the wound has healed	The scalp is very vascular and heals quickly; therefore, a dressing does not have to be in situ very long, and staples do not need to stay in beyond 5 days.	(1) Drain removed after 48 hours (2) Staples removed 5 days postoperatively

Problem	Goal	Nursing intervention	Rationale	Evaluation
		(2) Ensure that other wounds such as intravenous catheter sites are dressed using an aseptic technique and inspected regularly for signs of inflammation and infection	When the wound is healed it should be protected from the sun, and massaged twice daily to aid scar formation	(3) Wound well healed (4) Alison will examine wound regularly and massage it gently without oil or cream because John will be undergoing radiotherapy
John has already had one tonic–clonic seizure preoperatively	(a) To ensure John's safety during and after the seizure (b) To monitor the seizure and record the following: (i) time of start and end of seizure (ii) description of seizure (iii) presence of incontinence of urine or faeces (iv) duration of recovery period (v) oxygen saturation levels (c) To maintain a calm, efficient approach to the seizures and discuss with John and Alison their reactions to them	(1) Ensure John cannot fall from his bed (2) Record the data listed in (b)(i–v) on a seizure chart (3) Inform medical staff of seizures (4) Administer drugs prescribed for John's epilepsy (5) Support John and Alison during the seizure if it takes place in Alison's presence (6) If the seizures persist, long-term drug therapy and counselling should be provided	(1) Patients can harm themselves during falls associated with generalized seizures (2) Recording the patients' seizures accurately can assist in the diagnosis of the cause (3) Patients can also harm themselves by not being fully aware of their surroundings as they come around from their seizure (4) Patients and onlookers are often frightened by a generalized seizure. This can lead to social isolation	John had no further seizures postoperatively. Sodium valproate given as prescribed
Lack of information concerning diagnosis and treatment options	(a) To ensure that John is able to discuss the outcome of surgery (b) To ensure that the patient and his immediate family are given sufficient privacy in which to discuss the diagnosis, treatment and possible outcomes	(1) Offer John and Alison an opportunity to speak to the surgeon together and separately. (2) Provide a suitable environment for the interviews to take place (3) Listen to John and Alison's queries and anxieties as they arise (4) If appropriate, introduce them to the local Tumour Support Group	(1) The patient who is well informed is less anxious than a patient whose fear is imaginary (Cheetham, 1993; Leino-Kilpi et al, 1993) (2) Some patients are particularly frightened of diseases or damage to the brain	John and Alison were relieved that John had not only survived surgery but that he is conscious and they can speak to each other. John's main anxiety now is: • Will he regain the use of his arm? (Continued)

Table 9.2 (Continued)

Actual/potential problem	Nursing goals	Nursing action	Rationale	Outcome and evaluation
				Alison's main anxieties were: • Will John suffer more after surgery than he does now? • What will she tell the children and how? • How will she cope? John and Alison seen by the surgeons. John seen by the neuro-oncology team prior to accepting radiotherapy
John is at risk of inadequate personal hygiene due to deterioration in conscious level and left arm weakness	(a) To assist John in the maintenance of his personal hygiene (b) To encourage John to be independent	(1) Give John an assisted bath (2) Offer mouth care regularly and at least twice a day (3) Ensure that John is lying in a clean, tidy bed (4) Assist John to change his pyjamas when necessary (5) Ensure that John's nails are cut regularly	(1) Personal hygiene reduces the risk of infection and promotes the patient's sense of well-being. It also encourages a good self-image (Harris, 1994) (2) A clean mouth prevents dental caries and gum infection. It also improves taste and encourages a healthy appetite (Kelly, 1994)	First day after surgery John was given a bed bath. John's neurological condition improved sufficiently for him to be given assisted washes on the third postoperative day. His skin is in good condition. His nails are well manicured and he shaved himself with an electric razor on the third postoperative day
Poor nutritional status and fluid balance due to nausea and vomiting worsened by preoperative starvation	To ensure that John's nutritional state is maintained/improved postoperatively	(1) Administer antiemetics if John is nauseated (2) Record John's height, weight and calculate his body mass index (3) Refer to dietitian if necessary (4) Offer John small but nutritionally well-balanced meals high in protein and energy (5) Encourage John to drink	(1) Patients undergoing neurosurgery become hypermetabolic and hyperglycaemic. (2) Long periods of starvation before investigations or surgery add to the problem, as weight loss and muscle breakdown ensue (Chapman, 1996) (3) Gut motility is stimulated by the presence of food in the stomach	On day 3 post-operatively, John ate 3 meals a day, but left half of what was served. Liaised with dietitian to ensure appropriate diet

Problem	Goal	Nursing intervention	Rationale	Evaluation
John suffers from raised intracranial pressure and is at risk of reduced mobility and its complications	(a) Prevent pressure ulcers (b) Prevent deep vein thrombosis (c) Prevent hypostatic pneumonia (d) Prevent muscle contractures	(1) Turn or encourage John to turn himself 2 hourly (2) Use a pressure-relieving mattress (3) Encourage John to move his feet and contract his leg muscles frequently to prevent deep vein thrombosis (4) Sit John up in bed at an angle of 30–40° to assist his respiratory function and reduce raised intracranial pressure (5) Assist John out of bed as soon as his raised intracranial pressure is lowered and his condition improves (6) Assess John's risk from pressure ulcers using the Waterlow scale (7) Put John's joints through a full range of movements twice daily and position them in a neutral position in between	(1) Poor ergonomics and prolonged length of time in one position causes the formation of pressure ulcers (2) Prevention of pressure ulcers is promoted by frequent change of position and pressure-relieving ergonomic mattresses and cushions (Waterlow, 1988) (3) Muscle activity increases blood flow in deep veins and discourages the formation of deep vein thrombosis (4) Coordinate these activities so that all nursing care is not concentrated at one time, thus producing a rise in raised intracranial pressure	John was repositioned 2 hourly on a pressure-relieving mattress until his conscious level improved and he could turn himself. John was seen by a physiotherapist once a day and his limbs were put through a full range of movements. On the 2nd post-operative day John sat out in a chair. His skin is intact and he had no signs of deep vein thrombosis, chest infection or pneumonia. Waterlow score : 9
John has raised intracranial pressure and is at risk of urinary and faecal incontinence	(a) To prevent formation of pressure ulcers (b) To maintain John's dignity (c) To monitor John's urinary output and bowel movements	(1) Change John's bed linen if wet and/or soiled (2) Use incontinence aids to prevent soiling the bed linen and protect the skin (3) Maintain John's dignity and privacy (4) Ensure sufficient intake of fluid and diet to prevent kidney failure and constipation	Patients are more anxious about the possibility of incontinence than any other aspect of care. The patient has the right to privacy and dignity. Failure to maintain an adequate diet or fluid intake causes constipation and renal problems, including renal calculi and renal failure	John received 1.5 L of fluid per 24 hours and ate segments of orange during the day in addition to his small meals

The skills required to ensure a safe recovery from anaesthesia are described in Chapter 2.

ASSESSMENT AND CLINICAL MANAGEMENT OF RAISED INTRACRANIAL PRESSURE

Raised intracranial pressure after a craniotomy is likely to be caused by a haemorrhage into the wound site, cerebral oedema or hydrocephalus. Therefore, the patient must be assessed neurologically for signs of raised intracranial pressure, which have been described earlier (see p. 136).

There are many nursing and medical measures which can be used to reduce raised intracranial pressure. The head of the bed should be raised 30–40° to aid venous drainage from the head. The patient should also be positioned so that the chin and sternum are aligned. The shoulders should be aligned with the patient's ears. This not only aids venous drainage but also prevents abnormal synergies of large muscle groups, thus enabling the patient to be positioned more easily (Palmer and Wyness, 1988).

By pacing nursing activities in order to reduce the number of times that a patient is stimulated, the nurse can ensure that the intracranial pressure does not rise to dangerously high peaks of pressure (Chudley, 1994; March et al, 1990).

Deep tracheal suction, coughing and chest physiotherapy are all activities which greatly increase intracranial pressure (Crosby and Parsons, 1992). They should only be carried out when necessary and not for long periods at any one time.

Constipation should be prevented, as straining to pass faeces causes the intracranial pressure to rise, as will a distended urinary bladder. If the patient is in pain, this should be treated, because this too can contribute to the patient's unease and raise both blood pressure and intracranial pressure.

The neurosurgical patient requires a good oxygen supply and sufficient carbon dioxide to stimulate respiration without increasing vasodilatation. The ward should be well ventilated with fresh air, and the patient should receive a continuous oxygen supply. If blood gas analysis shows the patient to have a low PaO_2 the patient will be prescribed oxygen therapy. Pulse oximetry should be carried out regularly to measure peripheral oxygen saturations (Tremper and Barker, 1989).

Care should also be taken to protect the patient from the anxiety of others. The patient's relatives and friends may be very distressed at the patient's condition and prognosis at a time when the patient may not be quite so acutely aware of his situation. They will need much sympathy and understanding. However, if their distress is making the patient restless and anxious, then shorter visits may be suggested in order for both visitor and patient to rest. They should be allowed to participate in the less technical aspects of nursing care during the visit if this will help them to adjust to the situation.

In an attempt to reduce the amount of cerebral oedema, fluids should be restricted to 1.5 L in 24 hours by all routes following craniotomy, but currently this is limited to traumatic brain injury, and even this is under review. The only exception is for patients who have had surgery for cerebral aneurysm or arteriovenous malformation, when the fluids should be increased to 3 L in 24 hours in order to prevent vasospasm.

If the cerebral oedema is causing the patient's neurological state to deteriorate, then mannitol may be prescribed. Mannitol is an osmotic diuretic which has a particularly good effect on cerebral oedema (Davis and Lucatorto, 1994).

NURSING CARE PLAN – POSTOPERATIVE CARE

An example of the care required following craniotomy is shown in Table 9.2, which is based on the care of a patient who has had a craniotomy for the removal of a frontoparietal glioma. The care plan is divided into care which is required for a patient following any craniotomy, and that required for the potential sequelae of the problem for which a craniotomy was necessary. The patient is fictitious.

The academic care plan offered is based on the Roper, Logan and Tierney (1996) model of nursing. However, nurses may well find that when the patient is nursed in the intensive care unit immediately following surgery, the Mead model of nursing is used. The Mead model is based on the Roper, Logan and Tierney model and adapted for the specific needs of intensive care nursing (McClune and Franklin, 1987).

The patient scenario

We return again to John, who has now undergone surgery for the partial removal of a right-sided frontoparietal glioma. The postoperative care plan takes up the story when John has left the intensive care unit and is now on a neurosurgical ward.

Following his surgery he is drowsy but easily roused when he is spoken to. He obeys commands slowly and has a paralysed left arm. He has lost sensation in the left arm and neglects it.

Discharge planning and patient advice

Following neurosurgery, patients are usually transferred back to the referring hospital if hospital nursing care is still required. Some patients spend little time at the referring hospital or are discharged straight into the community. It is important to start the discharge planning process as soon as the patient is admitted, so that their return to the hospital or to home is not delayed. Discharge planning is a multidisciplinary activity, especially when the patient has physical or psychological deficits which require equipment and/or particular skills from the referring hospital or the community team.

Some of the discharge issues have been incorporated in the care plan (see Table 9.2), but there are other educational and professional issues. In the case of patients with malignant brain tumours there is fear of death and loss of mental clarity to consider. For many patients there is little time to adjust to the idea before surgery. Many patients benefit from the peer support and help of tumour support groups. As the patient's condition deteriorates, the principal carers need to be supported by other agencies such as social services, palliative care specialists and the general practice staff. The aim of care then is to provide the patient with good symptom control so that the last few months of life have quality.

Some patients may not be facing a poor prognosis but have to learn to live with major disability after surgery. Those disabilities can be obvious, such as difficulty in swallowing (dysphagia), or difficulty in the use of language (dysphasia). Motor and sensory loss can be a feature, as well as less obvious signs such as perceptual loss. The patient may be unable to visually recognize objects (agnosia), suffer memory loss, or be unable to carry out a pattern of movements such as picking up a cup and drinking (dyspraxia) or calculating (dyscalculia). There are many possible neurological deficits depending on the site and nature of the lesion. All of them are bewildering and distressing to the patient, and require the specialist knowledge and skills of the neuroscience nurse and the other members of the multidisciplinary team to help the patient/relatives to overcome their problems.

CONCLUSION

The lay public often feel that all neurosurgery leads to major disability and frequently death. The degree of disability and the likelihood of death are dependent on the cause and its position in the brain. Early diagnosis and the considerable technical advances in surgical technique and follow-up care give many patients a normal life expectancy with few or no disabilities today. Where there is a poor prognosis and/or major disabilities, then the neurosurgical nurse needs to liaise with other professionals and nurses specializing in a variety of neuroscience subspecialties such as neuro-oncology and neuro-rehabilitation. Other specialists such as palliative care nurses, transplant coordinators and epilepsy nurse specialists will also play a role in the care of these patients.

Summary of key points

- Knowledge of the underlying anatomy and physiology of the brain and spinal cord will assist in the understanding of the patient's signs and symptoms.

- A clear understanding of the mechanisms of raised intracranial pressure and its medical, surgical and nursing management is essential to all cerebral surgery and its pre- and postoperative management.

- Neurosurgical nursing requires a team approach. The disabilities and fears combined with a lack of understanding of the brain and the way it performs its complex and multiple tasks are the major causes of anxiety for patient and carers.

- Nurses play a key role in the assessment of neurosurgical patients and their care planning.

- Neurosurgical nursing also requires excellent communication skills.

References

Brenner, M. & Welliver, J. (1990) Pulmonary and acid–base assessment. *Nursing Clinics of North America* 25(4): 761–770.

British Association of Parenteral and Enteral Nutrition (2003a) *'Malnutrition Universal Screening Tool' ('MUST')* [Online] Available at http://www.bapen.org.uk/pdfs/Must/MUST-Complete.pdf (accessed on 17 April 2004).

British Association of Parenteral and Enteral Nutrition (2003b) *The 'MUST' Explanatory Booklet – A Guide to the 'Malnutrition Universal Screening Tool' (MUST) for Adults.* [Online] Available at http://www.bapen.org.uk/pdfs/Must/MUST-Explanatory-Booklet.pdf (accessed on 17 April 2004).

Cammermeyer, M. & Prendergast, V. (1997) Profiles of cognitive functioning in subjects with neurological disorders. *Journal of Neuroscience Nursing* 29(5): 163–169.

Chapman, A. (1996) Current theory and practice: a study of pre-operative fasting. *Nursing Standard* 10(18): 33–36.

Cheetham, D. (1993) Pre-operative visits by ITU nurses: recommendations for practice. *Intensive and Critical Care Nursing* 9(4): 253–262.

Chudley, S. (1994) The effect of nursing activities on intracranial pressure. *British Journal of Nursing* 3(9): 454–459.

Crosby, L. J. & Parsons, C. L. (1992) Cerebrovascular response of closed head injured patients to a standardized endotracheal tube suctioning and manual hyperventilation procedure. *Journal of Neuroscience Nursing* 24(1): 40–49.

Davis, M. & Lucatorto, M. (1994) Mannitol revisited. *Journal of Neuroscience Nursing* 26(3): 170–174.

Ellis, A. & Cavanagh, S. J. (1992) Aspects of neurosurgical assessment using the Glasgow Coma Scale. *Intensive and Critical Care Nursing* 8(2): 94–99.

Harris, M. (1994) The patient in need of rehabilitation. In: Alexander, M. F., Fawcett, J. N. & Runciman, P. J. (eds) *Nursing Practice: Hospital to Home: The Adult.* Edinburgh: Churchill Livingstone.

Hickey, J. V. (ed.) (2001) *The Clinical Practice of Neurological and Neuroscience Nursing*, 5th edn. Philadelphia: Lippincott.

Hinchliff, S., Montague, S. & Watson, R. (1996) *Physiology for Nursing Practice*, 2nd edn. London: Baillière Tindall.

Holtzclaw, B. J. (1990) Shivering: a clinical nursing problem. *Nursing Clinics of North America* 25(4): 977–986.

Juarez, V. J. & Lyons, M. (1995) Interrater reliability of the Glasgow Coma Scale. *Journal of Neuroscience Nursing* 27(5): 283–286.

Kelly, R. (1994) Disorders of the mouth. In: Alexander, M. F., Fawcett, J. N. & Runciman, P. J. (eds) *Nursing Practice: Hospital to Home: The Adult.* Edinburgh: Churchill Livingstone.

Kocan, M. J. (1988) Electrocardiographic changes following subarachnoid haemorrhage. *Journal of Neuroscience Nursing* 20(6): 362–365.

Leino-Kilpi, H., Iire, L., Suominen, T., et al (1993) Client and information: a literature review. *Journal of Clinical Nursing* 2(6): 331–340.

McClune, B. & Franklin, K. (1987) The Mead Model of Nursing – adapted from Roper, Logan and Tierney's Model for Nursing. *Intensive Care Nursing* 3(3): 97–105.

McCulloch, J. (1986) Mapping dynamic functional events in the central nervous system with 2-[^{14}C]deoxyglucose radioautography. In: Trimble, M. R. (ed.) *New Brain Imaging Techniques and Psychopharmacology.* Oxford: Oxford University Press.

March, K., Mitchell, P., Grady, S. & Winn, R. (1990) Effect of backrest position on intracranial and cerebral perfusion pressures. *Journal of Neuroscience Nursing* 22(6): 375–381.

North, B. & Reilly, P. (1990) *Raised Intracranial Pressure.* London: Heinemann Medical.

Ott, L. G. & Young, B. (1991) Nutrition in the neurologically injured patient. *Nutrition in Clinical Practice* 6(6): 223–229; 231–233.

Palmer, M. & Wyness, M. A. (1988) Positioning and handling: important considerations in the care of the severely head-injured patient. *Journal of Neuroscience Nursing* 20(1): 42–49.

Reimer, M., Conrad, B., Newcommon, N. & Annear, D. (1990) Validity and usefulness of cognitive functioning tools with patients hospitalized for head injury. *Journal of Neuroscience Nursing* 22(4): 252–253.

Reinhardt, H. F., Trippel, M., Westermann, B., et al (1996) Computer assisted brain surgery for small lesions in the central sensorimotor region. *Acta Neurochirurgica* 138(2): 200–205.

Roper, N., Logan, W. & Tierney, A. (1996) *The Elements of Nursing*, 4th edn. Edinburgh: Churchill Livingstone.

Rusy, K. L. (1996) Rebleeding and vasospasm after subarachnoid haemorrhage: a critical care challenge. *Critical Care Nurse* 16(1): 41–50.

Segatore, M. (1992) Vasospasm after aneurysmal subarachnoid haemorrhage: a review of pathophysiology. *Axon* 13(4): 129–131.

Taylor, M. P. (1996) *Managing Epilepsy in Primary Care.* Oxford: Blackwell Science.

Teasdale, G. & Jennett, B. (1974) Assessment of coma and impaired consciousness. *The Lancet* (July 13): 81–84.

Tremper, K. K. & Barker, S. J. (1989) Pulse oximetry. *Anaesthesiology* 70(1): 98–108.

Waterlow, J. (1985) Pressure sores: a risk assessment card. *Nursing Times* 81(48): 49, 51, 55.

Waterlow, J. (1988) Prevention is better than cure. *Nursing Times* 84(25): 69–70.

Woodward, S. (1995) Assessment of urinary incontinence in neuroscience patients. *British Journal of Nursing* 4(5): 254–258.

Further reading

Davies, E. & Hopkins, A. (eds) (1997) *Improving Care for Patients with Malignant Glioma*. London: Royal College of Physicians of London.

Guerrero, D. (ed.) (1998) *Neuro-oncology for Nurses*. London: Whurr Publishers.

Lindsay, K. W., Bone, I. & Callander, R. (1997) *Neurology and Neurosurgery Illustrated*, 3rd edn. Edinburgh: Churchill Livingstone.

Woodward, S. (1997) Neurological Observations, part 1 Glasgow Coma Scale. *Nursing Times* 93(45): 1–2 (Suppl.).

Woodward, S. (1997) Neurological Observations, part 2 Pupil response. *Nursing Times* 93(46): 1–2 (Suppl.).

Woodward, S. (1997) Neurological Observations, part 3 Limb responses. *Nursing Times* 93(47): 1–2 (Suppl.).

Woodward, S. (1997) Neurological Observations, part 4 Case studies. *Nursing Times* 93(48): 1–2 (Suppl.).

Chapter **10**

Patients requiring ophthalmic surgery

Biddy Knight and Sue Hart

Key objectives of the chapter

At the end of the chapter, the reader will be able to:

- understand the basic structure and function of the eye

- understand the causal relationship between altered physiology and patients' visual problems

- demonstrate an awareness of the special needs of patients undergoing ophthalmic surgery

- recognize the importance of continuity of care between hospital and the community

- acknowledge the need for effective patient education.

INTRODUCTION

Nursing patients with a real or potential visual handicap requires perception, patience and good communication skills as well as the implementation of good nursing care. Elective ophthalmic surgery is increasingly carried out on a day care basis, and a greater number of patients are having surgery under local anaesthesia.

Individual ophthalmic units have their own protocols regarding patient selection for day care or overnight stay, and there should be a specialist facility for those who need longer periods of care. The actual medical and nursing care that patients receive will also vary from unit to unit, and the following discussion is intended as a guide to key principles of care.

Many patients requiring ophthalmic surgery are in the older age group and may also have other medical conditions; these facts must be considered when planning their admission, care and discharge.

Surgery can take many forms, because within the eye there are many structures that affect vision and require surgical intervention to correct or halt a decrease in visual acuity. Knowledge of the structure and function of the eye and its component parts aids understanding of the abnormalities that can occur and the operations that are performed.

STRUCTURE OF THE EYE

Both eyes consist of a globe, cushioned by orbital fat within a cone-shaped bony orbit, and protected anteriorly by the lids, lashes and tear flow.

The eye has three layers:

- sclera and cornea – outer layer
- iris, ciliary body and choroid – middle layer, also known as the uveal tract
- retina – inner layer.

SCLERA

The sclera is an opaque, dense layer of tough fibrous tissue with a high collagen content which prevents light entering the eye inadvertently. The opaque nature of the sclera is due to the haphazard positioning of the collagen fibres. It is 0.6–1 mm thick except at the insertion of the recti muscles, where it is only 0.3 mm in depth. The blood supply comes from the posterior ciliary arteries in the elastic episclera that covers the sclera. The nerve supply is derived from the ciliary branch of the oculomotor nerve.

The weakest part of the sclera is the posterior area where it is pierced by the optic nerve fibres, resulting in a sieve-like structure known as the lamina cribrosa, and where the sclera becomes continuous with the dural layer of the meninges. Anteriorly, the sclera merges with the cornea at the limbus. The sclera is a protective layer; it is more elastic in children, becoming tougher with increasing age.

CORNEA

The cornea constitutes the anterior one-sixth of the eye; it is 0.5 mm thick centrally and thicker at the periphery; it averages 12 mm × 11 mm in adults.

It is a transparent layer with a convex anterior curve, allowing the passage of light rays to focus on the retina.

It can be divided into five layers:

- Epithelium is composed of five to six layers of squamous stratified epithelium which is continuous with the epithelium of the conjunctiva, and is the only regenerative layer. Damage results in bacteria being able to penetrate corneal tissue.

- Bowman's membrane is the anterior elastic membrane, consisting of a thin layer of collagen which is tough, forming a protective layer that does not regenerate if damaged, resulting in scarring.

- Stroma accounts for 90% of corneal tissue and consists of modified collagen fibres and keratinocytes.

- Descemet's membrane is the posterior elastic membrane, acting as a barrier against invasion by microorganisms, chemicals and changes in intraocular pressure.

- Endothelium is a single layer of cells that lines the posterior surface of the cornea and 'pumps' fluid from the cornea into the anterior chamber. Interference with this function results in corneal oedema and loss of transparency.

The cornea is essentially avascular; nutrition and oxygen is obtained from the vascular arcades of the anterior ciliary arteries at the limbus, the aqueous via diffusion at the endothelium and from atmospheric oxygen. Corneal nerve supply is derived from the ophthalmic division of the trigeminal nerve.

The cornea has several functions:

- protection
- refraction: it is the most powerful refractive part of the eye, and essential to this function is corneal clarity, which is maintained by:
  - avascularity
  - uniformity of structure
  - efficient epithelial function, maintaining clarity.

IRIS

The iris is a pigmented disc with a central opening, the pupil. It is situated in front of the lens and behind the cornea, so separating the anterior and posterior chambers, and is a forward extension of the ciliary body.

There are three layers:

- endothelium
- stroma, consisting of pigmented cells, blood vessels, nerves and muscles

pigmented epithelium, continuous with the pigmented epithelium of the retina.

The colour of the iris results from the presence of melanin and is genetically predetermined. Initially, babies only have pigment in the epithelial layer, but, over the first few weeks of life, pigment is laid down in the stroma and the eyes acquire their adult colour.

There are two muscle groups in the iris: the radial dilators and the central sphincter constrictor, the latter being the more powerful. The nerve supply is derived from the short ciliary branch of the oculomotor nerve for the sphincter pupillae and from the long ciliary branch of the trigeminal nerve for the radial pupillae. The arterial capillaries of the long posterior ciliary arteries and the anterior ciliary arteries join to form a circular vascular network.

The iris acts as a regulator, controlling the amount of light that reaches the retina, and this is determined by the environment, emotion and the intensity of surrounding light.

CILIARY BODY

The ciliary body is triangular in shape and lies between the choroid and the iris. It is continuous with the iris and has numerous folds on its inner surface, the ciliary processes, where secretion of aqueous takes place.

Most of the ciliary body consists of circular and longitudinal muscle fibres whose function is to alter the shape of the lens, i.e. accommodation, by exerting an equal force on the suspensory ligaments that run from the margin of the ciliary body to the periphery of the lens.

The ciliary body can be divided into three areas:

- The pars plicata contains the 70–80 radiating strips that constitute the ciliary processes and secrete aqueous into the posterior chamber.
- The pars plana is continuous with the pars plicata.
- The ciliary muscles are situated on the anterior surface of the ciliary body and are composed of circular and longitudinal fibres. They contract and relax to bring about accommodation, resulting in light rays being focused on the retina. Contraction of the ciliary muscles results in the relaxation of the suspensory ligaments, and the lens becomes more bulbous, so increasing refraction, as when viewing near objects.

The nerve supply is derived from the short ciliary branch of the oculomotor nerve. The blood supply is the long posterior ciliary artery and vein, the anterior ciliary artery and vein and the vortex vein. The ciliary body produces and secretes aqueous, as well as altering the shape of the lens.

THE CHOROID

The choroid is a pigmented, highly vascular layer lying between the sclera and the retina. It extends from its junction with the ciliary body, the ora serrata, posteriorly to the optic disc.

It is composed of four layers:

- suprachoroid – contains elastic tissue, pigment cells and collagen
- vascular layer – large and small blood vessels supported within a pigmented stromal tissue
- choriocapillaries – capillaries
- Bruch's membrane – a protective, supporting sheath.

The nerve supply is derived from the posterior ciliary branch of the oculomotor nerve. Blood supply is from the short posterior ciliary artery and is drained away by the choroidal and vortex veins.

The choroid provides nutrients for retinal cells adjacent to the choroid, especially the rods and cones. The pigment in the choroid prevents light rays scattering and causing internal reflection of light, so aiding focusing of light rays on the retina.

THE RETINA

The retina is a complex structure consisting of 10 layers of cells, divided into two separate parts. One part is made up of nine layers, the transparent neural division; this lies on the single pigmented epithelial layer which is adjacent to the choroid (Stollery, 1997). These two parts are firmly attached to each other only at the optic disc and the ora serrata.

Three specific areas of the retina must be considered:

- The macula lies in the central area of the retina, 3 mm to the temporal side of the optic disc, and is 1.5 mm in diameter. It consists mainly of cones, and in its centre is the fovea, an area consisting entirely of cones. Macular function is to give very precise, coloured, central vision, and it lies on the visual axis.

  The rest of the retina consists of a mix of cones and rods, the latter being responsible for the perception of light and dark.

- The optic disc is found at the point where the retinal veins and nerve fibres leave the eye and the retinal artery enters. There are no light receptors in this area, so it is insensitive to light and is consequently known as the 'blind spot'.

  Once a nerve impulse is initiated, it is transmitted along the visual pathway, via the optic nerve to the occiptal cortex. Impulses from the nasal fibres of each eye cross at the optic chiasma to the branch of the optic nerve on the other side of the brain.

- The ora serrata is the anterior edge of the retina, where the retinal pigmented layer merges with the ciliary epithelium and the neural layers end.

The blood supply of the retina is derived from two main sources: the anterior one-third is from the choriocapillaries of the choroid, and the posterior two-thirds is from the central retinal artery. The retina is one of the few areas in the body where the blood vessels can be viewed directly.

The retina reacts to the presence of light and initiates impulses that are then transmitted to the visual cortex of the brain for interpretation.

THE TRANSPARENT MEDIA OF THE EYE

This consists of the cornea plus the aqueous and vitreous humours and the lens.

Aqueous fluid

Aqueous fluid consists mainly of water, with some proteins and chlorides, and is produced by the ciliary processes of the ciliary body. It is secreted into the posterior chamber and flows around the lens, through the pupil and circulates around the anterior chamber before draining via the trabecular meshwork into the canal of Schlemm and so into the venous return of the eye. Aqueous also drains out through the ciliary body into the episcleral vessels, i.e. the uveal scleral route. The openings to the trabecular meshwork are located in the drainage angle of the anterior chamber, formed by the junction of the cornea and the iris.

The aqueous is responsible for maintaining intraocular pressure at approximately 15–20 mmHg (Stollery, 1997). It nourishes the lens and posterior surface of the cornea and provides a clear medium for refraction.

Lens

The lens is a biconvex structure measuring approximately 9 mm × 4 mm, which lies between the posterior surface of the iris and the anterior surface of the vitreous. It is avascular, is not innervated, and is held in position by the suspensory ligaments or zonules.

It is composed of three parts: the elastic capsule, epithelial cells on the anterior surface and the lens substance. Lens substance consists of a nucleus, layers of protein called crystallins arranged like an onion and 'Y' sutures that mark the junction of the protein fibres. Nutrition is provided by the aqueous, and the crystallins act as enzymes to convert sugar into energy. Depending on the position of the object being viewed, the lens 'accommodates', so allowing the light rays to focus on the retina.

Vitreous

Vitreous lies between the posterior capsule of the lens and the retina, in the posterior cavity, within the hyaloid membrane. The vitreous body consists of a semigelatinous substance that is produced during embryonic life and, if lost, cannot be replaced naturally. It is avascular, is not innervated and receives nutrition from the blood vessels of the choroid, retina and ciliary body. It is attached to the ciliary body at the ora serrata and to the retina at the optic disc. The vitreous holds the retina in place, helps to maintain intraocular pressure and preserves the shape of the eye. It also assists in refraction.

EYELIDS

The eyelids act as protection for the anterior portion of the eyes, and the epithelium of the lids is continuous with the conjunctiva lining the inner aspect of the lids. Their shape and strength is maintained by cartilaginous tissue forming the upper and lower tarsal plates; within these are found the meibomian glands that secrete sebum, a substance necessary to control tear flow, lubricate the lid margins and prevent excessive evaporation of tears from the surface of the eye.

Eyelashes are situated along the lid margins and act as protective filters; they are kept supple by sebum secreted directly into the lash follicles by the glands of Zeis.

There are two main muscle groups in the eyelids: a sphincter called the orbicularis oculae, responsible for closing the eye, and the levator palpebrae, whose function is to raise the upper lid. Movement of the lids may be both voluntary and involuntary.

The nerve supply to the orbicularis muscle is from the facial nerve (7th cranial), and the oculomotor nerve (3rd cranial) supplies the levator palpebrae. The blood vessels to and from the lids are the lacrimal artery and vein, the superior and inferior medial palpebral artery and vein, and the supraorbital artery and vein.

The functions of the eyelids are to:

- protect the eyes from excessive light
- protect the eyes from foreign objects
- lubricate the anterior surface of the eye
- prevent the anterior surface of the eye from drying out, even during sleep.

THE CONJUNCTIVA

The conjunctiva is a thin, transparent mucous membrane lining the lids; it reflects back over the anterior aspect of the eye and is continuous with the corneal epithelium. The point at which the bulbar and palpebral conjunctival layers meet is known as the fornix, and there is sufficient conjunctival tissue here to allow for movement of the globe.

The nerve supply is derived from the nasociliary branch of the trigeminal nerve. There is a rich blood supply from the anterior ciliary artery and vein, the superior and inferior medial palpebral artery and vein, and conjunctival artery and vein.

The conjunctiva:

- produces the mucin layer of the tear film, so reducing the rate of tear evaporation
- facilitates movement by moistening the surface of the eye and lids
- protects the eye against damage and infection.

LACRIMAL APPARATUS

The lacrimal apparatus consists of the lacrimal gland, ducts, superior and inferior puncta and canaliculi, common canaliculus, lacrimal sac and nasolacrimal duct.

Tears are produced in the lacrimal gland, which is situated in the upper outer quadrant of the orbit, and then drain via the tear ducts onto the anterior surface of the eye. Blinking causes the tears to be distributed across the cornea, towards the puncta at the inner aspect of the eye. They then drain into the canaliculi via the puncta and collect in the lacrimal sac before draining into the nose via the nasolacrimal duct. Tears consist of water, protein, glucose, sodium, potassium, chloride, urea and lysozymes. Mucin from the goblet cells of the conjunctiva, and an oily layer from the meibomian glands, facilitate movements, slow down evaporation and prevent overflow onto the cheeks.

The nerve supply to all parts of the lacrimal apparatus is from branches of the trigeminal nerve. The blood supply to the lacrimal gland is from the lacrimal artery and vein, whereas the rest of the system is supplied by the nasal artery and vein, and the superior and inferior medial palpebral artery and vein.

The lacrimal system produces tears which:

- aid refraction by providing an optically smooth corneal surface
- lubricate the anterior surface of the eye, so easing movement
- clean dust particles from the eye
- protect against infection by the action of lysozymes.

THE ORBIT

The eye is protected by being situated in a pyramid-shaped bony cavity – the orbit. It consists of seven fused bones:

- ethmoid
- sphenoid
- frontal
- lacrimal
- zygomatic
- palatine
- maxilla.

Anteriorly, the orbit is open and its apex is positioned posteriorly. Each orbit is described as having a medial wall on the nasal side, a lateral wall, a roof and a floor, the floor and the lower part of the medial wall being the thinnest.

The orbit contains the eyeball, six extraocular muscles, ophthalmic artery and vein, the 2nd (optic), 3rd (oculomotor), 4th (trochlea), 5th (trigeminal) and 6th (abducens) cranial nerves, lacrimal gland, lacrimal sac, orbital fascia, fat and ligaments. There are three openings within the orbital wall, the largest of which is called the foramen magnum or optic foramen, and it is here that the optic nerve and ophthalmic artery enter. The bony nature of the orbit acts as a very effective protection from most trauma, except anteriorly.

EXTRAOCULAR MUSCLES

There are six muscles concerned with the movement of each eye, and they work together to give the precise coordination of movement that is essential for good vision. They are mainly voluntary, and each one is involved in all ocular movement by a balance of contraction and relaxation.

All the muscles receive their blood supply from the muscular arteries, but innervation differs from muscle to muscle:

- superior rectus – oculomotor nerve
- inferior rectus – oculomotor nerve
- medial rectus – oculomotor nerve
- inferior oblique – oculomotor nerve
- lateral rectus – abducens nerve
- superior oblique – trochlea nerve.

ASSESSMENT OF THE EYE

Whenever anybody presents with an abnormality of vision, no matter how trivial it may seem, it can cause pain and a fundamental fear of losing sight. This means that the nurse has to use all their psychological skills to reassure the individual and gain their cooperation in order to make an accurate assessment of their vision and the condition of their eye. All information gained should be clearly documented, as a written recording of all findings is a legal requirement (Elkington and Khaw, 1999).

The first element of assessment should be the measurement of vision, unless this is not feasible because of the extent of injury, acute pain, or inability to participate, e.g. due to altered level of consciousness. This is done for medical, legal and diagnostic reasons, as visual acuity is a measure of macular function.

The most common way of testing visual acuity is with a Snellen's chart. This requires the patient to read letters of varying sizes on a chart 6 m away (this excludes all but a very small amount of accommodation). The letter size indicates at what distance a normal-sighted person should be able to see it; so:

- 6/60: normal-sighted person would
    see this 60 m away
- 6/6: normal-sighted person would
    see this 6 m away.

In younger people especially, vision may be better than this: e.g. 6/5, 6/4. However, if 6/60, being the largest letter on the chart, cannot be seen, then the person's ability to count the fingers on a hand held up a metre away (CF) or the appreciation of movement (HM) are recorded. If this is not achieved, then perception of a light source is determined and recorded as perception of light (PL) or no perception of light (NPL).

Each eye should be tested individually, the worst eye first, as there may be a degree of unconscious recall. A record should be made of whether glasses or contact lenses are being worn, as an apparent discrepancy in visual acuity may occur when it is recorded next time.

Improvement in visual acuity may be achieved by using a pinhole: the patient looks at the Snellen's chart through a small pinhole, which means that light only passes along the principal visual axis of the eye and so vision is less affected by any abnormality of refraction.

Assumptions must not be made about the patients' ability to read, especially if they appear to be able to see effectively, i.e. they have negotiated their way around obstacles with ease. They may be reluctant to admit they cannot read, but this can be overcome diplomatically by using a Snellen's chart based on the letter 'E' or with pictures rather than letters. Alternatively, use of a Logmar chart (logarithm of the minimum angle of resolution) gives a more effective and precise record of visual acuity.

Near vision is tested using ordinary printer's type. Colour vision can be assessed using the Ishihara colour plates.

Visual acuity should always be measured before instilling mydriatic drops, as many of them also have a cycloplegic effect and so paralyse the ciliary muscle and alter accommodation. This also applies when assessing a patient's visual field. If visual acuity is measured following instillation of mydriatics, this must be recorded in the notes.

A basic assessment of visual field can be done by asking the patient to say when they can see an object moving in from the side while focusing on a central object. More precise results can be obtained by using a perimetry machine, which plots peripheral vision by moving a target across a semicircle marked out in degrees. Computerized field analysers are also capable of interpreting results related to the intensity of light needed to stimulate retinal activity.

Mydriatics should not be used when raised intraocular pressure is suspected, as dilating the pupil decreases the amount of aqueous being drained and will increase intraocular pressure even more.

Intraocular pressure is measured most accurately by the use of an applanation tenometer attached to a slit lamp; as this requires the applanator head to be pushed against the cornea, local anaesthetic drops should always be instilled prior to use. Patients who cannot be positioned at a slit lamp can have their intraocular pressures measured using a handheld tonometer, such as a TonoPen. If this apparatus is not available, the presence of raised intraocular pressure may be identified by means of careful digital palpation, but this must be done with great care and never when a perforating injury is suspected.

Examination of the eye itself must be carried out systematically, and with the cooperation of the patient. If the patient is photophobic, a darkened environment will facilitate matters. The process of examination may be along the following lines.

1. The patient's head posture is noted, as abnormal positioning may indicate lid malalignment, squints or deficits of the visual field.

2. The actual appearance of the face must be observed for any asymmetry, lacerations, skin disorders or bruising.

3. The lids should be examined for signs of inadequate closure, abnormal tearflow, ability to open the eye, alignment of the lid margins, position of the lashes, swelling, and for any crusting or exudate along the lid margins.

4. The patient should be seated with their head well supported, and analgesic drops, e.g. proxymethocaine 0.5%, oxybuprocaine 0.4% or amethocaine 0.5–1% instilled if further examination would be difficult due to the level of ocular discomfort, and there are no other contraindications such as a possible perforating injury.

5. While the anaesthetic is taking effect, careful explanation of the examination should be given, and a detailed history of the condition/trauma must be obtained.

6. Once the eyes can be seen, their position within the orbits should be noted to ensure that there is no displacement and that both eyes are able to move together in parallel, horizontal and vertical planes. Any instance of double vision, i.e. diplopia, must be recorded and reported.

7. Once the patient is comfortable and able to open their eyes, a bright light source (using a slit lamp or a pen torch) is used to examine the eyes themselves, commencing with the less affected one.

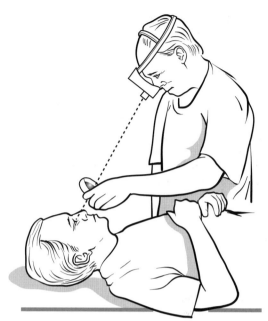

Figure 10.1   Indirect ophthalmoscopy.

Care must be taken to continue the systematic examination by beginning with the outer aspect of the eye and then going on to the internal structures, to ensure an accurate assessment of the condition of the eye.

- *Conjunctiva* – observe for lacerations, degree and position of vascular injection, oedema (chemosis), foreign bodies, naevus, pinguecula and pterygium.

- *Cornea* – note any lacerations, foreign bodies, surface anomalies and the degree of corneal clarity. Identification of superficial damage may be assisted by the instillation of fluorescein sodium 2% drops, as the damaged area will then appear bright green when illuminated. Rose bengal 1% drops may also be used, as they stain all dead corneal tissue pink. If the patient complains of seeing haloes around lights, this may indicate the presence of corneal oedema.

- *Anterior chamber* – by shining the beam of light in at an angle, it is possible to estimate the depth of the anterior chamber. It is also important to note whether the chamber is clear or contains red or white cells and, if these are present, whether they are settled with a specific level or diffuse throughout the chamber.

- *Iris* – it should be examined for any obvious bleeding points, any abnormal pigmentation, and to ensure that it is moving freely and equally in all directions, and is intact and in position.

- *Pupil* – both pupils should be examined to verify the existence of a consensual response and equality of

size. Their shape, size and briskness of movement should also be recorded. The pupil should be black in colour unless there is a reflection from the retina, in which case the pupil appears red. Sometimes the pupil may appear white, possibly indicating the presence of a cataract.

- *Retina* – the optic disc may be examined using a direct ophthalmoscope through a normal-sized pupil, but in order for the whole retina, especially the periphery, to be examined, the pupil needs to be dilated using mydriatic drops. The most efficient way of then examining the retina is with an indirect ophthalmoscope (Fig. 10.1).

Apart from the overall examination of the eye, more specific investigations may be carried out:

- Keratometry: measurement of the curvature of the cornea.
- Fluorescein angiography: injection of fluorescein dye, which allows the retinal vessels to be visualized.
- Gonioscopy: examination of the drainage angle.
- Biometry: measurement of the axial length of the eye.
- Ultrasound, which has a range of uses, including measurement of blood flow and exclusion of retinal detachment/tear or tumour in the presence of opacity in the transparent media obscuring direct observation.
- Corneal topography: maps the corneal surface.
- Pachymetry: measures the corneal thickness.

- Amsler grid test: monitors macular degeneration.
- Exophthalmometry: measures degree of proptosis.
- Refraction: determines strength of refractive elements of the eye.

PREOPERATIVE ASSESSMENT

An increasing proportion of ophthalmic patients are being cared for as day cases. The decision about whether patients are suitable for day surgery or will need to stay in hospital is made at the preoperative assessment clinic, and in most ophthalmic units these are now nurse-led sessions. Each day surgery unit has its own criteria for determining what care each patient will need, but some investigations and issues are common to all.

Most units require patients having day surgery to fulfil certain criteria (see Ch. 3). If the criteria are met, the patient's medical condition is monitored for suitability for local anaesthesia.

- The patient must be able to cooperate: for example, be capable of lying down and keeping still for a period of 30–40 minutes.
- Any medical condition, e.g. diabetes mellitus or hypertension, is well controlled.

Specific ophthalmic investigations will depend on the type of surgery being undertaken. For cataract surgery with lens implant, keratometry will be undertaken to measure the curvature of the cornea, and biometry to measure the length of the eye's axis. These two measurements allow the required strength of the implant to be determined. If the patient requires surgery for glaucoma, a series of recordings of their intraocular pressure may be taken. This is known as phasing and usually takes place over a 12-hour period.

Careful observation of the eyes should be made, especially with patients having intraocular surgery, as any local infection must be treated prior to admission. These assessments normally take place 2–4 weeks prior to admission, and any community support required postoperatively needs to be identified and arranged at this stage.

PRE- AND POSTOPERATIVE CARE OF PATIENTS UNDERGOING INTRAOCULAR SURGERY

Care needs to be planned systematically, either based around a nursing model such as Orem (1985), which emphasizes self-care, or Roper, Logan and Tierney (1996), which sees surgical intervention as an episode in life and looks for the actual and potential problems related to the activities of living, or increasingly through the use of integrated care pathways (ICPs). Planned ophthalmic surgery lends itself to ICPs, as the patient's journey is usually clearly defined and so fits Middleton et al's (2000:1) definition of an integrated care pathway:

> A multidisciplinary outline of anticipated care, placed in an appropriate timeframe, to help a patient with a specific condition or set of symptoms move progressively through a clinical experience to positive outcomes.

Well-designed integrated care pathways also make clear links between locally delivered care and the best-available evidence base (Clark, 2003).

The areas identified in the discussion on pre- and postoperative care are only meant as a guide (Tables 10.1 and 10.2), and focus on patients having their surgery under general anaesthesia, but they can be adapted to take type of anaesthesia, medical condition, degree of visual handicap and social background into account. The patient and carers should be involved if they so wish, and the design and use of care plans/ICPs should take into account the marked possibility that the patient may have difficulty reading, so time will be needed to discuss it with them.

CLEANING THE EYE

The eye should only be cleaned if there is exudate/secretions along the lid margins. The patient should be positioned comfortably, with their head well supported in a chair with a suitable head rest, or on a couch or bed.

If both eyes require cleaning, they are cleaned one at a time, and if there is any sign of infection, separate packs should be used for each eye, and the potentially infected eye should be cleaned second.

If a patient is known to have an infected eye, their eyes should not be cleaned until after all other dressings have been completed, and, if at all possible, they should be cared for by a nurse who is not responsible for any pre- or postoperative ophthalmic patients, so as to reduce the risk of cross-infection.

The cleaning is carried out using lint/gauze soaked in normal saline 0.9% or cooled boiled water. Sterile packs containing lint/gauze squares, cotton buds, gallipot and a paper towel are usually available. The towel is used to either dry the nurse's hands after washing or to protect the patient's clothing. The eye is cleaned using a lint/gauze square folded into four, with the fluffy side of the lint square innermost, so as to prevent strands being left in the eye, causing irritation.

Table 10.1   Preoperative care for patients undergoing intraocular surgery

Patient's problems	Intervention	Outcome
Communication		
New surroundings and unfamiliar routine	Introduce to staff and other patients. Orient patient and family to ward and explain expected course of events up to and including discharge	Well-oriented, relaxed patient; informed patient and family
Decreased vision and possible loss of independence	Explain that surgery may improve/maintain vision	Patient optimistic about outcome of surgery
Fear of anaesthesia and surgery	Explain exactly what is going to happen prior to, during and after surgery	Patient understands events
Maintaining a safe environment		
Potential risk of wrong operation	Check consent form has been signed and understood by patient	Correct operation performed
Potential risk of peri- and postoperative complications	Instil prescribed topical medication such as miotics, mydriatics or antibiotics. Give prescribed systemic premedication. Follow unit's preoperative protocol	Surgery is performed without complications
Potential risk of deterioration in a pre-existing medical condition	After consultation with medical/anaesthetic staff, give necessary medication, e.g. insulin, hypotensive agents. Initiate supportive therapy, e.g. physiotherapy. Facilitate patient's involvement in own care	No deterioration in medical condition
Risk of corneal abrasion due to loss of sensation, secondary to application of local anaesthetic drops	Keep the eye closed under a carefully applied eyepad. Examine for signs of corneal trauma	Cornea is not abraded

Table 10.2   Postoperative care following intraocular surgery

Patient's problem	Intervention	Outcome
Breathing		
Potential difficulty with breathing	Check that patient is able to maintain own airway. Position patient comfortably and encourage effective breathing	Adequate respirations and no acquired chest infection
Maintaining a safe environment		
Difficulty with maintaining own safety	Frequently assess orientation of patient, reorientate as required. Educate staff and visitors about the importance of keeping things in the same place and avoiding leaving objects around that may cause injury or confusion. Inform all appropriate departments and staff of patient's visual handicap. Adjust lighting to suit individual needs; dark glasses may be worn as required	Orientated patient, able to look after self
Potential problem of ocular pain/discomfort	Observe for signs of pain/discomfort. Offer prescribed analgesics. Monitor effect of analgesics. Report unrelieved or severe pain to the medical staff	Patient states that they are comfortable
Potential risk of delayed recovery due to ocular complications	Systematic examination of eye(s), identifying significant abnormalities.	Uneventful recovery

(Continued)

Table 10.2 (*Continued*)

Patient's problem	Intervention	Outcome
	Cleanse eye as required. Advise patient not to rub or wipe eye with used handkerchief/tissue. Instil, or educate patient/family to instil, prescribed eye medication. If necessary, apply 'shield' to eye to avoid inadvertent rubbing	
Risk of corneal abrasion due to loss of sensation secondary to application of local anaesthetic drops	Keep the eye closed under a carefully applied eyepad. Examine for signs of corneal trauma	Cornea is not abraded
Communication Difficulty due to poor vision reducing impact of non-verbal communication	Emphasize the importance of appropriate touch. Use tone of voice to reinforce message. Approach patient from the side with most vision and speak as approaching	To establish an effective rapport between nurse and patient. Patient is not startled
Anxiety regarding success	Adequate information is given and questions answered	Patient is aware of surgery
Mobilization Difficulty with mobilization due to: anaesthesia; visual acuity	Degree of mobilization varies, depending upon operation and surgeon's preference, but should be as soon as possible. Walking aids to be accessible and call bell within patient's reach	Preoperative level of mobility restored. Patient mobilizes safely
Eating and drinking Difficulty with eating and drinking due to: poor vision; effects of anaesthesia	Assist with selection of food and dietary intake. Observe for signs of nausea. Give antiemetic as required	Balanced diet eaten to facilitate healing. Patient does not vomit, and subsequent raised intraocular pressure does not weaken the incision
Working and playing Potential problem of being unable to return to normal lifestyle	With the involvement and cooperation of patient and family/carer, an effective discharge plan (see p. 186) is devised and implemented	Patient is confident to return home

The swab is held by the cut edges, the folded edges being used to actually clean along the lid margin. This further reduces the likelihood of particles being left along the margins.

The lid margins are cleaned from the inner canthus outwards, avoiding any potential infective agents being swept into the lacrimal drainage system via the puncti. Care should also be taken to avoid contact with the cornea, as this may cause the eyes to close involuntarily, due to pain, and may also result in corneal abrasion. Each swab is used once and then discarded; four to six swabs are usually sufficient for this procedure.

If an eyepad is required, the eye must be closed and the pad applied firmly, as contact between the cornea and the pad will result in a corneal abrasion. This is especially important if local anaesthetic drops have been instilled.

INSTILLATION OF EYE MEDICATION

Eye medications are usually prescribed in two main topical forms: drops or guttae (G.) or ointment or oculentum (Oc.).

Eye medication is usually instilled into the lower fornix, the 'gutter', which is formed by gently pulling down the lower lid. Drops are placed in the middle of the fornix, avoiding the puncti, as this can result in a dry mouth and unpleasant taste caused by the drops draining away via the lacrimal system. The eye dropper should not come into contact with the corneal surface, but should not be held too far away, as this increases the force with which the drop touches the eye, causing a sudden reflex squeezing which may increase intraocular pressure and so threaten the integrity of the incision, if present. This may also occur if the drops cause a stinging sensation, so the patient should be warned if the drops being instilled are known to sting.

Ointments are squeezed gently into the inner aspect of the fornix, being careful not to touch the eye with the nozzle of the tube. Only a small amount should be applied and the eye then closed gently; any excess should then be wiped away. Ointment may create a film across the surface of the cornea and so blur vision, which can concern the patient, so they should be made aware of this.

Contact between the dropper/nozzle and the cornea can result in a corneal abrasion, so any complaints of pain should be noted and the eye examined.

CORNEAL GRAFT (KERATOPLASTY)

A corneal graft is replacement of scarred or degenerative corneal tissue by healthy tissue. This is a less complicated procedure than organ transplant, because of corneal avascularity, although this may have been compromised by new vessel growth from the corneal margins.

Corneal tissue can be obtained in three ways:

- *Autogenous* – when the patient's other eye is blind, but has a healthy cornea, the eye can be enucleated to provide donor material.

- *Live donor* – when another patient has undergone enucleation, but the cornea is healthy, it can be used as donor material for someone requiring a graft.

- *Cadaver* – this is the most common and is the grafting of corneal tissue from donated eyes following death. Donated eyes should be removed within 24 hours of death and can be stored in short-term storage media for 3–7 days at 4°C, or for up to 30 days in an organ culture system at 34°C (United Kingdom Transplant Support Service Authority, 1995).

Removal of donor material is subject to the Human Tissue Act (DHSS, 1961).

Although most people are suitable donors, there are some exceptions, amongst which are:

- infections such as methicillin-resistant *Staphylococcus aureus*, HIV, hepatitis A, B and C, syphilis, and septicaemia
- unexplained neurological disease, because of the risk of infections such as Creutzfeldt–Jakob's disease
- leukaemia, lymphoma and myeloma
- eye conditions such as uveitis, retinoblastoma, history of intraocular surgery and malignancies of the ciliary body and iris
- jaundice
- death due to unknown cause, although donation may take place after a postmortem has been carried out.

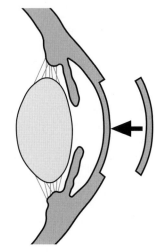

Figure 10.2 Lamellar keratoplasty.

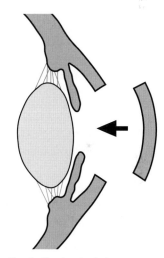

Figure 10.3 Penetrating keratoplasty.

Types of corneal graft

Lamellar
This is a partial-thickness graft that involves replacement of the opaque corneal tissue down to the level of Descemet's layer (Fig. 10.2). It is used when scarring is superficial or to maintain the integrity of the eye. The risk of rejection is decreased as the endothelium is not involved (Kanski, 2003).

Penetrating
This is the replacement of all five corneal layers (Fig. 10.3).

Reasons for corneal grafting

Reasons for corneal grafting are:

1. keratoconus
2. Fuchs' and other corneal dystrophies
3. bullous keratopathy
4. corneal scarring due to trauma or infection
5. herpes simplex keratitis
6. corneal melting syndromes/desmetocoeles
7. interstitial keratitis.

Specific preoperative care

Prior to preparing the patient for surgery, arrangements should be made with one of the eye banks, such as Bristol or Manchester, to check availability of donor material and arrange for its delivery.

Surgery is usually carried out under a general anaesthetic, and, provided the patient has attended for preassessment, they will be admitted on the day of surgery, having fasted for 4 hours. Patients may need considerable psychological support, as, for some of them, it may be the last chance of achieving useful vision. Topical medication consists of a miotic such as guttae pilocarpine 4% every 15 minutes for 1 hour. This constricts the pupil, and the iris acts as a protective barrier for the lens, so avoiding the risk of inadvertent cataract formation.

Specific postoperative care

The eye is examined before instillation of any topical medication, for the following:

- position of graft and integrity of sutures
- depth of anterior chamber
- presence of red cells, known as a hyphaema
- presence of white cells, known as a hypopyon
- clarity of cornea.

If the condition of the eye is satisfactory, prescribed medication may be given, but, if there is any cause for concern, medication should be withheld until medical opinion is sought.

Topical medication usually consists of:

- an antibiotic: e.g. guttae chloramphenicol 0.5% three to four times a day
- an anti-inflammatory: e.g. guttae dexamethasone 1% three to four times daily
- a mydriatic: e.g. guttae Mydrilate (cyclopentolate) 1% twice a day may be given, as this dilates the pupil and rests the eye.

When opacification has been due to viral infection, systemic antiviral agents may be prescribed to reduce the risk of recurrence (Kanski, 2003).

Provided the suture line is not leaking aqueous, no dressing need be applied, but the eye may feel uncomfortable because of the presence of the sutures, although the discomfort does decrease as the corneal epithelium regenerates over them. The level of discomfort can be reduced by wearing dark glasses or a cartello shield.

Discharge home may take place on the actual day of operation, providing the condition of the eye and home circumstances are acceptable.

Complications of corneal graft

1. Loose sutures lead to escape of aqueous. This can be proved by Seidel's test, which demonstrates the passage of fluorescein from the exterior to the interior of the eye, and also by the presence of a flat anterior chamber.
2. Damage to the lens at the time of surgery results in cataract formation.
3. Postoperative infection may occur.
4. Adhesions, known as synechiae, form between the iris and edge of the graft, and may result in blockage of the drainage angle, leading to postkeratoplasty glaucoma.
5. Iris prolapse can result if the iris herniates through the incision.
6. Rejection of graft may be 'early' or 'late' – 90% of grafts are successful and early rejection is unusual, but the highest risk is within the first 6 months (Kanski, 2003). The risk increases if the eye has been grafted before.
7. Astigmatism is caused by the tension of the sutures and size of the graft altering the curvature of the cornea. Rigid contact lenses may be prescribed following removal of sutures.
8. Growth of new blood vessels, neovascularization, around the graft can obscure vision if growth continues across the centre of the graft.

The cornea is avascular; therefore, healing takes considerably longer and the sutures may not be removed for up to 12 months. In the elderly, healing may take even longer. Removal of sutures is normally carried out under slit lamp illumination in the outpatient department, but if it is too uncomfortable for the patient, especially if a continuous suture has been used, then general anaesthesia may be considered.

REFRACTIVE SURGERY

The cornea and lens are the principal refracting structures of the eye. Until now, refractive errors have been corrected with lenses or spectacles, but, increasingly, people are opting to resolve the situation permanently, through surgery, as the procedure has become safer and more readily available in the last few years. The underlying principle involves altering the curvature of the cornea: flattening in myopia and making it steeper in hypermetropia, although the latter is less common.

The approaches are:

- radical keratotomy – involves making radial incisions in the peripheral cornea and is used for low degrees of myopia.
- laser in-situ keratomileusis (LASIK) – corrects refractive errors of hypermetropia, astigmatism and myopia.
- photorefractive keratectomy (PRK) – involves using a laser to remove specific areas of corneal tissue.

PENETRATING INJURIES

Any patient who gives a history of a sharp object entering the eye must be examined to exclude the possibility of a perforating injury, and lacerations to the globe need urgent admission to hospital and, usually, emergency surgery. Where possible, suspected perforating injuries should be treated in a specialist ophthalmic unit, as inexperience may result in a poorer visual outcome for the patient.

The commonest sites for such injuries are the sclera, cornea or corneoscleral junction, and they may range in severity from a slight puncture wound to a full-thickness laceration. Minor corneal perforations may heal themselves or resolve quickly following the application of a soft contact lens that acts as a 'bandage'. This has the advantage of maintaining the integrity of the eye without suturing, so reducing the risk of further scarring.

More severe injuries must be treated promptly, as they can potentially result in iris prolapse, damage to the lens, intraocular bleeding resulting in a hyphaema, and the possibility of secondary glaucoma, and infection. Scleral perforation may lead to uveal damage, and uveal and vitreous prolapse. Gross perforating injury often leads to damage to and disorganization of most of the contents of the eye. The most common causes of penetrating injury are broken glass or pieces of metal travelling at speed, as in hammer, chisel and lathe injuries, and this type of injury is 3 times more common in young males than females (Kanski, 2003).

The incidence has decreased since the mandatory wearing of seat belts and the advent of safety glass for windscreens, but even though the Health and Safety at Work Act (HSE, 1992) requires goggles to be worn when working with certain tools and machines, many people ignore the law. Some medical conditions may result in corneal perforation: for example, corneal ulceration and melting syndromes such as Mooren's ulcer.

The complications associated with perforating injuries mean that it is very important to take a detailed and accurate history and carry out a careful assessment. The latter may not be easy, as the eye is likely to be extremely painful; a local anaesthetic such as amethocaine drops can be given once the possibility of glass being present in the eye has been excluded. In some cases the pain may be so great that a systemic analgesic such as intramuscular morphine is necessary, and occasionally a full examination will only be possible under a general anaesthetic.

Sometimes, the perforation can be visualized, but the nurse or doctor carrying out the examination should also look for an anterior chamber that is shallower than the unaffected eye, indicating aqueous leaking out, hyphaema, abnormally shaped pupil or absence of part of the iris, amongst other things. The eye may also feel soft, and great care must be taken not to exert pressure on the eye, as this may increase the degree of damage.

It is necessary to determine whether the object that caused the injury is still in or on the eye. The person carrying out the examination cannot rely on the presence of a foreign body sensation, as this may be due solely to the damage to the corneal or scleral surface. If the object cannot be visualized, then an X-ray may be ordered to ascertain where the object is located, especially if there is reason to think it is in the eye itself. The X-rays should be taken at upward gaze, downward gaze and looking straight ahead, since, if there is an intraocular foreign body, it will move with the direction of gaze and so eliminate any radiological artefact. X-rays do not usually identify glass foreign bodies, unless the glass has a lead content. Once a definitive diagnosis has been made, then surgical intervention will probably be necessary to repair the perforation.

A metallic foreign body may be removed by using a magnet to draw the object back along its entry path; however, if the substance, from the history obtained, is thought to be inert, it may be left, as removal may cause more damage to adjacent structures.

At this early stage, the patient will need considerable psychological support, as it is extremely difficult to predict what the ultimate visual outcome will be. The cornea is an avascular structure, so it takes longer to heal, and consequently the lens or sutures used to close the perforation may be left in for up to 6 months. In cases where the perforation is relatively minor and does not affect other structures, mobilization and discharge will be quite rapid, provided that there is no sign of aqueous leakage.

Specific postoperative care

Following surgery for more extensive wounds, the treatment will vary depending upon the extent of the injury and the parts of the eye involved. Psychological care is very important, because vision may be affected by actual trauma, bleeding into the vitreous or aqueous, or by the local medication being used. However, nursing and medical intervention may include the following aspects:

- The eye may be padded for 12–24 hours, depending on the surgeon's instructions. It is inadvisable to keep the eye padded for any longer than is necessary, as this provides a warm, moist environment that encourages bacterial growth. Dark glasses or a plastic cartello shield may be worn for protection and to decrease photophobia. If the latter is a marked problem, then it may be possible to have subdued lighting in the bed area.

- Cleaning of the eye should take place as often as is necessary to maintain comfort, as an irritable eye may result in the patient rubbing it and causing further trauma.

- Examination of the eye should note if there is blood present in the anterior chamber, how deep the chamber is and whether the pupil is the shape that it was at the end of surgery. If any iris was found to be missing or had to be removed during surgery, this should be recorded in the notes, and the appearance of the eye can be checked against the operation notes.

- Medication will be both local and systemic and, in the case of eyedrops, is likely to be given intensively for the first 72 hours. The types of drug that may be given are:
  - antibiotics: e.g. cefuroxime or ceftazidime drops every hour. In severe cases, intravenous ceftazidime may be given for 5 days, otherwise oral ceftazidime, 750 mg twice daily for 5–7 days.
  - anti-inflammatories: e.g. dexamethasone drops decrease the swelling that results from the injury and the surgery and so reduce the risk of increasing intraocular pressure, decreases pain, and minimizes the risk of sympathetic ophthalmitis.
  - mydriatic/cycloplegic: e.g. drops such as atropine dilate the pupil and paralyse the ciliary muscle, so inhibiting accommodation and fixing the lens at distant focus, so resting the eye.

- If blood is seen in the anterior or vitreous chamber, the patient may be nursed sitting upright, or in a chair if they are more comfortable. This allows the blood to settle to the bottom of the chamber, a process that is much more rapid in the anterior chamber than in the vitreous, as is the actual absorption of the blood. Any signs of increased intraocular pressure, such as an increasingly hazy cornea, pain and redness around the corneal margin, must be reported, as blood cells can block the entrance to the trabecular meshwork and so decrease aqueous drainage. Sudden aggressive movement should also be avoided as this may cause a recurrence of the bleeding.

Irritation to the eye caused by inflamed conjunctival and corneal surfaces, plus the presence of minute sutures, can result in epiphora and excessive tear production, and the patient may feel the need to be constantly wiping the eye(s). This is potentially problematical, as it may lead to corneal abrasion, introduce infective organisms or put undue pressure on the wound. Patients should be educated to use disposable tissues once only, and to wipe below the lower lid, not on the eye itself. The problem can be eased by wearing dark glasses and the application of a small lint square/dental roll to the cheek immediately below the lower lid margin to act as a 'drip pad'.

Discharge arrangements

Discharge will be arranged when the wound is secure and bleeding has resolved and the level of pain can be controlled. The frequency of outpatient appointments will depend on the degree of injury and be determined by the consultant. The length of time for which these appointments carry on will depend upon the rate of recovery and the actual and potential risk of complications.

Complications of a penetrating injury

Complications include:

- *Panophthalmitis*: occurs when the intraocular infection involves the sclera (Lebowitz et al, 2001).

- *Cataract formation*: as a result of damage to the lens capsule, water is absorbed into the lens matter, which becomes opaque.

- *Corneal scarring*: the clear corneal tissue scars as a result of either the injury itself or the sutures used to repair the injury. Scarring is inevitable if the injury penetrates beyond Bowman's membrane (Trevor-Roper, 1974).

- *Astigmatism*: following injury and repair, the curvature of the corneal surface can be altered by scarring or suture tension, so disrupting refraction.

- *Retinal detachment*: this may result from direct retinal trauma, traction from a vitreous haemorrhage or a loss of pressure within the eye.

- *Secondary glaucoma*: a rise in intraocular pressure due to occlusion of the drainage angle by red blood cells, white blood cells or scar tissue, or damage to the trabecular meshwork/Canal of Schlemm.
- *Recurrent uveitis*: inflammation of the iris, ciliary body and choroid can be potentiated by the trauma itself, surgery or the presence of foreign bodies, or tissue material not normally in contact with the uveal tract.
- *Phthisis bulbi*: atrophy of the entire globe that is secondary to a non-functioning ciliary body, resulting in loss of aqueous production. The shrunken eye is sightless and painless.
- *Siderosis*: following injuries caused by iron fragments, deposits of iron are dissolved in the aqueous and vitreous and stain the surrounding tissues.
- *Sympathetic ophthalmitis*: this is a rare complication that may occur any time after the first 2 weeks following injury, even years later. It is a bilateral uveitis, probably resulting from an immune response to damage to the uveal tract, which exposes antigens unfamiliar to the body's defence mechanisms and so leads to their destruction; the same process then takes place in the uninjured eye (James et al, 2003).

Although these conditions are in order of probability (Kanski, 2003), incidence will depend on the site and severity of the injury. If an eye is very badly injured, with no perception of light, and cosmesis is a problem, enucleation within 9 days of the injury minimizes the risk of sympathetic ophthalmitis. If the condition does occur, then enucleation of the damaged, 'exciting' eye may be carried out.

CATARACT

A cataract is an opacity of the lens, which may interfere with vision. It results from denaturation of the lens protein, which may be caused by changes within the lens itself or by the lens capsule becoming no longer selectively semipermeable.

The lens epithelium continues to produce cell layers throughout life, so it increases in size. It is thought that, as the nutrients from the aqueous become less readily available to the lens nucleus, it hardens and accommodation becomes more difficult. This results in less efficient near vision, a condition known as 'presbyopia', which normally starts in middle age (Perry and Tullo, 1995).

In some people, lens changes continue, resulting in further deterioration of visual acuity, leading to loss of definition and colour appreciation, progressing to virtual blindness if not treated. During the development of the cataracts, vision may vary depending upon the light. Most difficulties arise in bright sunlight or at night, when headlights are being used. Cataracts are usually bilateral, one eye tending to be worse than the other and are generally painless, unless the lens absorbs enough water from the aqueous to cause a marked increase in size, which can result in an increase in intraocular pressure, i.e. secondary glaucoma.

Causes of cataract

There are several causes of cataract formation:

1. *Senile*: these are the most common, which are the result of the ageing process, and are more likely to develop in people with late-onset diabetes mellitus.
2. *Traumatic*: these can occur as a result of a 'blunt' injury, when a direct blow to the eye can cause a cataract by concussion; or after a penetrating injury, which results in perforation of the lens capsule, allowing aqueous to seep into the lens matter. Traumatic cataracts can develop very quickly, the opacity becoming apparent within 12–24 hours.
3. *Metabolic*: cataracts can develop quickly in individuals with insulin-dependent diabetes mellitus (Kanski, 1994). They may also occur in people with hypoparathyroidism, as a result of a rise in calcium levels in the lens.
4. *Inflammation*: local inflammation due to intraocular infection or chronic anterior uveitis causes changes in the lens function. Inflammation may also be secondary to skin disorders, e.g. rosacea.
5. *Congenital*: this can be secondary to maternal rubella, normally within the first trimester, or to the absorption of drugs across the placental barrier.
6. *Genetic*: this may be a manifestation of Down's syndrome or can be one of the consequences of an enzyme deficiency that causes galactosaemia.
7. *Drugs*: long-term medication using drugs such as steroids and thyroxine can lead to lens opacity.
8. *Radiation*: ionizing radiation, especially if the patient is undergoing treatment for malignancies of the head and neck.

Types of surgery

To re-establish normal visual acuity, it is necessary to remove the opaque lens and replace it with some means of optical correction. This can range from insertion of an artificial lens in the eye, usually in the posterior chamber, to the fitting of corneal contact lenses, or to the wearing of glasses. These methods all correct aphakia, the condition of having no lens; the intraocular lens (Fig. 10.5) is the most efficient, as the focal distance is not altered, whereas aphakic glasses give only a central field of vision and a considerable degree of magnification.

The type of surgery is categorized by the way in which it is carried out.

Lens aspiration/lensectomy

This is used for removing congenital cataracts, as they have a soft nucleus that allows the lens matter to be sucked out through an incision in the anterior lens capsule. Any remaining lens matter is absorbed by the enzymes in the aqueous, and the posterior capsule is left in place. The latter is initially clear, but may become opaque, in which case a capsulotomy is performed, using a YAG laser, to allow light rays to pass to the retina. This operation must be carried out as early as possible, as failure to do so can result in amblyopia.

Extracapsular extraction

This is the technique of choice, since, by leaving the posterior capsule in place, there is less risk of vitreous loss and subsequent retinal damage. An incision is made in the anterior lens capsule, and the hardened nucleus is lifted out and as much as possible of the soft lens matter is removed by irrigation with saline (Fig. 10.4).

Phacoemulsification is the most commonly used technique of extracapsular extraction and is the preferred method of cataract removal in the Western world (James et al, 2003). A 'stab' incision allows the phacoemulsifier to be passed into the lens, and high-frequency vibrations cause the hard nucleus to emulsify, allowing the lens contents to be 'sucked' out through an extraction tube which is part of the probe. The benefits of phacoemulsification, as opposed to a standard extracapsular extraction, are that healing is more rapid, less astigmatism occurs and improved vision is achieved in a shorter length of time (Kanski, 2003).

Intracapsular extraction

This used to be the most common method of cataract extraction, but due to advances in surgical technique, extracapsular is the preferred method, as the incision is smaller and there is less risk of postoperative complications.

The lens is removed in its entirety, and this is facilitated by the fact that, in an older person, the suspensory ligaments are weaker and can be easily broken to aid removal (Fig. 10.6).

Specific preoperative care

Surgery should be offered at the point at which the individual's lifestyle is affected by their decrease in visual acuity – although, in reality, it is usually at this time that patients are added to the waiting list for surgery.

Extracapsular cataract surgery (non-phacoemulsification)

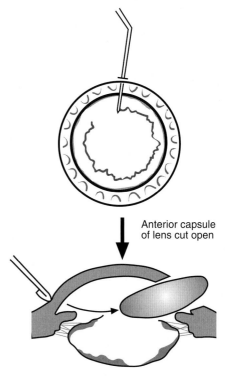

Anterior capsule of lens cut open

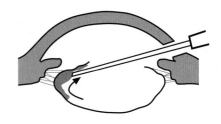

Nucleus of lens expressed from capsular bag

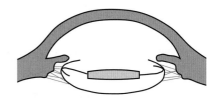

Lens remnants in capsule bag aspirated

Artificial lens implanted in capsular bag

Figure 10.4 Extracapsular extraction.

Patients may be treated as day cases or stay in overnight. If they are having surgery under a general anaesthetic, then local protocols are followed and the only specific care is that the pupil of the affected eye is well dilated, to facilitate access to the lens. This is done by using mydriatic drops such as Ocufen (flurbiprofen

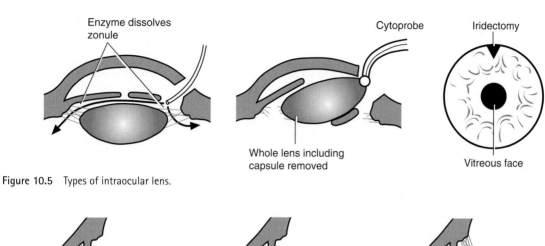

Figure 10.5   Types of intraocular lens.

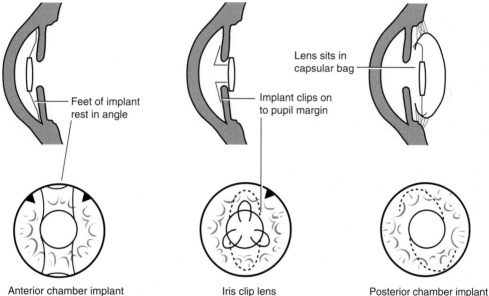

Figure 10.6   Intracapsular extraction.

sodium) 1%, mydrilate (cyclopentolate) 1%, phenyle-phrine 2.5–10% and homatropine 2% in varying combinations depending upon the surgeon's wishes. In addition, if local anaesthesia is used, drops such as amethocaine 1% may be administered topically, either on the ward or in theatre. Sedation may sometimes be given, but is avoided where possible, as there is a risk of the patient falling asleep and then waking with a 'start' during the operation.

Specific postoperative care

On return from surgery, blood pressure and pulse are recorded, and these observations are continued at the nurse's discretion. The patient may rest in whichever position they find most comfortable, unless specifically requested otherwise by the surgeon. Most patients can be mobile as soon as it is safe for them to do so; it is usually the effect of sedation that necessitates their resting for a period of time. Patients may eat and drink as soon as they like, unless they are feeling nauseated or the anaesthetist gives instructions to the contrary.

The eye is usually covered, either with a pad and shield, or simply with a shield. If the patient has had surgery to what is effectively their only eye, a transparent shield should be applied, so that they can still orient them to their surroundings. The patient should be educated not to rub their eye, as this may cause direct trauma to the incision, a rise in intraocular pressure or a corneal abrasion.

The timing of the first dressing will vary from unit to unit, on the surgeon and on the time of surgery, and may be done prior to discharge, at home the following day, either by the patient or by a nurse, or as an outpatient the following day. On removal of the dressing, the eye should be examined carefully and systematically

Table 10.3   Postoperative examination of the eye following cataract extraction

Element of examination	Possible findings
Dressing	Any exudate should be noted and recorded, special note being taken of colour that might indicate bleeding or infection
Lids	Excessive swelling and redness should be noted, as this may indicate signs of an allergy or infection. If the lid opening is small, this may make surgery more difficult, so a small cut may have been made at the outer junction of the lids. This is called a canthotomy, and its site should be checked. Normally, sutures are not required but, if present, are removed 5–7 days postoperatively
Conjunctiva	Any signs of a conjunctival haemorrhage or oedema are noted
Incision	The integrity of the wound should be checked, and any gap, loose sutures, or prolapsed iris tissue should be reported immediately. Prolapsed iris is recognized by the presence of a tongue of pigmented tissue protruding through the incision and may be accompanied by an updrawn pupil adjacent to the incision. The incidence of this is less if a corneal incision is used
Cornea	The clarity of this normally transparent structure should be checked. If the cornea is hazy, this may indicate corneal oedema and could be secondary to raised intraocular pressure, damage to the corneal endothelium or intraocular infection. This should be reported immediately
Anterior chamber	Using a pen torch beam, the depth of the anterior chamber is estimated. This can be quite difficult to establish, when the nurse has had little experience in eye examination. It is important, as a shallow or absent anterior chamber may indicate the incision is not secure or the aqueous lost during surgery has not been replaced. The unoperated eye can be used as an indicator of the individual's normal chamber depth, provided there has been no previous surgery. Visible accumulation of white blood cells, a hypopyon, indicates that a severe inflammation or infection is present. Occasionally, an accumulation of red blood cells, a hyphaema, indicates a blood vessel has ruptured. It is difficult to check the position of posterior chamber lenses without the aid of a slit lamp, whereas anterior chamber lenses can be seen on the surface of the iris
Iris	Sometimes there is a small triangular piece of iris missing at the periphery; this is known as a peripheral iridectomy, and is performed if there is a risk of the vitreous moving forward, resulting in pupil block and a sudden rise in intraocular pressure
Pupil	Its position, size and shape is noted, as an updrawn, peaked pupil may indicate an iris prolapse (see below), or it may be caused by a capsule tag or adhesion of vitreous through the incision

(Table 10.3), and provided the other eye is healthy, it is useful to use it for comparison. If the condition of the eye is satisfactory, no covering is necessary during the day, and patients complaining of photophobia are advised to wear dark glasses; but they may be recommended to wear a shield at night, to avoid inadvertent rubbing.

Medication will depend upon the surgeon's wishes, type of operation and unit protocol, but usually consists of topical antibiotic and anti-inflammatory agents. Any changes to optical prescriptions will only be carried out once all postoperative inflammation has settled, usually within 6 weeks and 6/12 vision or better is achieved in 80% of patients.

Long-term complications

1. *Iris prolapse*: the patient is required to return to the operating theatre to remove the prolapsed tissue and resuture the wound. This should be carried out

as soon as possible in order that the postoperative visual acuity is not affected.

2. *Raised intraocular pressure*: this is usually due to postoperative inflammation, impairing the flow of aqueous through the trabecular meshwork, and usually resolves with intensive topical medication. The regimen will depend upon the degree of raised pressure, but could include guttae Maxidex (dexamethasone) 2 hourly and acetazolamide 250 mg two to four times a day. Pressure may become raised as a result of 'pupil block', which occurs when aqueous is trapped in the posterior chamber, due to the forward protrusion of the vitreous or lens implant blocking the pupil.

3. *Panophthalmitis*: this is an infection that rapidly involves all the eye and its surrounding structures. Signs and symptoms include rapid reduction in visual acuity, acute intraocular discomfort,

lacrimation and severe intraocular inflammation. Incidence is rare, about 0.3% (James et al, 2003), but the consequences are severe.

4. *Retinal detachment*: when vitreous is lost or prolapses forward, this reduces the pressure that holds the retina in position, and so it may detach.

5. *Cystoid macula oedema/Irvine–Gass syndrome*: 2–3 months after surgery, the patient presents with decreased visual acuity and possible photophobia and ocular irritation. It is more common in patients with diabetes, hypertension and those who have had complications such as vitreous loss and iris prolapse. Although the exact cause of this condition is not known, some units now prescribe non-steroidal inflammatory drops both pre- and postoperatively, such as Acular (ketorolac trometamol) or Ocufen, (flurbiprofen sodium) as prostaglandins, have been identified as a possible mediator (Kanski, 1994).

6. *Posterior capsule opacification*: this occurs when remnants of the lens epithelium cells fibrose behind the implanted intraocular lens. It occurs in up to 50% of eyes following cataract surgery (Coombes and Seward, 1999). The subsequent loss of vision can be rectified by laser capsulotomy.

GLAUCOMA

Glaucoma is the name given to a group of conditions characterized by damage to the optic nerve, loss of peripheral vision and, commonly, an increase in intraocular pressure. Normal intraocular pressure is usually identified as being between 15 and 20 mmHg (Stollery, 1997), but it has become increasingly clear that relying solely on intraocular pressure readings is not advisable.

Cupping of the optic disc and loss of vision can sometimes be seen in people with a normal intraocular pressure; this is thought to be due to a decreased blood supply to the vessels near the optic nerve, which makes the area more vulnerable to damage from relatively small and usually normal variations in intraocular pressure (Gaston and Elkington, 1986).

Glaucoma is an age-related disease, and in Western countries primary open angle glaucoma occurs in approximately 1:100 people over 40 years of age (Chivers, 2003). There is a strong familial pattern with glaucoma: so much so, that in the UK free screening for glaucoma is available to the families of those diagnosed with glaucoma. Child (2003) found that patients with different types of glaucoma have different causative genes. The International Glaucoma Association (2004) suggests that the most significant risk is to siblings, followed by parents and children. The Royal National Institute of the Blind (2003) identified that people of African origin are more at risk, the disease having an earlier onset and increased severity.

The surgery to be described is that associated with glaucoma resulting in a high intraocular pressure, of which there are several types depending on the cause. Glaucoma can be subdivided into:

- primary
- secondary
- congenital.

Primary glaucoma

Primary glaucoma can be either acute or chronic in presentation.

Acute closed angle glaucoma

Acute closed angle glaucoma is an acute ophthalmic emergency and is due to obstruction of aqueous drainage by the closure of the angle formed by the iris and the cornea. It usually occurs in small, hypermetropic eyes with a shallow anterior chamber and narrow drainage angle and becomes more common as the lens ages, as it becomes hardened, larger and is less mobile. Kanski (2003) also says that it becomes more common with age, as in people over 40 the incidence is 1:1000, with women four times more likely to be affected.

As there is a strong familial pattern, screening is offered to the families of those diagnosed with acute angle closure. The condition is usually bilateral, but one eye supersedes the other (Stollery, 1997).

The attacks are episodic and, in between, the intraocular pressure is normal. An attack usually happens when the pupil dilates and the iris root moves forward to block off the entrance to the trabecular meshwork. An attack may be precipitated by emotion, a decrease in light such as the onset of evening or in the dark, or the instillation of mydriatic drops.

There is a subacute stage when the angle is not completely blocked, but the decrease in aqueous drainage causes a rise in intraocular pressure, resulting in corneal oedema. This causes the individual concerned to see haloes around lights and is often accompanied by mistiness of vision and frontal headaches.

If this stage is not recognized, then an acute attack is inevitable; the drainage angle becomes almost totally occluded, and the intraocular pressure rises massively to over 50 mmHg. This causes a sudden reduction in vision, severe pain in and around the eye, possible nausea and vomiting, photophobia and epiphora.

On examination the eye shows:

- a red, congested eye, worse around the limbus
- a hazy, green/grey cornea

- a shallow anterior chamber
- a moderately dilated immobile pupil, often irregular in shape.

The intraocular pressure must be reduced to within normal limits by intensive systemic and topical medical intervention, in order to prevent irreparable loss of vision before any ocular procedure is performed. The intraocular pressure should initially be monitored hourly and, once emergency treatment has finished, 4 hourly.

If topical therapy is not successful, oral glycerol and/or intravenous mannitol may be considered.

Open angle or chronic glaucoma

Open angle or chronic simple glaucoma normally occurs in both eyes in both men and women over the age of 65, and there is a recognized association with raised systolic blood pressure and a familial link (Stollery, 1997). One eye usually develops the condition before the other, and the effect on vision is so gradual that the individual may have significant visual field loss, unnoticed by the patient, before diagnosis is made.

Part of the problem is that the change in vision is wrongly attributed to changes due to ageing rather than a specific pathology. There are often no obvious signs and symptoms, although, on questioning, the patient may give a history of frontal headaches.

Examination may reveal a consistently raised intraocular pressure of above 21 mmHg (except in normotensive glaucoma), a cupped optic disc and a reduced visual field progressing to tunnel vision if not treated. Surgery is not indicated unless medical treatment fails to contain the rise in intraocular pressure, there is a continued reduction in the visual field or patient concordance with medical treatment is poor.

A range of surgically derived drainage procedures have been carried out in the past, but currently the most common are trabeculectomy and trabeculoplasty.

Trabeculectomy

Trabeculectomy entails raising a conjunctival flap and then a partial-thickness scleral flap (Fig. 10.7). A section of underlying sclera and trabecular meshwork is then removed, so making a larger, permanent opening into the Canal of Schlemm. This, plus removal of a piece of peripheral iris, an iridectomy, means that aqueous drainage should not be obstructed at any time. The scleral and conjunctival flaps are sutured back into position, but a small 'blister' of aqueous, a bleb, can be seen beneath the conjunctiva; this should result in a permanent maintenance of normal intraocular pressure.

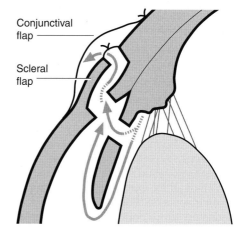

Figure 10.7 Trabeculectomy.

Specific preoperative care

Surgery is usually carried out when the visual field continues to deteriorate despite medical intervention. Patients may be treated as day cases or stay in overnight. If they are having surgery under a general anaesthetic, then local protocols are followed and the only specific care is that the pupil of the affected eye may be constricted in order to make sure the drainage angle is as open as much as possible and the intraocular pressure is within normal limits. This is done by using miotic drops such as pilocarpine 4% plus the patient's current medication.

In addition, if local anaesthesia is used, drops such as amethocaine 1% may be administered topically, either on the ward or in theatre. Sedation may sometimes be given, but is avoided where possible, as there is a risk of the patient falling asleep and then waking with a 'start' during the operation.

There is a risk that the development of scar tissue reduces the amount of aqueous drained, so sometimes steroids or antimetabolites such as 5-fluorouracil or mitomycin C may be given; however, the latter group should be used with caution (Fuller et al, 2002).

Specific postoperative care

Care is similar to that following cataract surgery (see p. 173), except that:

- Patients should be educated not to rub the eye, as this may cause direct trauma to the incision, resulting in a potentially damaging drop in intraocular pressure or a corneal abrasion.

- The timing of the first dressing will vary from unit to unit, on the surgeon and on the time of surgery and may be done prior to discharge, at home the

Table 10.4 Specific postoperative examination

Element of examination	Possible findings
Conjunctiva	The integrity of the flap is observed for the presence of a bleb, a small collection of aqueous under the conjunctiva. This may not always be visible to the naked eye. Signs of subconjunctival haemorrhage and/or oedema are also recorded
Anterior chamber	If a hyphaema is present, it is important to note whether the colour is bright red, a recent bleed, or dark, probably from the time of surgery. The hyphaema may also be diffuse, spread around the chamber, or may be settled, in which case the level should be recorded, as this will indicate whether it is resolving
Iris	In some types of surgery, a peripheral iridectomy may be seen

following day, either by the patient, carer or by a nurse, or as an outpatient the following day.

On removal of the dressing, the eye should be examined carefully and systematically, and, provided the other eye is healthy, it is useful to use it for comparison.

See Table 10.3 for details of postoperative examination and Table 10.4 for specific problems.

If the eye is satisfactory, the procedures followed are similar to those following a cataract extraction, except that a topical mydriatic may be prescribed in order to avoid the formation of synechiae (adhesions) between the iris and cornea or lens. This must be suspected if, on subsequent examination, the pupil becomes irregular and immobile. Mydriatic therapy may cause blurring of vision because some mydriatics have a cycloplegic effect, paralysing the muscles of accommodation. This must be discussed with the patient to prevent unnecessary anxiety being caused.

It is also essential that, if the second eye has not yet had surgery to correct glaucoma, the mydriatics prescribed for the operated eye are not inadvertently instilled into the wrong eye, so causing a rise in intraocular pressure. Current local and systemic therapy for the unoperated eye must continue.

Complications of surgery
- *Leaking wound*: if the situation is not rectified by application of a pressure dressing and mydriatic

therapy, synechiae formation, corneal endothelial damage and cataract may occur.
- *Choroidal detachment*: this occurs if there is excessive drainage via the bleb; this results in very low intraocular pressure and the eye may feel soft.
- *Panophthalmitis*: infection enters through the bleb and quickly spreads throughout the ophthalmic tissues, causing acute pain and a dramatic loss of vision. It is very difficult to treat, even if diagnosed early.
- *Hyphaema*: bleeding from the ciliary and iris vessels can result in the collection of red blood cells in the anterior chamber, which obstruct the drainage angle and cause a secondary rise in intraocular pressure.
- *Cataract formation*: during surgery, inadvertent contact with the lens epithelium can lead to increased permeability and cataract formation.

Trabeculoplasty

This is a procedure that is carried out as an adjunct to medical treatment, which is the first line of treatment in older patients, and consists of laser therapy to the trabecular meshwork, usually as an outpatient procedure. This procedure increases the aqueous drainage of the trabecular meshwork. It is not usually carried out on patients under the age of 25 years old, as its long-term effects are not known and it may only be a short-term solution (Kanski, 1994). Flammer (2002) identified a 60% success rate, although its effect is thought to be short-lived, perhaps for only 3 years.

Although this is a non-invasive procedure, it causes considerable local inflammation, which may result in a rise in intraocular pressure, so oral acetazolamide 250–500 mg may be given prophylactically. Acetazolamide is a carbonic anhydrase inhibitor that reduces the amount of aqueous produced.

Secondary glaucoma

This is a rise in intraocular pressure resulting from mechanical blockage of the drainage angle. Presentation is similar to that of acute glaucoma, and initial treatment is usually medical, but surgery may be indicated in some cases.

The most common causes are as follows:

Lens matter

Lens matter following extracapsular cataract extraction: in which case, treatment consists of acetazolamide and topical intensive anti-inflammatory therapy until enzymes in the aqueous absorb the lens material.

Lens protein may also leak out of a hypermature lens, in which case lens extraction is necessary. Extraction is also carried out when the lens is dislocated,

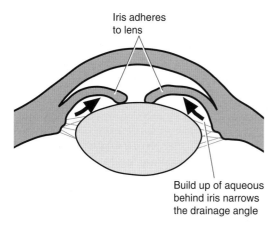

Figure 10.8   Iris bombe.

due to trauma or in Marfan's syndrome, as this may result in the lens either dropping into the posterior chamber and pushing the iris forward to obstruct the drainage angle, or into the anterior chamber, when there is direct obstruction of aqueous flow.

Haemorrhage

Red blood cells may be deposited in the drainage angle, following trauma or surgery. Surgery is not advocated, because of the risk of further bleeding, but an anterior chamber washout may be necessary if there is corneal involvement or synechiae formation that does not respond to medical intervention.

Uveitis

This inflammatory condition of the iris, ciliary body and choroid can cause secondary glaucoma by the presence of adhesions forming across the drainage angle and/or white cells in the aqueous (a hypopyon) collecting in the drainage angle. These are treated by intensive systemic and topical medications.

Adhesions may also develop between the posterior iris and the anterior lens surface, so obstructing the flow of aqueous into the anterior chamber and pushing the iris root forward to obscure the drainage angle. This is known as iris bombe (Fig. 10.8).

Infection

Infection can also result in the development of a hypopyon. Treatment is medical, with very intensive topical, subconjunctival and systemic antibiotic therapy.

Vitreous

Following cataract extraction, usually intracapsular or complicated extracapsular, the vitreous can move forwards and block the pupil, resulting in iris bombe.

Neovascularization

In conditions such as diabetic retinopathy and central retinal vein occlusion, in an attempt to establish a collateral blood supply, small blood vessels grow into the iris (rubeosis) and the drainage angle. The resultant rise in intraocular pressure is known as thrombotic glaucoma. Control is difficult to achieve and, in a last resort, the production of aqueous may be reduced by destroying part of the ciliary body by either freezing (cyclocryotherapy) or with laser (cycloablation).

Tumours

Indirect pressure from a tumour outside the eye or actual tumour infiltration can obstruct aqueous drainage. Treatment will depend upon the extent of spread and size of the tumour, but excision may be necessary.

Congenital glaucoma

Congenital glaucoma is due to the absence or malformation of all or part of the trabecular meshwork, resulting in aqueous drainage being severely reduced or absent. The nature of a child's scleral tissue allows the eye to increase in size – hence, the name 'buphthalmos' or 'ox eye', as the corneal diameter may be greater than 12 mm.

Surgery should be carried out as soon as possible and usually consists of a goniotomy, in which case a direct channel between the anterior chamber and Canal of Schlemm is opened up; this often needs repeating but has an eventual success rate of 85% (Kanski, 1994). Trabeculectomy and the insertion of aqueous shunts may also be carried out.

RETINAL SURGERY

Although small retinal breaks can be treated on an outpatient basis using laser therapy, more sophisticated, complicated surgery should be carried out in specialist units. Retinal breaks usually occur when the retinal tissue is ischaemic and breaks down. This can be due to tension on the peripheral retina, as in the case of myopia, or following trauma resulting in retinal bruising, known as commotio retinae. Breaks are usually found in the peripheral retina, immediately behind the ciliary body, as this is the least perfused area of the retina. They may also result from traction on the retina from the vitreous, especially if there has been intravitreal bleeding.

Breaks are treated depending upon their size and cause; if secondary to another condition, then that must be treated as well, but the break itself may be treated by laser therapy. This is usually an outpatient procedure, but the patient must be aware that they should not drive immediately following this treatment, as their pupils will have been dilated to allow good visualization of the retina, and the drops used can affect the ability to accommodate. Prior to the procedure, the patient should be warned that their eyes may feel slightly uncomfortable and may water; both these symptoms should resolve within 24–36 hours.

Retinal detachments

Breaks may not be significant in themselves, but there is a high risk of detachment if left untreated. The term 'retinal detachment' is misleading, as it is the retinal neural division that separates from the retinal pavement epithelial layer, not the entire retina from the choroid below.

Stollery (1997) uses the terms 'float', 'pulled' and 'pushed' to differentiate the basic causes of retinal conditions requiring surgery.

- *Float*: following the formation of a retinal break, subretinal fluid or vitreous penetrates the space between the neural retina and the pigmented epithelial layer and lifts off the former.
- *Pulled*: this happens when either fragile new blood vessels penetrate the normally avascular vitreous, as in diabetic retinopathy, or blood itself leaks into the vitreous, as in trauma. The fibrous strands formed in the vitreous as the blood 'organizes' itself, contract, causing tension on the retina, resulting in the neural layer being pulled off the epithelial layer.
- *Pushed*: the detachment occurs because of exudate from an inflamed choroid or because of the presence of an intraocular tumour, such as a retinoblastoma or choroidal tumour.

The person may complain of one or all of the following:

- seeing non-existent flashing lights, i.e. photopsia, due to separation of the neural layers
- black spots or threads, as blood leaks out into the normally clear vitreous.
- loss of visual field, or shadows across their vision, due to the lifting off and, if in a superior position, the dropping down of the detached retinal tissue, across the line of vision; the person will see this as loss of the opposing visual field, due to the normal inversion of the image in the visual process.

On examination, there may be no obvious external signs of visual pathology, and visual acuity may not have changed, unless the detachment is extensive enough to have obscured or directly affected the macula.

The pupils are dilated with mydriatic drops such as tropicamide 0.5–1%, to allow both retinae to be examined, as retinal changes are often bilateral. The most effective way of examining the retina is by using an indirect ophthalmoscope, as this makes it easier to see the periphery of the retina. The patient needs to have this procedure explained carefully, as the mydriatic drops may paralyse the muscles of accommodation and so reduce their vision, and the bright light from the ophthalmoscope can be difficult to tolerate.

Types of surgery/treatment

Laser Holes or tears are sealed by causing a localized inflammatory reaction that results in the layers adhering to one another, so preventing fluid seeping between them and pushing the layers apart. Where there is an actual detachment, laser therapy may be used to secure suspect areas around the periphery of the detached area.

Cryopexy This is the application of extreme cold to the affected area, using a probe chilled by the use of carbon dioxide under pressure. It causes an inflammatory reaction and so seals the layers together, but, again it is not effective when significant amounts of fluid are found between the detached layers, and so is often used to supplement other treatments.

Plombage/encirclement These are both methods of physically isolating the source of the detachment, especially from the macula. Plombage is the application of a single piece of inert silastic material, which is sutured to the surface of the sclera over the site of the retinal break. The sutures are tightened, so causing an indentation of the layers; this helps push the separated layers together by increasing the intraocular pressure and forming an intraocular barrier to prevent the detachment spreading.

Encirclement is used when there are several potential areas of weakness at the retinal periphery. Silastic straps, 2–3 mm, are used to encircle the eye and tightened fractionally to create an indentation all the way around, running underneath the extraocular muscles.

Subretinal fluid may be drained if it is felt that there is too much present for easy natural reabsorption, once its access to the potential space between the neural and pigmented layers has been closed.

Vitrectomy This entails making an incision(s) into the vitreous chamber, usually through the pars plana. This allows vitreous to be removed if it has been infiltrated by blood that has not subsequently been absorbed naturally. It is also useful if the source of the detachment is too far back for treatment by plombage or encirclement, as a specially adapted laser can be used to seal any breaks in the posterior retina.

Macular hole surgery In the majority of cases, the development of macular holes is idiopathic, more common in people over 55 years old and women

(70%), and results in the loss of central vision. Surgery is now resulting in better visual outcomes, with early intervention of early-stage disease having a 90% plus success rate (Jacobs, 2001).

Vitrectomy is often carried out in conjunction with other methods, such as the introduction of an intra-vitreal gas bubble, e.g. sulphur hexafluoride (SF), which is used to seal the break, the patient being posi-tioned so that the bubble (tamponade) lies immedi-ately next to the break and well away from the lens and cornea. This procedure carries a relatively high risk of retinal detachment and cataract formation.

Specific preoperative care

This will vary, depending upon the surgical procedure selected. The patient will have routine mydriatic drops, and further retinal examinations to allow the extent of the detachment to be accurately recorded, and a decision made about the type of surgery to be carried out. The patient may be encouraged to rest, lying in a certain position, depending upon the site of the detachment, as gravity may cause the area of detachment to increase.

It is important that the patient is told that certain pro-cedures, such as encirclement, may cause considerable pain and discomfort and that analgesics will be avail-able should they require them.

Specific postoperative care

Vitrectomy and intravitreal tamponade   Patients may have to stay in the required position for up to 2–3 weeks, which can be difficult, especially in the case of macular involvement, as they may have to lie on their front, with the head facing down, as much as possible. Conse-quently, they all need considerable care and support both from the nursing staff (Harker et al, 2002), and when discharged home. This is especially true of those with other medical conditions, such as chronic obstruct-ive airway disease. A support frame is available; this is designed to hold the patient's head in the correct posi-tion and may increase the patient's level of comfort.

Cryotherapy   The degree of reaction due to the appli-cation of extreme cold causes swelling and inflammation and may result in the eye being painful, so analgesics and an explanation of the cause of the pain must be given. Oral anti-inflammatory drugs such as ibuprofen 200–400 mg may also be given.

Encirclement   As the silastic strap encircles the whole eye, the subsequent swelling may cause an increase in intraocular pressure. The eye should be examined for any sign of corneal oedema, and complaints of increas-ing pain must be taken seriously. This is more likely

to occur if cryotherapy has been used as an adjunct. Acetozolamide can be given to control the pressure until the swelling is reduced.

Depending upon the extent of the surgery, the eye may become oedematous, especially the conjunctiva, when the degree of swelling (chemosis) may mean that the lids cannot shut properly and exposure keratitis is a possibility. There is also considerable lacrimation and the eye may required frequent cleansing.

Short-term complications
Anterior segment necrosis: the blood supply to the ante-rior part of the eye may be obstructed if the encircling band is applied too tightly. This requires total revision of the surgery, with loosening of the encircling strap.

Long-term complications
Extrusion of the plombe: over a period of time, the plombe may work loose and find its way forward under the conjunctiva. This is removed and careful examination made to ensure that there is no focus of chronic infection.

PRE- AND POSTOPERATIVE CARE OF PATIENTS UNDERGOING EXTRAOCULAR SURGERY

SQUINTS

Squint (strabismus) occurs when the axis of one eye is not parallel with that of the other, and it can result in double vision. It is usually horizontal, the two images being side by side, but can be vertical. Squints can also be divergent or convergent, the manifestation depend-ing on which muscles are involved: e.g. weakness of the lateral rectus will lead to a convergent squint. A child learns to control its eye movements in the first few years of life, and fusion of the images produced by each eye is brought about by a complicated, conditioned reflex.

The causes of squints fall into two main categories:

- *Concomitant* – where the sensory components of eye movement are not functioning, e.g. refractive error or mental deficiency. Concomitant squints are more common in children, the commonest refractive error implicated being hypermetropia (long sight).

- *Paralytic* – where the motor components of eye movement are not functioning: e.g. nerve or extra-ocular muscle damage, e.g. cerebrovascular accident. Paralytic squints are more common in adults.

The diplopia that results is compensated for in one of two ways:

- The image of one eye is suppressed completely, and, because of the subsequent lack of stimulus, the retina does not fully develop, resulting in amblyopia, the so-called 'lazy eye'.

- The images can be suppressed rapidly in turn, an alternating squint, meaning that full retinal development is achieved in both eyes.

In children, especially, treatment must be prompt, to prevent further deterioration in visual acuity, and in some cases simple correction of the refractive error is enough; however, if there is a risk of amblyopia, occlusion or 'patching' of the seeing eye may be necessary to improve the retinal function of the suppressed eye.

Every effort is made to correct the underlying cause of the squint before the child is of school age, as this increases the likelihood of a better visual outcome and because non-concordance can occur because of teasing at school. However, treatment is not always successful, and surgery may be necessary.

If the squint is paralytic in nature, the underlying cause should be identified and treated. Corrective surgery may be carried out if there is insufficient improvement in oculomuscular function.

In adults who have concomitant squints which are either untreated or require further treatment, this may be carried out for purely cosmetic reasons.

Specific preoperative care

An orthoptic assessment is carried out to identify the muscles requiring surgery and the degree of correction needed. Surgery is usually carried out on a day care basis, under general anaesthesia. The most common corrective surgery involves resecting a weak muscle, shortening it and so increasing its power, or recessing an overactive muscle. Recession involves moving the insertion of the muscle further back on the eyeball, so reducing its power.

The balance achieved by these two processes swings the eye back onto a parallel axis, although sometimes the patient may be concerned postoperatively that they still have some double vision; however, this is usually due to postoperative oedema.

Specific postoperative care

The eye may require cleaning quite regularly postoperatively, as the conjunctival sutures can cause irritation and the eyes may be 'sticky'. Irritation may be exacerbated by dusty, dirty environments.

The patient should be shown how to clean the eye using cooled, boiled water and moistened cotton wool. A sterile cleansing procedure is not required, as this is an extraocular operation and the risk of intraocular infection is minimal.

A combination of topical antibiotic and anti-inflammatory agents is given, according to the surgeon's preference. Mild analgesics may be required; this is especially so in the case of patients who have had previous surgery to the same area.

In more complex cases, such as thyroid eye disease or following a blowout orbital fracture, use of adjustable suture techniques can improve the long-term results. The sutures are adjusted the morning after surgery, with the patient conscious, but a local anaesthetic should be used (Kanski, 2003). This allows more precise adjustment of the extraocular muscles and a better visual outcome.

The patient may return to work as soon as the eye is comfortable, usually within a week. The continued use of eyepatches and spectacles needs to be specifically determined for each individual, and appropriate information given prior to discharge.

Complications of squint surgery

- *Infection*: if the eye becomes increasingly red, painful and purulent discharge is noted, this probably indicates the presence of an infection. In rare cases, this can extend to the lids; the patient may be pyrexial and sometimes orbital cellulitis is seen. Swabs must be taken for microscopy, culture and sensitivity and antibiotic therapy commenced, the route and frequency of administration being dependent on the severity and extent.

- *Stitch granuloma*: there is a persistent red swelling immediately over the suture. This can cause concern but usually resolves spontaneously. If not, a combination of antibiotic/anti-inflammatory topical agents is prescribed.

- *Over/undercorrection*: occasionally, muscles are recessed or resected inaccurately and further corrective surgery is required.

- *Breakdown of incision*: on the conjunctiva there may be gaping of the incision, either because of too few sutures or because they 'cheese wire' through the tissue. This may require insertion of further sutures. Sometimes the sutures securing the cut muscular surfaces tear out and result in abnormal ocular movement; this needs correcting as soon as possible.

DACRYOCYSTORHINOSTOMY

This operation is carried out to bypass an obstruction within the lacrimal drainage system. Obstruction results from chronic inflammatory changes secondary to recurrent infections in the canaliculi or nasolacrimal duct. The surgery should never be carried out during an acute episode of dacryocystitis, as this increases the risk of orbital cellulitis.

The operation bypasses the obstruction in the nasolacrimal duct by an anastomosis of the lacrimal sac itself to adjacent nasal mucosa, a small area of bone having been removed to make the necessary opening (rhinostomy). If the obstruction is at the level of the common canaliculus, the patency of the drainage ducts is threatened by postoperative inflammation and adhesions. Therefore, silicone tubes are inserted via the punctum, through the rhinostomy and into the nose, and left in place for 3–4 months.

Surgery becomes necessary when:

- epiphora (watering) is so excessive that it interferes with lifestyle, because it leads to continual wiping away of tears and excoriation of the skin below the affected eye
- there are recurrent episodes of dacryocystitis, which can be very painful
- congential obstruction is not cured by syringing and probing of the canaliculi and nasolacrimal duct.

Prior to surgery it is important to determine where the obstruction is sited, and this can be done by syringing the ducts and monitoring the outcome. If there is a clear obstruction, an X-ray in the form of a dacryocystogram, when radio-opaque dye is injected into the lacrimal drainage system via the punctum, may be used to locate it. In situations where the blockage is incomplete and not clearly identifiable, a scintigram may be undertaken using very small amounts of a radioactive source such as technitium (Olver, 2002).

Recently, endoscopic procedures via the nasolacrimal duct have resulted in less trauma to the lacrimal sac and the surrounding bone. However, the administration of topical steroids such as guttae Betnesol-N (betamethasone) is usually required postoperatively to reduce the degree of scarring and subsequent risk of blockage recurring (Yung and Hardman-Lea, 1998).

Specific preoperative care

Surgery is usually performed under a general anaesthetic, so the patient is usually admitted on the day of surgery, having fasted for 4 hours prior to admission. However, when endoscopic dacrocystorhinostomy is undertaken it may be carried out under local anaesthesia.

The preparation may vary according to surgeon's preference, and some patients have their noses packed with ribbon gauze soaked in a cocaine and adrenaline (epinephrine) solution to constrict blood vessels and reduce bleeding. This is usually done after induction of anaesthesia, but may be part of the ward preparation.

A systemic premedication is given, usually temazepam 10–20 mg, to reduce anxiety, and metoclopramide 10 mg is given to reduce postoperative nausea caused by the swallowing of blood draining from the nose in the immediate postoperative period.

The patient should be warned that they may feel light headed on mobilizing postoperatively, because of the use of hypotensive anaesthesia. It should also be made clear that marked bruising around the operation site is a possibility.

Specific postoperative care

As hypotensive agents are used during anaesthesia to assist in reducing the blood flow to the surgical site, the patient may be kept in overnight for observation.

Haemorrhage is a possible complication, so regular and frequent observations of blood pressure, pulse and swallowing pattern are essential. This may not occur immediately but as the blood pressure returns to within the individual's normal limits. Patients do not routinely return to the ward with an intravenous infusion in progress, but, if they do, then the cannula site should be observed for signs of extravasation, such as swelling and pain, and phlebitis, such as redness tracking along the course of the affected vein. The infusion is normally discontinued when the patient's blood pressure has returned to within normal limits and when the anaesthetist is satisfied with their condition.

A nasal bolster and/or pressure dressing may be applied in theatre, and this should be checked regularly for any signs of seepage. Any abnormal findings should be reported to the medical staff at once, as haemorrhage following a dacryocystorhinostomy is an ophthalmic emergency and may necessitate further surgery. In non-endoscopic surgery the dressing should be taken down the following day and the incision cleaned if necessary, skin sutures being removed 5–7 days postoperatively.

Medication following surgery does vary, but antibiotics and steroids are usually given, such as guttae betnesol-N (betamethasone) and broad-spectrum antibiotics systemically, such as flucloxacillin 250 mg four times a day for 1 week (Olver, 2002).

If silicone tubes have been inserted (Fig. 10.9), these are left in situ for 2–3 months, until all swelling has gone, and are removed in the outpatients department.

Patient education is important following dacryocystorhinostomy as patients should be discouraged from sniffing, blowing their nose and sneezing for the first week, as these actions may result in periorbital surgical emphysema. If tubes are in situ, patients should also be taught to check that they are positioned properly, since, if they slip up the nose and out

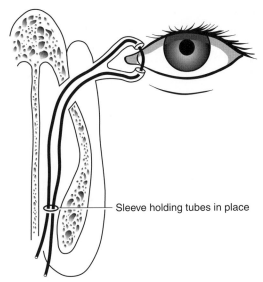

Figure 10.9   Position of silicone tubes following dacryocystorhinostomy.

through the lacrimal passages, the tube may encroach on the cornea and cause an abrasion. The incision between the nose and the inner aspect of the eye may cause discomfort for patients wearing spectacles, and they may initially require help to carry out the activities of living because of reduced visual acuity.

TUMOURS OF EYE AND ORBIT

There is a wide range of benign and malignant tumours that can occur in and around the eye; see Table 10.5 for some of the most common types.

Surgery for tumours of the eye and orbit

Enucleation
This entails removing the eye itself, and if a malignancy is diagnosed, part of the optic nerve.

Evisceration
This type of surgery involves removing the contents of the eye, but the scleral shell is left behind. It is usually carried out following severe ocular trauma to reduce the risk of sympathetic ophthalmitis, or following intraocular infection to prevent infection tracking back to the meninges.

Exenteration
This is radical surgery, involving removal of the entire contents of the orbit plus any bone suspected of having been infiltrated by the tumour.

Specific preoperative care

As all these operations will result in a degree of physical disfigurement, the psychological care of these patients is paramount. The amount of information given to each patient and their family will depend upon the individual, as some may find it very distressing to be given more information than they can absorb. It may be helpful for the patient to meet someone who has already had the type of surgery they are about to undergo.

Specific postoperative care

The amount of help and support the patient needs will vary from individual to individual and will also depend on the extent of the surgery and the reasons for it.

Initially, the socket may require frequent cleansing, using the same basic technique as following other ocular surgery, and antibiotic ointment/drops are instilled three to four times a day. A pressure dressing may be applied, in order to reduce bruising.

The size of the prosthesis will vary from a shell in enucleation/evisceration to a spectacle-mounted replacement of orbital bone and skin, plus an artificial eye in exenteration. The latter patient may need the help of other professionals, such as make-up therapists, in order to learn how to blend the prosthesis to the remaining facial structures.

The speed at which patients become proficient in caring for their prosthesis and socket will vary, and they must be allowed to take things at their own pace. This may mean that the community services have to be involved and may need education themselves in caring for patients following this type of surgery. The family should be encouraged to participate in the care, as they will be the main line of support following discharge.

The final prosthesis will not be made until all swelling has reduced and the wound is completely healed; the prosthetic technician plays an important part in restoring the patient's appearance and morale.

ORBITAL FRACTURES

The commonest orbital trauma is that of a 'blow-out' fracture. These occur when intraorbital pressure rises suddenly, due to a blunt injury to the eye, resulting in either the medial or inferior wall of the orbit breaking and being pushed out into the relevant sinus. The latter is the most common, and the patient may present with diplopia, restriction of elevation of the eye, decreased sensation over the maxilla and sinking of the globe further into the orbit (enophthalmos).

Table 10.5 Tumours of the eye and orbit

Location/type	Tumour	Description
Eyelids Benign	Xanthelasmata	These plate-like flat structures, often yellow tinged, are thought to be indicative of hypercholesterolaemia. They are usually removed by simple excision, as an outpatient, but may recur
	Papillomata	These small growths can be affected by the constant movement of the eyelid, becoming pedunculated. They are removed by excision, under a local anaesthetic, but may bleed and need cauterizing. These may also recur
Malignant	Basal cell carcinoma/ rodent ulcer	The majority of the patients presenting with these tumours are elderly. They need reassurance that, although the tumour invades surrounding tissues, it does not usually metastasize. It is the commonest malignancy of the eyelid, and there is usually a long history of the presence of a 'wart'. On examination, it has rolled edges and a crater in the centre covered by a scab and has grown slowly. These are treated by wide excision and/or radiotherapy. Pinch or Wolf skin grafts may be needed following more extensive surgery
	Squamous cell carcinoma	These present as a wart-like growth that can cause eversion and induration of the lid margins. They are not as sensitive to radiotherapy as basal cell carcinomata, and wide excision of the tumour may need skin grafting in order to preserve the function of the eyelid
Orbit Benign	Meningioma	These arise from the meninges surrounding the optic nerve and may cause loss of vision due to involvement of the optic disc, or there may be direct pressure on the optic nerve from the meninges in the ethmoid region. The most common presenting sign is exophthalmos, with diplopia and downward or lateral deposition. Depending on the speed of tumour growth, surgical excision or radiotherapy are treatment options
Uveal tract Malignant	Melanoma	These can arise from a pigmented naevus and can be found anywhere in the iris, ciliary body or choroid, as they arise from the pigment cells of the uveal tissue. The patient must be referred to a specialist centre, where treatment options vary, ranging from chemotherapy and radiotherapy to evisceration
Retina and Vitreous Malignant	Retinoblastoma	This is a tumour of the retinal layer that may be hereditary in origin, often affecting both eyes. It may also affect several members of the same family. If left untreated, it spreads to the orbital wall and surrounding structures

Perry and Tullo (1995) say that treatment should be conservative. However, if symptoms, especially diplopia and enophthalmos, persist, then surgical repair of the fracture, by insertion of silicone implant, is carried out. This is often done in conjunction with the maxillofacial surgeons.

THE EYELIDS

Entropion

The eyelid margins turn in, especially the lower lid, due to spasm of the orbicularis oculi muscle or to scarring of the conjunctiva, so the lashes come into direct contact with the cornea, which is excruciatingly painful and leads to corneal abrasion and scarring. Although temporary relief can be achieved by applying a strip of tape from the lower lid to the cheek, permanent improvement can only be achieved by surgery.

Treatment will depend on the cause of the entropion (Nerad, 2001). In the majority of cases, correction is achieved by excision of skin and/or muscle and/or the tarsal plate, effectively shortening the lower border of the eyelid and so pulling the upper aspect of the lid out. It is important not to overcorrect the entropion, as this can result in ectropion formation.

Ectropion

The eyelid margins turn out, usually due to loss of tone of the orbicularis oculi muscle or to scarring of the face near the eye. This causes a reduction in tear flow, as the puncta are no longer in apposition with the surface of the eye, and the tears flow down the cheek (epiphora), causing a red, uncomfortable eye due to exposure, and conjunctivitis caused by the ineffective tear flow and loss of lubrication of the ocular surface. If there is only a minor degree of ectropion, a small amount of cautery to the area of the conjunctiva below the lower punctum is enough to scar the area sufficiently to pull the lid back into its proper alignment.

Greater degrees of ectropion are resolved by excising a wedge of the tarsal plate and conjunctiva, so shortening the upper margin of the tarsal plate of the lower lid, pulling it back into place.

Postoperative care

Both these procedures are normally carried out under local anaesthesia. The eye is usually covered with an eyepad for 2–3 hours postoperatively, as there may be some bleeding. After the pad is removed, the patient applies antibiotic ointment two to three times a day for 4–5 days and returns to the outpatients department for the removal of sutures. The eye may need cleaning with cotton wool moistened with cooled, boiled water, with care being taken not to inadvertently remove the sutures.

Tarsorraphy

Tarsorraphy is performed when the patient is at risk of exposure keratitis and the use of lubricants and bandage contact lenses (large, soft lenses that have no other function than to protect the corneal surface and maintain the integrity of the eye) have been ineffective.

Ophthalmic conditions that may lead to tarsorraphy are exophthalmos, delayed healing of a corneal ulcer because of the constant blinking action of the upper eyelid disturbing the new corneal epithelium, and reduced ability to close the eye because of damage or malfunction of the facial nerve.

The patient is usually admitted for surgery, as this is usually the last resort of a planned course of treatment. They will need careful explanation of the procedure and may have some concern about their appearance

following the procedure, as the size of the palpebral fissure will be decreased. This alteration in appearance is more marked if a central tarsorraphy is planned, as this means the lids are joined centrally; this is only done in extreme cases of exposure keratitis and may be a temporary measure. The patients often find that the relief of pain outweighs the cosmetic effect.

During the operation, the conjunctival epithelium of the upper and lower lid margins is excised, usually at the lateral aspect of the lid. This causes two rough edges, which will adhere together as they heal. The lids are sutured together, the sutures being passed through small rubber sleeves, so preventing them 'cheese wiring' out under the pressure of lid movement. As these sutures usually stay in for a minimum of 10 days, the patient is taught how to clean them, and how to apply antibiotic ointment. If the presence of the sutures and rubber sleeves is unacceptable to the patient, dark glasses can be worn. If tarsorraphy is done on a temporary basis, it is easily reversed.

Ptosis

Ptosis can affect one or both eyes, be acquired or congenital, and means that the upper lid droops, sometimes resulting in loss of vision, or in the person developing an abnormal head posture, as they hold it back to allow them to peer out from under their lowered lids. It is usually due to a defective levator muscle, neural abnormality, or to abnormal weight upon the lid by oedema, tumour or scarring. Treatment will depend upon the cause.

Primary ptosis requires surgical intervention, but until this can be carried out the ptosis may be corrected by the use of hook glasses or benched contact lenses that lift the lowered lid back to its normal position.

If the condition is secondary to a neurological disorder such as myasthenia gravis, then the primary cause has to be identified and treated where possible. If it is due to trauma, then surgery is delayed until all oedema and inflammation has subsided and reassessment of the situation can be done.

The operation of choice is usually resection of the levator muscle, either via the conjunctiva or the lid. The degree of resection depends upon the severity of the ptosis, but must be carefully estimated, as overcorrection can lead to exposure keratitis, although the use of adjustable sutures has reduced this risk.

Chalazion/meibomian cyst

Sebum blocks the duct leading from the meibomian gland, resulting in stagnation of sebaceous secretions, which are then frequently infected by *Staphylococcus aureus*. This presents as a hard rounded lump, often on the under surface of the eyelid, causing irritation and may be large enough to obstruct the vision and/or cause astigmatism by pressing on the cornea and altering the curvature.

If the patient presents with recurrent infections, then diabetes mellitus should be ruled out. If the chalazion does not respond to antibiotic therapy, lancing and curetting of the infected gland is necessary, followed by antibiotic therapy.

DISCHARGE PLANNING

Length of inpatient stay has decreased dramatically over the last 10 years, and so effective discharge planning has become more important in order to ensure continuity of care and to reduce the risk of postoperative complications. Where possible, needs should be identified at preassessment clinic or on admission, especially if the community services are involved. The following factors need to be considered:

- *Medication*: nurses need to check that patients are capable of actually instilling their topical eye medication and understand the regimen to be followed for both topical and systemic drugs. If they are unable to give their own drops, then arrangements need to be made for this to be done by a carer or the community nursing service. Patients should also be told how to obtain further medication. Some devices to assist the instillation of drops are available, but some of these are not suitable for use on recently operated eyes, as they may compromise the integrity of the wound.

- *Follow-up*: details of appointments for the outpatients clinic should be given to the patient prior to discharge and any transport needs identified and arrangements made.

- *Care of the eye*: if this is necessary, patients or carers should be shown how to clean the eye and what they should use to do so. They should also be educated about recognizing possible complications and given a contact number to ring if advice is required. Patients may return next day for the first dressing, or they may be contacted by telephone to check there are no problems. Some ophthalmic units have nurses who visit the patient at home the following day, while others have short-term 'hotel' facilities and the patients return to the

unit the next day or the nurses visit them in this facility.

- *Transport*: patients are advised to arrange for transport on discharge, and, if they are unable to do so, then hospital transport can be arranged. It is inadvisable for patients who have had eye surgery to drive themselves home afterwards, as even minor treatments can affect their ability to judge distances and may reduce their peripheral vision.

- *Community services*: help such as home help and meals on wheels may need to be reinstated or initiated. Patients should be given a contact number for Social Services, in case there are any problems or circumstances change.

- *Carers*: they should be involved in the discharge planning and informed of all arrangements made and information given.

- *Activities of living*: the restriction on activities will be determined by the type of surgery and the surgeon's personal preferences.

All information should be given verbally and should be supported by patient education booklets/sheets. These must be designed to take the patient's degree of visual impairment into account. It is important to assess the patient and carer's understanding of the information given and to give further education if necessary.

CONCLUSION

This chapter has highlighted the needs of patients having both intra- and extraocular surgery and the specific care they require.

Ophthalmic nursing involves caring for a wide range of patients with a variety of problems and, to be effective, a holistic stance must be taken. The importance of taking into account the individual's psychosocial background cannot be underestimated. Care must not be planned in isolation; for example, in some cases the patient may themselves be a carer and feel unable to agree to treatment until arrangements have been made to support the family/friend.

Ophthalmic nursing care involves helping people who may have had their very independence threatened by the potential loss of vision, or, in a small number of cases, supporting those who have had to make some very fundamental changes to their lifestyle because of a visual handicap.

Nurses in this discipline need to be effective communicators and perceptive enough to recognize that even a situation that appears minor to them can be very frightening for the patient. This means that each patient should be seen as an individual – a process that may be difficult with the rapid throughput of patients in most ophthalmic units today. The effort that has to be put into supporting patients and carers is rewarded by seeing most people rediscovering their independence within the community.

Summary of key points

- A knowledge of the basic structure and function of the eye is necessary for the nurse to appreciate the problems patients may have.

- An awareness of the special needs of patients undergoing ophthalmic surgery is important in the planning of efficient and effective care.

- Recognition of the importance of continuity of care between hospital and the community leads to an appropriately planned and implemented discharge.

- Effective patient education can result in a well-informed patient and a reduction in the incidence of readmission.

References

Child, A. (2003) Genetic basis for primary open angle glaucoma. *Glaucoma Forum – International Glaucoma Association* 4: 22–23.

Chivers, J. (2003) Care of older people with visual impairment. *Nursing Older People* 15(1): 22–26.

Clark, A. (2003) Protocol-based care: 1. How integrated care pathways work. *Professional Nurse* 18(12): 694–697.

Coombes, A. & Seward, H. (1999) Posterior capsule opacification: IOL design and material. *British Journal of Ophthalmology* 83(6): 640–641.

DHSS (1961) Human Tissue Act 1961. London: HMSO.

Elkington, A. & Khaw, P. (1999) *ABC of Eyes.* London: British Medical Journal.

Flammer, J. (2002) *Glaucoma: A Guide for Patients, an Introduction for Care Providers, A Quick Reference*, 2nd edn. Toronto: Hogrefe Nad Huber.

Fuller, J., Bevin, T., Molteno, A., et al (2002) Anti-inflammatory fibrosis suppression in threatened trabeculectomy bleb failure produces good long term control of intraocular pressure without risk of sight threatening complications. *British Journal of Ophthalmology* 86(12): 1352–1355.

Gaston, H. & Elkington, A. (1986) *Ophthalmology for Nurses.* London: Croom Helm.

Harker, R., McLauchlan, R., MacDonald, H., et al (2002) Endless nights: patients' experiences of posturing face down following vitreoretinal surgery. *Ophthalmic Nursing: International Journal of Ophthalmic Nursing* 6(2): 11–15.

HSE (1992) *Guidance on the Personal Protective Equipment at Work Regulations.* London: HMSO.

International Glaucoma Association (2004) *The Risk to Relatives from Chronic (Primary Open Angle) Glaucoma.* [online] Available at http://www.iga.org.uk/servlet/ dycon/iga/iga/live/en/uk/About Glaucoma Fact Sheets (accessed 1 February 2004).

Jacobs, P. (2001) Macular hole. In: Taylor, R. H., Shah, P., Murray P. I. & Burdon, M. (eds) *Key Topics in Ophthalmology*, 2nd edn. Oxford: BIOS Scientific.

James, B., Chew, C. & Bron, A. (2003) *Lecture Notes on Ophthalmology*, 9th edn. Oxford: Blackwell Publishing.

Kanski, J. (1994) *Clinical Ophthalmology*, 3rd edn. London: Butterworth Heinemann.

Kanski, J. (2003) *Clinical Ophthalmology*, 5th edn. London: Butterworth Heinemann.

Lebowitz, D., Gurses-Ozden, R., Rothman, R. F., et al (2001) Late-onset bleb-related panophthalmitis with orbital abscess caused by *Pseudomonas stutzeri*. *Archives of Ophthalmology* 119(11): 1723–1725.

Middleton, S., Roberts, A. & Reeves, D. (2000) What is an ICP? [online] Available at: http://www.evidence-based-medicine.co.uk (accessed 11th July 2004).

Nerad, J. (2001) *Oculoplastic Surgery: The Requisites in Ophthalmology.* London: Mosby.

Olver, J. (2002) *Colour Atlas of Lacrimal Surgery.* Oxford: Butterworth Heinneman.

Orem, D. (1985) *Nursing: Concepts of Practice*, 3rd edn. New York: McGraw-Hill.

Perry, J. & Tullo, A. (eds) (1995) *Care of the Ophthalmic Patient: A Guide for Nurses and Health Professionals*, 2nd edn. London: Chapman & Hall.

Roper, N., Logan, W. & Tierney, A. (1996) *The Elements of Nursing*, 4th edn. Edinburgh: Churchill Livingstone.

Royal National Institute of the Blind (2003) *Understanding glaucoma.* [Online] Available at http://www.rnib.org.uk/ xpedio/groups/public/documents/PublicWebsite/ Public rnib (accessed 1 February 2004).

Stollery, R. (1997) *Ophthalmic Nursing*, 2nd edn. Oxford: Blackwell Science.

Trevor-Roper, P. (1974) *Lecture Notes on Ophthalmology*, 6th edn. Oxford; Blackwell Science.

United Kingdom Transplant Support Service Authority (1995) *Annual Report of the Special Health Authority (3rd Report).* Bristol: UKTSSA.

Yung, M. W. & Hardman-Lea, S. (1998) Endoscopic inferior dacrocystorhinostomy. *Clinical Otolaryngology and Allied Sciences* 23(2): 152–157.

Further reading

Brady, F. (1992) *A Singular View: The Art of Seeing With One Eye*. Toronto: Edgemore Enterprises.

Frith, P., Gray, R., MacLennan, S. & Ambler, P. (1994) *The Eye in Clinical Practice*. Oxford: Blackwell Scientific.

Ophthalmic Nursing: International Journal of Ophthalmic Nursing. London: TM & D Press.

Strominger, M. & Richards, R. (2000) Adjustable sutures in pediatric ophthalmology. *Journal of Ophthalmic Nursing and Technology* 19(3): 142–147.

Vaughan, D., Asbury, T. & Riordan-Eva, P. (1995) *General Ophthalmology*, 14th edn. London: Prentice Hall International.

Waldock, A. & Cook, S. D. (2000) Corneal transplantation: how successful are we? *British Journal of Ophthalmology* 84(8): 813–815.

Chapter 11

Patients requiring surgery to the ear, nose and throat

Julie Wain

CHAPTER CONTENTS

Key objectives of the chapter

The aim of this chapter is to provide an overview of ear, nose and throat surgery for nurses. At the end of the chapter the reader should be able to:

- describe the anatomy and physiology of the ear, nose and throat

- describe ear, nose and throat conditions that require surgical intervention

- demonstrate knowledge of nursing assessments specific to this specialty

- discuss pre- and postoperative nursing care

- provide professional and caring patient education, including safe discharge planning

- be familiar with the terminology related to rhinology, otology and laryngology

INTRODUCTION

The 19th century saw the establishment of ear, nose and throat (ENT) surgery as an independent specialty. Throughout the 20th century major advances were made: the development of microscopic, endoscopic and laser techniques; progress towards day case surgery; and innovative approaches shown in reconstructive head and neck surgery. These have all had enormous impact on nurses working within an ENT unit. Surgery can be a less traumatic experience for the individual, recovery rate can be faster and patient turnover is greater. In day surgical units, ENT surgery is now being performed on individuals who, having fulfilled certain criteria (as discussed in Ch. 3), are able to undergo general anaesthetic procedures and suffer only minimal disruption to their daily lives. The multi-disciplinary ear, nose and throat, head and neck team can now offer a more optimistic future and improved quality of life for those patients suffering from extensive and malignant disease of the head and neck.

The diversity within ENT surgery provides nurses working on an ENT ward with a wealth of opportunities and experience from which nursing skills and competencies can develop. It is hoped that the reader, upon following this chapter, will experience the rewards and challenges of oto-rhino-laryngology nursing care.

This chapter is divided into four sections:

- the ear
- the nose and paranasal sinuses
- the throat
- head and neck.

THE EAR

ANATOMY AND PHYSIOLOGY

The ear is divided into three parts:

- the external ear
- the middle ear
- the inner ear.

The external ear

The pinna, composed of fibroelastic cartilage and skin, acts by localizing and amplifying sound and protecting the auditory canal from the environment and from trauma. This canal efficiently self-cleans due to the continuous migration of epithelium from the inner to the outer aspect of its structure. Sound waves travel down the canal to the tympanic membrane, which transmits sound vibrations into the middle ear.

The middle ear

This is an air-containing cavity. It connects with the nasopharynx via the eustachian tube, which ventilates and equalizes pressure within the cavity. The middle ear contains three ear ossicles: the malleus, incus and stapes. These transmit sound vibrations from the tympanic membrane to the cochlea of the inner ear. Posterior to the middle ear lie mastoid air cells. The mastoid process is closely related to the cerebellum, temporal lobe and the labyrinth of the inner ear. Portions of the facial nerve (VII), which innervates facial movements,

and the chorda tympani nerve responsible for taste perception are also located here (Waddington et al, 1997).

The inner ear

The inner ear consists of two sections: the cochlea (hearing canal), and the vestibular apparatus (balance canal) contained within the labyrinth (Dart, 1997). Endolymph circulates in both canals to transmit sound and balance signals. The vestibulocochlear nerve (VIII) has two branches and functions: the cochlear/auditory nerve for transmission of electrical impulses to the cerebral cortex, where sound is perceived; and the vestibular nerve, which transmits impulses from the inner ear and semicircular canals to the cerebellum, conveying information about posture, movement and balance.

CONDITIONS OF THE EAR THAT REQUIRE SURGERY

There are a variety of conditions and diseases that benefit from surgical intervention. The following details the main examples, with types of surgery explained in Box 11.1.

- *Exostoses*: an overgrowth of bone in the external auditory canal. Repair is by canalplasty.
- *Perforated tympanic membrane*: due to trauma or otitis media (acute or chronic infection of the middle ear). Repair is by myringoplasty or tympanoplasty using a graft.
- *Ossicular discontinuity*: ossiculoplasty aims to repair the ossicular chain.
- *Otosclerosis*: an overgrowth of bone causing fixation of the stapes footplate and conductive deafness. This condition is familial, more common in women, and one which pregnancy appears to exacerbate. Repair is by stapedectomy.
- *Acoustic neuroma (schwannoma)*: a tumour of the vestibular element of the eighth cranial nerve. Its incidence is rare and progress can be slow; neurosurgeons and otologists often perform the surgical excision collaboratively.
- *Cholesteatoma*: a benign growth of squamous epithelial cells in the middle ear and mastoid air cells, which may lead to infection and suppuration, conductive and sensorineural hearing loss and facial nerve paralysis. Unless adequately treated, bony involvement (mastoiditis) occurs, which can lead to extra- and intracranial complications (Box. 11.2). Surgery to remove cholesteatoma is mastoidectomy; the extent of disease dictates the extent of surgery.
- *Ménière's disease*: aetiology is unknown. It affects the inner ear, causing vertigo, tinnitus and deafness.

Box 11.1   Types of ear surgery

- *Myringoplasty*: this is closure of a tympanic membrane perforation using a graft of temporalis fascia. The graft is tucked into place behind the membrane and is gently supported by pieces of Gelfoam, which are gradually absorbed over a few weeks. The graft is not completely stable until about 6 months later. There are two types of approach: endaural or postauricular. This procedure is also known as type I tympanoplasty.

- *Ossiculoplasty*: a connection is made between the stapes and malleus in order to improve ossicular conduction of sound. A myringoplasty may also be performed at the same time. This procedure is also known as type II tympanoplasty.

- *Mastoidectomy*: there are three types. A postauricular approach is used.
  - Cortical: mastoid air cells are removed; hearing is unaffected.
  - Radical: more extensive then cortical; the eardrum, bony ear canal wall, middle ear mucosa and ossicles are removed; hearing is greatly affected.
  - Modified radical: preserves as much of the eardrum and ossicles as possible; hearing is less affected.

- *Stapedectomy*: a window in the footplate of the stapes is made, and the diseased stapes is removed. A prosthesis is inserted which is mobile, to allow for the vibration and conduction of sound.

- *Saccus decompression*: the endolymph that fills the membranous labyrinth of the inner ear is drained, in order to alleviate vestibular disturbance.

- *Labyrinthectomy*: the entire structure of the labyrinth in the inner ear is destroyed, resulting in total hearing loss on that side.

Box 11.2   Potential progression of severe middle ear infection

Otologic complications:
- perforated tympanic membrane
- mastoiditis
- mastoid abscess
- labyrinthitis

Head and neck complications:
- neck abscess
- facial nerve palsy

Cerebral complications:
- extra dural abscess
- meningitis
- sub dural abscess
- cerebral abscess

Box 11.3   Causes of specific hearing loss

Conductive hearing loss
- impacted wax
- foreign body in ear canal
- damage to tympanic membrane
- otosclerosis
- cholesteatoma

Sensorineural hearing loss
- arteriosclerosis
- congenital
- ototoxic drugs
- acoustic neuroma
- trauma from ear/head injury
- overexposure to high-intensity noise
- presbycusis

Endolymphatic sac decompression is occasionally performed but a variety of medical treatments are first explored. No one treatment suits all Ménière's sufferers. Labyrinthectomy is performed if symptoms are severe and causing continued distress to the patient.
- *Profound sensorineural deafness*: may benefit from a cochlear implant.
- *Deafness*: a variety of deaf patients now benefit from Bone-Anchored-Hearing Aid (BAHA) – a permanently implanted hearing aid.

SPECIFIC INVESTIGATIONS

By a process of air conduction, sound waves pass through the ear canal to the ossicular chain. Bone conduction enables wave transmission to reach the inner ear, where sound energy is transformed into neural energy and interpreted by the brain. If a problem is identified within the external or middle ear, any hearing loss is termed conductive. If there is a cochlear, auditory nerve or central nervous system problem, hearing loss is sensorineural. Box 11.3 lists causes of specific hearing loss.

Clinical tests of hearing and ear disease

- *Simple audiometry*: i.e. use of tuning forks (Rinne and Weber tests): these distinguish between conductive and sensorineural loss. It is inexpensive, simple and portable.

- *Auriscopy*: an examination of the inner aspect of the ear canal and tympanic membrane, to visualize and diagnose conditions such as wax (cerumen) accumulation, perforation, foreign body, otitis externa/media, exostosis, cholesteatoma and mastoiditis.

- *Pure tone audiometry*: a formal measurement of hearing, usually conducted by an audiologist. The patient wears earphones and signals when a sound is heard. Results are plotted on graphs, reflecting air conduction and bone conduction of sound.

- *Impedence audiometry*: gives information about middle ear pressure, eustachian tube function and middle ear reflexes, and can provide measurement of any facial nerve dysfunction (Black, 1997).

- *Speech audiometry*: determines speech reception threshold and discrimination, and is effective in diagnosing sensorineural loss and evaluating for hearing aids.

- *Vestibulometry*: determines the functional state of the vestibular system; is useful in diagnosing dizziness.

- *Otoacoustic emissions*: assesses hearing in newborns to determine whether the cochlea is functioning. A probe with a speaker and a microphone is inserted into the ear canal. Tones are sent from the speaker through the middle ear, stimulating the hairs in the cochlea. The hairs respond by generating their own minute sounds, which are detected by the microphone. If there is a hearing loss, the hairs in the cochlea do not generate sound.

- *Brainstem auditory evoked responses*: measures the timing of electrical waves from the brainstem in response to clicks in the ear. Delays of one side relative to the other suggest a lesion in the 8th cranial nerve (such as acoustic neuroma) between the ear and brainstem, or the brainstem itself.

- *Radiology*: X-rays are useful to indicate stages of disease. Computed tomography (CT) and magnetic resonance imaging (MRI) scans are excellent diagnostic tools, particularly in determining middle ear, mastoid disease and acoustic neuroma.

- *Clinical test of balance*: the Romberg test is used to determine if a lesion is cerebellar or labyrinthine in origin. With feet together, the patient closes their eyes, standing erect. A labyrinthine lesion can cause the patient to sway to the side of the lesion, which is accentuated by closing the eyes. A cerebellar lesion may show symmetrical swaying unaffected by eye closure.

- *Clinical test of gait*: the patient walks in a straight line between two points and then quickly turns to return on the straight line. Patients with a labyrinthine lesion deviate to the side of the lesion. Marked imbalance on turning indicates a cerebellar lesion.

- *Clinical test of facial nerve*: the facial nerve is the main motor nerve to the facial muscles and the stapedius muscle in the middle ear, and enables taste on the anterior two-thirds of the tongue. Facial nerve function in ear disease should always be assessed.

In relation to hearing loss, the presence of any otalgia (earache), otorrhoea (aural discharge) and tinnitus also aid diagnosis. Observing for nystagmus is also important; the eye moves slowly away from the affected side and then rapidly flicks back (horizontal nystagmus). This is common in inner ear disease.

NURSING ASSESSMENT OF A PATIENT REQUIRING EAR SURGERY

On admission, the nurse gains a comprehensive assessment of the patient's physical and psychological status. A model of nursing such as that of Roper, Logan and Tierney (2000) provides the framework for this. Specific to a patient requiring surgery to the ear and the subsequent postoperative care is the assessment of the following activities of daily living: communicating; working and playing; expressing sexuality; eating and drinking; and eliminating.

Communicating

Hearing loss is a major disability that affects social, work and educational aspects of an individual's life. The nurse needs to assess the patient's hearing loss by addressing the following issues:

- Location and nature:
  - Which side is affected?
  - How severe is the loss?
  - Is there distortion of sound or tinnitus?
- Effects of the hearing loss:
  - on socializing
  - at work
  - with routine activities, e.g. shopping, telephoning
  - on body image and self-esteem.

Box 11.4   Nursing skills of communication for patients with impaired hearing

- Ensure a well-lit area to facilitate lip-reading and observation of facial expression.
- Ensure the patient's attention.
- Face the patient.
- Speak in a normal tone; shouting can cause distortion of sound.
- Speak clearly.
- Rephrase if misunderstood or misheard.
- Approach the better ear if not heard, but not too closely.
- Do not cover your face or lips, or speak with anything in your mouth.
- Write down anything that is not well understood.
- Do not rush the conversation or show annoyance or frustration; patients with hearing loss are often sensitive to facial expression.
- Encourage the use of the patient's hearing aid and give time for the patient to adjust it.
- Involve the patient in doctors' rounds; ensure all members of the multidisciplinary team are aware of the hearing loss; avoid talking over the patient, and check for understanding.

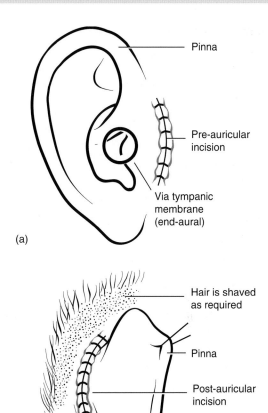

(a)

(b)

Figure 11.1   Types of incision in ear surgery.

- Methods used to improve hearing/communicating:
  - Is a hearing aid used?
  - Is the aid working properly? When was it last cleaned? Is it comfortable to wear?
  - Does the patient lip-read?

The nurse should endeavour to provide the optimum environment for effective two-way communication (Box 11.4).

Encouraging the expression of any fears or concerns about surgery and aftercare is essential. Some types of surgery, e.g. stapedectomy and mastoidectomy, carry some degree of risk to that side of further, or even total, hearing loss.

Working and playing

Establishing the patient's occupation and social situation helps the nurse to assess care and plan safe discharge. Some occupations involve exposure to high levels of noise, e.g. builders or disc jockeys, and this may have contributed to, or caused, the hearing loss. The surgeon may recommend changing occupation.

A certain amount of time (1–2 weeks) for full recovery is required in order to avoid complications. Arrangements will need to be made in advance for time off work and the caring of dependants if maximum rest is to be achieved. Home and work life needs must be addressed preoperatively.

Expressing sexuality

Body image and self-esteem can suffer if hearing loss interferes with the patient's life. Patients can feel sensitive, embarrassed, shy, and many lead isolated lives.

Scarring from surgery is minimal; incisions are either pre-auricular, via the tympanic membrane, or post-auricular (Fig. 11.1). The latter may involve shaving of hair, and this may cause the patient some concern.

Eating and drinking

Assessing the patient's normal diet and appetite is important. Due to labyrinth disturbance, postoperative complications may include dizziness, nausea and vomiting.

Eliminating

The patient's normal bowel and bladder function is discussed. Postoperative dizziness and bedrest, in addition to the effects of the anaesthetic drugs, can all make this activity difficult, particularly for older patients. Embarrassment about using the urinal or bedpan may add to this.

CASE STUDY

The following case study aims to demonstrate both pre- and postoperative care for an individual undergoing a stapedectomy for otosclerosis.

Mrs Susie Marsh is a 42-year-old housewife and mother of two children (aged 9 and 14 years old). Her husband, a businessman, works in France and returns home for weekends. Susie was electively admitted for a right-sided stapedectomy. Her symptoms include mild tinnitus and progressive right-sided hearing loss. Her two pregnancies may have exacerbated this loss.

Nursing assessment

Box 11.5 identifies the nursing assessment of Susie Marsh.

Specific preoperative preparation

The doctor admits and obtains informed consent from Susie. This includes a detailed discussion about any risks associated with surgery. The potential deterioration or total loss of hearing on her right side, due to failure of the prosthesis or surgical trauma, is of particular concern to Susie. The doctor seeks to allay such anxieties by providing realistic information and by confirming that Susie understands all aspects of the procedure.

Audiometry, unless performed within the previous 6 months, is repeated in order to obtain up-to-date information about the hearing function of the affected side.

Postoperative nursing care

Previous chapters have discussed general issues of postoperative care. For Susie, specific potential complications of surgery include displacement of the prosthesis, facial nerve palsy, dizziness, nausea and vomiting and difficulties in communicating. Box 11.6 details the plan of nursing care and evaluation of care given.

Discharge planning and patient education

The majority of patients who have undergone ear surgery are often discharged after 1–2 days, and some procedures are undertaken as day cases.

Box 11.5   Proeperative nursing assessment of a patient undergoing a stapedectomy

Maintaining a safe environment
- Observation of vital signs is performed: pulse, 72 beats per minute; blood pressure, 110/65 mmHg.
- Allergies: none known.
- Past medical history: caesarean section 9 years ago under general anaesthetic.
- Medication: Fybogel (fibre) sachet as required to maintain bowel regularity.
- Susie is anxious about surgery, in particular the potential but minimal risk to her existing right-sided hearing. She also expresses concern about speed of recovery, as her mother is caring for her children and her husband is away in France until the weekend (5 days away).

Breathing
- Respiratory rate: 14 respirations per minute.
- Susie smokes 10–15 cigarettes per day.
- Chest X-ray: no abnormalities.

Controlling body temperature
- Susie's temperature is 36.5°C.

Communicating
- Susie has normal vision.
- Normal hearing present on the left side.
- Susie has pronounced right-sided hearing loss; mild tinnitus is present; she finds socializing difficult, particularly with large, noisy groups of people. It causes her some embarrassment; a hearing aid is not used.
- Susie expresses concern about surgery and home commitments.

Eating and drinking
- Susie is petite: height 1.55 m; weight 50 kg.
- Susie has a normal appetite and diet.

Eliminating
- Susie is prone to constipation; bowels open every 2–3 days.
- She takes Fybogel to maintain this activity.
- Susie passes urine normally; urinalysis shows no abnormalities.

Personal hygiene and dressing
- Susie bathes every night and showers after exercise.

Mobility
- Susie is independent.
- Right-sided hearing loss makes her more cautious when driving, or out-and-about and in crowds.

Working and playing
- Susie is a housewife and mother; her husband is only at home at weekends, so she leads a very busy home life.
- Susie swims twice per week and walks the dog every day.
- Susie expresses concern about the family's summer holiday in 4 months' time; they plan to fly to Spain.

Expressing sexuality
- Susie is casual about her appearance and seems relaxed about the minimal expected surgical scarring.

Sleeping
- Susie sleeps well, about 7–8 hours per night.

Dying
- Susie feels a little apprehensive about the anaesthetic.

Box 11.6   Details of postoperative nursing care of a patient following a stapedectomy

Susie Marsh returns to the ward following a right-sided stapedectomy. She is orientated but drowsy. Oxygen therapy is in progress at 4 L/min. An intravenous infusion is in progress. Susie is allowed to take oral fluids if not nauseous.
A cotton wool plug sits in the external ear canal and is covered by a light gauze dressing; it appears to be moderately bloodstained. The surgeon has instructed flat bedrest with one pillow until the following morning in order to maintain the integrity of the prosthesis.

Breathing
- *Problem*: Potential loss of clear airway and respiratory distress due to anaesthetic, drowsiness and flat bedrest.
- *Goal*: Susie maintains a clear airway and normal breathing.
- *Care*:
  - Ensure oxygen is given at the prescribed rate; provide oral care to prevent a dry mouth.
  - Encourage Susie to lie in the recovery position, with operated ear uppermost, until fully awake, to maintain optimum airway; one pillow is allowed for comfort.
  - Frequently observe respiration rate, depth and rhythm (1/4–1/2 hourly for first 2 hours, reducing to 1–2–4 hourly as condition improves); also observe for cyanosis or respiratory difficulty and report at once to doctor.
  - Encourage deep breathing and coughing to clear secretions.
- *Evaluation:* Though drowsy for the first 2 hours, Susie showed no signs of respiratory distress. Oxygen therapy was stopped after the prescribed 4 hours. Though a smoker, her chest remained clear. Respiratory rate: 12–16 r.p.m.

Maintaining a safe environment
- *Problem*: Potential disturbance of middle ear prosthesis due to its initial vulnerability.
- *Goal*: To maintain integrity of prosthesis.
- *Care*:
  - Ensure Susie remains on flat bedrest as instructed; allow one pillow only.

- Ensure Susie does not fall out of bed as she will feel dizzy and drowsy for the first few hours.
- Place the call bell and necessities to hand, to minimize any inconvenience from the bedrest.
- Assist Susie in meeting her daily needs, but reduce physical activity to the minimum; ensure Susie knows not to move suddenly or jerkily; offer the slipper bedpan for toileting; facilitate taking of diet and fluids by providing soft foods and drinking straws.
- The following morning, ensure Susie mobilizes gently, at first with assistance in case of dizziness.
- Advise Susie not to perform highly strenuous activity for the next 6 months.
- *Evaluation*: Susie found flat bedrest tiresome but maintained it well despite a few episodes of nausea. She successfully used the slipper bedpan and took fluids easily with a straw. The next morning, Susie cautiously but safely mobilized. The doctors advised her to continue restful activity for the next 2 weeks and that flying to Spain in 4 months' time was acceptable.

- *Problem*: Potential facial nerve palsy due to surgical trauma to the facial nerve.
- *Goal*: To promptly detect the onset of any facial nerve defect.
- *Care*:
  - Perform facial nerve checks when taking vital signs:
    - Observe Susie's face at rest for asymmetry.
    - Ask Susie to raise both eyebrows.
    - Ask Susie to smile.
    - Ask Susie to close both eyes tightly.
  - If any weakness or deficit is noted, inform the doctor immediately and continue monitoring.
  - Reassure Susie that any weakness is more than likely due to postoperative swelling causing nerve compression and that this tends to resolve completely.
- *Evaluation*: Regular checks were maintained and no weakness was noted. Therefore, facial nerve function remained intact.

Eating and drinking

- *Problem*: Susie feels unable to eat and drink normally because of postoperative dizziness, nausea and flat bedrest.
- *Goal*: To alleviate nausea, any vomiting and dizziness; for Susie to gain adequate hydration and return to a normal diet.
- *Care*:
  - Administer intravenous infusion as prescribed and check patency and integrity of cannula and site.
  - Maintain accurate fluid balance chart until intravenous infusion is complete and Susie is drinking normally.
  - Administer antiemetic therapy as prescribed/required and monitor effect; encourage Susie to inform staff if feeling nauseous or dizzy, and also ask her how she feels frequently.
  - Oral fluids/diet are encouraged once nausea has subsided; then offer clear fluids and light bland foods as more easily tolerated; encourage relatives/friends to bring in favourite food and drink.
- *Evaluation*: Susie felt dizzy and nauseous upon returning to the ward. She felt nauseous at times. An antiemetic was given as prescribed, with good effect, though mild dizziness persisted. Susie then took oral fluids but declined diet until morning. The intravenous infusion was discontinued after breakfast was eaten. Susie was discharged home later that afternoon, once breakfast and lunch had been eaten and tolerated. She felt 'light-headed', but her family were there to take her home.

Communicating

- *Problem*: Susie states the hearing on her right side is worse than before surgery; she is anxious, particularly upon noting the bloodstained dressing.
- *Goal*: To alleviate Susie's anxiety.
- *Care*:
  - Reassure Susie that deterioration in hearing is normal; surgical oedema, aural packing and any middle ear drainage impairs existing hearing; effects of surgery are often not known for 2–6 weeks.
  - Some bleeding is expected; a moderate discharge of fresh blood onto the cotton wool can continue for the first 24 hours, and then this gradually declines.
  - Promote effective communication skills (see Box 11.4).
- *Evaluation*: Once the probable reason for Susie's worsened hearing was explained, she felt less anxious, and the postoperative visit by the surgeon was reassuring. Bleeding was moderate, and the cotton wool dressing was changed three times during the first 12 hours. By discharge, this had reduced to mild staining of slightly old blood. Susie was advised to change this three times a day for the next 2 days and then daily until discharge has stopped. Susie communicated with staff and visitors by relying upon her left ear for hearing.

Box 11.7   Discharge advice for patients following ear surgery

- Change the cotton wool in the opening of your ear canal every day. Take care not to remove the ear pack. If the pack falls out, contact the hospital for advice.
- A small amount of reddish discharge from the ear is normal. If this becomes offensive, appears yellow/green, or fresh bleeding is noted, contact the hospital.
- Protect the ear, when bathing/showering, with cotton wool dabbed with Vaseline. Keep water out of the ear canal for at least 1 month, as this can cause infection. Use a dry shampoo for 1 week, and do not go swimming for 1 month or as advised.
- If there are any stitches, you will be advised upon their removal.
- Mild dizziness is common for a few days. If this worsens, contact the hospital. Do not drive if dizzy, and refrain from working and any strenuous activity for 1–2 weeks, or as advised. If applicable, do not fly for at least 1 month, but clarify this with your doctor before you leave. Do not blow your nose or play wind instruments for 1 month. Sneeze with your mouth open. These precautions protect the ear and surgery from trauma.
- Hearing is often reduced for the first few weeks because of packing, swelling or discharge. Follow-up hearing tests will be performed.
- Pain is usually mild. If pain increases, contact the hospital.
- If concerned about any matter concerning recovery and aftercare, do not hesitate to contact the hospital.

Discharge planning and patient education begins in the preadmission clinic, and issues are reinforced throughout the patient's hospital stay. Written advice sheets are an invaluable source of education and reassurance, as patients often experience difficulty in absorbing all the verbal information given by nurses and doctors when on the ward. Box 11.7 illustrates discharge advice given to patients following ear surgery.

Outpatient follow-up varies depending on the nature of the operation, and it can be between 1 and 6 weeks. Any aural packing is removed at the outpatient appointment, as well as a repeat aural examination and audiometry.

THE NOSE

ANATOMY AND PHYSIOLOGY

The nose is the first section of the respiratory system, and is responsible for the sense of smell (olfaction). The nose also contributes major aesthetic features to the face (Behrbohm et al, 2002). The nasal passages link the face, the paranasal sinuses and the nasopharynx.

The external nose

The upper third of the external nose consists of two nasal bones, which are fused together. The lower two-thirds are cartilage, the tip of which is especially pliable and is protected by fibrofatty tissue.

The nasal cavity

This consists of twin passages, divided and supported by the osteocartilaginous septum. The anterior opening of each passage is the vestibule, and is lined with skin and hair. The posterior opens into the nasopharynx and is termed the choana. Turbinates line the lateral wall of each side; there are usually three – superior, middle and inferior. They function to maximize the surface area of mucous membrane, enabling the warming and humidification of inhaled air. The space between the middle and inferior turbinates contains the ostiomeatal complex, which functions to drain the sinuses (Daya and Crittenden, 1998). Cilia contained in the epithelium beat constantly in order to transport mucus posteriorly to the nasopharynx (Citardi, 2001).

Vascular supply

The rich arterial blood supply to the nose derives from the external and internal carotid systems serving the sphenopalatine artery and the anterior ethmoid artery. Venous drainage is via the sphenopalatine and ethmoid veins.

Nerve supply

The first cranial (olfactory) nerve innervates smell receptors in the nasal mucosa. Fibres of this nerve pass through the roof of the nasal cavity in the ethmoid sinus at the cribiform plate, and form the olfactory bulb in the brain. Secretory glands of the nose are controlled by the autonomic nervous system. Sensory innervation of the nasal cavity is via the ophthalmic and maxillary divisions of the trigeminal nerve (Ugwoke et al, 2001).

FUNCTIONS OF THE NOSE

Functions of the nose are:

- airway
- filtration and protection – by nasal hairs, mucus transport and cilia; and antibacterial action within the mucus
- humidification and warming – by blood and secretory glands
- olfaction
- resonance of sound.

The paranasal sinuses

The sinuses act as extensions of the nasal cavity. There are four pairs: frontal, sphenoid, ethmoid and maxillary. Sinus functions include:

- mucus production
- air-filled cavities to reduce the weight of the skull
- protecting the eye and brain from trauma
- aiding sound resonance.

CONDITIONS OF THE NOSE AND SINUSES THAT REQUIRE SURGERY

There are a variety of conditions and diseases that benefit from surgical intervention. The following details the main examples, with types of surgery explained in Box 11.8.

- *Disorders of the nasal lining*: e.g. allergic rhinitis, sinusitis and nasal polyps.
- *Disorders of the autonomic nervous system*: namely vasomotor rhinitis. An imbalance exists between parasympathetic and sympathetic nerve supplies to the nasal mucosa, resulting in increased vascularity of the turbinates and nasal obstruction.
- *Structural disorders*: e.g. deviated septum, septal haematoma, fractured nasal bones and irregular nasal bones.
- *Infection*: e.g. acute/chronic sinusitis. This is an inflammatory condition whereby the sinus ostia (natural sinus openings into the nasal cavity)

Box 11.8   Types of nasal and paranasal sinus surgery

Inferior turbinate surgery – for hypertrophy due to allergic/vasomotor rhinitis
- *Diathermy*: to scar/shrink mucosal lining of turbinate using bipolar, monopolar, laser or ablation methods
- *Turbinoplasty*: to reduce size of turbinate from within using a microdebrider
- *Turbinectomy*: partial or total removal – to increase airway patency
- *Outfracture*: to reduce size and function – to alleviate obstruction and symptoms of rhinitis

Septum surgery
- *Submucus resection of septum*: to straighten deviated septum, performed to increase nasal airflow
- *Septoplasty*: maximum septal cartilage is preserved; performed to correct septal deviation. Cartilage tissue may be reinserted, straightened, as supporting graft
- *Drainage of septal haematoma*: performed by either needle aspiration or formal incision

Nasal bones
- *Rhinoplasty*: external and internal bony and cartilaginous deformity is corrected, for aesthetic and functional reasons
- *Reduction of nasal fracture*: to restore patency of airway and aesthetics of nose

Sinus surgery
- *Polypectomy*: nasal polyps can be removed using a microdebrider or surgical forceps
- *Functional endoscopic sinus surgery (FESS):* aims to restore normal functional drainage of the sinuses; includes gentle removal of diseased mucosal lining and widening of natural ostium of each sinus
  - Maxillary antrostomy
  - Ethmoidectomy: posterior and anterior ethmoid sinuses gently debrided to improve mucus drainage
  - Sphenoid sinus surgery: sphenoid ostia opened to minimize further obstruction
  - Frontal sinus surgery: frontal recess opened to improve frontal sinus drainage
- *External ethmoidectomy*: an external incision is made to facilitate disease clearance. Improved endoscopic techniques have lessened the need to perform this surgery routinely. A good approach for tumour clearance
- *Antral washout*: saline is irrigated into the sinus via a cannula, and pus is expelled
- *Caldwell–Luc procedure*: the maxillary antrum is cleared of disease via an antrostomy made inside the upper lip. Endoscopic sinus surgery has diminished the need for this type of antrostomy

become blocked. Mucus accumulates in the sinuses, is unable to drain and may become infected. If normal sinus clearance is not restored, this can lead to chronic mucosal thickening and subsequent nasal obstruction, headache, facial pain and purulent discharge.

SPECIFIC INVESTIGATIONS

Physical examination and a thorough history need to be taken. Conservative treatment is the desired option, with the prescribing of topical nasal and sinus preparations. For some conditions, the following investigations are undertaken:

- allergy testing – to locate and eliminate allergens
- endoscopy – to visualize the problem
- rhinomanometry – objective measure of impaired nasal breathing
- X-rays – reveal bony pathology
- CT scan – gives a detailed image of bony and soft-tissue disease
- MRI scanning – valuable in malignancy.

NURSING ASSESSMENT OF A PATIENT REQUIRING NASAL/SINUS SURGERY

The majority of these procedures are performed as a day case or overnight admission. Referring to Roper, Logan and Tierney's model of nursing (2000), the following activities of daily living need to be assessed on admission.

Maintaining a safe environment

Because of the rich blood supply of the nose, there is a risk of haemorrhage following nasal and sinus surgery. Preoperative observation of the patient's vital signs gives an accurate baseline for postoperative reference. A full medical and drug history may reveal conditions or medications that can exacerbate bleeding, e.g. blood clotting disorders or anticoagulant therapy.

Breathing

Conditions and diseases of the nose and sinuses often lead to nasal obstruction, snoring, obstructive sleep apnoea (cessation of breathing for intermittent periods while asleep) and mouth-breathing. Assessment of the patient's respiratory rate, depth and rhythm is therefore indicated. The surgical insertion of nasal packing forces the patient to mouth-breathe, and this may be distressing. Chest conditions which may lead to respiratory difficulty are also noted, e.g. asthma.

Eating and drinking

Nasal packing makes this activity awkward, as a partial vacuum is created, and the patient may complain of a sucking sensation upon swallowing. Postnasal discharge, loss of sense of smell and the presence of blood in the mouth all hinder the desire to take diet and fluids.

Sleeping

Assessing the patient's normal sleep pattern is useful. As discussed, nasal and sinus conditions often cause nasal obstruction, and this interferes with the activities of breathing and sleeping. The patient may be a snorer, suffer from interrupted sleep and dry mouth and may complain of fatigue. Postoperative nasal packing, swelling and discharge will also affect the patient's ability to sleep; this tends to improve as recovery progresses.

Expressing sexuality

The presence of nasal dressings and/or nasal discharge can affect the patient's body image. Though present for only a short period, it can be distressing.

CASE STUDY

The following case study aims to demonstrate both pre- and postoperative nursing care for an individual undergoing a septoplasty.

Mr George Black is admitted to the ward at 10 a.m. as his surgery is planned for the afternoon. He is 52 years old, married and works as a chef. George suffers with a deviated septum, causing nasal obstruction and snoring. He is also asthmatic, controlled by inhalers, and for this reason he was admitted for an overnight stay.

Nursing assessment

Box 11.9 details the nursing assessment of George Black.

Specific preoperative preparation

George has been 'nil by mouth' since an early breakfast at 6 a.m. Because of his asthma, George has a chest X-ray to ensure fitness for anaesthetic and a peak flow to assess lung capacity. A premedication of three puffs of George's asthma medication is prescribed and administered.

Box 11.9 Preoperative nursing assessment of a patient undergoing a septoplasty

Maintaining a safe environment
- Observation of vital signs is performed: pulse, 80 beats per minute; blood pressure, 150/80 mmHg.
- Allergies: none known.
- Past medical history: asthma since childhood; admitted with bronchitis and exacerbation of asthma 5 years ago; never had a general anaesthetic.
- Medication:
  - Salbutamol inhaler – two puffs three times per day and as required
  - Becotide inhaler – two puffs twice a day.
- George is anxious about the surgery, as he has never had a general anaesthetic; he is also concerned that his asthma will flare up.

Breathing
- Respiratory rate: 16 respirations per minute.
- George gave up smoking 5 years ago when he required hospital admission and treatment for bronchitis and asthma.
- George breathes through his mouth due to nasal obstruction.
- Chest X-ray: lungs clear; anaesthetist satisfied.
- Peak flow rate: 480.

Controlling body temperature
- George's temperature is 36.8°C.

Communicating
- George wears glasses for reading.
- Bilateral hearing is good.
- As discussed, George expresses fears about the anaesthetic and the risk to his asthma.

Eating and drinking
- George is of stocky build: height 1.77 m; weight 81 kg.
- He has a healthy appetite and, as he is a chef, enjoys cooking and dining with friends.
- George is Jewish, so does not eat pork.

Eliminating
- George opens his bowels daily and passes urine normally.
- Urinalysis: nothing abnormal detected.

Personal cleansing and dressing
- George is smartly dressed. Bathes daily.

Mobility
- George is independent; avoids steep walks and climbing stairs because of his asthma.

Working and playing
- George works full-time as a chef in a busy restaurant. He has arranged for 2 weeks' time off to recuperate.
- He enjoys swimming twice per week and visiting his family.

Expressing sexuality
- George is apprehensive about the presence of internal splinting and its appearance.
- He is aware that there will be no external scarring.

Sleeping
- George breathes through his mouth, so awakes feeling very dry and uncomfortable.
- He snores and tends to have a restless night's sleep (about 6 hours), thus feeling unrefreshed.

Dying
- George is a little anxious about the anaesthetic.

Postoperative nursing care

Specific postoperative complications following septo-plasty, and most types of nasal/sinus surgery, are:

- haemorrhage
- infection
- haematoma: e.g. septal or periorbital, i.e. around the eye
- difficulty in eating and drinking due to nasal packing
- difficulty in breathing normally due to nasal packing.

Box 11.10 outlines the postoperative care plan for George.

Box 11.10   Postoperative nursing care of a patient following a septoplasty

George Black returns to the ward following septoplasty. Nasal packing and internal splints are in situ. The packs are to be removed 6 hours after surgery if bleeding is not excessive. The splints are to remain in place for 1 week. George is alert, orientated and receiving oxygen therapy at 2 L/min until the following morning. Moderate fresh blood is noted on the nasal bolster.

Breathing
- *Problem*: Potential loss of clear airway, and respiratory distress due to anaesthetic, nasal packing, splinting and asthma.
- *Goal*: George is able to maintain a clear airway and breathe normally.
- *Care*:
  - Maintain upright position to facilitate respiration and nasal discharge.
  - Ensure oxygen therapy runs to prescribed regime.
  - Observe respiratory rate, depth and rhythm, and for presence of wheeze/tightness so as to promptly detect any exacerbation of asthma and/or respiratory difficulty; adhere to appropriate frequency of observation.
  - Reassure George that mouth-breathing ensures adequate airflow; provide mouthwash and care to help prevent dry mouth.
  - Administer asthma medications as prescribed and monitor effect.
  - Reassure George that nose will feel blocked for 2–3 weeks due to surgical oedema.
- *Evaluation*: George maintained oxygen therapy until morning. His respiratory observations remained within normal limits. Mouth-breathing was tolerated well, though a dry mouth was a little uncomfortable. A mild wheeze was heard upon returning to the ward, and two puffs from his salbutamol inhaler eased this. George felt comfortable.

Maintaining a safe environment
- *Problem*: Potential haemorrhage following surgery to an area with a very rich blood supply.
- *Goal*: To minimize haemorrhage.
- *Care*:
  - Perform observations of vital signs as per recommended postoperative regime; hypotension and tachycardia are signs of haemorrhage.
  - Observe nasal discharge; change nasal bolsters as required and chart frequency of dressing change; check back of throat for postnasal bleeding.
  - Apply ice packs to forehead, back of neck and bridge of nose if bleeding heavily as this will vasoconstrict blood vessels.
  - Inform doctor if any of the above is apparent.
  - Remove packing as instructed (see p. 202) but, if bleeding heavily, do not remove packing until the doctor has reviewed George first.
  - Ensure George remains on bedrest until 1 hour after removal of pack, in order to minimize activity and risk of further bleeding; permit gentle mobility after that.
  - Reinforce no nose blowing or picking, and advise George to sneeze with the mouth open to reduce pressure within the nose.
- *Evaluation*: A steady moderate ooze of fresh blood continued for the first hour. An ice pack was applied, which appeared to reduce bleeding. After 4 hours, nasal discharge became minimal and haemoserous. Packing was removed as instructed without complication. Observations were within normal limits. George mobilized around the ward with no ill-effect.

- *Problem*: Potential infection of the nose due to surgery and week-long insertion of splints.
- *Goal*: To prevent infection.
- *Care*:
  - Observe for signs of infection: purulent discharge, pyrexia and inflammation; report to the doctor if any signs are apparent.
  - Administer antibiotic therapy as prescribed and ensure George knows to complete the course once discharged home.
  - Discourage contact with people with coughs/colds for 1 week once home.
- *Evaluation*: George showed no signs of infection. Antibiotic therapy was administered and 'take-home' medication was arranged and explained.

- *Problem*: Potential septal haematoma due to collection of blood between the septum and mucous membrane.
- *Goal*: To detect onset promptly.
- *Care*:
  - Advise George to inform staff if pain becomes worse and nasal blockage becomes severe after packing is removed.
  - Ensure splints remain in situ for 1 week as directed, to maintain septal position.
- *Evaluation*: There appeared to be no signs of haematoma. Pain was a mild discomfort (normal) that was relieved by paracetamol. Splints remained intact and were removed when George attended follow-up outpatient's clinic.

Eating and drinking

- *Problem*: Difficulty in swallowing due to the presence of nasal packs.
- *Goal*: To ensure adequate hydration/nutrition; for George to return to swallowing normally.
- *Care*:
  - Maintain intravenous infusion as prescribed if present; monitor cannula site for extravasation and signs of infection.
  - Encourage oral fluids/soft diet as able; provide supplement drinks if food is not taken.
  - Reassure that any difficulty in swallowing will pass once nasal packing has been removed.
  - Maintain an accurate fluid balance chart until intravenous infusion is completed and normal oral intake is achieved.
- *Evaluation*: George complained of a sucking sensation at the back of his throat whenever he swallowed. His oral intake was poor at first (350 mL water in 5 hours) and he only managed soup at supper. The intravenous infusion was maintained until complete at 9 p.m. Once the nasal packing was removed at 8 p.m., his swallowing returned to normal. A late sandwich was eaten.

NASAL PACKING AND SPLINTING

Nasal packing

As discussed previously, haemorrhage is the main postoperative complication following nasal and sinus surgery. For some types of nasal surgery, packs are inserted at the end of the operation, so that by exerting pressure against the mucosal wall the risk of haemorrhage is greatly reduced. However, it is now common for patients having nasal surgery to have no nasal packing postoperatively. Figure 11.2 illustrates types of nasal packing commonly used.

The surgeon determines when the packing is to be removed, and this may be 4, 12 or 24 hours later. Some fresh bleeding through the packs for the first 1–2 hours of recovery is normal. In order to monitor this, a nasal dressing (bolster) is applied, and this is changed as required. If the bleeding does not appear to be subsiding, the packing is left in situ and the doctor is contacted.

Nasal packing may be removed by the nurse. A basic dressing pack is prepared, as saline and gauze are used to gently clean the exterior of the nose once the packing has been removed. It is essential to outline the procedure to the patient in order to minimize anxiety. The patient needs to sit upright in the bed, as this facilitates pack removal and helps to avoid swallowing of any blood. The patient is then asked to breathe gently in and out in a steady rhythm; with each expiration the pack is slowly eased out of the nose with the aid of forceps. If both sides are packed, one alternates from side to side, removing a little at a time. At first, some fresh bleeding is common, in the form of a trickle of blood. Gentle pressure on the nose and the application of ice packs to the forehead, bridge of nose and the back of the neck will enhance vasoconstriction. A nasal bolster is applied, and monitoring of nasal discharge continues. It is normal for nasal secretions to decrease to a minimal amount of haemoserous discharge over 2–3 days.

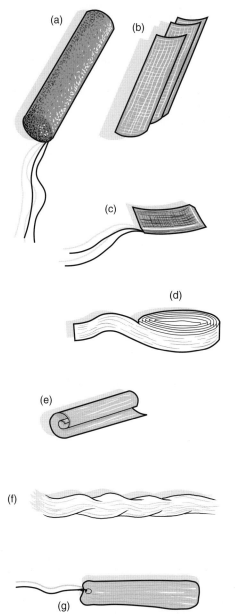

Figure 11.2   Examples of nasal packing: (a) Merocel (sponge); (b) Telfa Pack (paraffin non-adherent gauze); (c) Neurosurgical Patties; (d) BIPP (bismuth iodoform impregnated packing); (e) Merogel (absorbable hyaluronic acid sheet); (f) Kaltostat (calcium alginate wool); (g) gel-knit packs (hydrocolloid fabric).

Nasal splinting

Internal silastic splints may be inserted into each nasal cavity following septoplasty. The splints maintain septal position and remain in situ for 1–2 weeks. They are sutured in place, and the patient is advised not to touch

Box 11.11   Discharge advice for patients following nasal/sinus surgery

- The nose will feel more blocked due to swelling and can take 2–3 weeks to resolve. If prescribed, apply nasal drops to decongest the nose (see Fig.11.3 for correct method of instilling nasal drops).
- Scabbing within the nose may occur as it heals; douching with warm water may soften the scabs; do not pick the nose, as this may precipitate bleeding.
- Sneeze with your mouth open to reduce nasal pressure. Only wipe the nose, do not blow, until postoperative outpatients visit.
- Nasal discharge can continue for a few days and is normally lightly bloodstained.
- If fresh, steady bleeding occurs, pinch the fleshy part of the nose and lean forward; apply ice to the forehead and bridge of nose; avoid swallowing any blood as it can make you feel sick; if the bleeding does not stop after 15 minutes, ring the ward or casualty department for advice.
- For the first few days, avoid very hot drinks, meals, baths and showers, as these can increase the risk of bleeding.
- Avoid work and strenuous activity for at least 1 week or as advised.
- Avoid smoking, crowded smoky places and people with colds or coughs, as infection can be picked up in the nose.
- If nasal splints are in situ, do not touch; attend the outpatients appointment for removal.

them. The surgeon removes the splints in the outpatient's clinic.

If rhinoplasty is also performed an external splint may be applied, to support the new position of the nasal bones following repair of nasal fractures and septorhinoplasty. Splinting can be with layers of surgical tape, plaster of Paris, or a Thermoplast splint. The splint is removed by the doctor 1–2 weeks later, in the outpatient's clinic.

DISCHARGE PLANNING AND PATIENT EDUCATION

Both written and verbal discharge advice is given to the patient (Box 11.11). Outpatient follow-up varies from 1 to 6 weeks. Here, any nasal splinting is removed and examination of the nose and sinuses is performed. Assessing the benefits of the surgery is left until, at least, this time, as surgical swelling needs sufficient time to reduce.

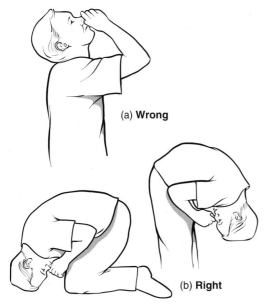

Figure 11.3 The correct method of instilling nasal medication. (a) If the wrong method is used, the nasal drops pass into the pharynx and avoid important internal nasal structures. (b) The correct method ensures the spread of nasal drops across important nasal membranes. *Drops*: staying with the head forward for a few minutes after instillation is advised. *Spray*: if medication is spray delivery, then upright position, no backward tilting, is recommended; the drug is delivered in a metered dose via a pump (Ugwoke et al, 2001).

THE THROAT

ANATOMY AND PHYSIOLOGY

The word 'throat' is ambiguous, as it can mean different things to different people. Within the speciality of ENT surgery, its components are:

- pharynx
  - nasopharynx
  - oropharynx
  - hypopharynx
- larynx
- salivary glands.

Pharynx

The functions of the pharynx are:

- to deliver food, saliva and mucus to the oesophagus
- to act as an airway from the nose and mouth to the larynx
- to resonate sound produced in the larynx.

The nasopharynx lies above the soft palate at the rear of the nose, is lined with mucous membrane and contains the eustachian tube orifice and the adenoids,

which are sacs of lymphoid tissue. The oropharynx lies between the soft palate and the hyoid bone. The hyoid is a small U-shaped bone that lies below and supports the tongue; muscles and ligaments secure its position. The palatine tonsils are located within the oropharynx on either side of the base of the tongue. Like the adenoids, they are lymphoid tissue and their function is to protect against infection.

The hypopharynx lies behind the larynx, and connects with the oesophagus.

Nerve supply to the pharynx is via branches of the glossopharyngeal (ninth cranial) nerve.

Larynx

The larynx is the organ of phonation, comprising rigid cartilage, ligament, muscle and membrane. The vocal cords consist of folds of mucous membrane, which adduct and abduct, producing controlled interference of airflow that results in audible vibrations, termed speech. The other important function of the larynx is to protect the tracheobronchial tree, and this is achieved by the following means:

- the *epiglottis*: a flap of cartilage and mucous membrane which occludes the larynx when swallowing.
- the *glottis*: the space between the vocal cords contained within the larynx, which can be closed in order to initiate a cough.

The vagus nerve supplies branches to the larynx, in the form of the superior and recurrent laryngeal nerve.

Salivary glands

There are three pairs of salivary glands:

- The *parotid glands* produce mainly serous saliva that secretes into the mouth via the parotid ducts near each second upper molar tooth.
- The *submandibular glands* produce seromucinous fluid that drains into the floor of the mouth via the submandibular ducts.
- The *sublingual glands* are principally mucous in nature and drain into the mouth via sublingual ducts.

Between 500 and 1000 mL of saliva is produced every 24 hours. The functions of saliva are listed in Box 11.12.

Blood supply

Arterial blood supply to the head and neck region derives from the arch of the aorta, to the internal and external carotid arteries. The internal carotid arteries deliver blood to the brain and the orbit of the eye; the external carotid arteries supply the more superficial tissues of the head and neck.

Box 11.12   Functions of saliva

- facilitates chewing and swallowing
- lubricates food
- aids taste
- protects the oral cavity from infection
- aids speech

Box 11.13   Types of throat surgery

- *Tonsillectomy*: surgical removal of the palatine tonsils.
- *Uvulopalatopharyngoplasty* (UPPP): surgical resection of the uvula, soft palate, ± tonsils is performed to widen the upper airway.
- *Repair of pharyngeal pouch*: an endoscope is used to visualize the pharyngeal hernia (Zenker's diverticulum), and is repaired using staples; traditional technique of repair involves external neck incision and pharyngeal repair.
- *Pharyngoscopy*: endoscopic examination of the pharynx.
- *Oesophagoscopy*: endoscopic examination of the oesophagus.
- *Laryngoscopy*: endoscopic examination of the larynx.
- *Tracheostomy formation*: a small window of cartilage is removed between the second and third tracheal ring in order to create airway patency. The chosen tracheostomy tube is inserted and initially sutured in place.

Venous blood from the face, neck and other superficial tissues drains into the external jugular veins.

There are many surgical procedures involving the structures of the 'throat'. The following two areas are discussed separately:

- surgical conditions of the throat
- surgical conditions of the head and neck.

CONDITIONS OF THE THROAT THAT REQUIRE SURGERY

The following are common examples of throat conditions that lead to surgery (Box 11.13).

Recurrent tonsillitis and peritonsillar abscess

Repeated bacterial infection, commonly streptococcal, can cause severe distress. Pain, pyrexia and difficulty in swallowing (dysphagia) are the problems experienced. The infection can localize over one of the tonsils, causing a peritonsillar abscess, known as a quinsy,

which if not adequately treated can lead to the complication of a restricted, oedematous airway. For both conditions a tonsillectomy is recommended.

Snoring and obstructive sleep apnoea

The temporary collapse of the upper airway on inspiration causes obstruction and snoring. The most common site of this problem is in the region of the soft palate.

Sleep apnoea is defined as 30 instances of stopping breathing, for at least 10 seconds each, over a period of 7 hours of sleep (Dhillon and East, 1994). Drinking alcohol, smoking and being overweight increase the risk of developing snoring and obstructive sleep apnoea, as they reduce pharyngeal muscle tone. Other factors include the following conditions: nasal polyps, deviated nasal septum, hypertrophied turbinates, enlarged adenoids and tonsils, floppy uvula and soft palate. Correcting these structural problems and addressing physiological obstruction should alleviate sleep apnoea and snoring.

The most common type of surgery for this condition is uvulopalatopharyngoplasty (UPPP) ± tonsillectomy, a procedure designed to improve the upper airway (Fig. 11.4).

Pharyngeal pouch

This is a hernia of the pharyngeal mucosa in which food debris collects. The pouch can enlarge to cause oesophageal compression, regurgitation and dysphagia. Endoscopic surgery can repair the pouch using a purpose-built diverticuloscope and a stapling device. The patient can commence fluids and soft diet the next day and may be discharged home the following day.

Foreign body

Fish, lamb and chicken bones are the most common foreign bodies lodged in the pharynx or oesophagus of adult patients. This can cause pain and dysphagia and be distressing. Endoscopy to retrieve foreign bodies may include pharyngoscopy and oesophagoscopy.

Airway obstruction

Acute or potential airway obstruction is serious and can be caused by the following:

- trauma to the trachea or larynx, causing oedema or structural injury
- oedema associated with head and neck surgery, and burns
- laryngeal incompetence (failure to function correctly)
- loss of gag reflex and therefore risk of aspiration into the lungs
- inability to expectorate lung secretions.

A tracheostomy is performed to restore or maintain a clear airway for the above conditions. If a patient is receiving long-term artificial ventilation, a tracheostomy is often performed, as endotracheal intubation can cause laryngeal and tracheal injury (Hooper, 1996).

Types of tracheostomy tube

The most common makes are Portex, Shiley and Silver Negus, and they all come in a variety of sizes. Silver Negus tubes are now uncommon as there are durable and more cost-effective alternatives. Tracheostomy tubes come in a variety of forms, as follows, and the patient's condition determines which type is used.

Plain or fenestrated A hole or fenestration in the upper aspect of the tube enables passage of air from the trachea through the larynx into the pharynx: i.e. it promotes the upper airway. Thus, when the end of the tube is occluded either with a finger or speaking valve, the patient can vocalize. Fenestrated tubes are therefore used in patients who have recovered from the acute period; have a functioning upper airway; have the functional ability to vocalize (laryngeal competence); and those who may be starting the process of weaning off the tracheostomy.

Plain tubes are inserted when the tracheostomy is initially performed. A plain tube has no hole; therefore, use of the upper airway or vocalization cannot be effectively achieved.

Cuffed or cuffless The cuff sits at the base of the tube and is inflated with air via a valve, which is visible on the outside of the tube. Its purpose is to prevent aspiration of gastric/oral secretions by closing off the upper airway. It is inflated for long-term ventilation, ensuring maximum oxygenation of the lungs by preventing air leaks. The cuff must be deflated, or the tube changed to a cuffless type if vocalization is desired, or if the process of weaning off the tracheostomy is to commence. Regular checks of cuff pressures when inflated are essential, as tracheal irritation and necrosis

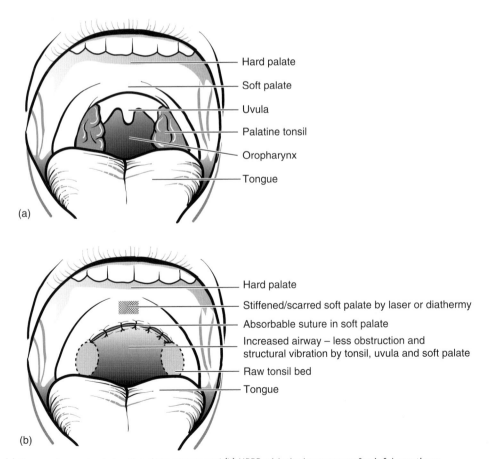

Figure 11.4 (a) The oropharynx in obstructive sleep apnoea and (b) UPPP with the large areas of painful raw tissue postoperatively, and the improved airway.

can occur with prolonged pressure; a specific manometer can measure this pressure.

With/without removable inner cannula Tubes with inner cannulae are widely preferred nowadays, as they promote safe practice: they can be removed as often as necessary in order to clear secretions; they reduce the frequency of suctioning, which is traumatic to the patient; and they reduce the risk of tube occlusion and associated respiratory distress. Tubes without inner cannulae tend to accumulate viscous secretions that are difficult to clear, and so carry a greater risk of tube occlusion.

Tracheostomy care
This is more fully discussed in the case study for laryngectomy. Common aspects of care include the maintenance of a clear airway, with suctioning and humidification, and communicating.

Boxes 11.14 and 11.15 outline key issues to be considered when caring for a patient with a tracheostomy.

Box 11.14   Specific issues of nursing care for tracheostomy patients

- *A tracheostomy is temporary.* Maintaining tube patency and security are essential in order to maintain airway. Sutures and/or tapes are used.
- *A tracheostomy bypasses the upper airway.* The body's natural humidification and warming systems of the mouth and nose are bypassed; so inhaled air is drier and cooler. Secretions become dry and viscous, and tracheal irritation can develop unless alternative methods of humidification and warming are applied, e.g. mechanical humidifiers, saline nebulizers and moist gauze veils.
- *A tracheostomy impairs the patient's cough reflex.* This causes an increase in tracheal irritation and sputum production. The ability to expectorate is reduced, so assistance is required in the form of physiotherapy and tracheal suctioning. Cleansing of inner cannula, if present, also clears secretions.
- *A tracheostomy impairs communication.* Patients can feel very anxious and isolated. Nursing them close to the nurses' station, having the call bell to hand, providing pen and paper and communication boards, and encouraging the use of mouthing and gesturing all alleviate difficulties in communicating. Patience and reassurance will establish the patients' confidence in their nurse's ability to care for them. Once a speaking valve can be used or the patient can vocalize by occluding the end of the tube with a finger, the patient may feel more at ease.
- *A tracheostomy can make swallowing uncomfortable.* If allowed to take diet, soft foods are offered for ease of ingestion. For conditions where swallowing is greatly impaired, e.g. loss of gag reflex and aspiration, enteral feeding is provided.
- *A tracheostomy can cause infection.* Wound infection can occur at the incision site; thorough attention to wound care prevents wound breakdown. Using an aseptic technique, the area around the tube is cleansed with saline using gauze and cotton buds; a dressing is then placed under the flange of the tube, e.g. Lyofoam. This is performed as required, and at least once per shift.

Box 11.15   Step-by-step suctioning of a tracheostomy tube

- Ensure functioning suction equipment is set up at the bedside in order to use promptly as required.
- Recognize signs for suctioning: ronchi (low-pitched gurgle), wheeze, dyspnoea, restlessness, restricted airflow felt on hand (Carroll, 1994).
- Discuss all care with patient in order to minimize anxiety.
- Remove inner cannula, if present, clear secretions and re-insert.
- If above signs persist, prepare equipment for suctioning.
- Attach suction catheter to tubing; its size has to be less than half the diameter of the tracheostomy tube, as too large a catheter removes too much oxygen and causes hypoxia.
- Turn suction on, pressure range being 80–120 mmHg; a high pressure can lead to hypoxia and trauma.
- Wear personal protective equipment – apron, goggles and gloves – to minimize risk of cross-infection.
- Remove catheter wrapping and insert catheter to only about one-third of its length, in order to minimize tracheal trauma.
- Apply suction by occluding the catheter porthole. This should only be done during its withdrawal, and for no more than 15 seconds. Inappropriate technique increases the risk of hypoxia and trauma (Hooper, 1996).
- Discard the catheter and gloves into infectious waste and rinse the suction tubing with sterile water. These actions maintain high standards of infection control.
- Assess the patient's airway and, if further suctioning is required, repeat the process.

SPECIFIC INVESTIGATIONS FOR PATIENTS REQUIRING SURGERY TO THE THROAT

The following investigations may be undertaken:

- sleep studies to ascertain degree of sleep apnoea
- endoscopy to visualize structural abnormalities, e.g. pharyngeal pouch, laryngeal oedema
- X-rays to demonstrate location and nature of foreign body
- CT/MRI scan for traumatic injury to throat or soft tissue lesions
- positron emission tomography (PET) scan to demonstrate cellular activity; also useful following radiotherapy
- barium swallow to reveal pharyngeal/oesophageal dysfunction, e.g. pooling in pharyngeal pouch.

The doctor takes a full history from the patient, and issues discussed include:

- frequency of tonsillitis/quinsy and if hospitalized for treatment
- severity of sleep apnoea and snoring, and their effect on sleep quality and relationship with partner
- nature of dysphagia, types of food tolerated and presence of any weight loss.

NURSING ASSESSMENT OF A PATIENT REQUIRING SURGERY TO THE THROAT

The following activities reflect the specific issues that need to be considered when assessing an individual admitted for throat surgery.

Breathing

Some types of throat surgery aim to improve the airway, e.g. UPPP and tracheostomy. Thorough assessment of the patient's respiratory status, chest condition and blood oxygen saturation levels are documented to obtain an accurate baseline for postoperative reference.

Assessing the techniques used by the patient to make any difficult breathing easier is essential in order to provide individualized patient care. Methods used may include sitting upright, leaning across a table, the use of nebulized drugs, oxygen therapy and relaxation techniques.

Maintaining a safe environment

For all patients, the nurse needs to preoperatively assess vital signs and assess past medical history and current/recent medication for any bleeding tendencies.

The patient may experience discomfort or pain following throat surgery, particularly so after a tonsillectomy/UPPP. Preparing a patient preoperatively,

with realistic expectations of postoperative pain, aims to improve recovery. Following tonsillectomy and UPPP, patients may experience various degrees of pain for up to 14 days.

Controlling body temperature

The swallowing of a foreign body, such as a sharply edged bone, carries a risk of pharyngeal/oesophageal perforation. The nurse performs a thorough assessment of the patient's temperature, pulse and comfort level; pyrexia, tachycardia and chest or upper back pain are signs of perforation (McCormick et al, 1992). If the perforation remains undetected and oral diet is allowed, the patient can develop serious and possibly life-threatening complications, e.g. mediastinitis and empyema (pus in the pleural cavity). Hence, a thorough assessment is of vital importance.

Eating and drinking

Assessing the patient's weight, body mass index, normal diet, fluid intake and general appetite are strongly indicated, as any condition of the throat affects an individual's ability to eat and drink. Repeated episodes of tonsillitis or quinsy may have led to weight loss, as can the dysphagia associated with a pharyngeal pouch and breathing difficulties. Obesity may be present in obstructive sleep apnoea patients.

Communicating

Assessment of this activity is particularly pertinent for patients admitted with breathing difficulties and who may require a tracheostomy. The patient may be too exhausted to speak. Relevant issues that need to be explored include the following:

- Does the patient speak, understand and write English?
- Are there any hearing problems?
- Does the patient need spectacles, and for which activities?

Based on the above, alternative methods of communicating can be planned, e.g. the use of pen and paper, communication boards, mouthing words and gesturing.

Sleeping

Obstructive sleep apnoea, snoring and respiratory difficulties often result in poor sleeping patterns; some patients are admitted to hospital exhausted. A sleep assessment is necessary to obtain information about the quality, duration and style of sleeping, including methods used by the patient to improve sleep.

POSTOPERATIVE NURSING CARE OF PATIENTS WHO HAVE HAD SURGERY TO THE THROAT

Specific postoperative complications following surgery to the throat involve the activities of breathing, maintaining a safe environment, controlling body temperature, and eating and drinking.

Potential loss of clear airway and difficulty in communicating

This applies especially to patients with airway obstruction or a tracheostomy. Specific aspects of nursing care focus upon the alleviation of the respiratory and psychological distress, and the maintenance of adequate respiratory function. It is essential to monitor the patient's vital signs and blood oxygenation levels, as the patient's condition can deteriorate rapidly. Box 11.14 outlines key issues concerning tracheostomy care.

Haemorrhage, infection and pain, particularly following a tonsillectomy

Postoperative haemorrhage is a potential complication of all surgery. Following tonsillectomy, raw, vascular areas may bleed without warning. Regular observation of the patient's vital signs is indicated; hypotension and tachycardia are signs of haemorrhage. It is good practice to perform hourly pulse monitoring throughout the first postoperative night (not applicable if the patient is a day case), as a raised pulse while asleep is a reliable indicator of bleeding. Haematemesis and repeated swallowing may indicate bleeding from the tonsillar sites.

Infection can also cause bleeding. The patient should eat and drink as normally as possible (three meals per day with snacks, consisting of textured food, plus 2 litres of fluids per day); the rationale being that this keeps the throat free of debris and infection, so minimizing the risk of bleeding.

Pharyngeal/oesophageal perforation following certain endoscopic procedures, including the retrieval of foreign bodies

As discussed earlier in the assessment process, close observation of vital signs is indicated. The surgeon dictates when the patient can commence oral fluids and diet; often only sterile water is allowed at first and, as long as the patient continues to demonstrate no signs of perforation, a soft diet is gradually introduced, usually by the next day.

Difficulty in eating and drinking

A patient with a tracheostomy may experience dysphagia due to oesophageal compression, so a soft diet

is recommended. Following pharyngeal pouch repair or removal of foreign body, a soft diet is also advised in order to allow the affected area to heal comfortably. By contrast, the recommendation is to eat a normal, textured diet following tonsillectomy, for reasons discussed below.

DISCHARGE PLANNING AND PATIENT EDUCATION

General advice is given to the patient regarding diet and pain control, and any take-home medication is explained. Patients having undergone a tonsillectomy receive written advice (Box 11.16) as a means of reinforcing important issues. Follow-up in the outpatient clinic ranges between 2 and 6 weeks.

Long-term patients with a tracheostomy are discharged with well-prepared community nursing support. Suctioning and nebulizing equipment may be delivered to the home, and the patient and family must have demonstrated competence in providing

---

Box 11.16   Discharge advice following a tonsillectomy

- Rest for 2 weeks and take time off work.
- Eat a normal diet, as chewing and swallowing textured food relieves pain and cleanses the tonsillar beds. This helps to prevent infection.
- Drink plenty of fluids (2–3 litres per day).
- Be strict with hygiene and use a mouthwash and gargle after meals.
- This is a painful procedure. Discomfort may increase between the 4th and 8th day, when a membrane loosens off the tonsil beds; this is normal. Take regular analgesics, especially prior to meals.
- You may suffer earache. This is normal, as the nerve supply to the tonsil area and ears is connected.
- Avoid smoking and being in crowded places; keep away from people with colds and coughs. This will help to prevent local irritation and infection.
- White spots at the back of the throat are normal and are part of the healing process.
- The above advice is important; it is vital to eat and drink normally in order to make a good recovery. If you experience any of the following symptoms contact the ward or hospital emergency department, as these are signs of infection and may require readmission to hospital:
  - severe and worsening pain
  - bleeding
  - a raised temperature.

total tracheostomy care before discharge. Often a trial at home, in the form of weekend or day leave, has been performed in order to assess the patient and family's ability to cope. Regular visits to the outpatient clinic are recommended, to facilitate tube change and assessment of the patient's progress (tube change is recommended on a monthly basis to prevent infection and tube occlusion). The patient and family are advised to contact the ward with any concerns or problems.

HEAD AND NECK

CONDITIONS OF THE HEAD AND NECK THAT REQUIRE SURGERY

This branch of ENT surgery covers a wide range of conditions, often malignant, which require surgery and/or radiotherapy treatments. The activities of breathing, communicating, eating and drinking, and expressing sexuality can be profoundly affected by both disease and treatment. Body image can be altered dramatically as a result of the disfiguring nature of the surgery. Nursing care is specialized, with the main aim of rehabilitating the patient to an altered way of life through education, and empathic support of the individual and family.

Head and neck neoplasms seem to occur more commonly in individuals who have been exposed to the following:

- smoking or snuff-taking
- alcohol
- hardwood dust
- heavy metals, e.g. chromium
- radiation
- viruses.

(Dhillon and East, 1994).

Because of the complex and, at times, extensive and reconstructive nature of head and neck surgery, it is not easy to tabulate the types of surgical procedure commonly used in practice today. The following gives a brief overview of head and neck disease and surgery offered.

Salivary gland neoplasm

The majority of salivary gland tumours are in the parotid glands and are benign; incidence of malignancy is greater in the submandibular glands.

Parotidectomy is removal of the parotid gland. The risk of damage to the facial nerve is explained to the patient; often facial weakness is temporary due to surgical swelling.

Submandibular gland excision carries the risk of injuring the submandibular branches of the facial nerve; this can be permanent.

Neoplasm of the ear

Chronic ear infection may induce malignant disease in the pinna, ear canal and middle ear. Sun overexposure may lead to external ear malignancy.

Surgery ranges from a wedge-shaped excision of the pinna, to radical and disfiguring resection of the total ear and surrounding tissues.

Neoplasm of the nose and sinuses

These are rare and may require ophthalmic, plastic, maxillofacial or neurosurgical collaboration. The close proximity to the eyes, face, jaw and brain requires delicate and precise resection, salvage and reconstruction. The ENT surgeon plays a key role in the management of these patients.

Nasopharyngeal neoplasm

Treatment for tumours arising in this region may involve surgical resection; clearance of disease is difficult, and radiotherapy may be a preferred treatment option.

Hypopharyngeal neoplasm

Benign tumours are rare. Typically, in malignant disease, patients are smokers and heavy drinkers of alcohol. The disease can develop without severe symptoms; a mild sensation of 'something in the throat' is often the earliest complaint (Dhillon and East, 1994). Upon diagnosis, the tumour has grown sufficiently to require surgery and/or radiotherapy. The larynx, pharynx and possibly part of the oesophagus are removed; the oesophagus may be reconstructed with jejunum (Singh and Soutar, 1993). Thirty per cent of those treated survive 5 years (American Cancer Society, 2003).

Oropharyngeal neoplasia

The posterior third of the tongue, the floor of mouth, epiglottis, soft palate, uvula, tonsils and pharyngeal wall can be affected by malignancy, commonly squamous cell carcinoma. Metastatic spread to lymph nodes occurs because of the rich lymphatic supply in these areas. Surgical resection may involve removal of the affected oropharynx, part of the mandible if disease involves the bone, and reconstructive repair using muscle and skin flaps. Postoperative radiotherapy aims to eliminate residual malignant disease.

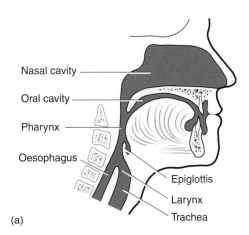

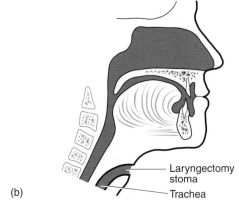

Figure 11.5   Altered anatomy following laryngectomy:
(a) before surgery; (b) after surgery

Laryngeal neoplasm

Benign tumours are rare, and squamous cell carcinoma is the most common malignant disease. Symptoms often include altered voice (dysphonia), dysphagia and, in advanced cases, breathing difficulties. Treatment may include endoscopic partial laryngectomy using a laser, or 'open' surgical removal of the larynx (laryngectomy) and neck dissection if neck nodes are affected. Postoperative radiotherapy may also be arranged. Figure 11.5 demonstrates the altered anatomy following a laryngectomy.

Neck lumps

Commonly, lateral neck lumps are metastatic malignant disease, i.e. the distant spread of a malignant carcinoma, with its primary site often within the structures of the pharynx and larynx. In order to ascertain full diagnosis, a thorough clinical investigation is required. The standard surgical procedure to remove a neck lump is neck dissection.

SPECIFIC INVESTIGATIONS FOR PATIENTS REQUIRING HEAD AND NECK SURGERY

Investigations include:

- Fine-needle aspiration of neck lump for cytology. This determines the nature of the carcinoma: e.g. squamous cell carcinoma.
- Radiology:
  - X-rays can demonstrate gross pathology
  - CT/MRI scanning reveal accurate images of disease and metastatic spread
  - PET scan if recurrence, and/or following chemotherapy/radiotherapy.
- Endoscopy, under general anaesthetic, ± biopsy of any abnormal lesions; this may include laryngoscopy, pharyngoscopy and oesophagoscopy. The diagnosis may be determined using the international TNM classification (Box 11.17).

Box 11.17   TNM classification

Head and neck cancer diagnosis and prognosis use the tumour–node–metastases classification (Sobin & Wittekind, 1997) to describe:

- Tumour T – size of primary
- Nodes N – if regional lymph nodes have cancer in them
- Metastases M – if cancer has spread to a different part of the body

The UICC (International Union Against Cancer) TNM classification promotes a consensus of one global clinically relevant staging classification for cancer.

NURSING ASSESSMENT OF A PATIENT REQUIRING SURGERY TO THE HEAD AND NECK

The following activities of daily living specific to the needs of individuals suffering with head and neck disease, who require surgery, need to be assessed.

Breathing

Assessing the patient's normal respiratory function is essential, as head and neck disease and surgery involves the risk of acute airway obstruction. The patient may be experiencing breathing difficulties due to the effects of the tumour on laryngeal function and patency of the airway.

Maintaining a safe environment

Because of the rich blood supply to the head and neck, haemorrhage and haematoma are potential postoperative risks. Assessing the patient's cardiovascular observations is performed preoperatively as a baseline. Some patients may be heavy drinkers or alcoholics: determining their weekly unit intake on initial assessment helps to prepare for any postoperative complications regarding alcohol withdrawal, and medication can be given in order to alleviate symptoms of withdrawal.

Controlling body temperature

The risk of postoperative infection requires assessment of the patient's temperature and ability to heal. Previous radiotherapy to the area can predispose to poor wound healing because of its effects on tissue integrity. Head and neck disease and major surgery can weaken the body's immune system, resulting in increased vulnerability to infections. Assessing for early signs of infection, e.g. chest (pneumonia) and mouth (oral thrush), is therefore routine practice.

Eating and drinking

Often patients are admitted having experienced dysphagia and weight loss for some time; they can be underweight and malnourished, so building-up with fortified foods and drinks is required to maximize well-being for surgery. All patients are weighed, and this continues on a regular basis (three times per week) until discharge.

Preparing the patient for difficulties in eating and drinking during the postoperative phase is also undertaken. The admitting nurse assesses the patient's understanding of the surgery and aftercare, in particular the need for prolonged 'nil by mouth' (approximately 7–14 days), enteral tube feeding and the need for soft or purée food once oral intake is permitted.

Eliminating

Assessment of the patient's normal bladder and bowel functions is performed. Poor fluid and food intake prior to surgery may cause constipation. Preoperative urinalysis is performed to detect any abnormalities.

Communicating

Preoperatively, patients may complain of a hoarse voice (laryngeal disease), and discomfort or pain in the affected area can make speaking arduous. The speech therapist performs a thorough assessment of the patient preoperatively, and this includes an evaluation for appropriate methods of speech restoration.

Expressing sexuality

Disfiguring disease and surgery of the head and neck often result in altered body image and low self-esteem. It is vitally important to prepare the patient as much as possible prior to surgery, and this includes an assessment of the patient's perception of disease and surgery, their effects on activities of daily living and the scarring involved.

Personal cleansing and dressing

As discussed previously, self-esteem is affected in patients with head and neck disease; the activity of cleansing and dressing is just as relevant. Any disfigurement may lead to a change in dress style, with the emphasis on covering up an unfortunate end-result. Therefore, it is important to assess patients' style and views on presenting themselves, as well as their perceptions of postoperative recovery and appearance.

Working and playing

Establishing the patient's occupation, social activities and home situation is essential for rehabilitation and discharge. For some, a long period of absence from work is required in order to allow for full treatment, which may include radiotherapy, and recovery. This could range between 2 and 12 months. Stopping work completely or changing occupation may be advised, as the surgery may irrevocably affect work performance, e.g. laryngectomy. Changes to an individual's lifestyle can be deeply distressing, both emotionally and financially. Assessing the need for social services is therefore indicated, and a referral can then be made to the appropriate services.

Dying

Fears of dying can be overwhelming when dealing with a diagnosis of cancer or when facing major surgery and months of rehabilitation. The nurse can explore such issues and provide realistic postoperative expectations; offering an empathetic and attentive approach when delivering nursing care and upon initial assessment helps to alleviate some of the fears.

CASE STUDY

A case study of a patient undergoing a laryngectomy for squamous cell carcinoma of the larynx is presented to demonstrate aspects of nursing care relevant to the field of head and neck surgery.

Mr Bill Warren is admitted to the ward for a total laryngectomy the next day. He was diagnosed with cancer of the larynx following a laryngoscopy 2 weeks earlier. Bill is 63 years of age, married with children and grandchildren, and took retirement from banking 3 years ago.

Nursing assessment

Box 11.18 details the assessment of Mr Warren upon admission for a laryngectomy.

Box 11.18   Preoperative nursing assessment of a patient undergoing laryngectomy

Maintaining a safe environment
- Observation of vital signs is performed: pulse, 76 beats per minute and regular; blood pressure, 155/85 mmHg.
- Allergies: none known.
- Past medical history: atrial fibrillation diagnosed 2 years ago; dental clearance under general anaesthetic 1 year ago; 4-month history of hoarse voice; laryngoscopy 2 weeks ago diagnosing laryngeal carcinoma.
- Medication: digoxin 125 μg daily; occasional paracetamol for throat discomfort.
- Bill is very anxious about surgery and his recovery: in particular, how he will cope with the laryngectomy stoma.

Breathing
- Respiration rate is 16 respirations per minute.
- Mild stridor (noisy breathing) noted.
- Oxygen saturation on air is 94%.
- Chest X-ray is satisfactory.
- Bill smoked 20–30 cigarettes per day for 35 years and cut down to 10–15 per day since hoarseness of voice began; still has 5 cigarettes per day since diagnosis.

Controlling body temperature
- Bill's temperature is 36.4°C.

Communicating
- Hoarseness of voice is apparent; Bill's voice gets tired easily.
- Glasses are worn for reading.
- Normal hearing is present.
- Bill states he is concerned that he will be unable to communicate after surgery, but he has come with a large pad of paper and pens. His son has made him a communication board to use while in hospital.
- Bill and his wife have met the speech therapist and discussed voice rehabilitation; he is to be a candidate for BlomSinger valve insertion, which he is pleased about.
- Bill and his family have been reading the laryngectomy booklets, and he has brought them with him.

Eating and drinking
- Bill manages a normal diet but avoids foods that require a lot of chewing, because of throat discomfort.
- Height is 1.84 m; weight is 82 kg.
- His appetite has become poor since diagnosis, due to apprehension.
- Bill admits to being a heavy alcohol drinker (about 40 units per week) for many years but he has cut down to about 10 units per week, mainly wine, since diagnosis of his cardiac condition.

Personal cleansing and dressing
- Bill dresses smartly. He requests to see the laryngectomy bibs and filters (devices worn over a laryngectomy stoma which protect the airway from airborne particles and help to humidify inhaled air). He takes a bath every night.

Mobility
- Bill is independent.

Working and playing
- Bill retired from banking 3 years ago and enjoys a busy, varied home life. He and his wife holiday abroad twice a year and regularly visit his children and their families.
- Bill's hobbies include gardening, golfing, socializing and amateur dramatics. He is saddened that he will no longer be able to perform on stage but hopes to continue with the drama club in a different way once radiotherapy after surgery is complete.

Expressing sexuality
- Bill is concerned that being dependent on nursing staff will compromise his masculinity, and he states that he is 'not looking forward to the baby food'.

Sleeping
- Sleep has been disrupted by the hoarseness of voice and mild stridor, particularly in the past month. Since diagnosis, his sleep pattern is more erratic; he tends to manage 6 hours sleep, though wakes four or five times.

Eliminating
- Bill opens his bowels daily, and micturition is normal; urinalysis shows no abnormalities.
- Bill knows that following a laryngectomy, regular bowel activity should be maintained, as the ability to close the glottis for straining is lost.

Dying
- Bill feels confident about having an anaesthetic.
- He does state that, for the first time since his cardiac condition was diagnosed, he is fearful for the future.

Specific preoperative preparation

In the outpatients department, the following procedure will be performed:

- CT scanning
- blood tests, electrocardiogram (ECG) and chest X-ray
- meeting the speech therapist and discussing speech rehabilitation
- meeting a laryngectomy patient (if the patient requests)
- preparation for surgery: i.e. discussion about surgery, altered anatomy, potential postoperative complications (difficulty in eating and drinking, and swelling) and the giving of information booklets.

Once admitted to the ward, psychological and physical preparations continue, both of the patient and family.

Postoperative nursing care of patients who have had head and neck surgery

The specific postoperative nursing care for the activity of breathing is explored in the care plan (see Box 11.19). The following aims to clarify other specific potential problems for a patient having undergone a laryngectomy.

Maintaining a safe environment
Continuous observation of the patient's vital signs for signs of haemorrhage is indicated, as surgery involves an area containing a very rich blood supply. The risk of haematoma is also present for the same reason, and, in order to minimize this risk, two Redivac drains are inserted, one on each side of the neck, which drain blood and tissue fluid from the surgical site. Chapter 4 discusses care of surgical drains and wounds in more detail.

The patient who has undergone a laryngectomy tends to experience moderate pain and discomfort during the postoperative period. Often there are areas of numbness in the neck region due to the loss of more superficial nerves during surgical resection. A patient-controlled analgesia (PCA) system is used for the first 2–3 days, after which regular analgesics are given until no longer required. Chapter 7 discusses pain control in more detail.

Controlling body temperature
Prolonged 'nil by mouth' may precipitate oral fungal infection, i.e. thrush, so assessing the mouth for early signs and providing hourly mouth care in order to keep the oral mucosa moist and clean are necessary.

The laryngectomy stoma and neck incision wounds need constant assessment, and dressings to these areas are minimal. Often, a transparent vapour-permeable film dressing (e.g. OpSite) is applied over the stapled areas of the neck, with light gauze in place around the drains.

Eating and drinking
Most types of head and neck surgery, except salivary gland or neck lump excisions, require a prolonged period of 'nil by mouth' in order to allow the affected areas to heal. Enteral feeding aims to maintain the patient's nutritional status until an adequate oral diet is taken. Feeding tubes come in a variety of forms: nasogastric, percutaneous endoscopic gastrostomy (PEG) or jejunostomy. Once an oral diet is permitted, soft or puréed food is recommended, as the muscles involved in chewing and swallowing, including the

Box 11.19   Postoperative nursing care of the activity of breathing for a patient having undergone a laryngectomy

Bill returns to the ward, orientated but drowsy. A tracheostomy tube (Shiley size 8, plain, cuffed and inflated) is in the laryngectomy stoma, secured with tapes; 40% humidified oxygen is in progress. Two surgical Redivac drains have been inserted, one on each side of the neck.

- *Problem*: Potential loss of clear airway and respiratory difficulty due to the effects of anaesthetic drugs, drowsiness, surgical swelling and the newly formed laryngectomy stoma.
- *Goal*: To maintain a clear airway and patent laryngectomy stoma. For Bill to adapt to the laryngectomy stoma and to learn self-care.
- *Care*:
  - Ensure the oxygen and suction equipment function correctly, as Bill relies upon them throughout his hospital stay.
  - Nurse Bill close to the nurses' station in clear view, in order to facilitate safe observation.
  - Bill has lost the ability to speak, so provide alternative methods for communicating: call bell at hand always, pen and paper and communication picture board; encourage Bill to mouth words and use gestures.

The first 72 hours

- Though it is a permanent structure, surgical swelling and secretions can occlude the laryngectomy stoma. To prevent this, ensure the tracheostomy tube remains in situ, well secured with tapes, until doctors instruct otherwise.
- Spare tracheostomy tubes (one the same type and size; the other, same type, one size smaller) and tracheal dilators should be kept at Bill's bedside, as this enables a rapid change of tracheostomy tube if the tube becomes irreversibly blocked or displaced. Having a lower size at hand is safe practice in case the laryngectomy stoma shrinks.
- Bill should be in an upright position with his head and neck well supported with pillows. These actions help to maintain a clear airway and to promote expectoration of secretions and surgical drainage; comfortable support reduces strain on the head, neck and surgical incisions.
- Bill has permanently lost the ability to humidify and warm inhaled air, due to altered anatomy; alternative methods must be provided:
  - Ensure the prescribed oxygen always runs through a mechanical thermohumidifier.
  - Administer nebulized saline as prescribed.
  - Ensure a tracheostomy mask is used, as facemasks are not suitable for the neck region.
  These actions ensure inhaled oxygen is humidified and warmed, and that secretions remain loose, thus preventing tracheal irritation.
- Perform observations of respiratory status 1/4–1/2 hourly for the first 2 hours and reduce regime to 1–2 hourly overnight if condition is stable and observations are within normal limits. Frequency can be reduced thereafter to 4 hourly if Bill is recovering well.
  Observations include those of:
  - respiratory rate, depth, rhythm
  - use of accessory muscles
  - signs of cyanosis or pallor
  - % saturations of blood oxygen
  - nature of tracheal secretions.
- Continually observe for accumulation of tracheal secretions, which will be apparent as any of the following signs:
  - rhonchi (low-pitched gurgling)
  - wheeze
  - dyspnoea
  - restlessness or anxiety
  - poor air flow on expiration (detected by placing a hand close to the tracheostomy tube entrance)
  - falling saturation levels of blood oxygen.
- If any of the above is noted, remove inner cannula of the tracheostomy tube and rinse away any secretions contained within, then dry and re-insert. Encourage Bill to cough (impaired now due to loss of larynx) and perform deep breathing exercises in order to assist expectoration of secretions.
- If Bill continues to show signs of respiratory difficulty, perform tracheal suctioning, following the recommended technique (see Box 11.15).

- Checking the inner cannula of Bill's tracheostomy tube and any suctioning should be performed every 1–2 hours until the next morning because secretions can accumulate without obvious signs. Thereafter, this can be reduced to 2–4 hourly or as required.
- Maintain inflation of the tracheostomy tube cuff; this prevents aspiration of any secretions from the surgical site and from the tracheo-oesophageal puncture; monitor cuff pressure every 4 hours using the cuff manometer; overinflation of the cuff causes tracheal irritation and necrosis.
- Deflate cuff with a syringe only on doctor's instructions (usually after 2–3 days); secretions will have accumulated on top of the cuff; in order to prevent their aspiration, perform immediate suction.
- Maintain a stoma care chart, recording the following information:
  - time of care given
  - description of secretions
  - episodes of checking and cleansing of inner tube and of suction
  - episodes of checking cuff pressure.

  This chart facilitates evaluation of Bill's progress, acts as an accurate reference for physiotherapists, doctors and nursing colleagues, and ensures thorough record-keeping.
- The next morning, refer Bill to the ward physiotherapist for assessment and input as required.

Days 3–7

- Perform care as already outlined, but reduce the frequency of observations (to 6 hourly); laryngectomy stoma care and suction are given as required.
- Liaise with the doctors regarding the removal of Bill's tracheostomy tube (once cuff is deflated), as prolonged use of the tube can cause tracheal irritation and mucosal breakdown.
- Upon the doctors' request, remove the tracheostomy tube and insert an appropriately sized stoma button (a small, tubular, plastic device) in order to support the stoma, prevent shrinkage and maintain airway.
- If the stoma button is prone to popping out, secure with neck tapes.
- Remove button as required in order to clean secretions; rinse it through, dry and re-insert.
- Continue to keep a spare tracheostomy tube and stoma button (of matching size) by Bill's bedside, in case of sudden respiratory difficulty or occlusion of airway.
- Once Bill's oxygen saturation levels appear within normal limits, tested when the oxygen is temporarily removed, and upon doctors' instructions, discontinue the humidified oxygen therapy, but continue to monitor oxygen saturations and respirations 6 hourly in order to detect respiratory insufficiency or difficulty.
- Continue to provide humidification by other means:
  - regular saline nebulizers, which are particularly effective in loosening tenacious secretions
  - saline-moistened gauze veils, which are secured with neck tapes and cover the laryngectomy stoma
  - moistened laryngectomy bibs.

  Observe secretions for amount, viscosity and colour – blood staining should have resolved.

Days 7 to discharge: the rehabilitation phase

- Begin to teach Bill stoma care; step-by-step, instruct Bill on how to clean the stoma with saline and gauze, how to cough and wipe away any secretions, and how to clean and insert the stoma button; adapt the teaching process to a pace that suits Bill and his family, as this will enable better understanding and absorption of information.
- Supervise Bill performing his own stoma care and give constructive feedback, including positive evaluation; reinforce the teaching process until Bill is competent and self-caring.
- Include the family as much as possible during this time, as they will be feeling very apprehensive about Bill's well-being and how to care for a laryngectomy stoma.
- If the stoma shows no evidence of shrinkage, and if the doctors instruct, remove the stoma button and leave the stoma exposed; the need for a button is indicated if the chin or neck flesh occludes the stoma, particularly more so at night when asleep.
- Remove stoma sutures as instructed (usually day 14); by then, the tracheal structure has healed in its new position.

Evaluation of care

Throughout, Bill was nursed near to the nurses' station, and close observation of his condition was possible.

Safe and effective communication was achieved by Bill writing things down, by using a picture board for the first day, as Bill soon preferred other means, and by gesturing basic requests. Soon he was mouthing words and staff often easily understood these. Bill kept hold of his call bell for the first 2 days, as he felt very anxious if it was out of sight. As his condition improved, Bill became more relaxed and confident about communicating with staff and visitors. Oxygen and suctioning equipment were checked every shift; no faults were found, and they functioned correctly.

The first 72 hours

Bill was very drowsy for the first 6 hours and was prone to slipping down the bed; two nurses strategically placed pillows (behind the head, neck, torso and each arm), and an upright position was achieved.

The tracheostomy tube was secure; tapes were changed every shift to prevent soiling and hardening.

Forty per cent humidified oxygen was continuously maintained. Saturation levels of blood oxygen ranged between 96% and 99%; after 2 days, random tests of oxygen saturations on air were performed, but results fell below 90% – indicating that oxygen therapy was required in order to prevent hypoxia. His respiratory rate ranged between 14 and 20 r.p.m. Cleansing of the inner cannula of the tracheostomy tube and suctioning was performed every hour until the next morning – secretions were bloodstained and loose. They then became more copious and viscous, but remained blood-stained for the next 2 days. Inner cannula care and suctioning was required frequently, often every 1/2–2 hours, in order to keep Bill's airway patent. Saline nebulizers were prescribed and given every 4 hours; secretions appeared looser as a result. Bill felt very anxious when secretions were building up, as he felt unable to breathe; he would use the call bell and gesture to the nurses frequently for assistance. As the amount of secretions reduced, Bill appeared to relax more.

On day 2, Bill suddenly became acutely distressed: his respirations were 25 r.p.m., oxygen saturation was 88%, and there was minimal air flow felt by the tracheostomy opening. The inner tube was clear, so immediate suction was per-formed, and on the third attempt a large, sticky plug of accumulated bloodstained secretions was removed. Bill's respi-ratory status returned to normal but he was very shaken by this episode. It was explained that mucous plugs could form from a combination of sputum, surgical secretions and under-humidification. Bill was comforted and reassured that his laryngectomy stoma was functioning well and that mucous plugs were not uncommon. Saline nebulizers were increased to 2–4 hourly in order to prevent under-humidification; this episode never occurred again. The cuff of the tracheostomy tube was checked every 4 hours in order to maintain safe pressure, and it was deflated, upon doctors' request, on day 3. A lot of stale bloodstained secretions were immediately suctioned out.

The physiotherapist assessed Bill the next morning and found his lungs to be mildly consolidated. Twice-daily input was therefore maintained for 3 days until his chest appeared clearer. Deep breathing and coughing exercises were taught, which helped Bill to expectorate more efficiently.

Days 3–7

The nature of secretions had improved by day 5 and were less viscous and clearer. The physiotherapist visited daily, mainly to check Bill's progress. Bill's suctioning needs were reduced to 3–4 hourly, as he was managing to expectorate more easily now into the inner cannula of the tracheostomy tube. Secretions were cleared more by cleansing the inner cannula than by performing suction. The intensity of humidification was reduced because the secretions were looser, and saline nebulizers were given 4–6 hourly.

The doctors instructed removal of the tracheostomy tube on day 5. The laryngectomy stoma was well formed and large; but, if Bill bent his head down, neck tissue, which was still swollen, occluded 50% of the stoma. A stoma button was inserted and secured with neck tapes, and this appeared to maintain stoma patency. Bill had found the tracheostomy tube cumbersome and uncomfortable, so felt happier with the button in situ.

The button was removed every 2–4 hours, and any secretions were rinsed away. Bill's suctioning needs reduced as the week progressed, and by day 7 his secretions were minimal and suction was only required once or twice per shift.

Days 7 to discharge

Bill and his family were keen to learn stoma care, so, once Bill's chest secretions had become minimal, they were taught the basics. His family brought in a large tabletop mirror for Bill to use when performing stoma care. Bill needed to wear his glasses in order to visualize his stoma clearly. Bill successfully managed to remove, clean, dry and re-insert the stoma button after only 2 days of instruction and supervision.

Bill found the cleaning of his stoma more difficult, partly because his very large hands and fingers blocked his view and made it awkward to retrieve any secretions. Bill's wife offered to assist him, and she quickly learnt the techniques involved. Secretions would often dry and form crusts near the opening of the stoma, and she was able to use forceps to pick these away. Bill remained enthusiastic and was determined to manage his own care so that he did not need to rely upon his wife. By his discharge, he had become more skilful and dexterous and was able to clean his stoma competently, though he left the picking of crusts to his wife.

By day 12, Bill was wearing the stoma button only at night, when support was required while asleep. There appeared to be no evidence of stoma shrinkage during the day. However, Bill and his family were advised to monitor stoma circumference once at home, as it could reduce over time, particularly while undergoing radiotherapy. Radiotherapy causes local inflammation and swelling to the neck and stoma and can persist for weeks once treatment is complete. If any shrinkage is apparent, Bill should wear the button all the time until side-effects settle.

By day 14, Bill rarely required suctioning (once per day maximum), but the ward had requested that the district nurses provide a portable suction machine for home in case of emergency. The need for saline nebulizers (6 hourly) continued, as Bill was prone to drying of secretions; again, the district nurses had arranged a nebulizer machine for home. Both these items of equipment were delivered prior to Bill taking day and overnight leave and then official discharge. Stoma sutures were removed on day 14; some sutures were deeply embedded, so, in order to make the procedure as comfortable as possible, surface anaesthetic cream (e.g. EMLA) was applied 1 hour prior to removal.

tongue, are often greatly affected. The speech therapist can perform a swallowing assessment upon request and provide invaluable advice for improving any difficulties in swallowing. Chapter 5 discusses nutrition and enteral feeding in more detail.

Eliminating

Postoperative enteral feeding can precipitate loose stools or diarrhoea, and, for some time after surgery, a urinary catheter may be in situ to facilitate micturition. Relying on commodes, bedpans or urinals can cause embarrassment to the patient, making this activity more awkward.

Communicating

Surgical removal of the larynx implies permanent loss of the ability to speak. Postoperative rehabilitation by the speech therapist occurs over a long period of time and can be a slow, frustrating process for the patient. The electronic larynx and the BlomSinger valve are examples of speech aids used. Preparations for the latter begin on the operating table with the formation of a tracheo-oesophageal puncture; this is a hole made in the tracheal wall which connects the trachea with the oesophagus, and which is large enough to initially house an enteral feeding tube (usually Ryles) and then the BlomSinger valve itself. The speech therapist inserts the valve in the outpatient's clinic, often weeks later, once radiotherapy and wound healing are complete. Until valve insertion occurs, the Ryles tube is used to keep the puncture site patent.

Expressing sexuality and cleansing and dressing

Some patients feel belittled by the presence of tube feeding and their dependency on nursing staff to meet their daily needs. Tubes and equipment hinder the ability to attend to independence and self-care; subsequently, patients may feel depressed and suffer with low self-esteem. Once discharged home, maintaining

intimate relationships can be awkward, and problems may arise. By providing thoughtful, caring and individualized nursing care, both in hospital and at home with community support, one aims to alleviate these negative emotions. Chapter 6 discusses issues surrounding body image in more detail.

DISCHARGE PLANNING AND EDUCATION OF PATIENTS WHO HAVE HAD HEAD AND NECK SURGERY

This commences in the preadmission clinic, continues throughout admission and after discharge home. Both the patient and family require a lot of support and preparation prior to leaving the ward for home. For patients who have undergone laryngectomy and other major head and neck surgery, it is good practice to have a trial at home, either as day or weekend leave, in order to assess the patient and family's ability to cope. Input from social services may be necessary, especially if the patient lives alone and requires assistance with the activities of washing, dressing, housework and shopping; any preparations required for this will have begun in the preoperative phase with the initial nursing assessment, and postoperative home visits may be undertaken to assess the patient's true needs.

Community nursing support is often required: district nurses can provide suctioning and nebulizing equipment if appropriate; supervision of stoma care and nutritional intake, including enteral feeding if this is continuing, can be maintained by community nurses; and athough direct physical care may not be indicated, the need for psychological support and care are required especially during the period of radiotherapy treatment.

Follow-up in the outpatients department ranges between 1 and 6 weeks. Radiotherapy treatment is often planned once the patient has settled back home and the wounds have healed.

CONCLUSION

This chapter has endeavoured to demonstrate the range of surgical procedures and patient care that represents the field of ear, nose and throat surgery. Recent surgical advances, including preservation of the hemilarynx, transoral laser surgery for pharyngeal and laryngeal malignancy, laser stapes surgery, bone-anchored hearing aids and transnasal endoscopic sinus, neurological and ophthalmic surgery all aim to provide the patient with the best result, using minimally invasive techniques that require an acute, shorter hospitalization and demand ENT nursing excellence.

The ENT ward is a dynamic and challenging environment in which to nurse, and has become an area of practice enriched with opportunities for professional development and fulfilment. Caring for a variety of individuals undergoing routine procedures and specialized complex surgery provides the practitioner with invaluable knowledge and skills, in particular concerning airway management, communication, nutrition and psychological care, which are of immense benefit in all healthcare settings.

Summary of key points

- Having an understanding of relevant anatomy and physiology enables the nurse to anticipate, plan and provide best practice.

- A comprehensive assessment of the patient's physical and psychological status forms the basis on which to plan, implement and evaluate nursing care.

- Clinical investigation of ENT disease encompasses patient history, audiometry, radiology, allergy testing, sleep studies, endoscopy and biopsy.

- Specific complications of:
  1. ear surgery, including further hearing loss, facial palsy or dizziness
  2. nasal/sinus surgery, including haemorrhage and infection
  3. throat surgery, including loss of a clear airway, dysphagia and reduced ability to communicate.

- Head and neck surgery encompasses a wide range of surgical techniques that aim to remove benign and malignant neoplasia, and as far as possible restore function to the affected area.

- Specialized nursing care is required for safe recovery and successful rehabilitation for the patient and his family.

- Discharge planning and patient education begins preoperatively in the outpatients clinic.

- A high standard of tracheostomy nursing care is imperative; knowledge of altered anatomy, variety of tracheostomy tubes and the implications of breathing, eating, drinking and communicating with a stoma are vital.

- Written advice sheets are an invaluable patient education tool, and should be given to most patients, especially day cases.

References

American Cancer Society (2003) Cancer Reference Information Website. http://www.cancer.org (accessed 26 January 2004).

Behrbohm, H., Hilderbrandt, T. & Kaschke, O (2002) *Functional and Aesthetic Surgery of the Nose*. Tutlingen, Germany: Endo-Press.

Black, B (1997) *An Introduction to Ear Disease*. Melbourne: Smith, Kline Beecham.

Carroll, P. (1994) Safe suctioning. *Registered Nurse* May: 32–36.

Citardi, M. (2001) *Brief Overview of Nasal and Sinus Anatomy*. American Rhinologic Society. http://www.american-rhinologic.org (accessed 26 January 2004).

Dart, C.M (1997) *Major Ear Surgery Resource Manual*, 2nd edn. Cherrybrook, NSW: CM Dart.

Daya, H. & Crittenden, G. (1998) *Inside ENT*. Herts: Schering-Plough.

Dhillon, R. S. & East, C. A. (1994) *An Illustrated Text: Ear, Nose and Throat and Head and Neck Surgery*. Edinburgh: Churchill Livingstone.

Hooper, M. (1996) Nursing care of the patient with a tracheostomy. *Nursing Standard* 10(34): 40–43.

McCormick, M. S., Primrose, W. J. & MacKenzie, I. J. (1992) *A New Short Textbook of Otolaryngology*, 3rd edn. London: Edward Arnold.

Roper, N., Logan, W. & Tierney, A. (2000) *The Roper–Logan–Tierney Model of Nursing.* Edinburgh: Churchill Livingstone.

Singh, W. & Soutar, D. S. (1993) *Functional Surgery of the Larynx and Pharynx.* Oxford: Butterworth-Heinemann.

Sobin, L. & Wittekind, C. H. (1997) *TNM Classification of Malignant Tumours,* 5th edn. Chichester: Wiley.

Ugwoke, M. I., Verbeke, N. & Kinget, R. (2001) The biopharmaceutical aspects of nasal mucoadhesive drug delivery. *Journal of Pharmacy and Pharmacology* 53(1): 3–21.

Waddington, C., McKennis, A. T. & Goodlett, A. (1997) Treatment of conductive hearing loss with ossicular chain reconstruction procedures. *AORN Journal* 65(3): 511–518.

Further reading and relevant websites

Bull, T. (1995) *A Color Atlas of ENT Diagnosis,* 3rd edn. London: Mosby-Wolfe.

Choate, K. & Barbetti, J. (2003) Tracheostomy: your questions answered. *Australian Nurses Journal* 10(11): 1–4.

Davidson, P. (1998) Voice restoration prosthesis: the options. *Nursing Times* 94(12): 56–58.

Depondt, J. & Gehanno, P. (1995) Laryngectomized patients' education and follow-up. *Patient Education and Counselling* 26: 33–36.

Hahn, M. J. & Jones, A. (2000) *Head and Neck Nursing.* Edinburgh: Churchill Livingstone.

Harris, L. & Huntoon, M. (2000) *Core Curriculum of ORL Nursing.* Florida. SOHN Society of Otorhinolaryngology Head and Neck Nurses.

National Institute on Deafness and Other Communication Disorders (1999) *Fact Sheet: Otosclerosis.* NIDCD. NIH Pub 99-4234.

Stammberger, H. (1998) *FESS Endoscopic Diagnosis and Surgery of the Paranasal Sinuses and Anterior Skull Base.* Germany: Verlag Endo-Press.

Steiner, W. & Werner, J. (2000) *Lasers in Otorhinolaryngology, Head and Neck Surgery.* Germany: Endo-Press.

http://www.entnursing.org British ENT nurses website (accessed 26 January 2004).

http://www.ciap.health.nsw.gov.au/specialties/OHNNG Australian Otolaryngology, Head and Neck Nurses Group (accessed 26 January 2004).

http://www.ifosworld.org Federation of worldwide Oto-Rhino-Laryngology medical societies (accessed 26 January 2004).

http://www.cochrane.org The Cochrane Collaboration ENT Newsletter (accessed 26 January 2004).

http://www.nidcd.nih.gov National Institute on Deafness, USA (accessed 26 January 2004).

http://www.cancer.org American Cancer Society (accessed 26 January 2004).

http://www.asohns.org.au Australian Society of Otolaryngology Head and Neck Surgeons (accessed 26 January 2004).

Chapter 12

Patients requiring thyroid surgery

Rosie Pudner

Key objectives of the chapter

At the end of the chapter the reader should be able to:

- describe the anatomy and physiology of the thyroid gland and related structures

- discuss the underlying conditions that require thyroid surgery

- explain the specific investigations required prior to thyroid surgery

- discuss specific issues related to nursing assessment

- discuss the relevant pre- and postoperative nursing care following surgery to the thyroid gland

- discuss the plan for a patient's discharge, including relevant patient education.

INTRODUCTION

Many people with a disorder of the thyroid gland will eventually require surgery, because of the effects on the body of an imbalance of the thyroid hormones, or due to malignancy. This chapter will explore issues related to the care of patients requiring thyroid surgery, recognizing issues related to the effect of an altered body image, and the potential complications that can occur.

ANATOMY AND PHYSIOLOGY

The thyroid gland consists of two lobes that lie either side of the trachea, and is situated in the anterior and lateral aspects of the neck, just below the larynx. The two lobes are joined by a band of tissue called the isthmus, which lies across the anterior surface of the trachea. The thyroid gland weighs approximately 20 g and is highly vascular. The arterial blood supply to the gland comes from the superior and inferior thyroid arteries, and venous drainage is through the superior, middle and inferior thyroid veins. Lymphatic drainage is via the deep cervical chain (laterally) and to the pretracheal and mediastinal nodes (inferiorly). The recurrent laryngeal nerves, which supply the vocal cords, lie posterior to the thyroid gland and are responsible for innervating many of the intrinsic laryngeal muscles, as well as playing a vital role in voice production and airway maintenance.

The primary function of the thyroid gland is to secrete various hormones: thyroxine, triiodothyronine and calcitonin. The lobes of the thyroid gland contain numerous follicles lined with epithelial cells. The follicles are filled with colloid, which is secreted from the epithelial cells. Thyroglobulin is a complex protein molecule that is also secreted from these epithelial cells. Iodine is an essential component for the synthesis of thyroxine and triiodothyronine. Production of the thyroid hormones is controlled by the thyroid-stimulating hormone (TSH) from the anterior pituitary gland and by thyroid-releasing hormone (TRH) from the hypothalamus. The thyroid hormones thyroxine (T4) and triiodothyronine (T3) are stored in the form of thyroglobulin in the follicles prior to their release into the bloodstream (Hinchliff et al, 1996). Thyroxine and triiodothyronine are essential for stimulating oxygen consumption of most cells within the body; regulating lipid and carbohydrate metabolism; normal growth and development; normal lactation; and the potentiation of the action of other hormones, e.g. insulin. Calcitonin is secreted by the parafollicular cells, in response to an increase in blood calcium levels. It plays a part in reducing the calcium concentration in body fluids, by promoting the excretion of calcium and phosphate in urine and movement into the bones.

The four parathyroid glands are attached to the posterior surface of the lateral lobes of the thyroid gland. The parathyroid glands secrete parathormone, a hormone which regulates the distribution and metabolism of calcium in the body. The blood concentration levels of calcium and phosphorus are regulated by its action on the intestine, bone and kidneys. It promotes the absorption of calcium in the intestine and the demineralization of bone and movement of calcium into the extracellular fluid. Undersecretion of the

hormone can lead to low calcium levels, which will result in muscle spasm, e.g. tetany.

DISORDERS OF THE THYROID GLAND

Thyroid disorders tends to occur as a result of over-secretion of thyroid hormones, i.e. hyperthyroidism; undersecretion of the hormones, i.e. hypothyroidism or myxoedema; or due to malignancy.

GOITRE

A goitre refers to an enlargement of the thyroid gland, and it can occur in response to demand on the gland, or because of a benign or malignant tumour of the gland. A deficiency of iodine in the diet can also lead to the formation of a goitre.

A goitre presents as a mass in the neck which moves on swallowing. This is because the thyroid gland is attached to the larynx by fascia. The mass may be situated on one or both sides of the trachea. In some instances the trachea may be displaced and compressed by the enlarged gland, which can lead to an alteration of tracheal, oesophageal and vocal function, and can compromise the patient's airway. On clinical examination, the doctor should be able to distinguish the shape and texture of the goitre. Goitres are often referred to as the following:

- smooth, non-toxic or physiological goitre
- nodular, non-toxic goitre
- smooth, toxic goitre (Graves' disease)
- toxic, nodular goitre (secondary thyrotoxicosis).

(Forrest et al, 1991).

HYPERTHYROIDISM

Hyperthyroidism, or thyrotoxicosis, can be caused by Graves' disease (an autoimmune disorder); toxic adenoma of the thyroid; and in multinodular goitres where the small thyroid nodules secrete excess thyroid hormone (Gillespie et al, 1992).

The clinical features of hyperthyroidism vary between individuals (Table 12.1) and are predominantly found in females, with a male-to-female ratio of 1:8 (Forrest et al, 1991). The symptoms are characterized by an excess secretion of thyroid hormones and are due to increased catabolism, increased heat production, autonomic lability and increased sensitivity to catecholamines, and increased gastrointestinal activity.

Graves' disease can cause distressing symptoms of altered body image, because of the patient's having a swollen neck, and the effect it has on the patient's eyes. This can range from the appearance of staring, to lid lag and lid retraction, and, in its severest form, exophthalmos. Exophthalmos (an abnormal protrusion of the eyeballs) and lid lag can result in corneal ulceration, which will cause visual disturbances, and in extreme cases can lead to papilloedema and an inability to move the eyeball (Gillespie et al, 1992).

HYPOTHYROIDISM

Hypothyroidism, or myxoedema, is a common disorder characterized by a hypometabolic state. It can occur at any age, but is often seen in the elderly. The deficit of thyroid hormones may be due to a disorder of the thyroid gland, e.g. Hashimoto's thyroiditis, or may result from a pituitary or hypothalamic disturbance. It can also occur following surgical removal of the thyroid gland. The clinical features are due to decreased production of the thyroid hormones, which results in a variety of manifestations (Table 12.2). The condition can be corrected by the patient taking the appropriate replacement drug therapy, e.g. thyroxine.

NEOPLASMS OF THE THYROID GLAND

Neoplasms of the thyroid gland can be benign, e.g. an adenoma, or malignant. Malignant neoplasms of the thyroid can be divided into four groups – papillary, follicular, medullary and anaplastic – and account for 1% of all cancers. The aetiology of thyroid cancer is

Table 12.1 Clinical features of hyperthyroidism (thyrotoxicosis)

Symptom	Problem
Weight loss Muscle wasting Increased appetite Intolerance of heat Pyrexia	Altered nutrition and metabolism
Tachycardia Raised sleeping pulse Palpitations Angina Possible atrial fibrillation Increased blood pressure Cardiac failure	Altered cardiovascular system
Shortness of breath	Altered respiratory activity
Moist, warm skin Increased sweating Hair loss Retraction of eyelids	Altered skin integrity

Weakness and fatigue
Tremor of hands
Increased muscle tone and
  reflexes
Shortness of breath on
  exertion
	Altered activity tolerance

Emotional lability Increased anxiety Restlessness Increased irritability Insomnia	Altered emotional and mental state
Diarrhoea Increased gastrointestinal motility	Altered bowel habits
Oligomenorrhoea or amenorrhoea Low sex drive Impotence	Altered sexuality

Table 12.2 Clinical features of hypothyroidism (myxoedema)

Symptom	Problem
Weight gain Poor appetite Sensitivity to the cold Decreased body temperature	Altered nutrition and metabolism
Decreased pulse rate Low blood pressure	Altered cardiovascular system
Decreased respiratory rate	Altered respiratory activity
Skin is dry, thick and pale Eyelids are oedematous Lips and tongue are enlarged Hair is coarse and sparse Interstitial oedema	Altered skin integrity
Weakness and fatigue Slow movements Dyspnoea Decreased muscle tone and reflexes	Altered activity tolerance
Slow mental processes Increased sleep and lethargy Speech is hoarse, slow and monotonous Mental disturbances Depression	Altered emotional and mental state
Decreased gastrointestinal motility Constipation	Altered bowel habits
Metrorrhagia Amenorrhoea Low sex drive Infertility	Altered sexuality

unknown, but risk factors include irradiation of the upper thorax, head or neck. Females outnumber males by a ratio of 2.5:1, and the rate is higher in Caucasians (4.4 per 100 000) than in African-Americans (2.3 per 100 000) (Moore and Haughey, 1997). The prognosis depends on the type and aggressiveness of the tumour and the presence of metastases, as well as the patient's age and overall health. Following investigations and staging of the disease, a thyroidectomy will be undertaken (British Thyroid Association/Royal College of Physicians, 2002).

CONSERVATIVE MANAGEMENT OF HYPERTHYROIDISM

Hyperthyroidism is initially treated conservatively by the use of antithyroid drugs, e.g. carbimazole or propylthiouracil. These drugs suppress the formation of the thyroid hormones and hopefully produce a euthyroid state, i.e. a normally functioning thyroid gland, and are also used in the preparation of a patient prior to thyroid surgery. If the patient has cardiac symptoms, a beta-adrenergic blocking agent may be used to decrease the heart rate, e.g. propranolol.

Radioactive iodine therapy is an effective treatment for patients over the age of 45 years. It avoids the prolonged use of drugs or the need for surgery, although there is a risk of causing hypothyroidism in the patient (Johnson, 1993). The patient swallows a solution of gamma-emitting radioactive sodium iodide, which destroys thyroid tissue and so reduces the production of the thyroid hormones T3 and T4.

SPECIFIC INVESTIGATIONS OF A PATIENT WITH THYROID DYSFUNCTION

A variety of laboratory investigations are undertaken to confirm the clinical diagnosis of hyperthyroidism, and will be performed prior to surgery.

BLOOD TESTS

Serum levels of the following are measured to evaluate thyroid function and distinguish between hyperthyroidism and hypothyroidism:

- thyroxine (T4)
- triiodothyronine (T3)
- thyroid-stimulating hormone (TSH)
- thyroid-releasing hormone (TRH)
- thyroid antibodies

- thyroglobulin
- calcitonin
- carcino-embryonic antigen (CEA)
- cholesterol.

RADIOACTIVE SCANNING PROCEDURES

This is useful in patients with a solitary autonomous toxic nodule, or toxic multinodular disease, but is of little value in the diagnosis of malignancy:

- thyroid isotope scan
- radioactive iodine uptake test.

OTHER IMAGING PROCEDURES

These will display any structural abnormalities within the thyroid gland, e.g. cysts or nodules:

- ultrasound of the thyroid gland
- duplex ultrasound scan
- computerized tomography (CT) scan
- magnetic resonance imaging (MRI)
- fluorescent scan.

(Wheeler, 1994).

NEEDLE BIOPSY

Fine-needle aspiration cytology, which allows an accurate diagnosis of the thyroid lesion to be determined, should be used in the planning of surgery for patients with thyroid cancer.

NURSING ASSESSMENT OF A PATIENT REQUIRING THYROID SURGERY

It is important to gain a comprehensive health history from the patient, as their health problems have often developed gradually over time and are often vague in nature. A knowledge of the effects of altered thyroid function enables the nurse to collect the relevant data and ask specific questions relating to the thyroid disorder. Using a model of nursing will also help to structure the assessment process (Box 12.1).

ASSESSMENT OF THE PATIENT'S VOICE AND TRACHEA

A chest X-ray is taken to ensure that the enlarged thyroid gland is not constricting the trachea, nor causing it to deviate to one side. As there is a risk of the recurrent laryngeal nerves being damaged during the surgical procedure, it is essential that the vocal cords are

Box 12.1 Nursing assessment of Joanna Sweet using the Roper, Logan and Tierney model of nursing (Roper et al, 2000)

Joanna Sweet is a 30-year-old married lady with three young children aged 2, 4 and 7 years of age. She works as a presenter for the local television station, and her husband is a journalist. She developed hyperthyroidism and has been managed conservatively, but it is felt that surgery is now an option as the thyroid gland is causing Joanna much discomfort on eating and she is concerned by the appearance of her swollen neck. She has been admitted for surgical removal of her thyroid gland.

Maintaining a safe environment
Joanna is very anxious regarding the outcome of the surgery and what will happen to her children while she is in hospital. She is concerned as to the appearance of the scar, and whether people will be able to see it.
     Observations of her vital signs are as follows:

- pulse: 86 bpm; sleeping pulse, 78 bpm; she says that she has had palpitations in the past
- blood pressure: 138/80 mmHg
- drug therapy:
  - carbimazole 15 mg daily for the past 6 months
  - propranolol 2 g three times a day
  - Lugol's solution 0.3 ml three times a day
- allergies: she is not allergic to anything that she knows of, and has had no problems with previous anaesthetics (she had an appendicectomy 10 years ago, and drainage of breast abscess 4 years ago).

Communicating
Joanna appears very anxious and asks lots of questions. She wears contact lenses as she is short sighted. She is concerned as to how her mother will cope with looking after the children and her husband while she is in hospital.

Breathing
Respiratory rate: 18 respirations per minute; regular. Joanna used to smoke 10 cigarettes a day before she became pregnant with her first child.

Eating and drinking
Joanna weighs 58 kg and is 1.62 m tall. Her body mass index is 22. She says that her weight had dropped to 50 kg even though she was always eating. Her appetite has now returned to normal and she is nearly back to her normal weight. She enjoys a glass of wine with her evening meal, or when she and her husband have friends around.

Eliminating
She usually has her bowels open once to twice a day. Urinalysis shows no abnormalities.

Personal cleansing and dressing
Joanna is very conscious of her appearance and dresses very smartly. She likes to shower at least twice a day. She has a Waterlow score of 7.

Controlling body temperature
Joanna's temperature is 36.8°C.

Mobility
Joanna has no problems with this activity.

Working and playing
Joanna is a presenter for a daytime programme with a local television company. Her two youngest children attend nursery, and her eldest child attends school. She has found that her tolerance of people has altered and she gets irritated very easily. She and her husband enjoy entertaining.

Expressing sexuality
Joanna takes pride in her appearance, and is very concerned as to how the scar will look after the surgery, and whether she will be able to conceal it from the viewers.

Sleeping
She usually sleeps 7 hours a night, but this varies, especially if she is stressed at work.

Dying
She expresses no fears about the anaesthetic.

assessed preoperatively. This is often undertaken in the outpatients department, where an indirect laryngoscopy is performed in order to assess the state of the vocal cords. Stojadinovic et al (2002) also suggest the value of undertaking a comprehensive voice analysis pre- and postoperatively, as they found that other factors besides laryngeal nerve injury may alter the voice post-thyroidectomy.

SPECIFIC PREOPERATIVE PREPARATION

The patient may be admitted on the day of surgery or a couple of days prior to surgery, depending on their condition. It is important for the patient to be kept as calm as possible and reduce any anxieties they may have. Giving the patient sufficient preoperative information can assist in reducing their anxiety. The patient will need to be made aware that they will probably have a sore throat postoperatively. They will be shown how to support their neck when moving their head, so as to reduce the strain on neck muscles and so reduce the stress on the surgical incision. The patient should be reassured that the surgical incision will be in the natural folds of the neck and so should not be too noticeable.

Lugol's solution may have been prescribed for 10 days preoperatively, in order to reduce the vascularity of the gland and to help maintain a euthyroid state. An electrocardiogram (ECG) will be performed to establish the patient's cardiac status if the patient has had previous cardiac problems, or is over 60 years of age. A full blood count will be taken, as well as blood for thyroid hormone levels and for typing and cross-matching, in case of haemorrhage peri- or postoperatively. Observations of the patient's temperature, pulse, respirations and blood pressure will be taken to ensure that the patient is in a euthyroid state.

SURGICAL INTERVENTIONS

A variety of surgical techniques may be undertaken, depending on the type and position of the nodules in the thyroid gland. The surgeon will always try to preserve a portion of the thyroid gland if possible, to allow continued production of the thyroid hormones, and in the hope of preventing problems with hypothyroidism postoperatively. It is also important to protect the parathyroid glands from damage or removal during the surgical procedure, as well as to prevent damage to the recurrent laryngeal nerves.

The use of the YAP laser has been found to enhance the safety of thyroidectomy, as it allows clean dissection of tissue while simultaneously coagulating smaller blood vessels. It has been found to reduce operative time, blood loss and possible injury to the recurrent laryngeal nerve, and, as the incision is small, causes less tissue trauma (Tyagi, 1993).

The more common surgical procedures are as follows.

THYROID LOBECTOMY

One lobe of the thyroid gland is removed; this is undertaken when a nodule or tumour which is benign is present in one lobe of the thyroid gland.

SUBTOTAL THYROIDECTOMY

Approximately five-sixths of the thyroid gland is removed, leaving the posterior portions of each lobe intact, so ensuring that the parathyroid glands are not removed. This is the usual procedure for patients with a goitre and/or a history of thyrotoxicosis. The advantage of this surgical procedure is that a small portion of the patient's thyroid gland is left intact, to allow thyroid hormone production, and in the hope of reducing the need for replacement thyroid hormones postoperatively.

TOTAL THYROIDECTOMY

Both lobes and the isthmus of the thyroid gland are removed; this is undertaken in patients with palpable carcinoma in both lobes of the thyroid gland (Moore and Haughey, 1997).

ENDOSCOPIC THYROIDECTOMY

This procedure is being considered by some surgeons for patients who do not have mediastinal, multinodular goitre or malignant thyroid lesions. Yamamoto et al (2002) undertook a small study and found there was significantly less blood loss using this technique, and better cosmetic results, as the incisions were made around the breast rather than in the skin folds of the neck.

SPECIFIC POSTOPERATIVE NURSING CARE

Postoperative care is the same as for any surgical patient, as has been briefly outlined in Chapter 2, and issues related to altered body image are outlined in Chapter 6. However, there are specific complications that can arise following this type of surgery which need to be closely monitored, i.e. obstructed airway, haemorrhage, damage to the recurrent laryngeal nerves, thyrotoxic crisis and tetany (Litwack-Saleh, 1992). These will now be discussed and are also illustrated in a postoperative care plan (Box 12.2).

POTENTIAL PROBLEMS FOLLOWING THYROID SURGERY

OBSTRUCTED AIRWAY

The patient's airway may become obstructed for a number of reasons:

- The trachea may have been damaged during surgery or compressed by a haematoma.
- The anaesthetic may have caused an increase in tracheal or bronchial secretions, or laryngospasm may occur because the trachea was irritated during intubation.
- A painful neck and sore throat may inhibit the patient's ability to expectorate any sputum.
- Damage to the recurrent laryngeal nerves during surgery can cause laryngeal paralysis, which will lead to respiratory difficulties, and may require an emergency tracheostomy. A loss of sensation above the vocal cords can lead to the patient's aspirating any secretions.

Box 12.2   Postoperative care plan following a subtotal thyroidectomy

This care plan illustrates the specific nursing care of a patient following thyroid surgery using the Roper, Logan and Tierney model of nursing (Roper et al, 2000).

Joanna Sweet has returned to the ward following a subtotal thyroidectomy for a benign nodule. She is conscious and is sitting in an upright position. She has an intravenous infusion in situ, but is able to take sips of water. The wound has been closed with staples and is covered with a postoperative dressing. A Redivac drain is placed close to the incision.

Breathing

- *Problem*: potential risk of respiratory difficulties due to anaesthesia, laryngeal spasm, damage to the recurrent laryngeal nerve, or the presence of a haematoma pressing on the trachea.
- *Goal*: Joanna is able to breathe normally.
- *Nursing actions and rationale for care*:
  1. Joanna should be sitting in an upright position, if her blood pressure allows, with her neck well supported with pillows. Supporting her head and neck ensures that Joanna is comfortable and that no strain is put on the incisional wound. Sitting upright also assists her to cough and expectorate.
  2. Joanna may be prescribed oxygen therapy in the immediate postoperative period. Ensure it is given at the prescribed rate, and that Joanna's mouth is moistened.
  3. Observe Joanna's respirations for rate, depth and stridor, and note any complaints from her of a choking sensation, or signs of cyanosis or respiratory distress. A change in these observations may indicate laryngeal paralysis or compression of the trachea by a haematoma, both of which require prompt intervention.
  4. Encourage Joanna to take deep breaths and to cough and expectorate any sputum several times an hour. Deep breathing aids full chest expansion, and with expectorating any sputum, helps to reduce the risk of chest infection.
- *Evaluation*: Joanna's respiratory rate was 18–20 breaths per minute, and she showed no signs of respiratory problems. Oxygen therapy was discontinued after 2 hours. She was experiencing some discomfort coughing, but was able to expectorate any sputum.

Maintaining a safe environment

- *Problem*: potential risk of haemorrhage.
- *Goal*: early detection of possible haemorrhage.
- *Nursing actions and rationale for care*:
  1. Ensure staple removers are by her bed, in case the staples need to be removed quickly, i.e. if a haematoma causes respiratory distress.

  2. Observe Joanna's pulse and blood pressure ¼ to ½ hourly initially. An increase in pulse rate and a falling blood pressure can indicate haemorrhage and should be reported immediately.
  3. Observe Joanna's respiratory state, as above, in order to detect any signs of respiratory distress which may be caused by the formation of a haematoma around the trachea.
  4. Observe the wound for signs of fresh bleeding, and check the side and back of Joanna's neck where blood may have collected. Fresh blood staining of the dressing and an increase in drainage will indicate haemorrhage.
  5. If the presence of a haematoma is suspected, remove Joanna's staples to release the haematoma, cover the wound with a sterile dressing and seek medical attention immediately.
- *Evaluation*: Joanna's observations remained within normal limits. There was no sign of excessive bleeding.

- *Problem*: potential risk of a thyroid crisis.
- *Goal*: early detection of this potential complication of thyroid surgery.
- *Nursing actions and rationale for care*:
  1. Observe Joanna's temperature, pulse, respirations and blood pressure at regular intervals. An increased temperature, pulse, respiratory rate or blood pressure could indicate a thyroid crisis.
  2. Observe Joanna for complaints of feeling hot or having palpitations, which could indicate the onset of this potential complication.
  3. Observe Joanna's mental state and monitor any periods of confusion or mania for the first 24 hours postoperatively to detect signs of a thyroid crisis.
  4. If any of these symptoms occurs, seek medical advice immediately.
- *Evaluation*: Joanna showed no signs of developing a thyroid crisis. Her observations remained within normal limits and she had no episodes of palpitations. She was alert and oriented to time and place.

- *Problem*: potential risk of tetany following her surgery.
- *Goal*: early detection of this potential problem.
- *Nursing actions and rationale for care*:
  1. Monitor Joanna for any complaints of numbness or tingling in her fingers and toes, which may indicate hypocalcaemia.
  2. Monitor Joanna for Trousseau's sign while taking her blood pressure, as seen by a contraction of her hand.
  3. Tap the side of Joanna's face over the zygoma bone to monitor any facial muscle twitching, i.e. Chvostek's sign.

4. Observe Joanna for a change in the pitch of her voice, as this may indicate spasm of her vocal cords.
5. Monitor Joanna for any complaints of stomach cramps, as this may indicate tetany.
- *Evaluation*: Joanna showed no signs of developing tetany during her postoperative recovery.

- *Problem*: Joanna has a painful neck following her surgery.
- *Goal*: to reduce her pain to an acceptable level.
- *Nursing actions and rationale for care*:
  1. Assess Joanna's pain using a pain assessment tool.
  2. Administer prescribed analgesics and monitor effectiveness after 30 minutes.
  3. Ensure Joanna is in a comfortable position, with her head and neck well supported with pillows. This should avoid tension on her neck, so allowing her neck muscles to relax and reduce tension on the wound. Encourage Joanna to support her head with her hands when moving, to ease the strain on her neck muscles.
- *Evaluation*: Joanna initially complained of severe discomfort in her neck and a sore throat, but this was effectively relieved with 10 mg morphine. The rest of the time her pain was relieved by taking 30 mg dihydrocodeine every 3 hours. She soon learnt the technique of supporting her head when moving, and was able to do this on her own.

Eating and drinking
- *Problem*: Joanna has difficulty in swallowing, because of a sore throat.
- *Goals*:
  1. Joanna's hydration and nutritional state is maintained.
  2. Joanna is eventually able to eat and drink normally.
- *Nursing actions and rationale for care*:
  1. Monitor the intravenous infusion, to check it is running at the correct rate and is not running into the surrounding tissue. This is to ensure that Joanna does not become dehydrated and that the cannula remains within the vein.
  2. Encourage Joanna to drink sips of water, and gradually increase this as she is able to tolerate it. Cool fluids are sometimes more suitable and better tolerated following thyroid surgery. Joanna should eventually be drinking 2 litres of fluid a day.
  3. If Joanna feels nauseated following the anaesthetic, offer prescribed antiemetics and monitor effectiveness.

4. Once Joanna is taking sufficient oral fluids, the intravenous infusion can be discontinued.
5. Joanna's fluid intake and output should be measured and monitored on a fluid balance chart, until she is taking an adequate fluid intake, and is passing sufficient amounts of urine.
6. Joanna can eat a soft diet, once she feels able to.
- *Evaluation*: Joanna was able to drink a glass of water within 2 hours of returning to the ward, and by the first postoperative day she was drinking cups of tea and tolerating a light diet. Her intravenous infusion was discontinued after 8 hours, as she was able to drink adequately and did not feel nauseated. Joanna passed urine within 5 hours of returning to the ward and thereafter was passing sufficient quantities of urine.

Communicating
- *Problem*: Joanna has a hoarse voice following her surgery.
- *Goals*:
  1. To detect signs of recurrent laryngeal nerve damage.
  2. To reassure Joanna that her voice should eventually return to normal.
- *Nursing actions and rationale for care*:
  1. Observe Joanna for a loss of phonation or respiratory difficulties, as this may indicate damage to the recurrent laryngeal nerves.
  2. Ensure Joanna has her vocal cords checked by the medical staff, to ensure that her cords are intact and have not been damaged during the surgery.
  3. Reassure Joanna that her voice will eventually return to normal, as most hoarseness is usually a temporary situation.
- *Evaluation*: Joanna had her vocal cords checked in the ENT outpatients department, and they were found to be intact. When she left the ward after 2 days, her voice was beginning to return to normal.

Cleansing and dressing
- *Problem*: Joanna has a surgical wound on her neck.
- *Goals*:
  1. The wound has healed when the staples are removed.
  2. There is no evidence of wound infection.
- *Nursing actions and rationale for care*:
  1. Observe the wound dressing for signs of bleeding and report to nurse in charge.
  2. Monitor the amount of drainage in the Redivac bottle, as excessive drainage may indicate haemorrhage. Ensure the Redivac drain is vacuumed at all times, to ensure the drainage system is patent.
  3. Once drainage is minimal, usually after 24 hours, the Redivac drain can be removed, and a small

absorbent dressing applied over the drain site.

4. Theatre dressing is removed after 24 hours, and if no exudate is present the wound can be left exposed. If the wound is still exuding, apply a light sterile dressing, so as to protect the wound from microorganisms.

5. Observe the wound for signs of redness, heat, tenderness and swelling, as this could indicate infection.

6. Monitor Joanna's temperature 4 hourly, as a pyrexia may indicate infection.

- *Evaluation*: Joanna's temperature remained within normal limits. The Redivac drain was removed after 24 hours and had collected 75 mL of haemoserous fluid. When the theatre dressing was removed, the wound was intact with no exudate present. However, Joanna felt very conscious of the wound, so a light gauze dressing was applied to it. As Joanna was discharged home after 48 hours, her staples were removed by the practice nurse after 7 days, where the wound edges were found to be united. Joanna was then encouraged to massage the scar with a gentle moisturizer daily, commencing 2 weeks after staple removal, so as to prevent contraction of the scar.

Mobility

- *Problem*: Joanna has difficulty in moving her head/neck following her surgery.
- *Goal*: Joanna has a full range of movement of her head/neck.
- *Nursing actions and rationale for care*:
  1. Ensure Joanna's head/neck is initially well supported with pillows, to relax her neck muscles.
  2. Encourage Joanna to support her head by placing her hands at the back of her head when she wishes to move.

3. Encourage Joanna to perform gentle head/neck exercises, i.e. forward and lateral flexion, hyperextension and rotation, once the surgeon gives permission. This is to ensure she does not get a stiff neck.

- *Evaluation*: Joanna was able to perform her head/neck exercises the day following her surgery, and had a reasonable range of movement by the time she was discharged home.

Expressing sexuality

- *Problem*: Joanna is concerned with the appearance of the scar, as she works with the media.
- *Goal*: Joanna feels comfortable with her body image.
- *Nursing actions and rationale for care*:
  1. Allow Joanna time to express her fears about her physical appearance.
  2. Give Joanna some ideas as to how she may camouflage the scar initially, until she becomes happy with it, e.g. use of scarves.
  3. Reassure Joanna that the scar should not be too noticeable, as it is in one of the natural folds of skin in her neck, and it will become flatter and paler as the healing process continues, and so will not be as noticeable.
  4. Inform Joanna of the need to gently massage the scar with a light moisturizer from 2 weeks after the staples have been removed, as this should prevent contraction of the scar.
- *Evaluation*: Joanna was concerned as to how her colleagues would react to her scar, and she felt happier wearing a light gauze dressing covered with a scarf. She said that she had met other people who had had this type of surgery and that their scars had faded over time.

HAEMORRHAGE

The thyroid gland is a highly vascular organ, and although the risk of haemorrhage should be at a minimum because of the preoperative preparation of the patient, it should be closely observed for, as blood may collect in the area surrounding the trachea, leading to respiratory difficulties. This is an emergency situation and removal of the sutures/staples should be immediately undertaken in order to allow the haematoma to be released. Surgical evacuation of the haematoma may be required if this has no effect on the patient's respiratory state.

The risk of haematoma formation is reduced if the surgeon can achieve good haemostasis during the surgical procedure. It is often thought that the insertion of a drain will also reduce the risk of haematoma formation, although Wihlborg et al (1988) found that drainage after uncomplicated thyroid surgery did not decrease the rate of complications due to postoperative bleeding. Wihlborg et al (1988) suggest that prophylactic drainage is not necessary in uncomplicated thyroid surgery, but may still be of value in patients where extensive dissection was undertaken, excessive haemorrhaging occurred or there were problems in achieving haemostasis.

RECURRENT LARYNGEAL NERVE DAMAGE

Damage to the superior laryngeal nerve will present as hoarseness, and the vocal cords may have a wrinkled appearance. Recurrent laryngeal nerve damage affects the patient's ability to speak. Damage to one side of the recurrent laryngeal nerve results in hoarseness and a paralysed vocal cord, while damage to both laryngeal nerves results in loss of speech and paralysed vocal cords, the latter causing respiratory problems. The damage may be temporary if due to swelling, i.e. laryngeal oedema, or permanent if the nerve is severed or damaged during surgery (Litwack-Saleh, 1992).

THYROID CRISIS

This may occur as a result of excessive amounts of thyroid hormones entering the circulation, causing an acute thyrotoxic state. It is thought to be due to handling of the thyroid gland during the surgical procedure (Gillespie et al, 1992), and is most likely to be seen 6–24 hours following surgery. The patient will become very breathless, feel very hot and complain of palpitations, and may also appear confused or manic. Due to the uncontrolled rise in metabolic rate, they will develop a hyperpyrexia, a noticeable tachycardia and become hypertensive. If this situation occurs, the patient should be given oxygen therapy, and prescribed sedatives and cool washes to reduce the hyperpyrexia, as well as having an intravenous infusion to correct dehydration and control hyperthermia. Intravenous beta-adrenoceptor blocking drugs, e.g. propranolol, antithyroid drugs, e.g. carbimazole, and glucocorticosteroids, e.g. hydrocortisone, will be given as an emergency treatment, as patients can die from cardiac failure.

TETANY

Damage or removal of the parathyroid glands during surgery can lead to a decrease in serum calcium concentrations – i.e. hypoparathyroidism causes hypocalcaemia – whereby the patient can develop tetany in the early days following surgery. This condition is commonly due to interference with the blood supply to the parathyroid glands, which occurs during surgery (Gillespie et al, 1992), or due to their inadvertent removal during a total thyroidectomy, and can be seen usually 24–72 hours postoperatively, although it can occur 1–3 hours postoperatively (Litwack-Saleh, 1992).

The patient may complain of numbness or tingling in the fingers and toes, and will also show evidence of carpopedal spasm, i.e. cramp in the hands and feet due to hypocalcaemia. Carpopedal spasm can be detected by observing for positive Trousseau's and Chvostek's signs (Litwack-Saleh, 1992). Trousseau's sign is where there is contraction of the hand induced by the application of a tourniquet around the upper arm, e.g. when taking the patient's blood pressure. A positive Chvostek's sign is seen by gently tapping the patient's face over the zygoma, which will produce spasm of the facial muscles. The patient's voice may become high-pitched and shrill, due to spasm of the vocal cords. Gastrointestinal cramps can also be associated with tetany. Initial treatment of tetany is with intravenous administration of calcium gluconate. If the parathyroid glands have been permanently damaged, the patient will need to receive oral calcium supplements.

DISCHARGE PLANNING AND PATIENT EDUCATION

Most patients undergoing thyroid surgery only stay in hospital for a short period of time, e.g. 1–2 days, so the amount of information they are given relating to their postoperative recovery is paramount if they are to make a full and successful recovery from surgery (see Ch. 8 for further information on discharge planning).

Prior to their discharge home, it is important that patients realize the need to rest once they are home, and that they may need some assistance, e.g. home help. Patients are not always aware of how tired they will feel once they leave hospital. They need to be made aware of this, and also informed that this is quite normal following any kind of surgery, as it can take 2–3 months before they are fully recovered from the surgery.

Clear written and verbal information should be given to the patient regarding the neck exercises that they should perform several times a day, and that these exercises should continue until they are able to freely move their head/neck without any feeling of pulling. The need to gently massage the scar with a gentle moisturizer should be reinforced, and should commence about 2 weeks following removal of the sutures/staples. Advice can also be given as to how to camouflage the scar if required, e.g. by use of a scarf.

Six weeks after surgery, the patient will be required to attend the outpatients clinic. This is to enable the medical staff to ensure that wound healing is progressing and that the patient has no problems with their voice or swallowing. Bloods are taken for thyroid hormone levels, to ensure the patient is not becoming myxoedemic. If the patient is suffering from hypothyroidism (myxoedema), they will need to be prescribed replacement thyroxine therapy, and if they have had a total thyroidectomy, they will need thyroid replacement therapy for life.

CONCLUSION

Surgery to the thyroid gland is only undertaken in cases of malignancy, or when drug therapy has failed to control the condition. Most of these patients are nursed in a general surgical ward, but some may be nursed in other units. A common problem facing patients undergoing thyroid surgery is the position of the scar following surgery, and how it may affect their body image, although this is always something the surgeon takes into consideration during the surgery. Postoperative nursing care is concerned with the early detection of specific potential complications, so that early intervention can be undertaken.

Summary of key points

- Thyroidectomy is undertaken for either malignancy of the thyroid gland or uncontrolled hyperthyroidism.

- Patients should be in a euthyroid state prior to surgery.

- Preoperative assessment of the vocal cords is essential.

- Postoperative care relates to careful monitoring for potential complications, e.g. obstructed airway.

- Many patients have a sore throat postoperatively.

- Some patients may require replacement thyroxine therapy, depending on their thyroid hormone levels.

References

British Thyroid Association/Royal College of Physicians (2002) *Guidelines for the Management of Thyroid Cancer.* Salisbury: Royal College of Physicians [Online] Available at http://www.british-thyroid-association.org (accessed 30 September 2003).

Forrest, A., Cartere, D. & Macleod, I. (1991) *Principles and Practices of Surgery,* 2nd edn. Edinburgh: Churchill Livingstone.

Gillespie, I., Ansari, N. & Zawawi, A. (1992) *Guide to Surgical Principles and Practice.* Edinburgh: Churchill Livingstone.

Hinchliff, S., Montague, S. & Watson, R. (1996) *Physiology for Nursing Practice,* 2nd edn. London: Baillière Tindall.

Johnson, J. K. (1993) Outcome of treating thyrotoxic patients with a standard dose of radioactive iodine. *Scottish Medical Journal* 38(5): 142–144.

Litwack-Saleh, K. (1992) Practical points in the care of the patient post-thyroid surgery. *Journal of Post Anesthesia Nursing* 7(6): 404–406.

Moore, S. & Haughey, B. (1997) Surgical treatment for thyroid cancer. *AORN Journal* 65(4): 710, 712, 714–716, 719–722, 725.

Roper, N., Logan, W. & Tierney, A. J. (2000) *The Roper–Logan–Tierney Model of Nursing.* Edinburgh: Churchill Livingstone.

Stojadinovic, A., Shaha, A., Orlikoff, R., et al (2002) Prospective functional voice assessment in patients undergoing thyroid surgery. *Annals of Surgery* 236(6): 823–832.

Tyagi, N. (1993) Contact tip YAP laser enhances safety of thyroidectomy. *Clinical Laser Monthly* 11(1): 7–9.

Wheeler, M. (1994) Investigation of the thyroid. *Surgery* 12(7): 145–147.

Wihlborg, O., Bergljung, L. & Martensson, H. (1988) To drain or not to drain in thyroid surgery. *Archives of Surgery* 123(1): 40–41.

Yamamoto, M., Sasaki, A., Asahi, H., et al (2002) Endoscopic versus conventional open thyroid lobectomy for benign thyroid nodules: a prospective study. *Surgical Laparoscopy Endoscopy & Percutaneous Techniques* 12(7): 426–429.

Further reading/websites

http://www.british-thyroid-association.org (accessed 30 September 2003). A society for health professionals in the UK involved in the management of patients with thyroid disease.

Chapter **13**

Care of the patient requiring cardiac interventions and surgery

Lindsey Ockenden and Christine Spiers

Key objectives of the chapter

At the end of this chapter the reader will be able to:

- describe the structure, function and blood flow through the heart

- identify the structural abnormalities that can affect the heart

- describe how to undertake a nursing assessment of the cardiac patient

- describe the procedure used for cardiac catheterization, its indications and the nursing management required by patients before and after catheterization

- describe the procedures used in the investigation and treatment of patients with cardiac arrhythmias

- identify the specific care required by patients requiring temporary and permanent pacing and internal cardiac defibrillators

- discuss the nursing management of the patient requiring open cardiac surgery

- identify the specific advice required by patients prior to discharge from hospital following cardiac investigations and therapy.

INTRODUCTION

This chapter aims to give an overview of the principles of the care required by patients undergoing a range of invasive investigations and treatments for cardiovascular disease. The more invasive cardiac procedures are reviewed in detail to enhance understanding of what is involved for the patient, so that the nurse is able to tailor information to meet the individual's needs. Although this chapter describes accepted day-to-day clinical practice, this may differ to local policy and guidelines and must be taken into consideration.

ANATOMY AND PHYSIOLOGY OF THE HEART

The heart lies behind the sternum, with two-thirds in the left side of the chest. It is composed of three layers: the inner layer is the endocardium; the middle muscular layer is the myocardium; and the outer layer is the epicardium. The epicardial surface is surrounded by a protective, inelastic fibrous sac called the pericardium, which contains a small amount of lubricating serous fluid.

The heart has four chambers: an atrium and ventricle separated by a valve on both the right and left sides, with the atria and ventricles being separated by the intra-atrial and intraventricular septa. The heart can be thought of as a low-pressure and a high-pressure pump in series. Deoxygenated blood flows from the body via the inferior and superior vena cavae into the right atrium. Blood flow from the right atrium to the right ventricle mainly occurs passively (about 70%) while the heart is relaxed and not contracting. This phase is called diastole. When the heart contracts (systole) the blood is propelled through the tricuspid valve into the right ventricle. When the ventricle contracts, the tricuspid valve closes and blood is expelled through the pulmonary valve into the pulmonary artery and into the pulmonary vascular system, where it is oxygenated in the lungs and carbon dioxide is removed. This is the low-pressure system.

From the lungs, oxygenated blood enters the left atrium via the pulmonary veins during diastole. Blood flows through the mitral valve into the left ventricle both passively and by contraction of the left atrium. When the ventricle contracts in systole, the mitral valve closes, the aortic valve opens and blood is ejected into the aorta. This is the high-pressure system, as the high pressure is necessary to propel the blood through the body. For this reason the left ventricle has greater muscle mass than the right ventricle. The blood then circulates around the body, becomes deoxygenated and returns once again to the right atrium via the vena cavae.

Contraction of the heart muscle (myocardium) needs to occur in a specific sequence, for these events to occur. This is achieved by the specialized conducting system within the heart. This consists of the sinoatrial (SA) node, which is found at the junction of the vena cava with the right atrium, and is the cardiac pacemaker that determines the heart rate. Impulses pass across the atria to the atrioventricular (AV) node at the base of the right atrium and thence to either ventricle via the bundle of His. In the normal heart this is the only route that can be taken by electrical impulses passing from the atria to the ventricles. Impulses are then conducted by the right and left bundle branches to a network of Purkinje fibres which supply the respective ventricles. For practical purposes, events can be regarded as happening simultaneously on both sides of the heart, so that identical volumes of blood flow through both the right and left sides of the heart. Heart rate and strength of contraction are affected by the autonomic nervous system. The heart is richly innervated by sympathetic nerve fibres, which on stimulation increase both the heart rate and speed of electrical transmission via the conducting system. This increases heart rate and strength of contraction. The vagus nerve of the parasympathetic nervous system also innervates the heart and has a broadly opposite effect – namely, slowing the heart rate on stimulation – and can therefore be considered as the heart's braking system.

Forward blood flow through the heart is maintained by the tricuspid and mitral valves, which prevent the blood flowing backwards from the ventricles to the atria, while the pulmonary and aortic valves prevent blood flowing backwards from the pulmonary artery and aorta into the right and left ventricles, respectively. Although these valves have similar functions, their structures differ. The tricuspid valve, positioned between the right atrium and ventricle, has three cusps, compared with two for the mitral valve, positioned between the left atrium and ventricle. The cusps are thin, strong and fibrous, and when opened are pushed against the ventricular wall to allow blood to flow through them. These valves are attached and stabilized within the heart by specialized parts of the cardiac muscle known as the papillary muscles, which are attached to the tricuspid and mitral valves via cords called chordae tendineae. The two semilunar valves positioned between the right ventricle and pulmonary artery (pulmonary valve) and the left ventricle and aorta (aortic valve) are anchored to the fibrous ring of the cardiac skeleton and do not have papillary muscles or chordae tendineae. Both the pulmonary and aortic valves have three cusps.

The myocardium receives its blood supply from the left and right coronary arteries. These arise from the aorta just above the aortic valve. The left main stem divides into the left anterior descending and circumflex branch. The left anterior descending artery supplies oxygenated blood to the interventricular septum and the anterior wall of the left ventricle; the circumflex branch supplies the lateral wall of the left ventricle. The right coronary artery supplies the inferior and posterior walls of the left and right ventricles. The myocardium receives its blood supply during the diastolic phase of the cardiac cycle. These vessels also supply the specialized conducting tissue with its oxygenated blood.

BASIC PATHOPHYSIOLOGY OF THE HEART

Any components of the heart can malfunction, either because of congenital abnormality or acquired disease. The heart can also be affected by conditions elsewhere in the body (Table 13.1).

Coronary heart disease is the most common cause of death in the UK, with 1 in 4 men and 1 in 6 women dying from the disease. Over 275 000 people suffer a heart attack each year and almost half of these are fatal. In 30% of cases, the patients die before they reach hospital. There is considerable variation in mortality from coronary heart disease across the UK. Death rates are higher in Scotland and lower in the south east of England. Death rates are also higher in manual workers than non-manual workers and higher in certain ethnic groups. However, death rates from coronary heart disease have fallen considerably in the UK, with a 40% reduction in the last 10 years. Although mortality rates are falling rapidly, the amount of morbidity is not falling. Over 2.5 million people in the UK are living with coronary heart disease, and approximately 2 million people have angina, which is the most common presentation of coronary heart disease (British Heart Foundation, 2003).

A variety of factors such as smoking, diabetes, sedentary lifestyle, diets high in saturated fats and obesity eventually cause the lumen of the coronary arteries to narrow, causing angina and possible myocardial infarction. The general name for this condition is atherosclerosis. The disease process causing this is due to a variety of complex mechanisms responsible for the accumulation of fatty plaques within the vessel walls and calcification of the vessels; this causes narrowing of the arteries. If the fatty plaques become ulcerated, thrombosis occurs, which may lead to vessel occlusion. The formation of atherosclerosis is essentially an inflammatory process and is caused by a variety of risk factors (Ross, 1999). This disease process reduces the blood supply to the myocardium, causing ischaemic chest pain (angina) and, if the artery occludes completely, results in heart muscle death (myocardial infarction). A myocardial infarction can cause additional complications if the valves or conducting system are affected.

There are two main problems which can affect each heart valve:

- if they cannot close properly they leak, which is called regurgitation
- when they cannot open properly they obstruct the flow of blood, and this narrowing is called stenosis.

Some of the disease processes affecting adults are due to degeneration through ageing of already damaged

---

Table 13.1 Diseases affecting the heart, in relation to cardiac structure

	Myocardium	Pericardium	Coronary arteries	Valves	Conduction system
Congential disease	Atrial/ventricular septal defects Hypertrophic obstructive myocardiopathies		Anatomical abnormalities Homozygous hypercholesterolaemia	Bicuspid atresia	Abnormal pathway Wolff–Parkinson–White syndrome Atrioventricular block
Acquired disease	Myocardial infarction Myocarditis Ventricular septal defect Cardiomyopathies	Pericarditis Tamponade Malignancy	Atherosclerosis Syndrome X	Rheumatic fever Infective Stenosis Regurgitation Papillary muscle rupture Chordae tendineae rupture	Atrioventricular block Sick sinus syndrome AV nodal re-entrant tachycardia

valves, with many patients not presenting until their fifth decade or later. An example of this is the 1% of the population born with a bicuspid aortic valve instead of a tricuspid valve (Swanton, 2003). This causes turbulent blood flow through the valve, which, over time, causes the cusps to become damaged and calcified, resulting in the valve being unable to open or close fully. This can cause either aortic stenosis or regurgitation, or both conditions can occur together. Similarly, rheumatic fever occurring in childhood can contribute to mitral valve disease in later life. Stenosis and/or regurgitation can also affect the other heart valves with similar results. The valves commonly affected by disease in adults are the aortic and mitral valves. Calcification of the valves due to repetitive mechanical stress can lead to stenosis and stiffening of the valve cusps, which partially obstructs blood flow, and so increases the workload of the heart (Blackburn and Bookless, 2002). If this is not corrected early enough it may eventually lead to heart failure. Myocardial infarction involving the papillary muscles or causing rupture of the chordae tendineae, results in acute mitral regurgitation. This may require urgent surgical repair and/or replacement of the valve.

The conducting system is also affected by a number of conditions which can affect rhythm, resulting in heart rates that can be dangerously fast or slow. Congenital abnormalities such as extra or anomalous conducting pathways (such as Wolff–Parkinson–White syndrome) provide an abnormal connection between the atria and ventricles, which allows the rapid transmission of impulses, causing tachycardia. Ageing, again, can cause fibrosis and calcification of the conducting tissue, which can produce rhythm abnormalities, including various degrees of heart block and slow heart rates. Conduction defects such as heart block may also be caused by coronary artery disease, as a result of occlusion of the artery supplying the conducting tissue with its blood supply.

Disease processes that affect the myocardium eventually interfere with the pumping action of the heart. This is a frequent cause of heart failure because the heart is no longer able to pump adequate amounts of blood to meet the body's oxygen demands. This may also lead to myocardial infarction. Heart failure may also result from valve disease, hypertension, pericardial or infective heart disease, or cardiomyopathy. Heart failure is a rapidly increasing problem in the UK, with over 650 000 people diagnosed with definite heart failure (British Heart Foundation, 2003). The condition is very serious, as many patients die within 3 months of initial diagnosis, and the 5-year mortality rate is nearly 60%, which contrasts with a less than 50% 5-year mortality rate for cancer (McMurray and Stewart, 2000).

The cardiomyopathies are categorized as:

- dilated cardiomyopathy
- hypertrophic cardiomyopathy
- arrhythmogenic right ventricular cardiomyopathy or dysplasia
- restrictive cardiomyopathy.

Dilated cardiomyopathy is the most common and has numerous causes from infective to toxic; but whatever the cause, it eventually results in congestive heart failure, which, when severe, may not respond to anti-failure drug therapy. Hypertrophic cardiomyopathy is thought to be genetically transmitted, resulting in thickening of the intraventricular septum, which eventually causes left ventricular obstruction and heart failure (Grech, 2003). Arrhythmogenic right ventricular cardiomyopathy or dysplasia is also an inherited disease; it is characterized by fibrofatty replacement of the right ventricle outflow tract. It predisposes individuals to serious ventricular arrhythmias and sudden cardiac death, and may eventually lead to right and then left ventricular failure. Restrictive cardiomyopathy is the rarest form and has numerous causes; it results in restricted ventricular filling and reduced ventricular volume. It also causes end-stage heart failure and serious cardiac arrhythmias. The principles of treating the cardiomyopathies include managing advancing heart failure, anti-arrhythmic therapy, insertion of pacemakers or internal defibrillators to manage potential sudden death events and heart transplantation for end-stage heart failure (O'Donoghue, 2002).

ASSESSMENT AND INVESTIGATIONS

Patients with heart disease may require extensive assessment and investigations to diagnose and establish the extent of the disease and its effects on body function. Cardiac assessment should be specific and focused, and may also include risk factor assessment and exploring family and social history. The cardinal symptoms of cardiac disease should also be investigated: in particular, questions should be asked about chest pain, breathlessness, palpitations, dizziness, loss of consciousness and ankle oedema.

CARDINAL SYMPTOMS OF CARDIAC DISEASE

Patients with coronary artery disease or aortic valve stenosis often experience angina or ischaemic chest pain. This type of pain is frequently described as a crushing or vice-like sensation across the chest wall, radiating into the jaw and down the left arm. Information should also be gained in regard to factors that provoke and/or ease the pain, as well as a description of the pain, its location, intensity, radiation and type.

Heart disease may cause cardiac arrhythmias and therefore the patient should be asked if they have experienced the following symptoms: palpitations, dizziness or blackouts. These symptoms may be associated with both fast and slow arrhythmias, such as ventricular tachycardia, varying degrees of heart block and atrial fibrillation. These slow or rapid rhythms can result in decreased cardiac output and lowered blood pressure (hypotension), which can if severe lead to cardiogenic shock.

Patients with left-sided heart disease often experience breathlessness, either on exertion or at rest. They will often give a history of being unable to lie flat for any length of time, and of wakening from sleep with an episode of acute breathlessness. In addition, the patient should be asked if they have a productive cough and to describe what the sputum looks like. If the patient is expectorating large quantities of frothy, clear/pinkish sputum, this may indicate the presence of heart failure and pulmonary oedema.

The nurse should enquire whether the patient has noticed any ankle swelling, which indicates the presence of oedema and possible right-side heart failure.

PAST HISTORY

Questions should be asked about past and recent medical history, as many seemingly unrelated conditions can be the cause of the current cardiac complaint. Enquiries about previous rheumatic heart fever should be made, as while the incidence of this disease is declining in the developed world, it remains the main cause of mitral stenosis (Swanton, 2003). Patients with diabetes mellitus have a substantially increased risk of coronary heart disease. This risk seems to be higher for women with type 2 diabetes mellitus, and these patients will often have other risk factors for coronary artery disease such as hypertension and obesity (Jowett and Thompson, 2003). Renal disease is often associated with hypertension; and hypertension, often referred to as the 'silent killer,' causes heart failure and acute coronary syndrome if left untreated. A history of recent invasive treatment will be of particular importance in a patient with known valvular abnormalities, as it may cause infective endocarditis. The classic 'invasive treatment' is usually dental but may also include any endoscopic procedure or even body piercing! (Swanton, 2003).

Social and family history

Many cardiac diseases have a familial or genetic component and tactful questioning may elicit this. A familial history of coronary artery disease is identified if there has been a death in a first-degree relative under the age of 55 years (Munro and Campbell, 2000). In addition, any sudden unexplained death at a young age in the family is significant, as it may lead to the patient being investigated for Wolff–Parkinson–White syndrome, hypertrophic cardiomyopathy or genetic abnormalities such as the long Q-T interval syndrome.

Occupational and functional status

Occupation is important, as cardiac disease can also be caused by certain occupations – for example, publicans may suffer with alcoholic cardiomyopathy, and organic solvents used in the dry cleaning industry are implicated in cardiac arrhythmias and cardiomyopathy. For medicolegal reasons, a diagnosis of cardiac disease can significantly limit if not completely curtail a career in the armed forces or police force, and limit the ability of an individual to hold a pilot licence or public service vehicle license (PSV) (DVLA, 2003).

Cardiac disease assessment should be made regarding the onset, duration and severity of any presenting symptoms. As cardiac disease is usually progressive, it is important to assess the development of the symptoms over a time span. Functional capacity should also be assessed, as patients may have deliberately reduced activities such as domestic duties, sporting or other hobbies to limit their symptoms (Munro and Campbell, 2000). Enquiries regarding the patient's ability to climb stairs or walk uphill (particularly into cold winds) are particularly revealing, as in some cases coronary artery disease presents predominantly with breathlessness on exertion, associated with climbing inclines.

RISK FACTORS

Cardiac risk factors can be divided into those which are modifiable and those which are non-modifiable. The predominant modifiable and non-modifiable risk factors are listed in Table 13.2.

Table 13.2 Cardiac risk factors

Non-modifiable risk factors	Modifiable risk factors
Age	Hypertension
Gender	Cigarette smoking
Race	Diabetes
Genetic predisposition	Obesity
Hyperlipidaemia	Alcohol
	Lack of exercise
	High blood cholesterol levels

Inquiry into the risk factors listed in Table 13.2 and also current drug therapy, including any recreational drugs, should be recorded as many treatments have cardiac side-effects. This will form a useful basis for any focused health education as part of the cardiac rehabilitation process. It is important to be non-judgmental regarding risk factors, as many patients are fully aware of the role of the risk factors in their current medical problem, and 'victim blaming' will only alienate the patient and will not serve as a useful basis for a therapeutic relationship.

PHYSICAL ASSESSMENT

General observation of the patient can reveal useful information such as shortness of breath at rest and ankle oedema.

The pulse and blood pressure serve as useful tools to assess cardiac output. Measurements of the blood pressure and pulse rate determine whether they are within the normal parameters of:

- pulse rate 60–100 bpm
- systolic blood pressure 100–140 mmHg
- diastolic blood pressure 60–85 mmHg.

A pulse rate below 60 or above 100 bpm may compromise cardiac output, resulting in low blood pressure and insufficient perfusion of body tissues. The quality of the pulse should also be assessed by noting strength and rhythm. Some patients may have an irregularly irregular pulse that could be the result of atrial fibrillation, or an irregular pulse that may indicate ectopic beats.

Further circulatory assessment involves palpating the radial, brachial, femoral, popliteal, dorsalis pedis and posterior tibial pulses to determine their presence and strength. Capillary refill can be used as an indicator of arterial sufficiency, evaluated by applying firm digital pressure to the nail bed to produce blanching; on release of pressure, blood flow should return in less than 3 seconds. This information can be used for comparison of circulatory status after cardiac catheterization.

Many cardiac abnormalities affect respiratory function and vice versa. A thorough respiratory assessment will establish the extent to which the respiratory system is affected. Respiratory assessment should include measurement of the respiratory rate, observation of the depth and rhythm of breathing and observation of the colour of mucous membranes. Patients having difficulty with breathing frequently use their accessory muscles. Accessory muscle use can be seen by observing for retraction of the skin on either side of the neck, just above the clavicles; if breathing difficulty is severe, the skin between the ribs retracts along with abdominal muscle movement. The patient should also be asked whether he experiences any breathing difficulty, and which factors cause/ease any breathing problems. Oxygen saturation levels (SaO_2) can be measured with a pulse oximeter, and is a useful indicator of the amount of oxygen bound to the haemoglobin of the blood, which is normally in the range 95–99% (Clinton, 2003). However, a patient with chronic obstructive pulmonary disease may have a normal level of less than 90% (Fox, 1996). The nurse should also enquire whether the patient has a cough, and if sputum is being expectorated, sputum colour, consistency and volume should be noted and recorded.

A detailed history of the patient's smoking habits should be undertaken, including the following: type and quantity of cigarettes smoked; the period of time of being a smoker; and when the patient has attempted to stop smoking in the past. This information will help in the formulation of a plan to help the patient give up smoking in the future.

MEDICAL INVESTIGATIONS

Some of these investigations are straightforward and, once explained, cause little discomfort for the patient. But the more invasive investigations such as cardiac catheterization can be uncomfortable and frightening and are associated with a number of risks. The following gives an overview of these investigations, followed by a detailed account of the more invasive investigation of cardiac catheterization and the care required by the patient following this procedure.

Chest X-ray

This non-invasive investigation demands little of the patient other than being able to take a deep breath and hold it for a few seconds, long enough for a radiograph to be taken of the chest wall and its contents. This investigation enables assessment of the lungs, heart and great vessels. No specific physical preparation is required, unless the patient is a woman within child-bearing age, in which case information will be required as to when she last menstruated, and whether there is any possibility of her being pregnant, as there is a potential risk that radiation exposure during the radiography could affect the developing fetus.

Blood tests

Blood samples will be obtained for a number of tests: these include estimation of urea and electrolyte levels, which can give an indication of renal function, and full blood count to assess for anaemia, polycythaemia and infection. Measurement of potassium is particularly important, since abnormally high or low levels may place the patient at risk of developing cardiac arrhythmias.

Clotting screening is necessary prior to any invasive investigation and treatment if the patient has been taking anticoagulant drugs. If clotting times are prolonged, the patient will be at risk of haemorrhage following any invasive procedure.

Serum cardiac markers are measured if there is suspicion of myocardial infarction. The enzymes and isoenzymes creatinine kinase (CK), myocardial-specific creatinine kinase (CK-MB) and related proteins myoglobin and troponin (troponin T and I) usually remain within the cell; however, if the cell is stressed or damaged, it releases these enzymes and proteins into the circulation. The presence of CK-MB, troponin T or troponin I in the blood is an indicator of heart muscle damage, thus making these blood tests invaluable diagnostic tools in myocardial infarction. The cardiac troponins are the best markers for definitive diagnosis and are also used to risk stratify patients with chest pain. Normal values for these enzymes can be obtained through individual hospital laboratories (Maynard et al, 2000).

Electrocardiography

Electrocardiography (ECG) involves attaching adhesive electrodes to the patient's skin in order to view the electrical activity of the heart. A 12-lead ECG involves the application of 10 electrodes – six to the patient's chest wall and four to the patient's limbs – to derive 12 'views' of the cardiac electrical activity. The 12-lead ECG gives information about congenital or acquired abnormalities of the heart, and disease of the pericardium, myocardium or endocardium. Most importantly, the 12-lead ECG gives information about myocardial perfusion, ischaemia and infarction, as these will alter the normal pattern of the ECG waveforms, most notably resulting in ST segment elevation or depression (Spiers, 2003). Careful placement of these electrodes is important, as minor alterations in lead placement can result in erroneous diagnosis, such as false patterns of right bundle branch block.

Exercise stress (tolerance) test

This is usually performed on a treadmill or bicycle. It employs a continuous 12-lead ECG and blood pressure recordings, and is an invaluable test to reveal cardiac symptoms or ECG changes which may not occur at rest. The test is also used to assess prognosis in patients with known cardiac disease and to evaluate treatments. It is not without risks and should always be performed by trained personnel, with resuscitation equipment nearby (Jowett and Thompson, 2003).

Ambulatory electrocardiography

Also referred to as Holter monitoring, this involves the patient wearing a small tape-recording unit which is attached to three ECG electrodes placed on the patient's chest wall. The tape recorder continuously records the patient's ECG for a period of 24–48 hours. The patient is able to activate an event marker that will indicate on the tape when symptoms have been experienced, which can be correlated with the recorded ECG. Holter monitoring is useful for patients who experience intermittent arrhythmias which may not be recorded during a conventional ECG, or for patients with silent ischaemia.

Echocardiogram

Transthoracic echocardiography is a non-invasive test which enables the cardiac anatomy and function to be assessed by producing images of the heart from recorded sound waves. The sound waves are recorded from the heart by moving a transducer over the anterior chest wall. Transthoracic echocardiography can identify structural changes of the heart. It can measure the size of the heart chambers, providing information about enlargement or constriction of the ventricle, as well as detecting such abnormalities as the presence of tumours or excess fluid within the pericardial sac (which if impairing the function of the heart is known as cardiac tamponade). It is also used to evaluate the functioning of the valves. The test is painless, lasting about 45 minutes, and on completion the patient can resume normal activity.

By comparison, transoesophageal echocardiography is more invasive and therefore associated with some risks. This involves introducing the transducer into the oesophagus, which provides a more direct view of the heart. This test is useful in identifying mitral regurgitation or prolapsed valve, and a dissecting aortic aneurysm. The patient should give informed consent before the procedure, as the procedure involves sedation, fasting and the application of an anaesthetic to the throat to assist insertion of the probe. The patient should therefore be recovered in the normal manner and carefully observed for potential arrhythmias during the recovery period.

Nuclear scans

Nuclear scanning is a rapidly evolving area of medicine and enables the assessment of myocardial perfusion, viability and ventricular function. It involves the intravenous injection of a radioactive substance such as technetium-99 or thallium-201. The substance is taken up by the heart, which is then visualized using a gamma-camera. The radioactive substances enable either myocardial damage (hot spot detection) or hypo-perfusion (cold spot detection) to be demonstrated. The techniques may be combined with exercise testing for a more accurate method of assessment. More recently, magnetic resonance imaging (MRI) and single-photon emission computed tomography (SPECT) scanning have been developed, but these techniques are not widely available in the UK (Jowett and Thompson, 2003).

Cardiac catheterization

This investigative procedure confirms and evaluates the extent of heart disease. The procedure involves gaining access to the heart via major blood vessels. Access to the left side of the heart is achieved by catheterizing either the femoral, radial or brachial artery, while right heart catheterization is performed via the venous route, usually the femoral vein, although the subclavian or jugular veins may also be used.

Information regarding cardiac function is gained by measuring intracardiac pressures, while X-ray visualization of the heart's pumping action and blood flow within the coronary arteries, aorta and pulmonary artery is achieved by injecting a radio-opaque dye during X-ray fluoroscopy. This enables visualization of any abnormalities within the chambers of the heart, as well as stenosis or occlusion in the coronary and pulmonary arteries.

Cardiac catheterization is used to confirm and evaluate the progression of the following disorders:

- coronary artery disease
- valve disease
- ventricular dysfunction
- pulmonary and aortic artery disease/disorders
- atrial and ventricular wall defects
- electrical conduction abnormalities.

Catheterization procedure

The procedure is performed under a local anaesthetic via the femoral, radial or less commonly the brachial artery: lidocaine (lignocaine) is injected subcutaneously around the right inguinal site over the femoral artery, or subcutaneously over the radial artery to numb/anaesthetize the skin. Both the femoral and radial approaches involve introducing a needle into the artery followed by threading a long, thin guide wire via the needle into the artery. The needle is removed, leaving the wire, over which an introducer sheath is inserted (Fig. 13.1). During this part of the procedure the patient will experience some discomfort, usually a feeling of pressure over the groin or wrist as the introducer sheath is inserted into the artery, and perhaps mild discomfort as the catheter is advanced along the artery. The patient's blood pressure and ECG is monitored closely throughout the procedure for any arrhythmias and ischaemic changes.

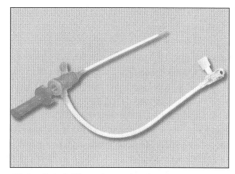

Figure 13.1   Arterial introducer sheath.

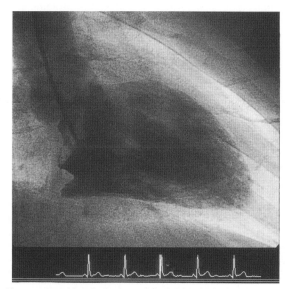

Figure 13.2   Ventriculogram of the left ventricle during cardiac catheterization.

The introducer sheath allows for repeated access to the artery and heart with different catheters. Within the sheath is a valve that prevents blood loss when the catheter is removed. A catheter can then be threaded up the descending aorta and the tip gently manipulated across the aortic valve into the left ventricle. Radio-opaque dye is injected rapidly into the ventricle (ventriculogram) so that its pumping action can be observed and recorded during X-ray fluoroscopy (Fig. 13.2). This will also identify the presence of abnormalities such as a ventricular aneurysm, valvular regurgitation or leakage via holes in the septal wall of the heart (atrial or ventricular septal defects).

During the ventriculogram the patient will experience a 'hot flushing' sensation, which may also include a feeling of urinary incontinence. This lasts for a few seconds and is due to the vasodilatory effects of the injected dye. The ventriculogram is followed by manipulating a different catheter into the opening of the coronary artery (Fig. 13.3). Once in position, a small amount of radio-opaque dye is injected into the coronary artery (Fig. 13.4). This will allow the arteries to be visualized by X-ray fluoroscopy and will show any irregularities within the artery, such as areas of stenosis or occlusion. During this part of the procedure, patients do not experience a hot flushing sensation; however, some patients experience angina during this part of the procedure due to partial obstruction of the coronary artery by the catheter and displacement of blood by the dye. The angina usually lasts for a few seconds only, but it is important that the patient informs the staff about the pain so that it can be monitored and treated with a vasodilator such as glyceryl trinitrate (GTN).

The average length of the procedure is between 15 and 30 minutes. On completion, the arterial introducer sheath is removed, and firm pressure is applied 1 cm superior and 1 cm medially to the femoral puncture site to prevent bleeding and promote haemostasis. Various measures are employed to achieve this; one method is to apply digital pressure for 10–20 minutes following arterial sheath removal. Various devices can also be used to promote haemostasis from the femoral artery site such as pneumatic devices (FemoStop), suturing devices (Perclose) and biodegradable devices which involve implanting a collagen seal into the arterial puncture site (AngioSeal and VasoSeal) (McLenachan, 2001). Although suture and biodegradable devices seal the puncture site rapidly and enable earlier mobilization than digital compression, the patient continues to require monitoring for complications, as Koreny et al (2004) found an increased risk of haematoma and pseudoaneurysm with these devices.

Haemostasis from the radial artery site can be achieved with digital pressure, or with various devices such as a pneumatic compression device (TR Band), or with a compression device (RadiStop) (Banchet and Cheron, 2003). One of these methods is usually used while the patient is still in the catheterization laboratory. Once haemostasis is achieved, the patient is transferred to the ward for further assessment and care.

Catheterization via the brachial artery differs in that a small skin incision is made over the artery in the antecubital fossa to expose the artery. On completion of the procedure, the arteriotomy is sutured followed by suturing of the skin incision. Otherwise, the procedure is the same as that described for the femoral approach.

Electrophysiological studies

Electrophysiology studies are used for patients with symptomatic arrhythmias to assess the conduction system of the heart, namely the sinoatrial node,

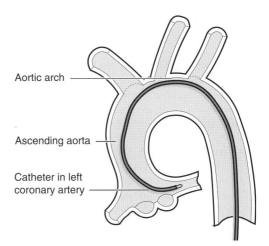

Figure 13.3 Diagram of a left Judkins-shaped catheter positioned in the ostia of the left coronary artery.

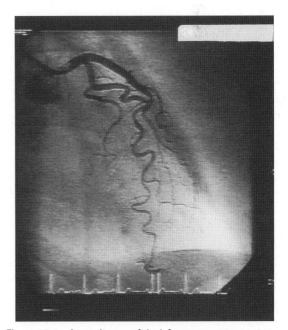

Figure 13.4 An angiogram of the left coronary artery system.

atrioventricular node and the Purkinje system. These studies are performed using right heart catheterization procedures similar to those described in the section on cardiac pacing. Electrodes are usually positioned in the right side of the heart via the venous system, and electrical signals can be ascertained from the left side of the heart by positioning an electrode in the coronary sinus. They are used to identify (and treat) the mechanism of an arrhythmia and the location of the anatomical abnormality (Kaye, 2003). Conditions investigated in this way include supraventricular tachycardias such as those caused by Wolff–Parkinson–White syndrome (WPW), atrial flutter and fibrillation, ventricular tachycardias or bradyarrhythmias. This procedure is used to obtain information about the electrical activity from within the heart, by recording and mapping intracardiac signals during normal sinus rhythm and during the induction of the patient's arrhythmia (Kaye, 2003). The electrical signals of the cardiac conducting system are recorded by electrodes, which can also pace the heart.

These studies can be lengthy, taking up to 4 hours to complete. The patient is usually conscious but may be lightly sedated during the study. Patients frequently find the procedure uncomfortable because of having to lie still for lengthy periods of time. In addition, patients frequently experience symptoms of their induced arrhythmia, which may be frightening and associated with symptoms such as dizziness, chest pain and palpitations. For a more detailed account of these studies, refer to Attin (2001).

Pre- and post-procedural care is similar to that for catheterization, except that patients may need to discontinue antiarrhythmic therapy some time before the study. Cessation of drug therapy leaves the patient without prophylactic protection against arrhythmias. This can cause some patients much anxiety during the period leading up to the study, as it may take many weeks before the body is cleared of some of the drugs.

PRE-PROCEDURE ASSESSMENT AND PREPARATION OF THE PATIENT PRIOR TO CARDIAC CATHETERIZATION

It should be documented whether the patient is aware of any allergies to contrast medium or iodine. Although rare, some patients are allergic to the iodine contained in the contrast medium, which may cause symptoms of allergy, anaphylaxis and, rarely, death. Patients taking a beta-blocker have an increased risk of allergic reactions to contrast media (Scanlon and Faxon, 1999).

Women within child-bearing age should be asked when they last menstruated and whether there is any possibility of them being pregnant, since the small dose of radiation from the X-rays could affect the developing fetus.

To enable the patient to give informed consent for cardiac catheterization, the procedure should be explained and consent obtained by the medical staff. Assessment of the patient's level of anxiety can be used as a gauge to establish the depth of information required about the procedure. Recording baseline observations provides a basis for post-procedure comparison. Assessment includes measuring blood pressure, pulse, ECG, temperature and respiratory rate. The rate and volume of pedal pulses for the femoral

approach and/or radial and ulnar pulses for the brachial approach should be assessed. These pulses can sometimes be difficult to find after catheterization, so a small pen mark can indicate their exact position. The colour and temperature of all limbs should be documented, noting the pulse strength and capillary refill times, as these can be useful indicators of arterial sufficiency following the procedure.

Body weight should be recorded, since the dose of many drugs is calculated according to weight: e.g. heparin, which is commonly given during catheterization.

It is necessary to ensure that blood results regarding the patient's coagulation status and blood chemistry are available prior to catheterization and that medical staff are informed of any abnormalities. A prolonged prothrombin time may result in bleeding after catheter insertion, whereas abnormal electrolytes may cause cardiac arrhythmias during or after the procedure.

Studies have suggested that patients whose coping mechanism is to actively seek information require information regarding the procedure and the likely sensations that will be experienced; by contrast, patients who seek little information may want information restricted to the procedure only (Davis et al, 1994).

The patient should be fasted for a minimum of 2–3 hours (fluids) and 4–6 hours for solids, if the patient has an increased risk of aspiration (Brady et al, 2004). Fasting will reduce gastric contents and the risk of inhaling vomit during the procedure, and reduce this risk in the event of complications requiring emergency surgery. Longer fasting periods cause patient discomfort, and dehydration, which can increase the difficulty of gaining venous access.

MANAGEMENT OF THE PATIENT FOLLOWING CARDIAC CATHETERIZATION

The main goals of care after catheterization are early detection of complications and to enhance patient comfort and safety. Major complications resulting from this diagnostic study include major vascular complications (<1%), arrhythmias (<0.5%), contrast agent reactions (0.23%) and death (<0.2%) (Kern, 2003).

Whatever the method used for promoting haemostasis, the patient will require regular assessment of vital signs, distal pulses and the skin puncture site for haemorrhage and haematoma formation.

Assessment for impaired circulation of the affected limb includes palpation of the radial and ulnar pulses if the radial or brachial approach was used, and the dorsalis pedis and posterior tibial pulses in the foot if the femoral approach was used. These pulses should be assessed every 15 minutes for the first hour (or according to hospital policy). Presence or absence of the pulse should be assessed as well as strength and rate. Doppler ultrasound may be useful when a pulse is weak or difficult to palpate. Pulse oximetry is another useful method of evaluating blood flow by attaching the sensor probe to the limb distally to the arterial puncture site. If blood flow is reduced, the pulse oximeter probe will show low saturation readings (Stoneham, 1995; Fox, 1996). The colour and temperature of the limb should also be observed; this may be done by feeling the limb or recording the temperature with an electrical peripheral probe. Capillary refill should be assessed for briskness and be less than 3 seconds.

A cool, pulseless, pale limb, with loss of sensation indicates poor or absent circulation due to interruption of blood flow by arterial occlusion. If an arterial compression device has been used to promote haemostasis, careful reduction of pressure (so as not to cause bleeding) over the puncture site may re-establish blood flow and pulse; otherwise, immediate medical attention and intervention should be sought.

The introducer site should also be observed regularly for signs of bleeding and/or haematoma formation. If either is evident, a sterile dressing and firm pressure should be applied a few centimetres above the puncture site for approximately 15 minutes or until haemostasis is achieved. Occasionally, large haematomas require surgical evacuation, although most are reabsorbed over a period of time.

Once haemostasis has been achieved, on average in 20–40 minutes, compression devices or manual compression can be discontinued and replaced by a small sterile dressing, e.g. a vapour-permeable film dressing which also enables observation of the puncture site.

Providing the patient has not had any arrhythmias during the procedure, continuous ECG monitoring may not be necessary. If arrhythmias or myocardial ischaemia have been a problem, the patient's ECG is continuously monitored for further signs of arrhythmias, ischaemic changes, infarction and bradycardia due to the vasovagal response (Barbiere, 1994). Vagus nerve stimulation may result in a decrease in pulse rate, myocardial contractility and vasodilatation, causing bradycardia and hypotension. If the heart rate is below 60 beats per minute and associated with hypotension, the immediate goal of care is to increase venous return and therefore blood pressure by positioning the patient in a supine position with the lower limbs elevated. If bradycardia persists the patient may be given atropine, which increases the heart rate and subsequently the blood pressure by inhibiting vagal stimulation.

Intravenous fluids may be given to increase intravascular volume and therefore blood pressure. The patient should then be closely monitored for any recurrence of bradycardia by regular assessment of pulse, blood pressure and ECG rhythm. Atropine may cause angina in some susceptible patients because of the increase in heart rate and subsequent increase in myocardial oxygen demand, but the need for atropine usually outweighs this complication.

Patients may experience discomfort from the needle puncture or incision site, as well as ischaemic pain due to angina. The patient's level of pain and discomfort should be assessed regularly using a pain scale. Prescribed analgesics should be given as required and their effects evaluated. Pain that is unresolved should be investigated further, as angina unrelieved by vasodilators may indicate myocardial infarction, which requires urgent medical intervention. Pain experienced in the affected limb may indicate haematoma formation, or reduced or occluded blood supply, both of which require immediate attention and appropriate intervention.

Providing the patient is neither nauseated nor drowsy, oral fluids and diet can be recommenced; if the patient's fluid intake is not restricted, an oral fluid intake of 2.5 L in 24 hours should be encouraged to counteract dehydration due to the diuretic effect of the contrast medium. Adequate fluid intake also increases renal excretion of the contrast medium, which can be toxic to the renal tubules and can cause acute renal failure (Scanlon and Faxon, 1999).

Bedrest and immobilization are required for patients after catheterization of the femoral artery, to ensure that haemostasis has been achieved and to minimize haematoma formation. During the period of bedrest the patient should be instructed to keep the affected limb straight and relaxed with minimal movement until haemostasis is established. Duration of bedrest following cardiac catheterization depends on local practice but need be no longer than 3–4 hours (Lehmann et al, 1999) and indeed may be as short as 2 hours or less if closure devices have been used (McLenachan, 2001). Shorter duration of bedrest improves patient comfort and independence, as well as decreasing nursing workload. Gentle mobilization can be commenced after the prescribed period of bedrest, providing there are no signs of bleeding or haematoma.

PREPARATION FOR DISCHARGE

Many patients are admitted for this investigation as day cases, whereas others may stay in hospital overnight. The patient will require the following information in preparation for discharge home:

- Minimize physical activity (including driving), and rest for 24 hours following the investigation (Montes, 1997).

- The patient should be advised not to lift anything that weighs more than 9 kg for 72 hours, to prevent bleeding from the arterial puncture site (Montes, 1997).
- If bleeding does occur, the patient should lie down and apply firm digital pressure over the puncture site for 15 minutes and contact their general practitioner or a telephone advice number given by the hospital if bleeding is not controlled.
- If the puncture site becomes red, swollen and painful, i.e. indicative of infection, the patient should contact their general practitioner as soon as possible.
- Ensure that the patient understands their diagnosis, future treatment options and any lifestyle changes that may be helpful in controlling the disease process. Advice should be given on giving up smoking, reducing weight if necessary and reducing dietary salt and saturated fat intake to improve cardiovascular health (De Backer et al, 2003).

The patient should be given information in regard to any drug therapy, which should include:

- why the drug has been prescribed
- name of drug(s)
- timing and dosage of drug
- potential side-effects and what actions the patient should take in the event of these occurring.

An informed patient is in a better position to make choices, is more likely to concord with therapy and will also probably be less anxious.

THERAPEUTIC CATHETERIZATION

Patients requiring percutaneous coronary intervention (PCI) and stent implantation or valvuloplasty should be prepared as for cardiac catheterization.

PERCUTANEOUS CORONARY INTERVENTION AND STENT IMPLANTATION

Percutaneous coronary intervention is a treatment for angina which eliminates or delays the need for coronary artery bypass grafts. The aim of the procedure is to dilate the stenosed or narrowed segment(s) of the coronary artery or, if the artery is completely occluded by thrombus and atheroma, the procedure aims to reopen the artery. Angioplasty and stent implantation widen the diseased vessel lumen, and improves blood flow, thus eliminating or reducing the symptoms of angina.

The procedure is similar to cardiac catheterization but differs in that a fine guide wire is introduced into a guiding catheter positioned in the opening of the affected coronary artery. The atraumatic wire is gently advanced into the artery and manipulated across the stenosed or occluded segment. Once the wire is in place, a tiny balloon measuring anything between 1.25 and 4 mm in diameter and between 10 and 30 mm in length (depending on the size of the artery and length of diseased segment) is threaded over the guide wire until it is positioned across the stenosed segment. Once the balloon is in place, it is inflated with a mixture of contrast medium and saline. Inflation of the balloon compresses the atheroma which may also crack, thus widening the vessel lumen; however, a side effect of this is local dissection of the arterial media layer (Roberts, 2001). Widening of the vessel improves blood flow to the myocardium, with cessation or reduction of angina.

The positive effects of balloon angioplasty alone are short lived, as elastic recoil of the vessel wall and dissected tissue can rapidly cause the vessel lumen to narrow or reocclude (Roberts, 2001). Following balloon dilation, the introduction of intracoronary stents helps to prevent occlusion. Stents are tiny tubes made of a wire mesh which when expanded by a balloon within them remain expanded and hold the artery open once the balloon has been deflated and withdrawn (Fig. 13.5). They measure between 2 and 5 mm in diameter, 8 and 38 mm in length and are made from metals such as stainless steel or cobalt-based alloys.

Stents provide structural support for the vessel wall by resisting elastic recoil and hold back any dissected tissue which could otherwise cause the artery to occlude immediately. Although stents have dramatically improved the angiographic results and halved the need for reintervention (Sigwart et al, 2001), they are associated with tissue hyperplasia, leading to instent restenosis. This becomes clinically apparent 3–6 months after the procedure, with approximately 20% of patients with simple lesions requiring repeat PCI. This tissue growth is caused by an inflammatory response, resulting in the proliferation of smooth muscle cells which migrate through the gaps in the stent and the production of an extracellular matrix, so reducing the lumen of the stent and causing the return of the

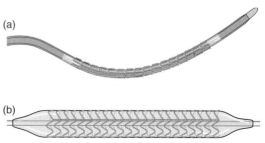

Figure 13.5 (a) Stent crimped onto a coronary angioplasty balloon. (b) A stent expanded by the balloon.

patient's original symptoms. Reintervention with PCI is as high as 50% in patients with diabetes, or those with small-calibre vessels (<3 mm in diameter), vein grafts or chronically occluded vessels (NICE, 2003). In an attempt to overcome in-stent restenosis, stents that are coated with a drug that inhibits tissue proliferation into the stent lumen have been developed. These are referred to as drug-eluting stents (DES) and are indicated for use in the patients described above (NICE, 2003).

The stent comes pre-mounted on a balloon catheter and is introduced into the coronary artery (see Fig. 13.6a). When the balloon is inflated, the stent expands and is embedded into the artery wall; the balloon is deflated and removed, leaving the stent behind. The stent remains in the artery for life to provide structural support, keeping the arterial lumen open (Fig. 13.6c). The patient remains conscious but sedated throughout the procedure, which can take as little as 20 minutes (although a complex procedure can take a few hours). During balloon inflation, patients often experience moderate to severe angina caused by total occlusion of blood flow. Pain lasts while the balloon is inflated (Fig. 13.7), usually 15–60 seconds, and subsides on deflation. This

is managed with vasodilating drugs such as glyceryl trinitrate. However, if the pain is severe, an opioid such as diamorphine may be given intravenously.

Pre-procedure preparation

Preparation of the patient is the same as that for cardiac catheterization.

To reduce the incidence of thrombus formation within the stent, patients undergoing PCI are prescribed a pre-treatment regimen of aspirin and clopidogrel which inhibits platelet aggregation; this reduces the incidence of acute stent thrombosis after the procedure (Starkey, 2001). Thrombus formation within the stent occurs in <1% of cases (Perrins, 2001), and is considered a medical emergency because it may cause myocardial infarction and in some cases death, due to abrupt occlusion of the stented artery.

The procedure should be explained and consent obtained from the patient. As additional procedures such as emergency coronary artery bypass surgery may be required, patients must also consent to this. The patient and their family must be informed of these potential complications, and the implications of this understood by them.

Post-procedure care and assessment

Assessment of vital signs and management postprocedure are similar to those for cardiac catheterization, except that the removal of the arterial introducer sheath from the femoral artery is delayed until the anticoagulant effects of heparin have worn off. Reversal of heparin is monitored by measuring activated clotting time (ACT), and the sheath is removed when this is <150 seconds (Lehmann et al, 1999). However, sheath removal may be done immediately after the PCI if a closure technique such as collagen implant or a suture device is used to seal the artery puncture site.

The patient should be placed in a supine position and instructed not to bend the leg at the hip, as this can cause kinking of the sheath, occlusion of the femoral artery or bleeding at the sheath site. To alter the patient's position, a 'log roll' procedure should be used. The sheath site should be observed regularly for bleeding and distal pulses assessed according to local guidelines. The temperature and colour of the affected limb should be assessed as above for signs of circulatory insufficiency, indicated by a cool, pale, pulseless limb.

The patient is continuously monitored by ECG to detect arrhythmias and waveform changes such as ST elevation or depression, which are indicative of cardiac ischaemia. Vital signs such as pulse, blood pressure and circulation are frequently monitored in the early post-procedure period, as described on p. 243.

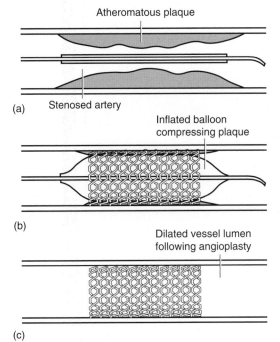

(a) Stenosed artery — Atheromatous plaque

(b) Inflated balloon compressing plaque

(c) Dilated vessel lumen following angioplasty

Figure 13.6 Percutaneous transluminal coronary angioplasty and insertion of an intracoronary stent. (a) Diagrammatic representation of a stenosed artery with a stent mounted on a balloon catheter within the artery lumen. (b) Angioplasty balloon inflated, expanding the stent within the artery wall. (c) Balloon removed, leaving behind the stent to maintain an open vessel lumen to improve blood flow.

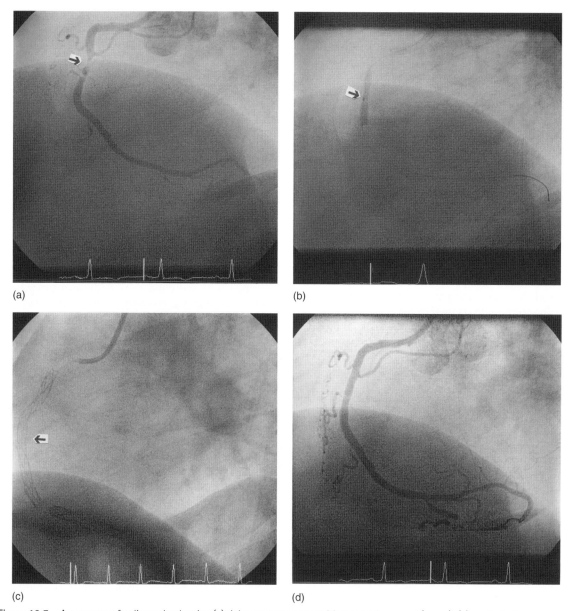

Figure 13.7 A sequence of radiographs showing (a) right coronary artery with stenosed segment (arrow); (b) angioplasty balloon inflated within the stenosed vessel; (c) a long stent within the vessel wall; (d) angiogram of the right coronary artery after angioplasty and stent implant.

Any procedure that breaches the body's protective skin barrier requires strict asepsis when the arterial sheath is removed. The sheath is removed by a doctor or nurse instructed in sheath removal (Penney, 1995; Schickel et al, 1996), once ACT <150 seconds. Haemostasis is achieved by applying firm pressure over the sheath site with digital compression or with a femoral artery compression device such as the FemoStop for 20–30 minutes. Some patients may continue to require the FemoStop for a prolonged period due to anticoagulation, but at a reduced pressure. Analgesics should be given prior to sheath removal to enhance comfort while firm groin pressure is required.

Patients are able to mobilize 3–4 hours after sheath removal, providing there is no bleeding and their vital signs are stable. Prolonged immobilization may be required for those with the following risk factors: anticoagulation therapy, obesity, advanced age,

Table 13.3   Potential complications associated with arterial catheterization

	Femoral neuropathy	Pseudoaneurysm	Retroperitoneal bleeding	Coronary artery/stent occlusion
Definition	Pressure around the nerve due to bleeding or excessive pressure from a compression device	Extravasation of blood within the artery wall, creating a pulsatile pouch of clotted blood	Puncture of the posterior artery wall, resulting in slow bleeding and severe bleeding	Occlusion of artery and/or with thrombus, resulting in myocardial infarction
Physical signs	Pain, tingling and numbness around puncture site or leg	Burning back pain. Pain, swelling and bruising around puncture site	Varying degrees of pain around back, groin, flank or lower abdomen	Crushing central chest pain; pale, clammy and nauseated; acute ST elevation on ECG
Nursing intervention	Reduce pressure over puncture site and monitor for return of colour and sensation. Investigate for signs of haematoma or pseudoaneurysm. Inform doctors if symptoms do not ease after 10 minutes	Monitor BP and pulse. Outline edges of bruising with marker; note skin thickness. Measure leg circumference 2 hourly. Apply firm pressure for 20–30 minutes to stop further bleeding. Inform doctor. Monitor distal circulation. Maintain bedrest	Monitor BP and pulse. Outline edges of bruising with marker; note skin thickness. Apply pressure to stop further bleeding. Inform doctor. Monitor distal circulation. Maintain bedrest	Monitor BP and pulse. Assess pain. Administer prescribed analgesics. Perform 12-lead ECG. Monitor ECG continuously. Inform doctor of any changes
Medical intervention	May require surgical intervention to remove haematoma or stop bleeding responsible for nerve compression	If unresolved, prepare for surgical removal of haematoma and repair	Blood transfusion and volume expanders to reverse hypotension. Surgical repair if bleeding continues	Prepare patient for emergency cardiac catheterization/ angioplasty/antiplatelet therapy to dissolve thrombus. May require urgent coronary artery bypass grafts

Source: adapted from Davis et al (1997).

large-diameter sheath, thrombolytic therapy and infection (Jones et al, 1995a).

There are a number of additional potential complications that can occur at varying times in both the immediate and late post-procedure period, such as:

- *Retroperitoneal bleeding* due to bleeding from the posterior wall of the artery (potentially serious complication). This manifests within 24–48 hours post-procedure with hypotension, back, flank or abdominal pain and skin discoloration.
- *Femoral neuropathy* due to excessive pressure from the haemostasis device (early complication).
- *Stent thrombosis or coronary vessel occlusion* (early/ delayed complication): coronary artery spasm and occlusion can occur at any time after the procedure. Spasm and restenosis are more common after PCI when a stent has not been used. The patient should be monitored for chest pain and ischaemic ECG changes.
- *Pseudoaneurysm* due to damaged or ruptured vessel wall, resulting in bleeding into the surrounding tissue, and indicated by an enlarging, painful haematoma and widespread bruising (Jones et al, 1995a).

In view of these complications, the nurse's role is to monitor the patient closely to detect these early and minimize their effects (Table 13.3).

Following stent implantation, patients are prescribed clopidogrel and aspirin for their antiplatelet effects. Clopidogrel is prescribed for about 4 weeks after implant of a bare metal stent and for approximately 6 months following DES implants, and aspirin is prescribed indefinitely (Gershlick, 2001). These drugs prevent stent thrombosis whilst protective endothelial tissue grows over the stent; endothelialization takes longer on drug-eluting stents, so longer periods of antiplatelet therapy are required. It is essential that the patient has a good understanding of and is concordant with this drug therapy. Poor concordance may result in thrombosis and occlusion of the vessel, causing myocardial infarction or death. Once endothelialization is complete, the risk of thrombosis reduces and the antiplatelet drugs can be stopped, although aspirin is continued for life.

Care of the puncture site is much the same as for that described in the cardiac catheterization section (see p. 242).

Patient education

Dietary advice is pertinent to any patient with a history of atherosclerosis. A reduction in salt, sugar and saturated fat is recommended. Saturated fats should be replaced by polyunsaturated and monounsaturated fats, while an increased intake of fibre in the form of fresh fruit and vegetables, and replacement of fatty red meat with fish and chicken, should be advised (De Backer et al, 2003).

Time spent teaching the patient and relatives is valuable, helping to clarify information, reduce fears and increase concordance in treatment regimens. Written information helps to reinforce the advice and serves as a reference after discharge (Gardner et al, 1996).

CARDIAC TREATMENTS

The following therapies involve catheterization of the right side of the heart via the venous system. Veins commonly used are the cephalic, subclavian, jugular and the femoral vein. Electrodes may be inserted for:

- temporary or permanent pacing
- an implantable cardioverter defibrillator (ICD)
- ablation of intracardiac conduction pathways
- mitral valvuloplasty.

CARDIAC PACING

Cardiac pacemakers are battery-powered devices that electrically stimulate the heart to contract (capture) when the patient's heart rate is abnormally slow. Pacemakers have two major functions: to sense the cardiac rhythm and to pace the heart. If the rhythm slows, the pacemaker will sense this and pace the heart at a pre-programmed rate. If the rhythm is faster than the programmed rate, the pacemaker is inhibited until the heart rate slows again. This is known as demand pacing and maintains a stable heart rate. Biventricular pacing has recently been introduced, which involves insertion of an additional pacing wire into the coronary sinus at the base of the right atrium. This acts as the left ventricular pacing lead and has proved extremely effective in improving cardiac output in patients with chronic heart failure and left bundle branch block (Chow et al, 2003).

Temporary pacemakers consist of a battery outside the body (pacing box), which is attached to an electrode positioned within the right atrium and/or right ventricle of the heart. Permanent pacemaker batteries are implanted under the skin of the chest wall. The indications for cardiac pacing and antiarrhythmia devices have recently been reviewed (Gregoratos et al,

2002). Pacing systems are indicated for the following reasons:

- to support the conduction system following cardiac surgery (usually temporary)
- following myocardial infarction complicated by atrioventricular block (usually temporary but may require permanent pacing)
- prophylaxis during general anaesthesia for patients with slow heart rates or asymptomatic atrioventricular block (usually temporary)
- conduction disturbances resulting in sinus arrest and ventricular standstill; bradycardia associated with a low cardiac output (usually permanent)
- overdrive pacing for tachyarrhythmias (permanent pacemakers with antitachycardia functions)
- when a permanent pacing system has failed or become infected (temporary).

Cardiac pacing is usually done under local anaesthesia, and involves introducing a pacing electrode (wire) via the cephalic or subclavian vein into the right ventricle for single-chamber pacing, or into both the right atrium and ventricle for dual-chamber pacing. The heart can then be electrically stimulated to contract by an external temporary or permanently implanted pacemaker. An electrical impulse is initiated by the pacemaker, via the pacing electrode, which stimulates the heart muscle to depolarize and contract.

Preparation for cardiac pacing

Temporary pacing is often performed as an emergency procedure, with little time to prepare the patient psychologically, whereas permanent pacing is usually performed electively, allowing adequate time for patient preparation.

The patient should not eat for 4 hours prior to the procedure, but may be able to take oral fluids up until 2 hours before (according to local hospital policy) (Brady et al, 2004), as dehydration and subsequent collapse of the veins causes difficulty in cannulation for insertion of the pacing electrode. Blood pressure, pulse, temperature, respiratory rate and 12-lead ECG are recorded.

Informed consent should be obtained by the medical staff, but this may not be possible during an emergency. The patient's understanding of the procedure and his need for information should be ascertained. An explanation of why pacing is required and what to expect during and immediately after the procedure should be given.

Postoperative care and assessment

Caring for the patient following temporary or permanent pacing is similar, except that, with temporary pacing the pacing box is external and will require intermittent checks to ensure correct functioning.

The ECG is monitored for rhythm, rate and presence of pacemaker-induced beats, which are preceded by an artefact called the pacing spike. The pacing spike either appears before the P wave in atrial pacing or before the QRS wave in ventricular pacing. Patients with temporary pacemakers require the dressing to be inspected to ensure that it is secure, and that the pacing electrode is taped to prevent movement and accidental removal. It is important to check that the electrode is securely attached to the pacing box, which is positioned safely to prevent it falling. The pacemaker settings, such as rate, pacing mode, and energy output, should be recorded in the patient's nursing notes. Vital signs should be monitored closely for the first hour (or according to hospital policy), because although complications are uncommon it is important that they are detected early and treated (Pavia and Wilkoff, 2001). Complications include:

- *Pneumothorax/haemothorax* (1–2%): frequently asymptomatic, caused by air or blood entering the pleural space during subclavian vein cannulation. Respiratory status is monitored for dyspnoea, increased resting respiratory rate, unequal chest movement, tachycardia, hypotension and reduced oxygen saturation. If symptomatic, treatment with an intercostal chest drain may be required.

- *Cardiac perforation:* caused by the electrode penetrating the heart during the procedure. This is often asymptomatic and resolved by repositioning the electrode. Rarely, this can result in the serious complication of cardiac tamponade, where blood leaks into the pericardial space. Blood compresses and reduces the size of the ventricles and compromises ventricular filling and cardiac output, resulting in hypotension and tachycardia. This emergency is managed by inserting a needle through the chest wall into the pericardial space to aspirate the blood and relieve the tamponade.

- *Pacemaker pocket haematoma:* caused by inadequate haemostasis within the pocket or by backflow from around the pacing electrode in the vein. Haematomas frequently resolve without the need for intervention and are slowly absorbed; however, the pocket wound should be monitored for pain and haematoma formation. In cases where the haematoma expands rapidly, surgical evacuation may be required; this is necessary in 1–2% of patients (Pavia and Wilkoff, 2001).

- *Infection:* 2–8% of pacemaker systems become infected and may require removal and replacement.

Infection causes appreciable morbidity and mortality (Pavia and Wilkoff, 2001). Strict asepsis during and after pacemaker implantation is essential to prevent this; if infection does occur, early detection and treatment are important.

These complications can occur with temporary or permanent pacing, following electrophysiology studies and ablation, and require immediate treatment.

Pacemaker dysfunction

The ECG should be monitored for pacing failure as indicated by the following:

- *Oversensing*: pacemaker senses, and is inhibited from pacing by non-cardiac signals such as skeletal muscle contraction. These extra signals switch the pacemaker off, causing an absence of pacing, with the heart rate dropping below the set demand rate of the pacemaker. To remedy this fault, it may be necessary to decrease the sensitivity level of the pacemaker, or remove any ungrounded electrical equipment which may be interfering with the pacemaker.

- *Undersensing*: pacemaker is unable to sense the patient's underlying rhythm and so paces regardless, which may initiate ventricular tachycardia if a pacing stimulus coincides with the vulnerable phase of the heart's relative refractory period. Undersensing may be caused by the following:
  - loose connections (temporary pacemaker), requiring tightening of the lead connections
  - loss of electrode contact with the myocardium, or lead fracture requiring repositioning or replacement of the lead (temporary or permanent pacemaker)
  - low battery, necessitating pacemaker replacement
  - pacemaker sensitivity levels set too low (Witherell, 1994).

- *Failure to capture*: pacemaker fails to capture or pace the heart, indicated by a pacing spike that is not followed immediately by a QRS complex. Possible causes for this fault are similar to those causing under- or oversensing.

The threshold of temporary pacemakers should also be checked daily. The threshold is a measure of the minimum amount of energy required to pace or depolarize the heart continuously (Attin, 2001). It is normal for the threshold to rise slightly during pacing. This is due to inflammation that results from the repetitive electrical stimulation of the heart by the pacemaker, although some metabolic disturbances such as acidosis and hyperkalaemia will also increase the threshold. This will also rise if the electrode has moved or become displaced within the ventricle. If there is a considerable threshold increase, large levels of energy will be required to pace the heart, which may be beyond the energy output of the pacemaker, resulting in pacing failure (Witherell, 1994).

Threshold is measured by a cardiac technician or nurse with the appropriate training. A continuous pacing rhythm must be present; to achieve this it may be necessary to increase the pacing rate above the patient's intrinsic heart rate. Caution should be exercised if the patient's intrinsic rate is high, as pacing at a higher rate may cause ventricular tachycardia or fibrillation. Once a pacing rhythm is detected on the ECG monitor, the voltage output switch is slowly reduced until the pacing rhythm is interrupted (Attin, 2001). This is the pacing threshold. The pacing output should then be reset to a level two to three times greater than the threshold. This allows for subsequent threshold increases, and the pacing rate to be reduced to the prescribed level. If the pacing threshold has increased dramatically, the medical staff should be informed, since the pacing electrode may require repositioning to prevent pacing failure.

Patient education

Generally, patients recover quickly from pacemaker insertion and experience an improvement in physical activity and confidence due to cessation of pre-pacing symptoms (Jones et al, 1995b).

Patients with permanent pacemakers need to be educated about their pacemaker prior to discharge home. It is essential that the patient understands the need to attend regular pacemaker clinic appointments, where pacemaker functions can be checked using non-invasive techniques. This involves placing a small device called a programmer (specialized computer) on the skin surface over the pacemaker site, enabling the technician to obtain information such as pacing thresholds and battery level. It is also possible to change pacing parameters, such as the rate, with the same device.

Some alteration in lifestyle may be required, and the patient is given the following information:

- Patients should be advised not to make vigorous arm movements for a few weeks following implantation of the pacemaker. This prevents dislodgement of the pacing electrode from the heart (British Heart Foundation, 2001). After this period, scar tissue develops and holds the electrode firmly within the heart.
- Pacemaker manufacturers provide patient information sheets with advice about electrical equipment to be avoided: e.g. mobile phones should be held on the opposite side to the pacemaker (Myerson and

Mitchell, 2003) and shop alarm systems and security systems at airports may be activated by the metal components in the pacemaker.

- Pacemaker patients must not have MRI scans (British Heart Foundation, 2001).
- The patient is advised to seek medical advice if the original symptoms return so that the pacemaker function can be checked.
- The patient should be given information on how to recognize signs of wound infection, and actions to take in the event of this.
- The patient should be encouraged to always carry a pacemaker identification card.
- Pacemakers have a life span of 6–10 years (Jones et al, 1995b), so patients should be aware that the pacemaker will eventually need to be replaced because of a flat battery.
- Patients should not drive a vehicle until after their first pacemaker check, which will ensure that it is functioning correctly (usually 1 week after insertion) (DVLA, 2003).

Patients should be reassured that pacemakers are very reliable (Skehan, 1996) and encouraged to resume their pre-pacing lifestyle. Useful patient information about pacing and cardiac procedures can be obtained from the British Cardiology Society website (http://www.bcs.com).

IMPLANTABLE CARDIOVERTER DEFIBRILLATOR

Implantable cardioverter defibrillators (ICDs) were introduced in the late 1980s. These devices have numerous functions, as described below, but are essentially used for patients at risk of sudden cardiac death due to malignant ventricular cardiac arrhythmias. Implantable cardioverter defibrillators act in a similar way to pacemakers in sensing cardiac rhythms, triggering anti-tachycardia pacing, providing bursts of pacing impulses and, if necessary, delivering high-energy defibrillation to revert ventricular fibrillation. The use of these devices was not routinely considered until the introduction of the NICE guidelines in 2000, a summary of which is listed in Table 13.4.

The implantable cardioverter defibrillator looks very similar to a pacemaker except that it is larger and heavier, weighing 78 g rather than about 30 g (Nisam, 1997) (Fig. 13.8); it is implanted in the same way as a pacemaker.

The ICD has a number of functions: it is able to detect life-threatening tachyarrhythmias and terminate these by either overdrive pacing, cardioversion or defibrillation. When the ICD detects a fast rhythm, it

Table 13.4 Indications for implantable cardioverter defibrillators (NICE, 2000)

Secondary prevention (in absence of a treatable cause)	Primary prevention
Cardiac arrest due to ventricular tachycardia or ventricular fibrillation	Non-sustained ventricular tachycardia on Holter monitoring
Spontaneous sustained ventricular tachycardia, causing syncope or haemodynamic compromise	Inducible ventricular tachycardia on electrophysiological testing
Sustained ventricular tachycardia, without syncope or cardiac arrest, with reduced cardiac function	Familial cardiac conditions causing sudden cardiac death, such as long QT syndrome, arrhythmogenic right ventricular dysplasia (ARVD)

Source: NICE (2000).

will attempt to slow it down by initiating a short burst of rapid pacing that may interrupt the tachycardia, thus slowing the rate. If this is unsuccessful, the ICD will either cardiovert the rhythm with a low-energy shock, or if the rhythm degenerates into ventricular fibrillation, the ICD will defibrillate the heart with a higher-energy shock. The ICD is also able to pace the heart in the event of the recovering rhythm being too slow (NICE, 2000; Houghton and Kaye, 2003).

Specific pre- and post-implant care

Physical preparation and post-implant care of the patient are the same as for pacemaker implantation. The patient may, however, require a higher level of psychological preparation and support before and after the procedure. The ICD does not cure the patient's arrhythmia, it merely controls it. The shocks emitted from the ICD are sudden and painful, whatever the energy level of the shock. The shocks can

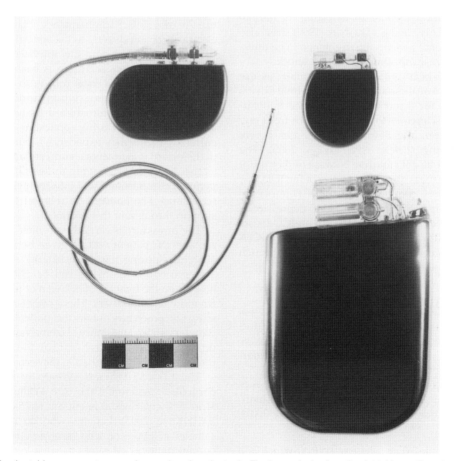

Figure 13.8 Implantable permanent pacemakers and pacing electrode. The larger device is an implantable cardioverter defibrillator with pacing functions.

bring into sharp focus the fact that the patient has probably just experienced a life-threatening arrhythmia. Some patients may lose consciousness prior to the shock, due to interruption of cardiac output as a result of the tachyarrhythmia.

Patient education

Dunbar (1993) identified a number of things that should be discussed with patients to help them adjust to living with an ICD. These include giving the patient the opportunity to talk about the meaning of the shocks, which will involve honest discussion regarding the seriousness of the arrhythmia. The patient must be prepared for the fact that the shocks may be painful and sudden, which has been described by some patients as like being kicked in the chest by a horse. Both patient and relatives need to be reassured that the shock will not be felt by anyone else touching the patient during the shock.

Considerable time may need to be spent with both the patient and relatives, helping them to understand the implications of having an ICD, and helping them regain confidence in their ability to resume the normal activities of daily living. Dunbar (1993) has also reported that some patients are frightened to be physically active in case movement initiates a shock.

Patients with heavy goods vehicle or public service vehicle licences lose these automatically; normal drivers may not drive for 6 months following the implantation, and subsequently they must be free from any intervention from the device for 6 months before resuming driving (Petch, 1998; DVLA, 2003). The patient will not be able to drive because of the risk of losing consciousness during activation of the ICD.

Anxiety is very common following ICD implantation, affecting up to 87% of patients, and depression is reported in up to 33% of patients with an ICD (Sears and Conti, 2002). Many centres which insert ICDs offer considerable support for their patients through patient-led support groups.

CARDIAC ABLATION

When abnormal conducting tissue is discovered during electrophysiology studies, cardiac ablation may be considered; this involves the destruction of the abnormal conducting tissue.

A variety of conduction abnormalities causing symptomatic and potentially life-threatening tachyarrhythmias are indications for this procedure (Gilbert, 2001), and include:

- *Wolff–Parkinson–White syndrome (WPW)* which is a congenital abnormality where the atria and ventricles are connected by abnormal conducting muscle

fibres other than the AV node, known as accessory pathways. Impulses can travel along these pathways very rapidly, causing tachycardia.

- *Atrioventricular nodal re-entrant tachycardia (AVNRT)* occurs when there are slow- and fast-conducting pathways in the AV node or perinodal tissue. Impulses normally travel via the fast pathway. If the patient has a premature atrial ectopic, this conducted impulse may find the fast pathway blocked, or refractory to further stimulation, and so is conducted via the slow pathway. If the fast pathway has recovered sufficiently, the impulse can then return via this route to re-excite the atrium, causing a re-entrant tachycardia. This type of tachycardia can be treated by partially destroying the AV node (Swanton, 2003).

- *Atrial fibrillation*, *flutter* and *ventricular tachycardia* may also be treated by ablation.

Ablation of the abnormal conduction pathway is carried out using radiofrequency electric current or cryoablation that destroys the tissue by freezing it to −70° or −85°C. Radiofrequency ablation delivers an electrical current directly to the abnormal endocardial tissue via the catheter; the interface between the catheter and the endocardium is heated to temperatures over 47°C until focal cell death occurs (Grubb and Furniss, 2001). This results in the disappearance of electrical activity in the ablated tissue (Guaglianone and Tyndall, 1995). During application of the electrical current, patients may experience a burning sensation in their chest (Guaglianone and Tyndall, 1995), as well as the discomfort of having to lie still for prolonged periods, as movement will interfere with intracardiac recordings. The patient will require reassurance and support throughout this treatment.

The procedure is carried out under local anaesthesia, and the patient will be given both sedation and analgesics during this often lengthy and uncomfortable procedure. Catheters can be positioned in the heart from the femoral, subclavian or jugular veins, or from the femoral artery. These catheters are removed after the procedure while the patient is still in the catheterization laboratory. Haemostasis is achieved through the application of firm pressure over the insertion sites, as described in the section on p. 243.

There is a 95–98% success rate for this procedure, particularly for Wolff–Parkinson–White syndrome and atrioventricular nodal re-entrant tachycardia (Gilbert, 2001; Kaye, 2003). Patients who do not respond to catheter ablation, or who have a subendocardial re-entrant pathway causing recurrent ventricular tachycardia, may be candidates for surgical ablation. This involves open heart surgery with endocardial tissue resection and cryotherapy of the arrhythmogenic tissue (Swanton, 2003).

Pre-procedure preparation

Physical preparation of the patient is the same as that for pacemaker insertion, although psychological preparation should be tailored to helping the patient understand the treatment and likely sensations that will be experienced during the ablation. There is a 2% risk of complete heart block, resulting in the need for a permanent pacemaker (Swanton, 2003).

Post-procedure management

On return to the ward, the patient should be monitored for early detection of the original arrhythmia (Guaglianone and Tyndall, 1995). Vital signs should be monitored closely in the immediate post-procedure period for complications such as pneumothorax and tamponade associated with catheter insertion. Vascular puncture sites should be observed for bleeding and haematoma formation. If the artery was cannulated during the procedure, perfusion of the affected limb should also be monitored as described on p. 242.

Providing the patient is well and has not had any complications, discharge from hospital usually occurs the following day. Prior to discharge, the patient should be given advice about puncture site management and educated about the drug therapy.

Patients who receive clear, informative and relevant information tailored to their individual needs are more likely to adapt better to any constraints of their illness, and are in a position to make informed choices.

MITRAL VALVULOPLASTY

Mitral valve stenosis is a progressive disease which is usually fatal without some form of intervention that will enlarge the valve orifice enough to allow adequate cardiac output. Stenosis occurs when the valve cusps thicken and there is fusion of the commissures, which interferes with normal valve opening and closing. This disease process usually occurs as a result of a previous episode of rheumatic heart disease, which primarily affects women (Carabello and Crawford, 1997).

Percutaneous balloon mitral valvuloplasty (PBMV) is the treatment of choice for the majority of patients with symptomatic mitral stenosis (Prendergast et al, 2002). The preparations for valvuloplasty are similar to those of cardiac catheterization. The patient remains conscious, although sedated throughout the procedure. Although the mitral valve is in the left side of the heart, an Inoue balloon catheter is introduced into the right side over a pre-positioned guide wire via the femoral

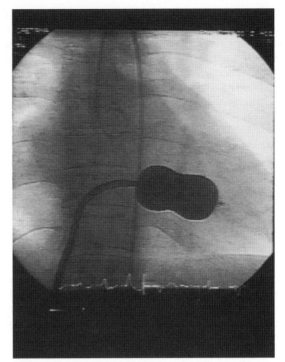

Figure 13.9 An X-ray of an inflated valvuloplasty balloon dilating a stenosed mitral valve.

vein (Fig. 13.9). Access to the left atrium and ventricle is obtained by puncturing the atrial septum from inside the heart with a transeptal needle. This part of the procedure is usually well tolerated by the patient. Once the balloon is positioned within the valve opening, it is inflated with diluted contrast medium, which dilates the stenosed valve. This interrupts blood flow through the left side of the heart for a short period, which may cause the patient to feel faint and dizzy (Carter and Lamerton, 1996).

On completion of the procedure the balloon and other catheters are removed, and the vascular introducer sheaths are removed once the anticoagulant effects of heparin have reversed, as described for cardiac catheterization. The patient should avoid moving the affected limb to assist haemostasis, and should remain on bedrest until haemostasis has been achieved and vital signs are stable (Carter and Lamerton, 1996).

Pre- and post-procedure care is similar to the care described for patients undergoing cardiac catheterization. However, the patient should be closely monitored for the first few hours for any arrhythmias, and for signs of tamponade caused by compression of the heart's chambers by fluid in the pericardial space (Bines and Landron, 1993). This may occur if the guide wire or catheter puncture the myocardial wall and cause blood to leak into the pericardial space. This results in hypotension, low cardiac output, tachycardia and tachypnoea, and requires immediate medical intervention to prevent irreversible shock and death. Patients are discharged home the following day providing there have been no post-procedure complications.

Balloon valvuloplasty can also be carried out in patients with aortic valve stenosis, but with less success, and it is therefore used for palliation only. Patients with severe stenosis gain greater benefit from valve replacement (Carabello and Crawford, 1997).

CARDIAC SURGERY

Cardiac surgery is required for a number of disorders that cannot be controlled or treated by conservative management. Coronary artery disease and valvular disease are the most common conditions requiring open cardiac surgery. A proportion of patients will require heart transplantation due to end-stage heart failure where other treatments are no longer effective in controlling their heart failure.

Prior to cardiac surgery, patients have usually undergone a series of investigations and treatments, as discussed above. The patients and their family typically attend a pre-admission clinic 1–3 weeks prior to admission so that the appropriate blood tests and other investigations can be carried out. Preoperative education is given either on an individual or group discussion basis. Not surprisingly, patients are often very anxious prior to cardiac surgery and it is often difficult to balance the need to explain the procedure without unduly alarming them; it must be recognized that the patient's extreme anxiety state may preclude any meaningful learning (Margereson and Riley, 2003). On admission to hospital, a nursing assessment is performed, as described earlier. Physical preparation for surgery is as for any surgery (see Ch. 2). Psychological preparation for surgery plays an important role postoperatively, as anxiety and pain may be reduced; these can cause hypertension, which increases the risk of postoperative bleeding.

CORONARY ARTERY BYPASS SURGERY

A number of patients do not get symptomatic relief from PCI, or if their coronary artery disease is extensive they may require coronary artery bypass grafting (CABG). A small number of patients require this surgery urgently, either due to acute deterioration or following complications from cardiac catheterization or percutaneous transluminal coronary angioplasty. This is a major procedure and postoperative care in the intensive care unit may be required; however, stable patients are increasingly extubated early and 'fast tracked' back to high dependency areas, so reducing the pressure on intensive care beds.

The traditional procedure involves exposing the heart through a median sternotomy and placing the patient on cardiopulmonary bypass (CPB), which takes over the function of the heart and lungs during surgery. This is followed by excision of a portion of a donor vessel, which is then anastomosed to the aorta and distally to the coronary artery below the obstruction, thus re-establishing blood flow via the graft.

The most common donor grafts used include the long saphenous vein, or the radial artery. An alternative technique is to use the internal mammary artery (IMA). In this case the artery is detached distally and the free end anastomosed to the coronary artery below the blockage. Use of the internal mammary artery is now the 'gold standard' graft in CABG, and is used in the UK in over 90% of patients undergoing CABG (Taggart, 2002). The internal mammary artery is used because it remains patent for a longer time than other grafts; this appears to be due to its resistance to atheroma formation. Bilateral internal mammary artery (BIMA) grafts are also being used in carefully selected individuals and initial results are encouraging (Taggart, 2002). The use of the IMA is not, however, without risk, as its use may lead to delayed sternal healing; respiratory complications may be more common due to the concomitant increase in pain associated with this procedure. The use of IMA grafts and in particular BIMA grafts is usually avoided in heavy smokers, diabetics and patients with chronic respiratory disorders (Margereson and Riley, 2003).

Recovery from surgery obviously takes longer than from percutaneous techniques; as well as the sternal wound there may also be wounds in the thigh and/or wrist if the saphenous vein or radial artery have been used. If the saphenous vein is used, the wound may take longer to heal than the sternal wound for a number of reasons; these include anaemia, oedema and reduced blood supply to the lower limb because of the presence of peripheral vascular disease (Flynn, 1996). When the radial artery has been used rather than the saphenous vein, mobilization tends to be earlier; however, circulatory problems in the hand, such as numbness and tingling, may occur, and these will need close monitoring (Wolff et al, 1997).

NEWER APPROACHES

Recent years have seen discussions regarding the safety of the conventional approach of full sternotomy, CPB and induced cardiac arrest. There is particular concern about the manipulation of the aorta when the patient is first put on CPB, as it increases the risk of microemboli in the general circulation. In addition, CPB may cause a total inflammatory response, due to contact of the blood with the artificial surfaces of the CPB circuit (de Jaegere and Sukyer, 2002). As a result, CPB may be responsible for causing many of the postoperative complications: myocardial ischaemia, arrhythmias, respiratory distress syndrome, acute renal failure, cerebrovascular accident and post-pump psychosis (de Jaegere and Sukyer, 2002). Consequently, less interventional surgery such as minimally invasive coronary artery surgery using a mini-thoracotomy incision has been developed. This reduces the risks associated with sternotomy and improves postoperative recovery. Off-pump, or beating heart surgery, using a device known as an octopus to stabilize and immobilize a portion of heart tissue during graft anastomosis, is an alternative approach to this problem (Margereson and Riley, 2003).

VALVE REPLACEMENT

Patients with symptomatic valve disease will eventually require surgery, since without this progressive heart failure will develop, leading to death. Valves may either become regurgitant or stenosed. Depending on the severity of the dysfunction, the valve can either be repaired or replaced. Three types of prosthetic valve are used: animal valves (xenografts); mechanical valves; or valves from a cadaver (homografts). An example of a mechanical valve is the St Jude, a bileaflet valve (Fig. 13.10a) (Davis and Small, 1995). Animal valves are commonly harvested from the pig: e.g. a Carpentier–Edwards valve, which can be treated for human use (Fig. 13.10b). Cadaver valves are used less commonly (Brecker, 1996). Each valve has advantages and disadvantages. Mechanical valves are at risk of thrombosis and therefore obstruction. This means that the patient has to take anti-coagulants for the rest of their lives. Infection is another problem. However, if neither of these complications occur, these valves are very durable, lasting for many years (Prendergast et al, 1996). Animal and cadaver valves are associated with less thrombogenesis and therefore only require a limited period of anti-coagulation. However, they are not as durable as mechanical valves and are vulnerable to wear and tear (Brecker, 1996; Prendergast et al, 1996). Obviously, it is important that the patient is involved in the decision-making process. For some patients it may not be feasible to accept a xenograft or homograft, for religious, moral or ethical reasons, while other patients may baulk at long-term anti-coagulation. One result of the number of patients undergoing successful valve replacement is that more 'redo' replacements are now being performed.

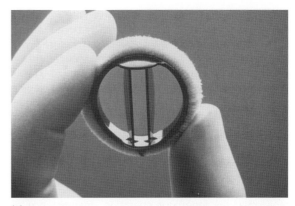

(a)

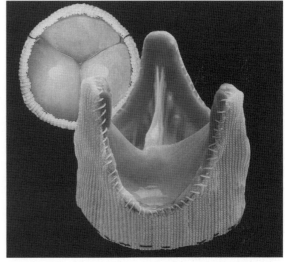

(b)

Figure 13.10   Examples of prosthetic valve: (a) St Jude medical bileaflet valve; (b) Carpentier–Edwards porcine valve (xenograft).

Patients with a prosthetic valve may require future replacement because of the valve developing faults. All patients with prosthetic valves need to take precautions against infection. Prophylactic antibiotics must be taken prior to any invasive surgical or dental procedure (The Task Force on Infective Endocarditis of the European Society of Cardiology, 2004). There is also a risk of developing infective endocarditis, particularly in the first 2 months after surgery, which can damage the anastomosis, causing life-threatening valve failure (Brecker, 1996).

POSTOPERATIVE MANAGEMENT FOLLOWING OPEN HEART SURGERY

Traditionally, patients undergoing open cardiac surgery have been considered as being critically ill, and have therefore remained in intensive care for 24–48 hours postoperatively. This has recently been reduced to only a few hours, or an overnight stay, before being transferred back to a high dependency area within a ward where close monitoring can be continued. This is known as the 'fast track approach'. This evolved as a result of advances in surgical and anaesthetic techniques and the need to streamline cardiac services, with the increased demand for cardiac surgery. At pre-assessment, some patients will be identified as suitable for 'fast tracking'; factors taken into account are the patient being fit preoperatively, with no abnormalities of renal, liver or lung function. As well as the preoperative risk, the length of operation, maintenance of haemodynamic stability and early extubation have to be taken into account (Fisher et al, 2002). This group of patients spend less time in intensive care and return to the ward as soon as they are haemodynamically stable, i.e. when blood pressure, pulse rate and rhythm, and central venous pressure are normalized and stable. Blood loss from chest drains should also be minimal, and the body temperature should have risen to 37°C from its previously induced hypothermic state. The patient should also be breathing spontaneously, although probably still requiring oxygen, and maintaining satisfactory arterial blood gases and oxygen saturation levels.

Once the patient is transferred back to the ward after being 'fast tracked', the continuing goals of care in the postoperative period are to maintain adequate spontaneous ventilation, oxygenation and haemodynamic stability, which will in part be achieved if the patient is comfortable and pain free.

Cardiac rhythm disturbances

ECG monitoring is required for early detection of atrial/ventricular arrhythmias; atrial fibrillation is one of the commonest arrhythmias, occurring in over 50% of valve patients postoperatively (Ommen et al, 1997). Arrhythmias are common due to electrolyte derangement resulting from CPB and the induced hypothermia as part of the procedure. Rhythm disturbances can compromise blood pressure, so appropriate drug therapy will be prescribed. The patient may develop bradyarrhythmias, which can also affect blood pressure and require temporary cardiac pacing via the epicardial pacing electrodes inserted during surgery (Bernat, 1997).

Fluid balance disturbances

The central venous pressure (CVP) is monitored for pressure increases (indicating hypervolaemia) or decreases (indicating hypovolaemia). Central venous pressure is also an indicator of right ventricular function,

with raised pressure indicating some degree of impairment. Frequent blood pressure monitoring is required (for early detection of hypotension and/or hypertension). Hypotension may indicate vasodilatation due to elevated core temperature, or hypovolaemia due to blood loss or inadequate fluid replacement. Hypertensive episodes (systolic pressure >150 mmHg) may cause rupture or blood leakage at the graft suture lines. Prevention of these complications requires treatment with an intravenous vasodilator such as glyceryl trinitrate, which is titrated against the patient's blood pressure to maintain normotension. Nurses frequently manage fluid balance using integrated care pathways that detail which medications or intravenous infusions should be given to optimize the patient's fluid balance (Fisher et al, 2002). Hypertensive episodes may be caused by pain and therefore require effective analgesia. Anxiety may be reduced by the nurse reassuring the patient and perhaps involving relatives in the patient's care; if these measures fail, anxiolytic treatment may be required.

Chest drains are inserted at the time of surgery into the pleural, mediastinal and pericardial spaces; these must be closely monitored and blood loss recorded (see Ch. 14). Suction is commonly applied to the chest drains to encourage drainage. In the immediate postoperative period, measurement of drainage will be carried out regularly and if excessive (>100 mL/h) reported to the medical staff (Margereson and Riley, 2003). If drainage does not diminish, it may indicate complications such as rupture of the suture line or a clotting disorder due to anticoagulants given during CPB, and requires immediate medical management. Once drainage has been minimal (<10–20 mL/h) for a few hours, the drains can be removed (Margereson and Riley, 2003). Chest drains can be a source of pain, and nursing care should ensure that the drains neither restrict patient mobility nor pull on the patient's skin.

Pain management

In the immediate postoperative period, pain will be controlled with intravenous or intramuscular opioids, and many patients benefit from controlling their own pain with a patient-controlled analgesia (PCA) pump (Margereson and Riley, 2003). Pain must be well controlled to enhance patient comfort, prevent episodes of hypertension and enable the patient to breathe deeply and expectorate, thus preventing lung infection and alveolar collapse. Painful procedures, such as removal of chest drains, may require additional boluses of opioids or nitrous oxide and oxygen (Entonox). The need for opioids diminishes over time, but effective pain control remains a priority to enable the patient to regain mobility, and thus prevent the many complications associated with immobility, such as deep vein thrombosis and chest infection.

A number of patients experience psychological disturbance in the early postoperative period, referred to as post-cardiotomy psychosis or post-pump psychosis (Bernat, 1997). This results in behavioural disturbance, manifestations of which range from confusion and disorientation to visual and auditory hallucinations. Nursing patients with post-cardiotomy psychosis can be both difficult and challenging, posing a threat to the patient's safety, since the patient may be aggressive and uncooperative with treatment. This condition is also very alarming for the patients themselves and their relatives who may observe behaviour that is uncharacteristic of their loved one. Psychological disturbance is usually transient, lasting a day or so (Bernat, 1997), but may necessitate the need for sedation if the patient is at risk of self-harm.

Sternal and leg wounds should be observed daily for signs of infection and impaired healing. Dressings are removed the day after surgery; if the wounds are clean and dry, they can be left exposed. If the wound is oozing or open, it should be managed aseptically and covered with an appropriate dressing. Wounds are generally closed with a soluble suture material, which does not need to be removed, although loose ends of the suture may need to be trimmed close to the skin.

Neurological complications such as stroke or behavioural changes may be seen postoperatively; these are due to disruption of the atheromatous plaque with the release of debris when the aorta is clamped during surgery. Careful neurological assessment of the patient in the early postoperative period will detect any neurological disturbance (Bernat, 1997).

The patient should be monitored closely in the immediate postoperative phase for breathing difficulties due to pneumothorax or haemothorax (see Ch. 14) and hypoventilation due to pain (Thornlow, 1995). The patient's lungs are also vulnerable to areas of collapse (atelectasis) where the lung has not fully expanded after being collapsed during surgery and having undergone a period of mechanical ventilation postoperatively.

Respiratory assessment involves monitoring and recording respiratory depth and rate for hypoventilation or hyperventilation, and pulse oximetry for reduction of oxygen saturation indicated by a saturation level (SaO_2) of <95%. Humidified oxygen should be given to maintain SaO_2 levels at >95%. The patient should be reminded to take 8–10 deep breaths with a 3–5 seconds inspiratory hold every hour while awake. This helps to prevent lobar infection, consolidation and collapse. Once the patient begins mobilization, the frequency of deep breathing exercises can be reduced (Brooks-Brun, 1995).

Body temperature should be monitored 4 hourly for elevation >37°C which may indicate the presence of infection.

Patients usually require an intravenous infusion for the first 24 hours postoperatively to maintain fluid balance until they are able to resume oral fluid intake. Oral fluids can be gradually given as nausea subsides, and once the patient is drinking normally the infusion can be discontinued.

Patients frequently experience a loss of appetite postoperatively and need to be encouraged to start eating as soon as possible, to facilitate wound healing and to regain strength. Regaining a normal dietary pattern may take time, and will need to be built up slowly with small, light nutritious meals. Patients who have been advised to lose weight and reduce their saturated fat intake should not change their dietary pattern in the early postoperative period, but should wait until they begin to feel well and are ready to make changes.

The majority of patients will have a urinary catheter for up to 48 hours postoperatively. This enables urinary output and renal function to be monitored. Urinary output should be measured and recorded hourly. If output is less than 0.5 mL/kg/h, it may indicate that the patient is hypovolaemic and/or the kidneys are poorly perfused due to hypotension, which will require immediate medical attention to prevent acute renal failure.

A high standard of urinary catheter hygiene, maintenance of a closed system (Winn, 1996) and high fluid intake will help to reduce the risk of catheter-related infection. Patients with a prosthetic heart valve who develop a urinary tract infection may be at risk of developing infective valvular endocarditis (Hudak and Gallo, 1994). Providing the patient makes an uncomplicated recovery, the catheter may be removed earlier than 48 hours to reduce this risk.

Urinalysis should be performed daily to detect occult blood in those patients with prosthetic heart valves who are receiving anticoagulant therapy.

Patients are usually exhausted after cardiac surgery and have to contend with pain and bruising from sternal and leg wounds. Gentle mobilization is encouraged the day after surgery, providing the patient's condition is stable. This will start with getting out of bed with assistance and sitting in a chair, followed by gradually increasing activity from walking around the bed area to longer excursions around the ward. Active limb exercises help to prevent deep vein thrombosis, along with early mobilization, which also helps in the prevention of chest infection and pressure ulcers, and increases the patient's self-esteem and enhances recovery from surgery.

PREPARATION FOR DISCHARGE

Providing the patient has had an uncomplicated recovery, they are discharged home on/about the seventh postoperative day. Prior to discharge, the patient will require the following information:

- Nutritional information should be given to optimize wound healing, maintain ideal body weight and reduce cholesterol levels if elevated. Patients should be taught about healthy eating, avoiding foods high in sugar and saturated fats. They should also eat plenty of fresh fruit, vegetables, cereals, pulses, fish and lean meat. Foods high in saturated fats should be eaten in moderation or avoided completely. Salt intake is associated with hypertension and should also be reduced to <6 g daily (De Backer et al, 2003). Simple measures such as not adding salt to food can help to reduce intake.

- If the patient has a leg wound, advice should be given about contacting their general practitioner if the wound becomes red, painful or swollen. The patient should also be told that ankle swelling at the end of the day is not uncommon. This can be minimized by elevating the leg, wearing a support stocking and avoiding crossed legs when sitting.

- Sternal wounds tend to heal quicker than the leg wounds but still require observation for signs of infection and poor healing. Although the incidence of sternal wound infection is low, the risk of infection is increased in those who have a tracheotomy. This is due to the proximity of the tracheotomy to the sternal wound and associated risk of contamination from respiratory pathogens. When the internal mammary artery has been used in revascularization, the blood supply to the sternum may have been interrupted during dissection and this may cause delayed sternal healing (Kuo and Butchart, 1995).

- The patient should be informed that chest discomfort may take a few weeks to settle. It is tempting for the patient to sit in a hunched position, which may worsen aches and stiffness and reduce air entry to the lungs. Lifting heavy weights greater than 7 kg should be avoided for up to 3 months after surgery, as well as certain sporting activities such as tennis. These activities can stress the sternal would and may interfere with healing (Possanza, 1996).

- Some patients may develop chest pain a number of days to weeks after surgery, because of post-pericardiotomy syndrome. This is an inflammatory condition of the pericardium which causes fever, pain, dyspnoea and a pericardial or pleural friction rub. This syndrome usually responds to analgesics, anti-inflammatory agents and diuretics (Dziadulewicz and Shannon-Stone, 1995).

- Physical activity should be positively encouraged because this may reduce blood pressure, cholesterol levels and body weight. Patients should be encouraged to exercise at least four times a week, but preferably daily for a period of 30 minutes (De Backer et al, 2003). Exercise does not need to be complex or competitive; a daily walk is sufficient to gain health benefits.

- Patients who have had valve replacements require additional verbal and written information about protecting their prosthetic valve from infective endocarditis which will result in valve damage or death. Dental infections can affect the valve, so it is important that the patient understands the importance of oral hygiene and visiting a dentist regularly. Prophylactic antibiotics are required prior to any dental treatment, including scaling and polishing, and other surgical procedures (The Task Force on Infective Endocarditis of the European Society of Cardiology, 2004).

- Patients with mechanical prosthetic valves will require warfarin anticoagulation for life to prevent valve thrombosis and embolism. Effective education and information are required to enhance understanding of and concordance with drug therapy.

HEART TRANSPLANTATION

A number of patients will deteriorate so much that conventional therapies are no longer effective in controlling their heart failure. These patients are severely limited physically, often requiring continuous oxygen therapy and a cocktail of drugs, and these measures may maintain life for about a year. Many patients in the UK require heart transplants, but due to a limited supply of donor organs, less than 300 transplants occur a year. Unfortunately, some patients suitable for transplantation will die before a suitable heart becomes available (British Heart Foundation, 2000).

There are a number of heart conditions causing end-stage heart failure. The most common are dilated cardiomyopathy (45%), coronary heart disease (38%) and congenital heart disease (6%) (Anyanwu et al, 2002).

Before being selected for transplantation, patients undergo a rigorous selection procedure which aims to establish whether all other treatment options have been exhausted. Secondly, it must be established that the patient does not have any pre-existing conditions such as renal failure that may increase the risk of the transplanted heart failing and being rejected. Those not selected for transplantation may require a great deal of emotional support to help them accept this disappointment and come to terms with their impending death.

Survival after transplant has improved over the years because of an improvement in the management of rejection and infection. The 1-year survival rate is now 80%, with the highest failure rate for transplants occurring during the first postoperative month (Anyanwu et al, 2002). Transplantation both prolongs and improves quality of life; so much so that 39% of patients have returned to work and 90% have regained full activity with no physical limitations (Hosenpud et al, 1997).

Patients deemed suitable for transplantation have a vigorous work-up prior to surgery, and after this may have to wait anything from a few days to over a year before a suitable heart becomes available. During this time the patient will require both physical support to maintain optimum health before surgery, and psychological support to help the patient come to terms with issues surrounding being the recipient of a donor heart.

Immediate postoperative care of the transplant patient is similar to that for any patient undergoing cardiac surgery, except that because the patient is receiving immunosuppressant drugs, signs of infection may be masked. Thorough health education enables patients to adjust to lifestyle changes required to keep their hearts healthy. In addition, the patient may have to cope with alterations in body image, induced by anti-rejection therapy; these include an increase in weight and body hair.

Any transplanted tissue will be rejected by the body's immune system in the absence of immunosuppressant therapy. When rejection occurs, the transplanted heart is attacked by the immune cells and thus begins to fail (Dressler, 1993). Drugs that suppress this immune response have to be taken for life.

Immunosuppressive drugs also suppress the body's ability to fight infection, which causes an added burden for the patient, potentially leaving them vulnerable to serious infections that increase morbidity and mortality. The drugs also have a number of other side-effects which may reduce patient concordance.

Typical anti-rejection therapy revolves around the following drugs: corticosteroids, azathioprine, ciclosporin A, FK506 (tacrolimus), cyclophosphamide and mycophenolate mofetil (Cox, 2002). Steroids may be prescribed for a limited period only, but the other drugs will be taken for life. Corticosteroids inhibit the production of interleukins 1 and 2; these are chemical mediators which help to enhance the immune response. There are a number of side-effects of these

drugs, resulting in altered fat distribution across the shoulders, causing a hump, and in the face, causing a rounded appearance or 'moon face'. Corticosteroids also reduce bone density, leading to osteoporosis, so increasing the risk of fractures. They can also induce diabetes mellitus, which may require insulin therapy to control elevated blood glucose levels. In addition, they can cause mood changes (Dressler, 1993). Side-effects of these drugs can be unpleasant and may affect patient concordance, especially if the patient is an adolescent, when altered body image may be perceived as being important.

Azathioprine suppresses the bone marrow with inhibition of lymphocyte production, thus reducing the number of immune cells responsible for rejection. Because all cells made by the marrow are suppressed, patients may become anaemic and thus lethargic (Dressler, 1993).

Ciclosporin A suppresses T-cell production and activation; these cells are responsible for the destruction of transplanted tissue. Ciclosporin can alter appearance, increasing body hair growth and enlarging gums, which may affect patient concordance with this drug. It also causes hypertension, which requires additional drug therapy with anti-hypertensives to prevent associated complications such as stroke and left ventricular failure (Dressler, 1993).

The overall aim of the drug therapy is to maintain a fine balance between preventing rejection and not suppressing the immune system too much so that the patient is unable to fight infection.

In spite of immunosuppressant therapy, patients still experience episodes of acute rejection which places the heart at risk of being destroyed by their own immune system. Episodes of acute rejection are difficult to diagnose because there are few reliable clinical signs to indicate its presence, so endomyocardial biopsy will need to be performed regularly (Levine et al, 1996). This involves the insertion of a bioptome catheter into the right ventricle via the subclavian or jugular vein, so that small samples of heart tissue can be removed for histological examination.

Acute rejection episodes decline with time and the patient's immune system develops some tolerance to the transplanted tissue. However, the majority of patients experience chronic rejection, which is manifested by a diffuse form of coronary artery disease which gradually narrows the coronary arteries, causing the myocardium to become ischaemic. Coronary artery disease is the main cause of death in those surviving more than 1 year after transplantation, but, because the donor heart is denervated as a result of surgery, the majority of patients do not experience angina. However, about 12% do, which suggests that reinnervation of the heart occurs (Tsui and Large, 1998). Additionally, long-term immunosuppressive therapy (azathioprine being particularly implicated) is associated with an increased risk of malignancy, such as cutaneous tumours (Cox, 2002). Clinical evaluation of new immunosuppressants is underway which may have less unpleasant side-effects than current therapy (Tsui and Large, 1998).

Transplant patients are therefore faced with many changes that require them to make a number of adaptations; regular hospital appointments are required to monitor organ function. This involves a range of tests from simple blood tests, echocardiography and ECG, to the more invasive endomyocardial biopsies which initially may be as frequent as monthly and then every 4–6 months for the next 2–5 years.

Monitoring chronic rejection may require annual cardiac catheterization and coronary angiography, to monitor for the development of coronary artery disease (Dressler, 1993).

Patients also need to understand that good hygiene in both personal care and food preparation is required to prevent infection. In addition to this, the patient needs to know how to monitor themselves for signs of infection, so that early antibiotic therapy can be given. The patient must be shown how to take their temperature; this should be done twice a day and recorded. If abnormalities indicating infection or a possible rejection episode are detected, patients must consult their general practitioner or return to hospital.

Patients also need to be fully educated in what they can do for themselves to maintain a healthy heart. This should centre on healthy eating, aimed at preventing weight gain, which increases the heart's workload, and maintaining blood cholesterol at normal levels to slow down the disease process that causes coronary atherosclerosis and subsequent myocardial infarction (Grady and Jalowiec, 1995). Healthy eating involves avoiding foods high in saturated fats, sugar and calories, and eating foods such as fresh fruit, vegetables, white meat and oily fish (De Backer et al, 2003). There

is a tendency for the diet to become less healthy over time. This is in part due to patient's feeling healthier and experiencing an increase in appetite, but also, because the patient feels healthy, they may feel that there is less reason to follow a healthy diet regime (Grady and Jalowiec, 1995).

Exercise is another important factor in the maintenance of a healthy heart and needs to be maintained throughout life (Ellis, 1995). The American College of Sports Medicine (ACSM) guidelines (1993) state that the individual will benefit from daily bouts of aerobic exercise totalling 30 minutes. Normally, heart rate is increased rapidly by stimulation of the sympathetic nervous system, but because this is no longer present in the transplanted heart it has to rely on the slower release of catecholamines to increase heart rate and blood pressure with exercise. Conversely, it takes longer for the heart rate to fall after exercise, since it takes about 15 minutes for the catecholamines to be broken down and for their effect to be reduced. Consequently, any exercise programme devised by the physiotherapist will involve a 10–15 minute warm-up and cool-down period. This allows the denervated heart to increase its heart rate in response to the release of catecholamines such as adrenaline (epinephrine) and noradrenaline (norepinephrine). During the cool-down period patients will be aware of an increased heart rate for longer than expected; the 15 minutes of cool-down exercise allows the rate to return to normal (Ellis, 1995).

CONCLUSION

Cardiac surgery is now a common treatment for conditions involving specific structures such as the coronary arteries, valves or the conduction system. Heart transplantation is the ultimate option when other treatments are no longer effective; however, the number of patients receiving heart transplants is limited by the scarcity of donor hearts.

Summary of key points

- Nursing cardiac patients requires an extensive knowledge of the heart's function and the effects of its dysfunction on the body.

- The nurse needs to be able to carry out a comprehensive assessment to establish the effects of heart disease on the individual's

physical and psychological function and well-being.

- Cardiac care is constantly changing as knowledge of heart disease progresses and innovative therapies develop. This requires the nurse to be an informed and knowledgeable practitioner.

References

American College of Sports Medicine (1993) *Resource Manual for Guidelines for Exercise Testing and Prescription*, 2nd edn. Philadelphia: Lea & Febiger.

Anyanwu, A. C., Rogers, C. A. & Murday, A. J. (2002) Intrathoracic organ transplantation in the United Kingdom 1995–99: results from the UK cardiothoracic transplant audit. *Heart* 87(5): 449–454.

Attin, M. (2001) Cardiac aspects of critical care: electrophysiology study: a comprehensive review. *American Journal of Critical Care* 10(4): 1–23.

Banchet, F. & Cheron, E. (2003) Equipment designed for or adapted to transradial interventions. In: Hamon, M. & McFadden, E. (eds) *Transradial Approach for Cardiovascular Intervention*. France: Europa Stethascope Media.

Barbiere, C. (1994) Malignant vasovagal syncope after percutaneous transluminal coronary angioplasty: a potential for disaster. *Critical Care Nurse* 14(1): 90–93.

Bernat, J. B. (1997) Smoothing the CABG patient's road to recovery. *American Journal of Nursing* 97(2): 23–27.

Bines, A. S. & Landron, S. L. (1993) Cardiovascular emergencies in the post-anaesthetic care unit. *Nursing Clinics of North America* 28(3): 493–505.

Blackburn, F. & Bookless, B. (2002) Valve disorders. In: Hatchett, R. & Thompson, D. (eds) *Cardiac Nursing: A Comprehensive Guide*. Edinburgh: Churchill Livingstone.

Brady, M., Kinn, S. & Stuart, P. (2004) Preoperative fasting for adults to prevent perioperative complications (Cochrane Review). In: *The Cochrane Library; Issue 1*. Chichester: John Wiley and Sons.

Brecker, S. (1996) The leaking prosthetic valve. *British Journal of Hospital Medicine* 55(7): 415–418.

British Heart Foundation (2000) *British Heart Foundation Coronary Heart Disease Statistics Database: Annual compendium*. London: BHF.

British Heart Foundation (2001) *Pacemakers: Patient Information*. [online] Available at: http://www.bcs.com (accessed 27th March 2004).

British Heart Foundation (2003) *British Heart Foundation Statistics Database*. London: BHF.

Brooks-Brun, J. (1995) Post-operative atelectasis and pneumonia. *Heart & Lung* 24(2): 94–111.

Carabello, B. A. & Crawford, F. A. (1997) Valvular heart disease. *New England Journal of Medicine* 337(1): 32–41.

Carter, L. & Lamerton, M. (1996) Understanding balloon mitral valvuloplasty: the Inoue technique. *Intensive & Critical Care Nursing* 12(3): 147–154.

Chow, A. W. C., Lane, R. E. & Cowie, M. R. (2003) New pacing technologies for heart failure. *British Medical Journal* 326(7398): 1073–1077.

Clinton, H. (2003) Haemodynamic monitoring in theatre. *British Journal of Anaesthetic and Recovery Nursing* 4(1):10–16.

Cox, W. (2002) Cardiac transplantation. In: Hatchett, R. & Thompson, D. (eds) *Cardiac Nursing: A Comprehensive Guide*. Edinburgh: Churchill Livingstone.

Davis, J. & Small, B. (1995) Advances in the treatment of aortic stenosis across the lifespan. *Nursing Clinics of North America* 30(2): 317–332.

Davis, T. M. A., Maguire, T. O., Haraphongse, M. & Schaumberger, M. R. (1994) Undergoing cardiac catheterisation: the effects of informational preparation and coping style on patient anxiety during the procedure. *Heart & Lung* 23(2): 140–149.

De Backer, G., Ambrosioni, E., Borch-Johnsen, K., et al (2003) European guidelines on cardiovascular disease prevention in clinical practice. *European Journal of Cardiovascular Prevention and Rehabilitation* 10(4: suppl 1): S1–S78.

de Jaegere, P. P. & Sukyer, W. J. L. (2002) Off-pump coronary artery bypass surgery. *Heart* 88(3): 313–318.

Dressler, D. K. (1993) Transplantation in end-stage heart failure. *Critical Care Nursing Clinics of North America* 5(4): 635–648.

Dunbar, S. B. (1993) Internal cardioverter device discharge: experience of patients and family members. *Heart & Lung* 22(6): 494–501.

DVLA (2003) *At a glance*. [Online] Available at: http://www.dvla.gov.uk/at_a_glance/ch2_cardiovascular.htm. (accessed 1 May 2004).

Dziadulewicz, L. & Shannon-Stone, M. (1995) Post-pericardiotomy syndrome: a complication of cardiac surgery. *AACN Clinical Issues* 6(3): 467–470.

Ellis, B. (1995) Cardiac transplantation: a review and guidelines for exercise rehabilitation. *Physiotherapy* 81(3): 157–161.

Fisher, S., Walsh, G. & Cross, N. (2002) Nursing management of the cardiac surgical patient. In: Hatchett, R. & Thompson, D. (eds) *Cardiac Nursing: A Comprehensive Guide*. Edinburgh. Churchill Livingstone.

Flynn, M. B. (1996) Wound healing in critical illness. *Critical Care Nursing Clinics of North America* 8(2): 115–123.

Fox, K. (1996) Hypertension and heart disease. *Nursing Standard* 10(23): 52.

Gardner, E., Joyce, S., Iger, M., et al (1996) Intracoronary stent update: focus on patient education. *Critical Care Nurse* 16(2): 65–71.

Gershlick, A. (2001) Anti-thrombotic pharmacology and angioplasty. In Norell, M. S. & Perrins, E. J. (eds) *Essential Interventional Cardiology*. London: WB Saunders

Gilbert, C. J. (2001) Common supraventricular tachycardias: mechanisms and management. *American Association of Critical Care Nursing*. 12(1): 100–113.

Grady, K. L. & Jalowiec, A. (1995) Predictors of compliance with diet 6 months after heart transplantation. *Heart & Lung* 24(5): 359–367.

Grech, E. D. (2003) ABC of interventional cardiology: non-coronary percutaneous intervention. *British Medical Journal* 327(7406): 97–100.

Gregoratos, G., Abrams, J., Epstein, A. E., et al (2002) *ACC/AHA/NASPE 2002 Guideline Update for Implantation of Cardiac Pacemakers and Antiarrhythmia Devices*. [Online] Available at http://www.americanheart.org (accessed 2 June 2004).

Grubb, N. R. & Furniss, S. (2001) Radiofrequency ablation for atrial fibrillation. *British Medical Journal* 322(7289): 777–780.

Guaglianone, D. & Tyndall, A. (1995) Comfort issues in patients undergoing radiofrequency catheter ablation. *Critical Care Nurse* 15(1): 47–50.

Hosenpud, J., Bennett, L., Keck, B., et al (1997) The registry of the International Society for Heart and Lung Transplantation; fourteenth official report. *Journal of Heart & Lung Transplant* 16(7): 691–712.

Houghton, T. & Kaye, G. C. (2003) ABC of interventional cardiology: implantable devices for treating tachy-arrhythmias. *British Medical Journal* 327(7410): 333–336.

Hudak, C. M. & Gallo, B. M. (1994) *Critical Care Nursing*. Philadelphia: Lippincott.

Jones, C., Holcolb, E. & Rohrer, T. (1995a) Femoral artery pseudoaneurysm. *Critical Care Nurse* 15(4): 47–51.

Jones, J. V., MacConnell, T. J. & Evans, S. J. (1995b) Pacemakers. *Care of the Critically Ill* 11(2): 53–55.

Jowett, N. & Thompson, D. (2003) *Comprehensive Coronary Care*, 3rd edn. London: Elsevier Science.

Kaye, G. C. (2003) ABC of interventional cardiology: percutaneous interventional electrophysiology. *British Medical Journal* 327(7409): 280–283.

Kern, J. M. (2003) *The Cardiac Catheterization Handbook*, 4th edn. Philadelphia: Mosby.

Koreny, M., Riedmüller, E., Nikfardjam, M., et al (2004) Arterial puncture closing devices compared with standard manual compression after cardiac catheterization: systematic review and meta-analysis. *Journal of the American Medical Association.* 291(3): 350–357.

Kuo, J. & Butchart, E. (1995) Sternal wound dehiscence. *Care of the Critically Ill* 11(6): 245–248.

Lehmann, K. G., Heath-Lange, S. J. & Ferris, S. T. (1999) Randomized comparison of haemostasis techniques after invasive cardiovascular procedures. *American Heart Journal* 138(6 part 1): 1118–1125.

Levine, A., Clarke, S. C. & Forty, J. (1996) Cardiac transplant. *Hospital Update* 9: 386–391.

McLenachan, J. M. (2001) Femoral artery complications and the use of closure devices. In: Norell, M. S. & Perrins, E. J. (eds) *Essential Interventional Cardiology.* London: W. B. Saunders.

McMurray, J. J. & Stewart, S. (2000) Epidemiology, aetiology and progress of heart failure. *Heart* 83(5): 596–602.

Margereson, C. & Riley, J. (2003) *Cardiothoracic Surgical Nursing: Current Trends in Adult Care.* Oxford: Blackwell Science.

Maynard, S. J., Menown, I. B. A. & Adgey, A. A. J. (2000) Troponin T or Troponin I as cardiac markers in ischaemic heart disease *Heart* 83(4): 371–373.

Montes, P. (1997) Managing outpatient cardiac catheterisation. *American Journal of Nursing* 97(8): 34–37.

Munro, J. F. & Campbell, W. (2000) *Macleod's Clinical Examination*, 10th edn. Edinburgh: Churchill Livingstone.

Myerson, S. G. & Mitchell, A. R. (2003) Mobile phones in hospital. *British Medical Journal* 326(7387): 460–461.

National Institute for Clinical Excellence (2000) NICE: *Guidance on the Use of Implantable Cardioverter Defibrillators for Arrhythmias.* Technology Appraisal Guidance No 11. [Online] Available at: http://www.nice.org.uk/pdf/Defibrillators_A4_summary.pdf (accessed 2 April 2004).

National Institute for Clinical Excellence (2003) *Guidance on the Use of Coronary Artery Stents.* Technology Appraisal 71. October 2003. [Online] Available at: http://www.nice.org.uk/pdf/TA71_coronaryarterystents_fullguidance.pdf (accessed 2 April 2004).

Nisam, S. (1997) Technology update: the modern implantable cardioverter defibrillator. *Annals of Non-Invasive Electrophysiology* 2(1): 69–78.

O'Donoghue, A. (2002) Cardiomyopathies. In: Hatchet, R. & Thompson, D. (eds) *Cardiac Nursing: A Comprehensive Guide.* Edinburgh: Churchill Livingstone.

Ommen, S., Odell, J. & Stanton, M. (1997) Atrial arrhythmias after cardiothoracic surgery. *New England Journal of Medicine* 336(20): 1429–1434.

Pavia, S. & Wilkoff, B. (2001) The management of surgical complications of pacemaker and implantable cardioverter-defibrillators. *Current Opinion in Cardiology* 16(1): 66–71.

Penney, C. (1995) Learning how to remove femoral sheaths. *Nursing 95* 25(5): 32QQ–32SS.

Perrins, E. J. (2001) Intracoronary stenting. In: Norell, M. S. & Perrins, E. J. (eds) *Essential Interventional Cardiology.* London: W. B. Saunders.

Petch, M. C. (1998) Driving and heart disease. *European Heart Journal* 19(8): 1165–1177.

Possanza, C. (1996) What you should know about coronary artery bypass graft surgery. *Nursing 96* 26(2): 48–50.

Prendergast, B. D., Banning, A. P. & Hall, R. J. C. (1996) Valvular heart disease: recommendations for investigation and management. *Journal of the Royal College of Physicians of London* 30(4): 309–315.

Prendergast, B. D., Shaw, T. R. D., Lung, B., et al (2002) Contemporary criteria for the selection of patients for percutaneous balloon mitral valvuloplasty. *Heart* 87(5): 401–404.

Roberts, D. H. (2001) Pathology of balloon dilatation and restenosis. In: Norell, M. S. & Perrins, E. J. (eds) *Essential Interventional Cardiology.* London: W. B. Saunders.

Ross, R. (1999) Atherosclerosis – an inflammatory disease. *New England Journal of Medicine* 340(2): 115–126.

Scanlon, P. J. & Faxon, D. P. (1999) ACC/AHA guidelines for coronary angiography. *Journal of the American College of Cardiology* 33(6): 1756–1824.

Schickel, S., Nones, S., Mize, A. & Voelker, C. (1996) Removal of femoral sheaths by registered nurses: issues and outcomes. *Critical Care Nurse* 16(2): 32–36.

Sears, S. F. & Conti, J. B. (2002) Quality of life and psychological functioning of ICD patients. *Heart* 87(5): 488–493.

Sigwart, U., Prasad, S., Radke, P. & Nadra, I. (2001) Stent coatings. *Journal of Invasive Cardiology* 13(2): 139–140.

Skehan, J. D. (1996) Advances in pacing. *British Journal of Hospital Medicine* 55(1–2): 41–43.

Spiers, C. (2003) The normal 12-lead ECG. *British Journal of Anaesthetic and Recovery Nursing* 4(4): 12–15.

Starkey, I. R. (2001) Patient investigation, work up and preparation. In: Norell, M. S. & Perrins, E. J. (eds) *Essential Interventional Cardiology.* London: W. B. Saunders.

Stoneham, M. D. (1995) Uses and limitations of pulse oximetry. *British Journal of Hospital Medicine* 54(1): 35–41.

Swanton, R. H. (2003) *Cardiology*, 5th edn. London: Blackwell Publishing.

Taggart, D. P. (2002) Bilateral internal mammary artery grafting: are BIMA better? *Heart* 88(1): 7–9.

The Task Force on Infective Endocarditis of the European Society of Cardiology (2004) Guidelines on prevention, diagnosis and treatment of infective endocarditis. Executive summary. *European Heart Journal* 25(3): 267–277.

Thornlow, D. (1995) Is chest physiotherapy necessary after cardiac surgery? *Critical Care Nurse* 15(3): 39–48.

Tsui, S. L. & Large, S. (1998) The current state of heart transplantation. *Care of the Critically Ill* 14(1): 20–24.

Winn, C. (1996) Basing catheter care on research principles. *Nursing Standard* 10(18): 38–40.

Witherell, C. (1994) Cardiac rhythm control devices. *Critical Care Nursing Clinics of North America* 6(1): 85–101.

Wolff, C. A., Scott, C. & Banks, T. A. (1997) The radial artery: an exciting alternative conduit in coronary artery bypass surgery. *Critical Care Nurse* 17(5): 34–39.

Further reading

http://www.bcs.com. British Cardiology Society (accessed on 27 April 2004).

Chapter **14**

Care of the patient requiring thoracic surgery

Emma Gardner

Key objectives of the chapter

Upon completion of this chapter, the reader should:

- have revised the anatomy and physiology of the respiratory system and the fundamental principles of breathing

- have an understanding of the disease processes that require patients to undergo investigative and operative procedures related to the chest

- understand the principles of respiratory assessment

- understand the rationale for the nursing care of postoperative thoracic surgical patients, and associated research, including the management of chest drains

- be able to plan for the patient's discharge with the inclusion of appropriate patient education.

INTRODUCTION

Respiratory disease kills more people than coronary artery disease, and accounted for £2.5 billion of the NHS budget for the year 2000; 7% of the UK adult population have a long-term respiratory complaint and it is the main cause for absenteeism from work. Between 1999 and 2000, 10 500 thoracic surgical procedures were performed, of which 45% were for cancer (British Thoracic Society, 2001).

It is essential for nurses working within the speciality of thoracic surgery to understand the anatomy and the physiology of the respiratory system, the relationships between the structures of the ribs, pleura, lungs, chest wall and diaphragm, together with the associated structures of the mediastinum. An appreciation of the mechanics and regulation of breathing is also important when considering changes in respiratory pattern.

This chapter will commence with an overview of respiratory anatomy and physiology. Respiratory disorders requiring surgical intervention, the care required by patients undergoing surgical intervention and the associated nursing care will then be examined.

AN OVERVIEW OF THE RESPIRATORY SYSTEM AND THE MECHANICS OF BREATHING

The primary function of the respiratory system is the efficient transfer of oxygen from the atmosphere, through the respiratory tract to the alveoli within the lungs, and the elimination of carbon dioxide in the opposite direction. This function is facilitated by the process of breathing. Breathing can be described as an automatic, rhythmic process, which is centrally regulated within the brainstem and results in contraction and relaxation of the skeletal muscles of the diaphragm, rib cage and abdomen, with the consequent movement of gas in and out of the pulmonary alveoli.

Respiration is the overall process (which includes breathing) of controlled oxidation of carbohydrates and fat, to generate energy within all cells of the body, and the production of carbon dioxide as a waste product.

This section will consider the structure and function of the respiratory system and the manner in which ventilation and gaseous diffusion takes place.

STRUCTURE AND FUNCTION

The thorax contains two lungs, each consisting of airways, an extensive blood supply and elastic connective tissue. The right lung consists of three lobes and the left lung has two, but with a division of its upper lobe called the lingula, arguably corresponding to the right middle lobe. The airways, which are the conducting passages for air flow into and out of the lungs, commence with the nose and mouth and include the pharynx and larynx (see Ch. 11 for details of anatomy and physiology). The trachea, the beginning of the lower respiratory tract, commences below the larynx

and continues into the mediastinum, where it divides into the right and left main bronchi. The adult trachea averages 2–2.5 cm in diameter, and ranges from 10–12 cm in length. The trachea remains patent through the support of 16–20 C-shaped cartilaginous rings. Posteriorly, situated directly behind the trachea, a thin muscle extends between the open ends of the cartilage, which stretches to allow the passage of food down the oesophagus. A bolus of food passing down the oesophagus temporarily decreases the lumen of the trachea.

At the point of tracheal bifurcation into the right and left main bronchi, there is a sharp dividing cartilage, the carina. The carina helps to divide airflow to the right and left sides, minimizing turbulence. The right main bronchus angles off the midline at 20–30 degrees, with the left main bronchus deflecting at a sharper angle of 45–55 degrees. The consequence of this difference is that inhaled or aspirated objects in upright subjects tend to follow the straighter course into the right main bronchus. In supine subjects, aspirated or inhaled objects go into the dependent segments of the lung.

Functionally, the lungs can be divided into two zones: the conducting airways and the respiratory zone. The conducting airways (referred to as anatomical dead space) do not contain alveoli, and therefore do not participate in gaseous exchange. The respiratory zone is the alveolar-containing regions of the lung, where gaseous exchange takes place, and accounts for most of the lung volume.

THE CONDUCTING AIRWAYS

The right and left main bronchi subdivide into lobar and then segmental bronchi. Terminal bronchioles, the smallest airways without alveoli, are the product of smaller subdivisions. These airways become progressively narrower, shorter and more numerous as they penetrate the lung. The terminal bronchioles subdivide further into respiratory bronchioles, which contain some alveoli within their walls, and therefore enter the respiratory zone.

By convention, the conducting airways can be broadly categorized into two distinct types: cartilaginous bronchi and membranous bronchioles. The trachea, main bronchi and subsequent divisions of the bronchi contain supporting cartilaginous plates within their walls. The cartilaginous plates maintain patency in the large airways, and enable the bronchi to dilate or constrict independently of lung volume. As the bronchi progressively subdivide, the cartilage gradually disappears. In airways of 1 mm diameter and less, i.e. terminal bronchioles and further subdivisions, the cartilage disappears completely.

Additionally, the bronchi are characterized by a pseudostratified columnar epithelium on spiral bands of smooth muscle and ciliated, mucus-producing epithelium. The 'mucociliary escalator' is a significant function of the respiratory system, trapping dust and other inhaled particles in the mucus, which along with scavenging macrophages are swept up to the larynx by the cilia and coughed out, swallowed or removed by nose blowing. This mechanism may contribute to airway obstruction when patients are unable to cough adequately to clear secretions, either because of tracheal intubation, poor cough reflex or pain following thoracic surgery.

THE RESPIRATORY ZONE

The respiratory bronchioles contain some alveoli within their walls and subdivide finally into the alveolar ducts, which are completely lined with alveoli. These airways, lined with a simple cuboidal epithelium, contain no cartilage within their walls. An important functional difference between the bronchi and the bronchioles is that the latter are embedded directly into the connective tissue framework of the lungs, and, with no cartilage support, their diameter is dependent on lung volume.

The alveoli are thin-walled sacs, each approximately 0.3 mm in diameter and covered in a network of fine capillaries. The surface tension of the thin film of liquid within the alveoli would tend to cause inward collapse of the air space, but is prevented by a secretion from the cells lining the alveoli. The secretion contains surfactant, which lowers the surface tension, thereby preventing alveolar collapse. Collapse of these small air spaces remains a potential problem, and frequently occurs in respiratory disease.

PLEURA

The shape of the lungs conforms to that of the thoracic cavity, through a balancing of tensions within the thorax, held in balance by the pleura. The pleura is a double membrane: the visceral pleura covers the surface of the lung and doubles back as the parietal pleura, which covers the internal surface of the chest wall. The visceral pleura is devoid of a sensory nerve supply, but the parietal pleura receives innervation from the intercostal and phrenic nerves, providing pain and sensation properties.

The two pleura function as one unit because of the small volume of pleural fluid existing between the two layers. This fluid acts as a lubricant to permit the sliding of one layer across the other during respiratory movements, but does not allow the pleura to be pulled apart (rather as two plates of glass with a small drop of water between them cannot be separated except by sliding apart). The pleura, acting together, permit the transfer of movement from the respiratory muscles of the chest wall to the lungs, facilitating the variations of intrathoracic pressure, which are vital for respiratory function.

The tendency of the lungs to pull away from the chest wall and collapse is due to the natural elasticity of the pulmonary connective tissue, and the surface tension in the fluid lining the alveoli. The negative intrapleural pressure balances these tensions throughout the entire respiratory cycle. The negative intrapleural pressure is a consequence of the external forces on the pleura in the form of the inward pull of the lungs away from the chest wall, and outward movements of the chest wall.

REMOVAL OF INHALED PARTICLES

Filtration of inspired air is accomplished by large hairs within the nose and by the nasal mucosal membrane, which traps inhaled particulate matter. The direction of the inspired air stream changes abruptly at the nasopharynx, causing particulate matter to land on the back wall of the pharynx. The tonsils and adenoids located nearby provide the immunological defence against biologically active inspired material. Smaller inhaled particles may reach the lower airways, some of them lodging in the mucous epithelium, and are removed via the mucociliary escalator, or by reflex coughing or sneezing. Some small particles remain suspended as aerosols and are simply exhaled. Alveoli are not ciliated, and particles that deposit there are engulfed by macrophages, and removed from the lung via the lymphatic system or the blood flow.

Nasal breathing is the normal mechanism for air entry because of the additional pulmonary defence mechanisms it provides. Mouth breathing is necessary during colds (when the nasal passages are congested) and when large volumes of air need to be moved in and out, e.g. during exertion. Mouth breathing is a basic physiological response to dyspnoea, since the nasal turbinates create twice the resistance to air flow through the nose, compared with air flow through the mouth. Oral breathing bypasses the protective mechanisms of the nose, thereby allowing unwarmed, unfiltered, dry air to enter the tracheobronchial tree.

INSPIRATION AND EXPIRATION

The rate and depth of respiration is a complex activity regulated by the respiratory centre in the medulla oblongata within the brainstem. Breathing is regulated to some extent through voluntary (behavioural) control, where breathing may be temporarily suspended or altered. The main regulation is through metabolic (automatic) control. Voluntary control of breathing allows ancillary actions related to breathing to occur: e.g. talking, singing, swallowing, straining, sneezing and coughing. Metabolic control serves the basic body requirements for oxygen.

The respiratory centre receives sensory input from many sources, including chemoreceptors and proprioceptors. Chemoreceptors are receptors that respond to changes in the chemical composition of blood or other fluid. Central chemoreceptors are found on the brainstem surface surrounded by brain extracellular fluid. They are sensitive to changes in hydrogen ion concentration (pH), where an increase, i.e. a fall in pH, stimulates ventilation. Carbon dioxide dissolved in cerebrospinal fluid causes a fall in pH, and is a powerful stimulus to respiration. Peripheral chemoreceptors are located in the carotid bodies at the bifurcation of the common carotid arteries, and in the aortic bodies above and below the aortic arch. The peripheral chemoreceptors respond to decreases in arterial oxygen concentrations – $PaO_2 < 10\,kPa$ and $pH < 7.3$ – and increases in arterial carbon dioxide levels ($PaCO_2$). These receptors are responsible for the increase in ventilation that occurs in response to arterial hypoxaemia. A fall in oxygen concentration is a stimulus to respiration, but only a weak one. It becomes more important in chronic obstructive pulmonary disease where there is tolerance to an established rise in levels of carbon dioxide.

The rhythmicity of respiration is controlled by the pneumotaxic centre in the pons, responding to impulses from the proprioceptors, or lung stretch receptors, which are believed to lie within the smooth muscle of the bronchi and possibly the bronchioles. They respond to distension of the lung, which dilates and stretches the airways and alveoli, with the effect of inhibiting further inspiratory activity. The opposite response is also seen: i.e. deflation of the lungs tends to initiate inspiratory activity. The stretch receptors help to prevent overinflation of the lung, and, in the presence of airway narrowing or slow inspiration, their delayed activation allows inspiration to last longer until an adequate tidal volume is achieved.

Irritant receptors are thought to lie between epithelial airway cells, and are stimulated by noxious gases, cigarette smoke, inhaled dusts and cold air. They are similar to receptors found within the nose, nasopharynx, larynx and trachea. Various responses may be initiated such as sneezing, coughing and bronchoconstriction. It is possible that these receptors play a role in the bronchoconstriction of asthma, as a result of their response to released histamine.

THE MECHANICS OF BREATHING

Gas flows from a region of higher pressure to one of lower pressure. When the total pressure in the alveoli is equal to atmospheric pressure, there is no air flow. For inspiration to occur, alveolar pressure must be less than atmospheric pressure, and the reverse for expiration. There are two ways of creating the pressure difference necessary for inspiration to occur: alveolar pressure can be lowered, as in natural breathing, or airway pressure can be raised, as in positive pressure ventilation by mechanical ventilators.

Inspiration is the active phase of breathing, during which time the diaphragm and external intercostal muscles contract. The contraction of the diaphragm forces the abdominal contents downwards, and the contraction of the intercostal muscles produces elevation of the ribs. This results in expansion of the thoracic cavity, and lowering of the pressure in the pleural space surrounding the lungs. As the pressure falls in the pleural space, the distensible lungs expand passively, causing the required pressure drop within the alveolar ducts and air spaces. As the pressure decreases, air flows down the airways into the alveolar spaces until the pressures are equalized, marking the end of the inspiratory phase.

During expiration, which is generally the passive phase, the diaphragm and intercostal muscles relax, allowing the elastic recoil of the lungs to occur, which increases the alveolar pressure, and gas flows out of the lungs. During exercise and voluntary hyperventilation, expiration may become active rather than passive. The significant muscles of expiration are the muscles of the abdominal wall, including the rectus abdominis, the internal and external oblique muscles and the transversus abdominis. When these muscles contract, intra-abdominal pressure is raised, and the diaphragm is pushed up.

Other muscles which may be used to assist respiration are the accessory muscles in the neck and shoulders, the scalene muscles which elevate the first two ribs, and the sternomastoid muscles which raise the sternum. There is very little or no activity in these muscles during quiet breathing, but during exercise or laboured breathing they may contract vigorously.

The exchange of carbon dioxide and oxygen between alveolar air and the pulmonary capillaries occurs by a simple process of diffusion from areas of high concentration to areas of relatively low concentration. The large surface area of the lungs provided by the alveoli is estimated to be $50–100\,m^2$, and with the extremely thin blood–gas barriers of the alveolar membrane and capillary membrane, create the ideal environment for gaseous diffusion to occur. Carbon dioxide is highly soluble and diffuses much more rapidly than oxygen across the membranes.

BLOOD GAS CONCENTRATION

Oxygen is carried in the blood in two forms: dissolved and in combination with haemoglobin. The amount of dissolved oxygen is proportional to the partial pressure of oxygen, but is insufficient alone to meet the demands for oxygen by the tissues. Oxygen transported in combination with haemoglobin, i.e. oxyhaemoglobin, is the significant mode of oxygen carriage, and ensures that the dissolved oxygen within the plasma can be continuously replenished, for uptake by the tissues. Oxygen forms an easily reversible combination with haemoglobin, and will combine or separate from the haemoglobin depending on the relative partial pressures of the surrounding plasma. Differences within the amino acid chains within the haemoglobin can produce variants of haemoglobin with diminished oxygen-carrying capacity, e.g. haemoglobin S or sickle cell.

Oxygen saturation is defined as the ratio of the concentration of oxyhaemoglobin to the concentration of desaturated (or reduced) haemoglobin, and is expressed as a percentage. Normal haemoglobin levels are approximately 15 g haemoglobin/100 mL of blood and the normal oxygen saturation level of arterial blood is 97% when all the haemoglobin is carrying oxygen to full capacity. The oxygen saturation of venous blood is about 75%, reflecting the uptake of oxygen by the tissues, and a large reserve of remaining oxygen. Arterial blood gas analysis measures the plasma concentration of oxygen (PaO_2), where the normal range is 11.5–13.5 kilopascals (abbreviated to kPa).

LUNG VOLUMES

For the purposes of measurement and description, the total volume of air in the lungs is divided into volumes and capacities, where a capacity is considered to be the combination of two or more volumes (Fig. 14.1). While breathing at rest, the volume of air moved in and out, i.e. tidal volume, TV or V_T, approximates to 500 mL. The volume of air remaining in the lungs at the end of tidal expiration is the functional residual capacity (FRC), which is composed of the expiratory reserve volume (ERV) and the residual volume (RV), this being the volume of air remaining in the lungs at the end of a full expiration. The ERV is required when increases in breathing are needed, e.g. during exercise. From knowledge of the FRC, other volumes may be assumed. The inspiratory capacity (IC) is the maximum volume that can be inspired, and consists of the tidal volume and the inspiratory reserve volume (IRV). The latter, like the ERV, is the additional volume

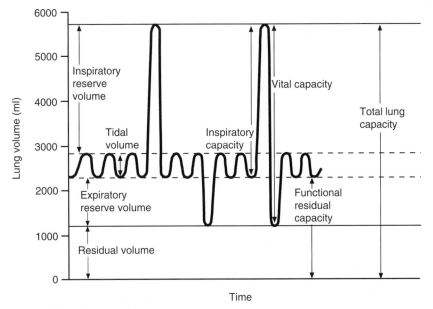

Figure 14.1   Lung volumes. (From Foss, 1989.)

available during exercise, or other increased levels of breathing.

At maximum inspiration, the total volume of air is the total lung capacity (TLC). The RV, the TLC and the FRC cannot be measured directly without complex equipment. However, the vital capacity can be efficiently measured, and indicates the difference in volume between the TLC and the RV. In considering these facts, it is obvious that the lungs have large reserve volumes and capacity for increased ventilation. The consequences of lung resection, therefore, may not greatly limit respiratory function if the remaining lung tissue is healthy and the reserve capacity can be utilized.

RESPIRATORY ASSESSMENT

Respiratory assessment is a vital part of the care of patients undergoing thoracic surgery to gain a clinical impression of the respiratory function or dysfunction, severity of symptoms to confirm the need for medical interventions and highlight subject areas for subsequent patient education.

ASSESSMENT OF BREATHING

Rate, depth and quality determine the pattern of breathing. Respiratory rate is calculated by counting the number of chest movements per minute. One rise and fall of the chest is one full respiratory cycle. The normal respiratory rate at rest is 12–18 breaths per minute (in adults); it is faster in infants and children. The ratio of pulse rate to respiration is approximately 5:1. The depth of respiration is the volume of air moving in and out with each breath: i.e. the tidal volume = approximately 500 mL. The quality of breathing is compared with normal relaxed breathing, which is effortless, automatic, regular and almost silent.

Breathing patterns

Hyperpnoea
Hyperpnoea is an increased respiratory rate, being a normal physiological response, e.g. to exercise.

Tachypnoea
Tachypnoea is an increased respiratory rate, e.g. seen in fever as the body tries to rid itself of excess heat. Respirations increase by approximately seven breaths per minute for every 1°C rise in temperature. Respiratory rate also rises in pneumonia, obstructive pulmonary diseases, respiratory insufficiency and lesions in the respiratory centre of the brainstem.

Bradypnoea
Bradypnoea is a decreased, but regular respiratory rate, e.g. caused by depression of the respiratory centre in a response to opioid drugs or a brain tumour.

Dyspnoea
Dyspnoea is difficult and laboured breathing. Dilated nostrils are often apparent and the entire chest wall and shoulder girdle are raised and lowered in an exaggerated manner. Dyspnoea is a subjective complaint, being an unpleasant awareness of inappropriate effort required for breathing and can be caused by obstruction to air flow.

Orthopnoea
Orthopnoea is breathlessness which occurs when a patient is lying flat. The condition is relieved by adopting a more upright position; the number of pillows required may give a rough indication of the degree of dyspnoea experienced.

Hypoventilation
Hypoventilation is an alteration in the pattern of respiration which becomes irregular or slow and shallow in depth, as a result of drugs, carbon dioxide narcosis or anaesthetic agents.

Hyperventilation
Hyperventilation is an increase in the rate and depth of respiration, e.g. in fear, anxiety, hysterical states, hepatic coma, midbrain lesions of the brainstem, and acid–base imbalance such as diabetic ketoacidosis (Kussmaul's respiration).

Cheyne–Stokes respiration
Cheyne–Stokes respiration is a cyclical pattern in which respirations gradually increase in rate and depth and then decrease over a cycle of 30–45 seconds. Periods of apnoea (20 seconds) alternate with these cycles. This type of breathing pattern is associated with increased intracranial pressure, severe congestive heart failure, renal failure, meningitis and drug overdose. It is also commonly associated with the dying patient.

Apnoea
Apnoea is the total absence of respirations. It may be periodic or cyclical.

Respiratory noise heard without the aid of a stethoscope

Additional information about respiratory status can be determined by listening to the breathing of the patient. Descriptions of respiratory noise heard without the aid of a stethoscope are given below.

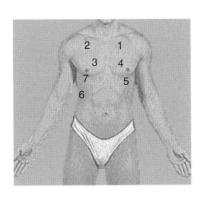

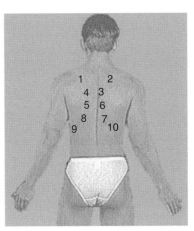

Figure 14.2   Chest auscultation. The numbers represent the order in which to listen.

Stertorous

These noisy, snoring-type respirations usually caused by excessive secretions in the trachea or bronchi are commonly heard in the unconscious patient.

Stridor

Stridor is a loud, harsh, high-pitched sound on inspiration, usually caused by laryngeal obstruction. It tends to be louder and harsher than a wheeze.

Wheeze

A wheeze is a high- or low-pitched sound mainly heard on expiration. Wheezes are generated by the vibration of the walls of narrowed airways as air travels at high velocity through them. The diameter of the airway may be reduced by bronchospasm, mucosal oedema or by foreign objects. The pitch of the wheeze is unrelated to the length of the airway, but is directly related to the degree of airway compression, i.e. the tighter the airway, the higher the pitch.

Respiratory auscultation

Respiratory auscultation is heard with the aid of a stethoscope (Fig. 14.2).

Rales/crackle

Rales or crackles are discontinuous noises that can be differentiated into fine, medium or coarse crackles. The sound is like the crackling of tissue paper at the end of the stethoscope. It is believed that crackles are moist sounds produced by excess liquid in the airways, and are significant in pneumonia, pulmonary fibrosis and congestive cardiac failure.

Pleural rub

Pleural rub is characterized by a rough grating sound heard in both inspiration and expiration, caused by inflammation of the pleural surfaces. The pleural rub is associated with breathing but unaffected by coughing.

ADDITIONAL OBSERVATIONS

Additional observations may contribute further to the assessment of respiratory status.

Cyanosis

Cyanosis is a bluish discoloration of the skin caused by a relative decrease in oxygen saturation within the capillaries of the skin. Generally, cyanosis is said to occur when more than 5 g of deoxygenated haemoglobin is present per 100 mL of blood, i.e. when the haemoglobin level is within normal limits. Patients who are anaemic do not appear cyanotic unless they are severely hypoxaemic, and polycythaemic patients require considerably lower percentages of deoxygenated haemoglobin to display cyanosis. Cyanosis, when present in fingers, toes and ear lobes, i.e. peripheral cyanosis, is usually related to circulatory problems, such as heart failure. Central cyanosis is present when the patient's more central regions are affected, e.g. the tongue and lips, and the trunk. This is related to a lack of oxygenation of arterial blood through the pulmonary system.

Clubbing of the digits

Clubbing of the digits is a significant manifestation within chronic cardiopulmonary disease, although the mechanism is unknown. It is identified most commonly in patients who have bronchogenic carcinoma, chronic obstructive pulmonary disease and cystic fibrosis. It is characterized by a painless enlargement of the terminal phalanges of the fingers and toes, and a widening and deepening of the nail bed.

Cough

Coughing is the most common symptom in patients with pulmonary disease and can be initiated by inflammatory, mechanical or thermal stimulation of the

Table 14.1   Evaluation of cough

Evaluation of cough	Possible causes and indications
Throat clearing	Postnasal drip
Dry and hacking	May be due to nervousness, viral infections, bronchogenic carcinoma or congestive cardiac failure
Loud and harsh	Irritation in the upper airway
Wheezing	Associated with bronchospasm
Severe, or changing in character or with position	May be bronchogenic carcinoma
Loose	Indicates problems in peripheral bronchi and lung parenchyma
Painful	May indicate pleural involvement, or chest wall disease

Table 14.2   Types of cough

Type of cough	Description of cough
Effective	Strong enough to clear the airway
Inadequate	Audible but too weak to move the secretions
Productive	Mucus expelled as a result of the cough
Dry	Moisture or secretions not produced
Barking	Like a seal bark, indicative of a problem in the upper airways, e.g. croup, laryngotracheal bronchitis
Brassy/hoarse	Harsh, dry cough, associated with upper airways disorders, e.g. laryngitis, laryngotracheal bronchitis
Hacking	Frequent brief periods of coughing, or clearing the throat. The cough may be dry, as a result of smoking, a viral infection or postnasal drip

Source: adapted from Wilkins et al (1995).

receptors located in the pharynx, larynx, trachea, large bronchi and even the lung and visceral pleura.

The character of a cough should be evaluated using the descriptions in Table 14.1, and assessed in terms of relationship to time, patient's position and environmental exposure. Coughs of recent onset suggest probable infection and those most noticeable on wakening suggest bronchitis or a suppurative lung disease. Nocturnal paroxysms of coughing may be indicative of asthma or left-sided heart failure. Coughs that worsen on lying down may be due to bronchiectasis or a postnasal drip from sinusitis, and those associated with food intake to aspiration of food into the trachea. Types and descriptions of coughs are shown in Table 14.2.

Table 14.3   Description of sputum

Description of sputum	Possible causes/indications
Clear or mucoid	Viral infection, chronic bronchitis, postnasal drip
Yellow or green	Primary or secondary bacterial infections
Rusty	May indicate bacterial pneumonia
Malodorous	Due to lung abscess, infection from anaerobic organisms
Frothy and pink	Acute pulmonary oedema

Source: adapted from Brunner and Suddarth (1992).

Sputum

Sputum is the substance expelled from the tracheo-bronchial tree, pharynx, mouth, sinuses and nose. The term phlegm refers strictly to secretions from the lungs and tracheobronchial tree; phlegm may contain mucus, cellular debris, microorganisms, blood, pus and inhaled particulate matter. Normal secretions of up to 100 mL are produced daily, removed by the mucociliary escalator and swallowed unnoticed. Sputum may be described as thin, thick, viscous (i.e. gelatinous), tenacious (i.e. extremely sticky), frothy, mucoid or mucopurulent. Other observations of sputum include colour, odour and quantity (Table 14.3).

Haemoptysis

Haemoptysis is the expectoration of blood, ranging from sputum-containing flecks of blood, to expectoration of large amounts of frank blood. The source of blood may be from the mouth, nose, airways or lung tissue. Careful questioning may help to differentiate haemoptysis from haematemesis. Massive bleeding can occur with pulmonary tuberculosis, lung abscesses, pulmonary embolism and pulmonary infarction, bronchiectasis and bronchogenic carcinoma. Haemoptysis can also occur following lung surgery, lung biopsy or bronchoscopy, and so the patient should be warned of these possibilities.

Chest pain

Thoracic pain is associated with a number of cardiac and pulmonary disorders. Careful assessment of precipitating factors, type and quality of pain, and the location and duration of the pain is required to distinguish between them.

Chest pain of pulmonary origin involves the chest wall and parietal pleura, the major airways, diaphragm and mediastinum. Pain arising from the chest wall is well localized and very sharp, increasing with deep breaths and coughing. It is often referred to as pleuritic pain because of the similarity to the pain experienced with pleurisy. Pleuritic pain is a knife-like pain in the chest, particularly associated with a deep intake of breath. Pain associated with neoplasms of the lungs or major bronchi is less well defined, being less localized and dull. Diaphragmatic pain is experienced as referred pain in the shoulders.

COMMON DISORDERS REQUIRING SURGICAL INTERVENTION

CONDITIONS AFFECTING THE PLEURA

Recurrent pneumothorax

Pneumothorax is a condition in which air enters the pleural space for a variety of reasons and causes collapse of the underlying lung. Air entry into the pleural space disrupts the surface tension of the fluid film that holds the two pleura together, with loss of negative intrapleural pressure. The two pleura separate and no longer function as one unit. The underlying lung collapses, since the elastic recoil forces of the lung are now greater than the intrapleural pressure. Small pneumothoraces may go unnoticed. Pain may accompany the occurrence of the pneumothorax, particularly if parietal pleural irritation also occurs, due to the innervation of the parietal pleura. With a large pneumothorax the patient appears acutely dyspnoeic, tachypnoeic and tachycardic, with reduced chest movement on the affected side. The diagnosis is confirmed by chest X-ray.

Pneumothoraces can be broadly categorized into three main types: spontaneous, traumatic and tension.

Spontaneous pneumothorax
Spontaneous pneumothorax can occur with (primary) or without (secondary) pulmonary pathology. Primary pneumothorax commonly occurs in tall, thin, young men. Possible explanations may be due to the rupture of alveoli or bullae, which disrupts the visceral pleura (bullae are air cavities within the lung tissue which are created when alveoli rupture). Secondary pneumothorax can be a consequence of chronic lung disease, e.g. severe asthma, emphysema or cystic fibrosis, and also arises from the rupture of alveoli or bullae.

Traumatic pneumothorax
Traumatic pneumothorax occurs when air enters from outside the chest wall, e.g. following chest wall trauma such as stab wounds or fractured ribs. Thoracentesis, pleural biopsy or the insertion of a central venous catheter or pacemaker can likewise result in pleural rupture. Thoracic surgery itself creates a pneumothorax because of the necessity of entering the pleural cavity to reach the lung tissue. Positive pressure ventilation, particularly when positive end-expiratory pressure is used, can also cause a pneumothorax since it involves raised airway pressure throughout the entire respiratory cycle. Rupture of the oesophagus can also allow air to enter the pleural space.

Tension pneumothorax
Tension pneumothorax is a serious and potentially fatal condition, caused by air entering the pleural space on inspiration, which cannot escape during expiration, resulting in progressive compression of the underlying lung. If left untreated, a tracheal and mediastinal shift towards the unaffected lung can occur, compromising both the ventilation of that lung and venous return to the heart, resulting in shock and potential death.

Small pneumothoraces usually resolve spontaneously because the air is reabsorbed from the pleural space. Larger pneumothoraces may require the insertion of an underwater seal chest drain, or Heimlich valve, to facilitate air drainage and consequently the resolution of the surface tension within the pleural spaces as the lung re-expands. Recurrence of spontaneous pneumothoraces may result in consideration for surgical intervention, i.e. pleurodesis or pleurectomy.

Pleural effusion

Pleural effusion is an abnormal accumulation of fluid in the pleural space because of changes in hydrostatic pressure. Causes of pleural effusion include malignant disease, infection, congestive heart failure, hypoprotein states, atelectasis and following radiotherapy.

The size of the effusion will influence the patient's presenting symptoms: i.e. the degree of dyspnoea experienced (ranging from mild to severe) and the degree of pain experienced (chest or referred shoulder pain). The pulmonary symptoms result from the space-occupying effects of the fluid within the pleural space and may include cough, fever, sweats and sputum production. A fluid volume of 300 mL or more can be seen on X-ray along with a mediastinal shift, depending on the volume of fluid collection.

Thoracentesis
Thoracentesis will provide a definitive diagnosis, and small effusions may be effectively drained in this way. Larger or recurrent effusions may require the insertion of a chest drain, since repeated thoracentesis can cause loculation, whereby the fluid collects in multiple pockets caused by adhesions from repeated aspiration attempts. Palliative surgery, such as pleurodesis, may

be required in malignant disease where repeated collections of fluid are problematic, thus preventing further accumulations.

Empyema

Pleural empyema, i.e. pyothorax, is a collection of infected or purulent fluid within the pleural space. It represents the end stage of a pathological process starting with a contaminated pleural effusion following bacterial pneumonia, the rupture of a lung abscess into the pleural space, or from a subphrenic abscess. Bronchopleural fistulae, traumatic penetration of the pleura and the necessity for prolonged use of chest drains can likewise result in infection. Empyema classically starts as an infection of low-viscosity pleural effusion with an underlying lung that is fully expansible. The progression of the empyema will eventually reduce lung capacity because of increasing viscosity of the fluid and the development of a thick, fibrous walled cavity surrounding the infected fluid.

Patients with empyema can experience pleural pain and fever. Initial treatment of the empyema may be conservative, with attempts to drain the empyema using chest drains and antibiotics. Chronic, cavitated empyema requires surgical intervention because drainage alone will not prevent recurrence of a collection of infected fluid within the cavity. The surgical procedure includes decortication and drainage of the fluid.

Malignant disease of the pleura

Primary malignancy of the pleura is rare and is associated with exposure to asbestos. Of the primary pleural tumours that do occur, most are mesotheliomas of which there are two types:

- *Pleural fibroma*: a localized fibrous mesothelioma which may be treated by surgical excision.
- *Diffuse malignant mesothelioma*: a thick fibrous sheet producing rapidly occurring high-volume pleural effusions. It carries a poor prognosis and surgery is purely palliative in an attempt to prevent further effusion forming.

MALIGNANT DISEASE OF THE LUNG

Bronchogenic carcinoma refers to a malignant tumour of the lung arising within the wall or epithelial lining of the bronchus. The lung is also a common site for metastatic spread from cancer elsewhere within the body.

Lung cancer is the most prevalent form of cancer, with approximately 40 000 cases diagnosed a year (British Thoracic Society and Society of Cardiothoracic

Surgeons of Great Britain and Ireland Working Party, 2001). The extraordinary rise in the incidence of lung cancer in the 20th century is attributed to cigarette smoking. It is still more common in men, who account for nearly 80% of cases, although the male/female ratio is falling due to the increased uptake of smoking among women. The reduction in coal fires and urban air pollution, however, is contributing to a slowing of the epidemic (Kadri and Treasure, 1993).

Histological types of lung cancer

There are four histological types of lung cancer:

- *Squamous cell carcinoma* (incidence is 40–70%): it arises in the epithelium of large bronchi and so the tumour is therefore located centrally in the lung fields. Five-year survival following diagnosis is 16–18%. Squamous cell carcinoma is a slow-growing tumour which has a greater potential for operability than other cell types (Margereson and Riley, 2003).

- *Small cell carcinoma* (incidence is 20%): it develops in the central airways from the epithelium of large bronchi – a common cause is smoking. The 5-year survival rate is very poor, owing to its high potential for rapid growth and early metastases. It is an aggressive tumour with very poor potential for surgery, because it is usually unresectable on presentation and associated with widespread dissemination. In contrast to other forms of cancer, this type of carcinoma responds moderately well to chemotherapy (Margereson and Riley, 2003).

- *Adenocarcinoma* (incidence is 5–15%) and *large cell carcinoma* (incidence is 7%): both of these arise peripherally, have the potential to form metastases and respond poorly to systemic treatment. They are occasionally operable (Margereson and Riley, 2003).

The poor survival rates of patients with these cancers are due to its insidious development, with symptoms becoming evident only later in the progress of the disease. Occasionally, the presence of a tumour is detected early as part of X-ray screening for routine medical examinations. These patients may feel fit and well and have difficulty accepting that such a diagnosis has been made.

An international coding system for stage grouping is used in the diagnosis of lung cancer, which enables the medical team to optimise therapeutic interventions. Three areas are considered:

T = tumour size
N = nodal involvement
M = possible metastatic spread

- Stage IA (T1, N0, M0): tumour <3 cm, involving the lung or visceral pleural without nodal involvement or metastatic spread.
- Stage IB (T2, N0, M0): tumour >3 cm, with involvement of the main bronchus more than 2 cm distally to the carina. No nodal or metastatic spread despite some pressure or obstructive problems.
- Stage IIA (T1, N1, M0): tumour <3 cm, with associated involvement of the hilar nodes but without metastatic spread.
- Stage IIB (T2, N1, M0) tumour >3 cm, with involvement of the main bronchus, visceral pleura and obstructive problems but no metastatic spread.

(Adapted from Margereson and Riley, 2003.)

SPECIFIC INVESTIGATIONS REQUIRED PRIOR TO SURGERY

Many investigative procedures are dependent upon patient cooperation for their success, with the evident need for clear explanations and informed consent. The period of investigation is one of extreme anxiety for the patient, because of the uncertainty about diagnosis, treatment and possible outcomes. Many of these investigations are performed with the outcome of malignancy as a possibility.

CHEST X-RAY

Chest X-ray can be used to observe the progression and detect alterations within the lungs caused by disease processes; determine the position of chest drains and central venous lines; and evaluate the effectiveness of treatment. Chest X-rays do not allow definitive diagnoses to be formed except in the case of pneumothorax.

Standard chest X-rays are taken in two directions:

- *Posteroanterior (PA) view*: the patient stands in front of the film and is X-rayed from behind. As the heart is in the anterior half of the chest, this view produces less cardiac magnification. The patient stands with their hands on their hips so that the scapulae are displaced to the sides of the chest and do not overlap the lung fields.
- *Lateral view*: generally, a left lateral film is taken where the patient stands with their left side against the film. This view provides less cardiac magnification and a sharper image of the left lower lobe, which is partially obscured on the posteroanterior view by cardiac shadow. Similarly, a right lateral film will produce sharper images of a right-sided lesion.

Portable films are required in the immediate postoperative phase or while the patient is critically ill. A portable film is taken with the film behind the patient and is therefore an anteroposterior view. Interpretation of the film requires skill due to the shadows superimposed by sheets, nightclothes and any tubes, etc. The scapulae may also be evident.

Chest X-rays are usually taken with the patient maintaining full inspiration. Expiratory films may be helpful when detecting small pneumothoraces, because the lung volume is reduced while the volume of pleural air remains the same but occupies a greater percentage of the thoracic volume.

COMPUTERIZED AXIAL TOMOGRAPHY

Computerized axial tomography (CAT) scanning is invaluable in the investigation of pulmonary disorders because the clarity of the images is superior to that of those produced by conventional radiography. The non-invasive cross-sectional views create images that will confirm chest wall invasion by tumour involvement, metastatic spread or small metastic nodes.

POSITRON EMISSION TOMOGRAPHY

Positron emission tomography (PET) is a nuclear medicine technique that measures biochemical and metabolic activity of cells following the injection of a positron-emitting isotrope. PET scanning is useful in the detection and staging of malignant cells.

MAGNETIC RESONANCE IMAGING

Magnetic resonance imaging (MRI) is a non-invasive procedure whereby the patient is placed within a magnetic field and microwave radio signals are passed over the body, interacting with hydrogen. An image is then generated because the hydrogen atoms absorb the image.

LUNG (PULMONARY) FUNCTION TESTS

Lung function tests are a means of assessing the functional status of the lungs. Measurements can determine tidal volumes, rates of gas flow and the stiffness, i.e. compliance, of the lungs and chest wall. The diffusion characteristics of gas movement across the alveolar–capillary membrane can also be demonstrated.

Lung function tests are not a diagnostic tool. They are, however, of value in distinguishing between a restrictive defect within the lungs, e.g. pleural effusion or rib fractures, and an obstructive defect, e.g. asthma or emphysema. The importance of lung function testing in the context of surgery lies within the assessment of the degree of pulmonary involvement in the diseased lungs, and the assessment of pulmonary function prior to anaesthesia.

The primary tool in lung function tests is the spirometer, which is designed to measure lung volumes and gas flows. Spirometry is now also performed with small, portable, hand-held devices. The tracings from spirometry show the ratio between the volume of air expired in one second (FEV_1) compared with the total volume of expired air (FVC). Normal lung function would show an FEV_1/FVC ratio of 75–80%. A ratio of less than 70% is found in patients with air flow obstruction. In restrictive disorders the FVC is reduced but the FEV_1 is normal, which may show a ratio of over 80% (Kendrick and Smith, 1992).

Peak expiratory flow rate (PEFR), commonly known as peak flow, is also used to determine functional status of the lungs, since it determines the maximal flow of air from the lungs during forced exhalation. It correlates closely with the FEV_1 described above, and provides a readily available measure of lung function.

OXYGEN SATURATIONS

Non-invasive assessment of oxygen saturation can be performed by pulse oximetry. This technique measures the absorption of selected wavelengths of light passed through a finger, toe or earlobe. As blood loses oxygen in the capillary beds, it becomes less permeable to red light. The oximeter measures the differences in light absorption and converts the value to a percentage, representing the level of oxygen saturation of the haemoglobin. False readings may be obtained when patients have received intravascular dyes, in jaundiced patients who have raised plasma bilirubin levels or if the patient is wearing coloured nail polish (Hatchett and Thompson, 2001).

SPUTUM EXAMINATION

Respiratory secretions may be sent for bacteriological or cytological examination to ensure appropriate treatment is prescribed. Cytological examination is appropriate if malignancy is suspected, because malignant cells may be shed into the airways. However, a negative result is not necessarily indicative of a diagnosis of non-malignancy.

ARTERIAL BLOOD GAS ANALYSIS

Arterial blood gas analysis provides precise information concerning the acid–base balance and the level of oxygen and carbon dioxide present in arterial blood. Accurate interpretation of the results requires knowledge

Table 14.4	Arterial blood gas measurements
Parameter	Range
pH	7.35–7.45
PO_2	11.5–13.5 kPa
PCO_2	4.5–6.0 kPa
HCO_3	25–30 mmol/L
Saturation	95–99%
Base excess	−2 to +2

Source: Hatchett and Thompson (2001).

of the patient's total clinical picture, including treatments. Arterial blood is used for the sample, as it contains levels of oxygen and carbon dioxide that are determined by the lungs. Venous blood does not reflect lung function.

The arterial samples are commonly obtained from the radial artery, the femoral artery and occasionally the brachial artery. Alternatively, arterial samples may be taken from an arterial line if the patient has one. Normal gas measurements of arterial blood are shown in Table 14.4.

BRONCHOSCOPY

Bronchoscopy is an endoscopic view of the tracheo-bronchial tree using either a flexible fibreoptic, rigid or laser bronchoscope. A bronchoscopy can be diagnostic, or therapeutic, i.e. for alleviation of stenosis or removal of a foreign body, and is performed under a local or general anaesthetic.

The procedure involves the passage of a bronchoscope through the larynx and the trachea into the major airway branches. The bronchial walls can be visualized, and biopsies, brushings and aspirate taken for examination, and non-surgical interventions applied. The patient is placed in a recumbent position or an upright position, supported with pillows. The bronchoscope is then advanced into the trachea either through the nose or the mouth (Fig. 14.3). Six hours of fasting is required prior to the procedure to reduce the risk of aspiration should the patient vomit.

Rigid bronchoscopy

This is a palliative procedure usually performed under general anaesthesia for the relief of airway obstruction within the tracheal and main bronchi. Rigid bronchoscopies are also performed for biopsies and for the retrieval of inhaled foreign objects. Stenting, laser ablation, and bronchial brachytherapy, a delivery of high

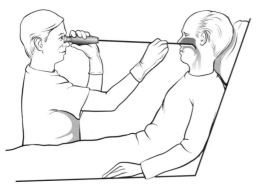

Figure 14.3   Fibreoptic bronchoscopy (pernasal). The patient adopts a sitting position. The bronchoscope is passed directly backwards through the nose, into the nasopharynx. (From Stradling, 1991.)

doses of radiation over a short period of time without damaging healthy tissue, can be implemented via this route. Complications following this procedure include haemorrhage and pneumothorax (Seijo and Stenman, 2001).

Fibreoptic (flexible) bronchoscopy

The patients are required to fast prior to the procedure to prevent potential aspiration should the patient vomit, because the larynx and upper airway are anaesthetized prior to the insertion of the bronchoscope. The patient is placed in a recumbent or upright position, supported with pillows. The bronchoscope is advanced into the trachea either through the nose or mouth in order to visualize the upper airways and airways distal to the main bronchial tree.

Potential complications following bronchoscopy

Complications following bronchoscopy are rare. However, pneumothorax, bleeding, cardiac arrhythmias and worsening hypoxia may occur (Margereson and Riley, 2003). Post-procedure care includes maintenance of the airway and observation for laryngeal spasm (which usually resolves spontaneously but may require a high concentration of humidified oxygen until it does so). Fasting is required following local anaesthetic until the effects have worn off. The gag reflex can be tested with sips of water, and this should precede free drinking and eating. Fluids can be taken approximately 2 hours post procedure because topical anaesthetic is sprayed into the throat. It is common for sputum to be bloodstained following a bronchoscopy, especially if biopsies have been taken.

TRANSTHORACIC/PERCUTANEOUS NEEDLE BIOPSY

This investigation is used when peripheral lung lesions are present, particularly unresectable lesions, in order to determine the choice of treatment: i.e. chemotherapy or radical radiotherapy. A biopsy needle is inserted into the lungs to gain aspirate for cytology or tissue samples for histology. Pneumothoraces can be a complication of either procedure. A chest X-ray is performed following the procedure and it may be required for the patient to stay in hospital overnight.

Contraindications for this procedure include coagulopathies, multiple emphysematous bullae, haemoptysis or air embolus. An open lung biopsy under a general anaesthetic may be required when transthoracic/percutaneous or bronchoscopy methods have been unsuccessful. The biopsy will therefore need to be obtained via a small thoracotomy incision (Margereson and Riley, 2003). The procedure may be performed with a view to proceeding with resectional surgery, following confirmation of histology by examination of a frozen section.

MEDIASTINOSCOPY AND MEDIASTINOTOMY

This is a diagnostic technique to establish the histology of enlarged mediastinal lymph nodes found by chest X-ray or imaging. The approach is via an incision midway between the bottom of the sternal notch and the cricoid cartilage, allowing the examination of the mediastinum and obtaining a biopsy. The mediastinoscope is passed through the incision into the tract made by finger dissection through the pretracheal fascia (Fig. 14.4). Complications of the procedure include haemorrhage and hoarseness due to damage of the recurrent laryngeal nerve and pneumothorax.

Anterior mediastinotomy is an alternative approach used to reach nodes that are inaccessible by mediastinoscopy. Nodes around the aortic arch to the left of the tracheal bifurcation and anterior mediastinal nodes on either side of the chest can be accessed via this route. The incision is made over the second cartilage/intercostal space, and may involve opening of the pleura in order to inspect the hilum.

THORACOSCOPY

A rigid thoracoscope is inserted into the pleural space, unless pleural adhesions are present to obstruct the passage or view of the thoracoscope. Access is gained via the intercostal spaces. Other procedures can also be performed through the thoracoscope: for example,

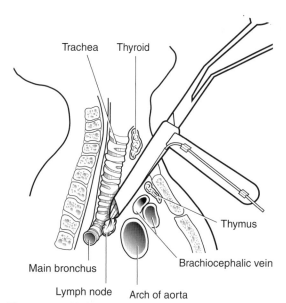

Trachea   Thyroid

Thymus

Brachiocephalic vein

Main bronchus

Lymph node   Arch of aorta

Figure 14.4   Mediastinoscopy. Diagram of a mediastinoscope in position, anterior to the trachea, allowing biopsy of a lymph node in the region of the main carina. (Reproduced from Crompton, 1987, with permission of Blackwell Science Ltd.)

pleurodesis by poudrage (using powder), biopsy or pleurectomy. A chest drain is usually inserted following the procedure to reinflate the lung.

PREOPERATIVE CARE

The psychological stress of patients awaiting surgery is well documented in the literature. In particular, classic studies have shown that detailed preoperative information tends to effect a reduction in stress and anxiety (Mitchell, 1997) and a reduction in the requirement for postoperative analgesics (Hayward, 1975). However, the specific needs of thoracic patients awaiting surgery are not well defined. It is known that patients who are in good physical health, but who require admission for surgery, have higher levels of anxiety than those who are ill on admission (Livingstone et al, 1993). This is of particular relevance to thoracic patients, since those waiting for surgery for conditions such as persistent pneumothorax, or those who have been found to have a malignancy on a routine medical examination, often feel well when admitted electively. The patient will also be anxious about the possibility of malignancy and whether their condition is operable because the surgeon cannot guarantee that resection is possible until surgery is underway. In these circumstances, the

patients fear that they will recover from the anaesthetic to learn that the surgeon has been unable to proceed. Patients will often attend a preadmission clinic, which provides an opportunity for both patients and their relatives to discuss the implications of surgery, as well as allow the patient to undergo other preoperative investigations (Mitchell, 1997).

The role of the nurse in the preoperative phase is to obtain a comprehensive nursing assessment taking into account any personal, social, medical, psychological, spiritual or cultural needs. The nurse will also ensure that the patient is fully prepared for their procedure, and that the appropriate and relevant information is provided to meet individual need. Some regional centres have written their own information booklets, supporting the verbal information provided.

Assessment of the patient prior to surgery may include some or all of the investigations described earlier, some of which may have occurred in the outpatient setting. Occasionally, investigations such as chest X-rays may be repeated to observe for disease progression. The preoperative phase will also include the recording of a 12-lead electrocardiogram (ECG) to assess fitness for general anaesthesia, and blood testing for haemoglobin levels, clotting screen and cross-matching. Usually 2 units of blood will be requested to be made available for the surgery and immediate postoperative period.

During the preoperative phase, a physiotherapist will assess the patient and discuss the breathing exercises that need to be performed postoperatively. Other multidisciplinary personnel may need to be involved: e.g. the dietician if the patient is undernourished or has lost weight through disease progression. The patient will be required to fast preoperatively, according to the protocol of the unit, and to undergo skin preparation which may include bathing and hair removal from the operation site.

THORACIC SURGICAL PROCEDURES

THORACOTOMY

Thoracotomy is the normal surgical approach to the lungs and pleura, although exposure of the anterior mediastinum may be made via a median sternotomy. This latter approach may also be utilized when there are bilateral pulmonary lesions, or to perform bilateral pleural surgery.

Thoracotomy incisions, approximately 20–22 cm long, are made along the line of the fifth intercostal space, with the underlying chest muscles being incised in layers. Thoracotomy approaches may be made in several ways, but, commonly, are either an anterolateral incision, which is situated more to the front of the chest, or a posterolateral incision, which is placed more towards the back. The patient is positioned into the lateral decubitus position.

Following the incision, access to the thoracic organs is facilitated through the spreading of the ribs and entry of the pleura is accomplished. The patient is ventilated throughout the procedure with a double-lumen endotracheal tube, which enables the anaesthetist to ventilate selectively through the right or left main bronchus. While the surgery is in progress, the operated lung is deflated and the patient is ventilated entirely through the other lung. Prior to closing the chest, the affected lung is reventilated and inflated, allowing the surgeon to check the security of any suture lines, testing their ability to withstand the pressure changes occurring throughout the respiratory cycle, and one or two intercostal drains are then inserted.

The thoracotomy approach allows several surgical procedures to be performed, and these are detailed below.

PULMONARY RESECTION

Resectional surgery is performed to remove malignant or infected portions of the lung. Resectional surgery usually follows the anatomical divisions of the lungs and may involve:

- removal of a whole lung: pneumonectomy
- removal of one or two lobes of a lung: lobectomy
- removal of a segment of a lung: segmentectomy
- removal of lung tissue without reference to anatomical divisions: wedge resection

(Margereson and Riley, 2003).

The extent of the resection depends upon several factors: the size, location and cell type of the tumour. A tumour which does not cross a fissure within the lung, and is located within one lobe, may be treated by lobectomy or possible segmentectomy. Tumours which cross the fissures and affect more than one lobe will require more extensive resection. Tumours which affect the hilum of the lung may require pneumonectomy since removal of the entire tumour may not be otherwise possible.

Pulmonary function may demand a more limited resection than is desirable, in order to conserve adequate lung function following surgery. This would be particularly relevant in patients with limited lung function due to asthma or emphysema.

Resectional surgery may also be performed using bronchoplastic procedures, which aim to preserve lung tissue while removing a diseased section of the bronchus. The free ends of the bronchus are then anastomosed together. An example of this type of surgery is a sleeve resection, where an upper lobe is removed with a sleeve of main bronchus, and the remaining lower lobe is then anastomosed by its bronchus to the trachea.

Segmentectomy

Segmentectomy is indicated for patients with limited pulmonary reserve. The procedure involves a blunt dissection and resection of the bronchopulmonary segment. Chest drains are inserted following the procedure to aid lung reinflation and drainage of haemoserous fluid.

Lobectomy

Lobectomy is the removal of a lobe of the lung as a result of benign/malignant tumours.

Pneumonectomy

Pneumonectomy is the removal of one lung because of a primary carcinoma or infection.

The pneumonectomy space

Changes occur in the pneumonectomy space following resection of the whole lung. The space is reduced by diaphragmatic elevation to less than that previously occupied by lung tissue. In the immediate postoperative period the space is filled with air (during the final stages of surgery centrality of the mediastinum is ensured by regulation of the volume of gas in the space). Occasionally, patients develop dyspnoea and deteriorating oxygen saturation levels following surgery and a chest X-ray may reveal deviation of the trachea and mediastinum, usually away from the space, compromising existing lung function. Correction can be achieved through removal of a volume of air or blood from the space, with a repeat chest X-ray to check tracheal alignment.

Bleeding into the space occurs within the first 36 hours following surgery, producing a visible fluid level above the diaphragm on chest X-ray. In some centres, the volume of fluid accumulating within the space may be regulated for the first 24 hours with a chest drain, which is kept clamped, but released for 1 minute every hour. This procedure allows fluid to accumulate slowly and any increase in the rate of blood loss to be observed. The volume of gas within the space gradually lessens, as firstly the carbon dioxide and then the oxygen within the air is reabsorbed. Over the ensuing days the fluid volume is increased by an inflammatory exudate, and it gradually changes in nature from a fluid state to become a more solid substance by changes within the fibrin content. The final changes in the space occur slowly, involving the reabsorption of nitrogen and the development of a negative pressure with a slight shift in the centrality of the mediastinum. This promotes the formation and accumulation of a low-protein fluid, effectively filling the remainder of the space (Foss, 1989).

The space remaining following lobectomy is much smaller. Filling of this space is achieved by elevation of the diaphragm, and expansion of the remaining lobes of the lung.

PLEURAL SURGERY

Indications for pleural surgery are spontaneous and recurrent pneumothoraces.

Pleurectomy

Pleurectomy involves stripping the parietal pleura away from the apex and posterolateral surface of the lung via a small posterolateral thoracotomy incision or a less-invasive, keyhole approach using video-assisted thoracic surgery (VATS) (Society of Cardiothoracic Surgeons, 2002). Complete pleurectomy is impossible since the parietal pleura cannot be stripped from the diaphragm. The ensuing inflammatory response, as a result of stripping of the pleura, causes adhesion of the visceral pleura (with underlying lung) to the chest wall. Where parietal pleura remains, adhesion is achieved by mechanical abrasion to produce the required inflammatory response. The surgery is completed with the insertion of chest drains.

Pleurodesis

Pleurodesis involves stimulating an inflammatory response to promote the formation of adhesions, by either the instillation of iodized talc, i.e. chemical pleurodesis, or by mechanical abrasion of the pleural surfaces, in an attempt to promote pleural adhesion via a VATS or thoracotomy incision. This procedure is useful in preventing the recurrent pleural effusions associated with malignant disease. One or two chest drains are inserted at the close of the procedure.

Procedures involving the pleura are very painful and careful attention to pain control is required following surgery to ensure that the patient can breathe easily. Unresolved pain will cause the patient to minimize breathing, so compromising lung expansion.

THORACOSCOPY

Advances in thoracoscopic techniques have resulted in the use of telescopes and video-assisted devices that project magnified images onto video-recording monitors, enabling the surgeon to perform pulmonary and mediastinal resections, biopsies, thymectomies and drainage of pericardial and pleural effusions. In many cases, thoracoscopic procedures have replaced the need for thoracotomy, with consequent benefits of greatly reduced incisions, i.e. two to four small puncture sites of 5–7 mm instead of a thoracotomy incision, less pain and less restricted muscle activity in the shoulder (that results from dissection through muscle in thoracotomies).

Thoracoscopic procedures still necessitate the insertion of chest drains at surgery, but these seldom remain in situ for longer than 2 days.

DRAINAGE OF EMPYEMA AND DECORTICATION

This technique involves the removal of the thick fibrous crust from the surface of the lung and the chest wall via a post lateral small thoracotomy, in order to allow the underlying lung to re-expand. The surgery often causes a large blood loss, which may continue following surgery. Chest drains will be inserted to monitor the severity of blood loss following the procedure.

Some patients may not tolerate decortication, so open drainage may be considered. This option necessitates a rib resection to facilitate the insertion of a large-bore chest drain. The drain is cut short and the end inserted into a stoma bag for drainage. It may be left in situ for long periods of time, as necessary. This drain is an exception to other intercostal drains in that an underwater seal is not required. The empyema cavity is sealed by the fibrous coating with no connection to the pleural space. An open drain is therefore possible without the danger of pneumothorax.

LUNG VOLUME REDUCTION

This procedure is performed via a median sternotomy to allow the excision of 25–30% of volume from each lung, in an attempt to improve elastic recall and reduce respiratory workload as a result of severe empyema.

THYMECTOMY

The thymus gland lies retrosternally within the mediastinum (see Fig. 14.4), and enlargement of the gland may cause respiratory embarrassment due to exerted pressure. Tumours of the thymus may be benign (e.g. cysts or teratomas) or malignant (e.g. carcinoma or sarcoma). The prognosis following surgical resection is directly related to the aggressiveness of the lesion and the associated systemic disorder. Myasthenia gravis is an autoimmune disorder of neuromuscular transmission, characterized by weakness and fatigue of voluntary muscles. Many patients with myasthenia gravis have pathological changes within the thymus gland. In these cases thymectomy may influence the clinical course of the disorder. Thymectomy is usually performed via a median sternotomy and a chest drain is inserted postoperatively.

LUNG TRANSPLANTATION

Lung transplants have been successfully completed for over two decades. Between 1991 and 2001, 1095 lung transplants were carried out within the UK and Ireland, averaging 125–169 a year (British Heart Foundation, 2003). Initially, lung transplantation was limited to patients with pulmonary vascular disease, but it is now used successfully in those with end-stage parenchymal lung disease, including cystic fibrosis (Murday and Madden, 1996). The main indications for lung transplantation include severe respiratory failure despite maximal medical therapy (in practice the FEV_1 is usually less than 30% of the predicted value); severely impaired quality of life; and a positive attitude of the patient towards transplantation. Single lung transplantation is performed via a posterolateral thoracotomy,

with the anastomosis being made at the level of the main bronchus (Murday and Madden, 1996). Immuno-suppressive medication will need to be taken to suppress any graft rejection.

Survival rates post-transplantation are as follows, with infection and obstructive lung disease being the main cause of death (British Cardiac Society, 2003):

- 1 year – 76%
- 3 years – 57%
- 5 years – 42%.

POSTOPERATIVE CARE

The priorities of nursing care following thoracic surgery are broadly similar, irrespective of the type of surgery that the patient has undergone: i.e. assessment and maintenance of respiratory and haemodynamic status and provision of adequate pain control. Table 14.5 illustrates the postoperative care for a patient following thoracic surgery.

Table 14.5 Postoperative care following thoracic surgery

Nursing priorities	Rationale
Haemodynamic monitoring Following surgery the patient will need to be closely observed and monitored.	To observe the postoperative recovery of the patient.
Assessment of temperature, pulse, blood pressure and respiratory rate are performed initially half hourly and reduced in frequency as the patient becomes stable.	To assess for any haemodynamic changes that may indicate bleeding, shock, respiratory distress or infection.
A chest X-ray may be required within a few hours of surgery.	To observe for centrality of the mediastinum and reinflation of the lung.
Following pneumonectomy, cardiac monitoring may be required.	Possibility of cardiac dysrhythmias following pneumonectomy if the pericardium has been opened.
Respiratory assessment Careful observation of oxygen saturations is required, either by continuous monitoring or at the time of other vital signs measurement.	To ensure that the patient is receiving oxygen at an adequate percentage, particularly if pneumonectomy or other resection has been performed.
Some routine arterial blood gas samples may be taken in the early postoperative stages.	To monitor all respiratory parameters, including PO_2 and PCO_2.
Oxygen, set at the prescribed rate, and using a delivery system that humidifies and permits precise oxygen percentages, should be utilized.	Humidification facilitates expectoration of sputum by maintaining the moisture within the secretions.
Pain control Careful attention to the patient's experience of pain is required, to minimize the pain as far as possible.	Patients who are in pain will be reluctant to breathe deeply and cough, increasing their risk of chest infection. They will also be reluctant to move around in bed, increasing risk of pressure ulcers and deep vein thrombosis.
Several methods of pain control are available: Patient-controlled analgesia (PCA) is becoming	Patient-controlled analgesia facilitates patient involvement, allowing them a degree of control over their pain.

(Continued)

Table 14.5   *(Continued)*

Nursing priorities	Rationale
increasingly popular following thoracic surgery, and is an effective method of pain control if the patients are adequately prepared preoperatively in its use. PCA utilizes opioid analgesics and commonly an antiemetic. Use of any opioids necessitates careful respiratory monitoring.	Careful preoperative teaching is required, as the patient may not wish to be bothered to learn following surgery. Opioid analgesics can cause depression of the respiratory centre.
Some centres use epidural analgesia, again an effective means of pain control, but this may hinder mobility of the patient.	The patient is generally on bedrest until the epidural catheter has been removed. Some urinary retention may also be observed, due to reduced sensation.
Continuous intravenous infusion of opioid analgesics	An effective delivery system; controlled by the nurse.
Pain control needs to be continually reviewed, particularly as intravenous forms are changed to oral preparations.	Continuous assessment is necessary to ensure that the patient's pain is effectively managed.
Pain levels may be significantly reduced following removal of the chest drain.	The chest drain is a significant factor in the pain experienced by the patient.
Fluid balance Maintenance of crystalloid fluid will be prescribed.	To prevent dehydration of the patient, and to replace any small volume blood loss.
Fluid balance will need to be maintained in accordance with: • blood loss	Larger volume blood loss will need to be replaced with plasma expanders or blood, to sustain blood pressure and to maintain the oxygen-carrying capacity of the blood.
• blood pressure	To maintain a blood pressure that sustains systemic perfusion.
• urine output	Low urine output may indicate a dehydrated state.
• central venous pressure (CVP).	In the absence of urine output, a CVP measurement will indicate whether the patient is dehydrated and needs fluids, or whether the patient is volume overloaded and needs diuretics to stimulate renal function.
The patient will be able to commence small volumes of fluid and progress to a light diet when able, unless any oesophageal surgery has been performed, or an anaesthetic spray applied to the throat.	To encourage drinking and eating as tolerated by the patient. Oesophageal surgery will require the patient to be nil by mouth to allow anastomoses to heal. Anaesthetic throat spray can cause the patient to aspirate while swallowing.
Chest drain Most thoracic procedures will result in one or two chest drains being inserted.	Chest drains facilitate lung re-expansion by the drainage of blood and air from the pleural space.
The chest drains will be connected to an underwater seal drainage unit.	The underwater seal acts as a one-way valve, permitting air draining from the chest to bubble through the water, but it cannot return to the chest.
A low vacuum suction may be applied.	A low vacuum encourages drainage from the chest, and therefore re-expansion of the lung.
Blood loss into the drainage bottle should be recorded at least hourly for the first 24–48 hours. Observe the drain for swinging of the fluid level within the tube.	To monitor rate of blood loss, and to ensure large losses are replaced. Swinging corresponds to pressure changes within the lungs during respirations but may be absent if the drain becomes blocked, or if suction is applied. The fluid will move towards the patient on inspiration and away from the patient on expiration. This movement may be masked in the presence of suction. If the patient is ventilated by positive pressure ventilation, the pattern will be reversed, i.e. moves away from the patient during inspiration.
Observe the drain for bubbling.	Bubbling corresponds to the drainage of air from the chest during expiration and coughing. It signifies a patent drain. Bubbling may be vigorous, particularly if suction is applied, and may be continuous with

(Continued)

Table 14.5   (*Continued*)

Nursing priorities	Rationale
	suction. In the absence of suction, bubbling will be associated with expiratory activity and coughing. Both bubbling and swinging may diminish as the lung becomes fully inflated.
Ensure that the chest drain bottle remains lower than chest level. See text for differences in the care of pneumonectomy drains.	Facilitates drainage of fluid from the chest. Prevents siphoning of fluid back into the pleural space.
Chest physiotherapy The aim of physiotherapy is to promote deep breathing, coughing and mobility. Initially, the patient is encouraged to sit upright. The physiotherapist, who was involved preoperatively, sees the patient soon after surgery.	This will help to facilitate re-expansion of the lung. To facilitate optimum lung expansion. To encourage the patient to take deep breaths and cough, to ensure the operated lung is quickly restored to full expansion and to remove any retained secretions. This will also help to prevent a chest infection.
Between the physiotherapist's visits the nursing staff continue to encourage deep breaths and coughs. As the postoperative course progresses, the physiotherapist will be involved in helping the patient to mobilize.	Mobility, as exercise, is an effective means of encouraging good lung expansion.
Mobility Pressure area relief must be provided while the patient is in bed. The patient is encouraged to sit out of bed on day 1 following surgery. Progressive mobilization is encouraged on the following days, particularly once the chest drains are removed. The patient is encouraged to begin mobilizing to the bathroom initially, and then to go for longer walks. The patient will be observed climbing a flight of stairs prior to discharge. Mobility of the affected shoulder is encouraged through exercises provided by the physiotherapist.	Thoracic patients tend to predominantly sit upright, causing a lot of pressure on the skin of their sacrum. Early mobilization is encouraged to prevent complications of bedrest. Progressive mobility, to maintain lung expansion, challenge the breathing to a slight degree of dyspnoea to improve exercise tolerance. To restore normal range of a range of movement and to prevent a frozen shoulder.
Wound care Theatre dressings are observed regularly in the early postoperative phase. Theatre dressings are left intact for 48 hours (or according to unit protocol). Wound observation and care according to unit protocol. Removal of staples/sutures according to protocol.	To observe for bleeding from the incision. To prevent wound infection. The wound should be regularly observed for signs of exudate or infection. The staples/sutures are commonly removed prior to discharge, or arrangements made with the community team to remove them following discharge.

POTENTIAL COMPLICATIONS FOLLOWING THORACIC SURGERY

Respiratory failure

Respiratory failure is the inability to maintain adequate gaseous exchange. Causes include surgically induced haemopneumothorax, pneumonia, atelectasis and occasionally the administration of opioids for pain relief. This will be indicated by shortness of breath, reduced respiration rate, decreased oxygen saturation levels, abnormal arterial blood gases, reduced lung expansion, respiratory sounds and cyanosis. Upright positioning of the patient, use of prescribed oxygen therapy, titrated against oxygen saturations levels, and provision of reassurance should be included in patient management.

Haemorrhage

Blood loss can become more apparent following surgery, when blood pressure stabilizes and small vessels begin to bleed, which were previously prevented from doing so either by vasoconstriction or by hypotension. More serious bleeding can occur from larger vessels such as the pulmonary artery or vein, and will require further surgery to repair the defect. Management of haemorrhage includes oxygen and fluid administration and correction of any coagulation problems by either returning to theatre or drug administration, depending on the cause of bleeding.

Sputum retention

Sputum retention is the accumulation of secretions in the lower tracheobronchial tree, and can be detected as airway obstruction, with hypoxia and respiratory acidosis due to retained carbon dioxide and inadequate oxygenation. The nursing management includes administration of humidified oxygen or nebulized saline and bronchodilators; bronchoscopy to remove the plug of sputum; or mini-tracheotomy to permit airway suction.

Chest infections

Chest infections can occur in patients who are unable to mobilize effectively, or cannot tolerate physiotherapy due to poor pain tolerance. They are more common if the patient was a smoker prior to surgery. Effective pain relief to permit mobilization and breathing exercises is vital to prevent this occurring.

Cardiac arrhythmias

Postoperative arrhythmias, atrial fibrillation or supraventricular tachycardia are experienced by 9–33% of patients following thoracic surgery (Amar, 1997). The use of oral or intravenous antiarrhythmic medication may be considered should the patient become compromised.

Bronchopleural fistula

A bronchopleural fistula is a communication between the airways and the pleura following surgery, and may be due to problems at the time of surgery involving disease of the bronchial stump, or stump breakdown at a later stage due to lack of healing or infection. It can occur following lobectomy, but is more common following pneumonectomy, and symptoms include the expectoration of pneumonectomy space fluid, and the potential for contamination of the remaining lung with infected fluid. Small fistulae may heal spontaneously, but may require the insertion of a chest drain to prevent movement of fluid into the airways. Surgery to the bronchial stump may include excision of infected or necrotic tissue and repair with pericardial or intercostal tissue.

Surgical emphysema

Surgical emphysema may be a consequence of a bronchopleural fistula, but not exclusively so, because it can also accompany a pneumothorax. Surgical emphysema indicates the presence of air in the subcutaneous tissues, particularly in the neck, chest wall and head. If the air leak in the chest is extensive, the surgical emphysema can be very debilitating, including complete closure of the eyelids through swelling, with consequent temporary blindness for the patient, and requirements for skilled nursing care. The subcutaneous air usually reabsorbs spontaneously when effective chest drainage is established.

NURSING MANAGEMENT OF INTERCOSTAL CHEST DRAINS

Intercostal (chest) drainage is required following surgery, to facilitate the drainage of air and blood from the chest, and to allow the lung to re-expand fully. Some nursing observations of the drain are noted in Table 14.5.

Chest drains are attached to a sterile water chamber, providing a one-way valve to allow air removal in

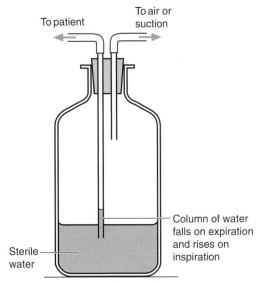

To patient   To air or suction

Column of water falls on expiration and rises on inspiration

Sterile water

Figure 14.5   Intercostal chest drainage bottle.

expiration (column of water falls or bubbling may occur) and prevention of air re-entry on inspiration (column of water rises) (Fig. 14.5). External suction can be added to the system to provide a greater negative pressure draw to assist in the expansion of the lung.

Clamping of the drains should be avoided, because air will build up within the thoracic cavity, creating an increase in positive pressure and thus increasing the potential for a tension pneumothorax. The stripping or milking of drains is an extremely controversial issue, and is strongly discouraged because of the associated increase in intrathoracic pressure and risk of pneumothorax.

Patients whose drains become disconnected are best treated by swift reconnection of the tubing, and, secondly, coughing to dispel any air, followed by a chest X-ray to assess for a change in condition should be undertaken.

Removal of the chest drain should only be considered when the lung has reinflated or the drainage has stopped. A modified Valsalva manoeuvre is employed while the drain is being withdrawn, i.e. the patient takes a full inspiration and holds their breath in order to diminish the risk of air entry into the pleura. Analgesics will be required prior to removal of the drain. The purse string suture ensures skin closure as the drain is removed. The suture is removed approximately 2–5 days later, or according to unit protocol. A small dressing is usually sufficient to absorb any local blood loss and can be removed the following day. Application of paraffin gauze (thought to prevent air leaks through the skin) is unnecessary; any obvious air leaks should be referred immediately to the medical team. A chest X-ray is usually advised following drain removal, to ensure that the lungs remain fully expanded (Laws et al, 2003).

SPECIFIC HEALTH EDUCATION/PATIENT TEACHING AND PREPARATION FOR DISCHARGE

Many people who have undergone pulmonary resection for lung cancer regard the surgery as curative and expect a fairly rapid return to good health. Those who have had a pneumonectomy may find that initially they are quite short of breath, due to reduced lung capacity and, if unprepared for this fact, may become quite disheartened. Careful preparation of each patient for discharge should include realistic expectations of exercise tolerance and how this may be improved. The physiotherapist will be closely involved in this aspect of discharge.

Patients preparing for discharge will require advice on a number of issues, including pain control, wound care, resumption of sexual activity, dietary advice and sports. The advice will need to be tailored according to the patient's age, surgery and presurgery fitness, as well as being specific to the individual unit policies.

The majority of patients will not return to work until they have been seen by the surgeon, i.e. 6–8 weeks postoperatively. Similarly, patients will be advised not to drive until after the appointment, and they need to inform their insurance company of their surgery.

Advice about smoking cessation may also be pertinent. Specific advice may be sought by some patients concerning permission to fly, and individual airlines will be able to give advice. It is difficult to be prescriptive concerning health education, since each patient has differing needs and levels of understanding, but attempts should be made to offer individualistic health education as appropriate.

CONCLUSION

Thoracic surgery is a rapidly expanding speciality, challenging the nurse working within this field. It is therefore essential that nurses should fully understand the anatomy and physiology of the respiratory system and associated surgical procedures.

This chapter has examined the respiratory system and reviewed current thoracic therapies in an attempt to ensure development of theoretical knowledge and advancement in clinical competence.

Summary of key points

- Knowledge of the normal physiology of the lungs is essential to an understanding of the altered physiology consequent to disease or surgery.

- Breathing is normally an automatic, rhythmic process that continues without conscious effort. Respiratory disease or thoracic surgery can disrupt this process to one of painful effort.

- Respiratory assessment is fundamental to the nursing care of respiratory patients undergoing surgery.

- Knowledge of the disease processes that alter respiratory anatomy and function will be important in assessing the resultant symptoms affecting the patient.

- Understanding of the investigative procedures that precede thoracic surgery is vital in order to prepare patients physically and psychologically. Sensory and procedural information are both important.

- The role of the nurse in the preoperative phase is essential in recording a comprehensive nursing assessment, taking account of personal, social, medical, psychological, spiritual and cultural needs.

- Thoracic surgical procedures are very painful and require skilled nursing care to alleviate pain and maintain optimum respiratory effort.

- Knowledge of postoperative nursing care and potential complications are vital to the safe recovery of the patient.

- Specific health education and health promotion opportunities should be actively sought, in order to ensure that the patient is fully informed to their satisfaction throughout the perioperative period.

References

Amar, D. (1997) Prevention and management of dysrhythmias following thoracic surgery. *Chest Surgery Clinics of North America* 7(4): 817–829.

British Cardiac Society (2003) http://www.bcs.com (accessed 20 April 2004).

British Heart Foundation (2003) http://www.bhf.org.uk (accessed 20 April 2004).

British Thoracic Society (2001) *The Burden of Lung Disease*. London: British Thoracic Society.

British Thoracic Society, Society of Cardiothoracic Surgeons of Great Britain and Ireland Working Party (2001) Guidelines on the selection of patients with lung cancer for surgery. *Thorax* 56(2): 89–108.

Crompton, G. (1987) *Diagnosis and Management of Respiratory Diseases*, 2nd edn. London: Blackwell Scientific.

Foss, M. (1989) *Thoracic Surgery*. London: Austen Cornish.

Hatchett, R, & Thompson, T. (2001) *Cardiac Nursing – A comprehensive Guide*. London: Churchill Livingstone.

Hayward, J. (1975) *Information – A Prescription Against Pain*. London: RCN.

Kadri, M. & Treasure, T. (1993) Malignant disease of the lung. *Cardiothoracic Surgery* 11(6): 421–424.

Kendrick, A. & Smith, E. (1992) Respiratory measurements 2: interpreting simple measurements of lung function. *Professional Nurse* 7(11): 748–754.

Laws, D., Neville, E. & Duffy, J. (2003) BTS guidelines for the insertion of a chest drain. *Thorax* 58(5) (suppl 2): ii53–ii59.

Livingstone, J. I., Harvey, M., Kitchen, N., et al (1993) Role of pre-admission clinic in a general surgical unit: a six month audit. *Annals of the Royal College of Surgeons of England*. 75(3): 211–212.

Margereson, C. & Riley, J. (2003) *Cardiothoracic Surgical Nursing. Current Trends in Adult Care*. London: Blackwell Science.

Mitchell, M. (1997) Patients perceptions of pre operative preparation for day surgery. *Journal of Advanced Nursing* 26(2): 356–363.

Murday, A. & Madden, B. (1996) Surgery for heart and lung failure. *Surgery* 14(1): 18–24.

Seijo, L. M. & Stenman, D. H. (2001) Interventional pulmonology. *New England Journal of Medicine* 344(10): 740–749.

Stradling, P. (1991) *Diagnostic Bronchoscopy: A Teaching Manual*. Edinburgh: Churchill Livingstone.

Wilkins, R., Krider, S. & Sheldon, R. (1995) *Clinical Assessment in Respiratory Care*, 3rd edn. London: Mosby.

Further reading

Brunner, L. & Suddarth, D. (1992) *The Textbook of Adult Nursing*. London: Chapman & Hall.

Finkelmeier, B. A. (2000) *Cardiothoracic Surgical Nursing*, 2nd edn. Philadelphia: Lippincott.

Scanlon, C., Spearman, C. & Sheldon, R. (1995) *Egan's Fundamental Principles of Respiratory Care*, 6th edn. London: Mosby.

Society of Cardiothoracic Surgeons (2002) http://www.scts.org (accessed 20 April 2004).

West, J. (1990) *Respiratory Physiology – The Essentials*, 5th edn. London: Williams & Wilkins.

Wilkins, R., Krider, S. & Sheldon, R. (1995) *Clinical Assessment in Respiratory Care*, 3rd edn. London: Mosby.

Chapter **15**

Patients requiring gastrointestinal/ colorectal surgery

Fiona Hibberts and Emin Carapeti

Key objectives of the chapter

At the end of the chapter the reader should be able to:

■ describe the basic anatomy and physiology of the gastrointestinal system

■ briefly explain specific investigations

■ briefly explain causes, conditions and surgical interventions

■ give examples of assessment procedures for patients undergoing gastrointestinal surgery

■ highlight specific pre- and postoperative management

■ give a case study example and evidence-based care planning

■ assist in the education and discharge planning of patients.

INTRODUCTION

This chapter will provide information for nurses who are caring for patients on a surgical ward that specializes in gastrointestinal/colorectal surgery. It will focus on surgical interventions that are carried out when all other methods of treatment have been ineffective, or are indeed inappropriate. This chapter will also include endoscopic practice, and both diagnostic and therapeutic procedures will be outlined.

It must also be remembered that there are many different techniques and practices in the field of gastro-enterology. Therefore, surgical procedures may have slightly different names, according to their origin. It is important to use this book in conjunction with current evidence-based practice and research.

Each organ will be addressed in distinct sections of this chapter, and the associated anatomy and physiology will be discussed, followed by details of specific nursing assessment. However, the specific investigations will be addressed together at the beginning of the chapter in order to avoid repetition.

Nursing assessment refers to the collecting of data, reviewing or analysing the data, and identifying problems. It is essential that a comprehensive history is taken from the patient or their family to serve as a baseline for assessment. Assessment can be completed through interviewing, i.e. asking questions related to the patient's condition, observation for any non-verbal indications of discomfort or distress, and measuring through use of tools of assessment, e.g. pain assessment chart. It is a continuous process and needs to be frequently reviewed. For the purpose of this chapter the framework is based on the Roper, Logan and Tierney model of nursing, as described in Holland et al (2004) and Holloway's (1993) care planning, as this remains best practice in the ward environment. The generalized pre- and postoperative management remains the same as for any patient undergoing upper and lower abdominal surgery, and only specific problems will be highlighted following the discussion of the disease or organ dysfunction.

OVERVIEW OF THE ANATOMY AND PHYSIOLOGY OF THE DIGESTIVE SYSTEM

The digestive system refers to the organs, structures and complementary glands of the digestive canal that together are involved in the breaking down of food constituents into smaller components for absorption and final utilization by the cells. The digestive system, therefore, consists of the gastrointestinal tract, which is a continuous musculomembranous tube lined with mucous membrane, which is approximately 9 m long. This tube extends continuously through the body cavity from the mouth to the anus, and includes the mouth, pharynx, oesophagus, stomach, small intestine, large intestine, rectum and anus.

There are four basic activities that take place in the digestive system: ingestion – taking the food into the body (eating); movement of the food along the gastrointestinal tract (peristalsis); absorption of nutrients into the cells for use; and finally defecation, the elimination

of waste products. Two methods of digestion are employed – chemical and mechanical digestion. Chemical digestion is where large carbohydrates, proteins and lipid substances are broken down by chemical reactions. Ancillary organs which produce and store digestive enzymes are involved in this process. These include the salivary glands, liver, gallbladder and pancreas, and are external to the digestive tract. Mechanical digestion is where the food is physically moved, for example chewing, and mixing or churning the contents in the stomach with the digestive enzymes.

INVESTIGATIONS

There are many investigative procedures that a patient may undergo in order to diagnose the disorder and enable the surgical team to plan the relevant course of action or surgical intervention (Table 15.1). It is often a process of elimination by considering differential diagnosis.

The patient requires a full explanation of the proposed investigation, in order to make an informed decision about whether to go ahead with the test or not. Patients will be required to give verbal and often written consent. Informed consent will involve a discussion with the patient, outlining what the test will look at

Table 15.1 Investigations of the gastrointestinal or biliary tract undertaken prior to surgical intervention

Investigation	Surgery
Abdominal X-rays	GI tract/biliary tract
Fluoroscope	GI tract/biliary tract
CT scan	GI tract/biliary tract
Barium meal	Upper GI tract
Barium swallow	Upper and lower GI tract
Barium enema	Lower GI tract
Cholecystogram	Biliary tract
Cholangiogram	Biliary tract
Cholangiography	Biliary tract
Oesophagogastroduodenoscopy (OGD)	Upper GI tract
Colonoscopy	Lower GI tract
Sigmoidoscopy	Lower GI tract
Proctoscopy	Lower GI tract
Endoscopic retrograde cholangiopancreatography (ERCP)	Biliary tract
Percutaneous transhepatic cholangiography (PTC)	Biliary tract
Ultrasound	GI tract/biliary tract
Endoscopic ultrasound	Upper GI tract
Proctography	Lower GI tract
Transit study	Lower GI tract

specficially, the risks involved and the potential outcomes of the test and indeed not having the test at all. The Department of Health have a new initiative called 'Good practice in consent' which outlines the issues (DOH, 2001). The most common investigations are briefly described below.

Abdominal X-rays

Under normal circumstances, dense material may be penetrated by X-rays which give an outline of the organs or bones under investigation. When investigating the soft tissue and organs of the abdominal cavity, it is often necessary to use a contrast medium such as barium sulphate, to highlight the spaces and cavities in the gastrointestinal (GI) tract. X-rays use ionizing radiation and therefore carry a degree of risk, particularly during rapid cell division.

Nursing issues The most at-risk patients are therefore female patients during their reproductive life, as there is an increased possibility of affecting a fetus through pelvic X-rays. Therefore, any abdominal or pelvic radiography should be carefully monitored and only carried out if absolutely essential. A 10-day rule applies to all radiological examinations of the lower abdomen for female patients of reproductive age. This rule requires the examination to be carried out within 10 days following the first day of the menstrual cycle. There may be some exceptions to this rule for those women who have been sterilized, are menstruating or are not sexually active. Abdominal X-rays are useful in detecting gallstones (approximately 10% of gallstones are radio-opaque) and abdominal fluid levels. Bowel gas, constipation and obstruction can also be seen on abdominal X-rays.

CAT scan (computerized axial tomography)/CT scan

This scan provides a computerized picture of a part of the body, which is achieved by combining fine X-rays often with a contrast medium. 'Slices' of the abdomen are produced and are useful for detecting irregular anatomy, including tumours.

Barium studies

A radio-opaque contrast medium called barium sulphate is used for radiological studies of the gastrointestinal tract. It is a fine, milky contrast medium that can be taken orally or given rectally, to allow detection of small alterations in the stomach, small bowel, colonic and rectal mucosa.

Barium swallow and barium meal

This test is usually undertaken to highlight the oesophagus, stomach and upper intestinal tract, therefore assisting in detecting any exacerbation of oesophagitis, dysphagia, gastric or duodenal ulcers, Crohn's disease, or the presence of abnormalities such as hiatus hernia, strictures, obstruction or fistulas.

Barium meal and follow through

The barium is followed through the digestive system by X-ray studies, known as fluoroscopy. This form of investigation is particularly useful in detecting strictures and narrowing of the small intestine that is associated with Crohn's disease.

Nursing issues It is advisable for the patient not to have anything to eat or drink for a period of 6–8 hours prior to the investigation, as the examination is more successful if the stomach and small bowel are empty. Smoking is also discouraged, as it has the effect of increasing gastric motility.

Barium enema

Barium sulphate is introduced into the rectum and retained by the patient while the radiological studies are undertaken to detect disorders of the rectum and large intestine. It is particularly useful in diagnosing diverticular disease, strictures, obstruction, polyps and tumours, but contraindicated where there is a fistula present or potential risk of perforating the bowel.

Nursing issues When barium is used for radiological studies in the rectum, special attention should be paid to ensure that the rectum is emptied prior to the procedure, and that constipation following the procedure is avoided by increasing the fluid intake, and removing the contrast medium by a cleansing enema.

Proctogram

Barium sulphate paste is introduced into the rectum and the patient is given barium sulphate to drink. This will highlight the presence of an enterocele, rectocele and any anatomical disorder of the rectum.

Transit studies

In order to investigate the amount of time food takes to work its way through the gastrointestinal tract, radio-opaque markers in capsules are given to the patient and swallowed. After 5 days, a plain abdominal X-ray is taken and the markers can be traced. Slow gut transit, resulting in constipation, can be diagnosed.

Cholecystogram

A cholecystogram is an X-ray showing the gall bladder following the introduction of a radio-opaque contrast medium containing iodine. This may be introduced by ingestion or injection, and the technique is usually undertaken to detect gallstones or biliary obstruction, or to assess the ability of the gall bladder to fill and empty. It is now largely superseded by ultrasonography and other investigations.

Cholangiogram or cholangiography

The radio-opaque contrast medium is injected directly into the biliary tract or intravenously. The procedure is carried out during biliary surgery to detect any abnormalities or blockages, as it allows the bile ducts to be viewed on X-ray film. A cholangiogram can also be performed some days postoperatively in order to check the patency of the common bile duct following exploratory surgery and removal of any residual gallstones (sometimes the common bile duct can become oedematous and inflamed). The contrast medium is introduced through the indwelling T-tube inserted during the surgical procedure.

Nursing issues The postoperative cholangiogram should be carried out and results reviewed by the surgical team prior to the removal of the T-tube. The nursing role will be discussed later in this chapter.

Endoscopy

The cavities or interior of the gastrointestinal tract can be investigated through the use of an endoscope, which is a luminous fibreoptic instrument that can be inserted through a natural orifice for viewing cavities and internal organs, then relaying them to a television screen. The fibreoptic endoscope is often used to reach areas previously inaccessible with other instruments, as it has greater flexibility. Instruments can also be passed through the special tube of the endoscope to obtain biopsies or perform other procedures such as polypectomy.

Oesophagogastroduodenoscopy

For examination of the upper gastrointestinal tract, it is necessary to wait for the stomach to be empty, for visualization and prevention of aspiration. Oesophagogastroduodenoscopy (OGD) is usually performed to detect and diagnose ulcers and tumours. It is also used to establish the cause of upper gastrointestinal bleeding and to obtain biopsy samples. It may also be referred to in the chapter as gastroscopy.

Nursing issues It is necessary for the patient to have nothing orally for approximately 6 hours prior to this procedure, in order to ensure that the stomach is empty. During the procedure, an anaesthetic spray is often used to anaesthetize the throat. Therefore, following the procedure, it is usual to wait for throat sensation to return to normal prior to drinking. This takes approximately 1 hour, after which the patient may eat or drink normally. Sometimes fluids are withheld following an oesophageal dilatation until X-rays have been taken, in order to rule out any damage or trauma caused by the procedure.

Colonoscopy, sigmoidoscopy, proctoscopy

For this investigation to be successful, the bowel should be clear. Therefore, an enema, aperient or suppositories may be given to remove faecal contents. More commonly, one or two sachets of bowel preparation may be given prior to the investigation. This procedure is usually performed to detect any abnormalities of the colon, investigate rectal bleeding, changes in bowel pattern, anaemia or the cause of an obstruction, e.g. a cancer.

Nursing issues Cleansing of the lower colon may be contraindicated in lower rectal carcinoma and colonic inflammatory disease. The patient may also feel uncomfortable, with a bloated sensation, associated wind pains and, occasionally, nausea.

Endoscopic retrograde cholangiopancreatography

Endoscopic retrograde cholangiopancreatography (ERCP) views the biliary tree endoscopically. It can be purely diagnostic or also used for therapeutic purposes. The endoscope with a fine catheter is passed via the oesophagus, stomach and duodenum to the duodenal papilla. There, the pancreatic and common bile ducts are injected with the contrast medium introduced through the ampulla of Vater. Any irregularities will be viewed on the screen, and biopsies and cytology specimens may be taken. The investigation is usually performed to aid diagnosis of obstructive jaundice, chronic pancreatitis or pancreatic carcinoma, biliary colic, and can also facilitate the removal of gallstones.

Nursing issues The patient should be nil by mouth for at least 6 hours prior to the procedure. An anaesthetic throat spray may be used, as may sedation. Following the procedure the patient is usually unable to eat or drink for a few hours. Observations should include blood pressure and pulse for indications of bleeding or perforation. This procedure may be contraindicated in patients with cardiac and respiratory disorders (Hibberts and Barnes, 2003).

Percutaneous transhepatic cholangiography

In percutaneous transhepatic cholangiography (PTC), heavily concentrated contrast medium dye is injected straight into the biliary tree, enabling all parts of the biliary system to be viewed. This is done through a needle and catheter introduced transcutaneously under ultrasound guidance. It is particularly useful for investigating persistent symptoms related to the biliary system of those patients who have already undergone a cholecystectomy or gastrectomy and cannot have an ERCP.

Nursing issues   As in ERCP.

Ultrasound

High-frequency sound waves are transmitted by the ultrasound probe and echoes are received from various organs outlining them. It is safe, as it is non-invasive, and does not use ionizing radiation. It is used in gastroenterology to investigate and detect abnormalities of the biliary system, pancreas, liver and spleen.

Nursing issues   If the ultrasound is carried out for investigation of the gall bladder or pancreas, it may be necessary for the patient to stop eating for up to 12 hours, and drink clear fluids only, prior to the procedure. This will ensure that the gall bladder will be fully enlarged due to the retention of bile.

Stool specimens

These are usually obtained and cultured to detect infective organisms, occult bloods or faecal fats collection. The stool specimen may be a single sample or be part of a series of specimens.

UPPER GASTROINTESTINAL DISORDERS

MOUTH

Anatomy and physiology

This chapter will not discuss disorders of the mouth but will highlight the importance of a healthy mouth in the role of digestion. The mouth contains structures that are involved in the preparation of food for passage through the gastrointestinal tract. These structures are the tongue, teeth, hard and soft palates and salivary glands. The act of biting and chewing requires the ability of the extrinsic muscles of the tongue to move the food from side to side, and the intrinsic muscles of the tongue to alter the shape of the food for swallowing. This act of chewing is also variable according to the dental pattern and shape of the mouth of the individual and the type of food ingested.

The formation and assisted passage of the bolus requires the secretion of saliva from the parotid, submandibular and sublingual salivary glands, which secrete mucus and amylase. The flow of saliva is dependent on the stimulus initiated from taste and pressure in the mouth. Saliva is also responsible for keeping the mouth clean and removing food particles through keeping it moistened (Rutishauser, 1994).

It is therefore important that individuals have moistened, clean mouths and regular dental check-ups to assist and facilitate the function of chewing, forming and swallowing the bolus of food.

OESOPHAGUS

Anatomy and physiology

The oesophagus, sometimes called the gullet, is approximately 24 cm long, and is a muscular canal which is collapsible. It runs from the base of the pharynx, behind the trachea, through the opening between the thoracic cavity and abdominal cavity, terminating at the lower oesophageal sphincter of the stomach. It comprises of four layers:

1. The tunica adventitia (outer layer).
2. The muscularis – longitudinal and circular muscles that aid propulsion of food via the action of peristalsis. These muscles graduate from voluntary or striated muscles at the upper, pharyngo-oesophageal sphincter to involuntary or smooth muscles at the cardiac sphincter.
3. The submucosal layer, containing blood vessels and tissue.
4. The mucosal layer, which aids passage of the food bolus along the oesophagus through the secretion of mucus from special glands.

The function of the oesophagus is to transport the food bolus along the canal by the involuntary action of peristalsis (contractions and waves). The whole process takes 1–8 seconds, depending on the consistency of the food bolus. The two sphincters, i.e. pharyngo-oesophageal and gastro-oesophageal, control the flow of the bolus by relaxing, so as to allow the passage of the food through, and contracting, to prevent backflow of contents.

Oesophageal dysfunction

Dysfunction refers to any condition that disrupts or affects the normal function of the oesophagus, resulting in uncomfortable symptoms. Symptoms may include acute pain (odynophagia) and difficulty in swallowing (dysphagia), obstruction of food, and feeling the passage of liquids when swallowing, and often the patient will be able to point to the locality of the problem. Some of the conditions, causes and interventions are shown in Table 15.2 and are described below.

Oesophageal diverticulum

Oesophageal diverticulum refers to a weakness in the muscle wall of the oesophagus where a pouch of mucosa and submucosa can slip through causing a protrusion. Diagnosis is through barium swallow and X-rays.

Table 15.2 Oesophageal dysfunction – causes and surgical interventions

Cause	Intervention
Oesophageal diverticulum	Oesophagomyotomy
Oesophageal trauma/ perforation	Gastroscopy/OGD/reconstructive surgery
Oesophageal achalasia	Oesophagomyotomy or dilatation
Oesophageal stricture	Dilatation, insertion of a stent
Oesophagitis	Dilatation, oesophagastrostomy, fundoplication, vagotomy and pyloroplasty
Oesophageal cancer	Oesophagectomy, insertion of a stent

OGD = oesophagogastroduodenoscopy.

Gastroscopy or passing of a nasogastric tube is not undertaken, as there is an increased risk of perforation.

Intervention   Intervention is by removal of the pouch surgically. Because of its position, care must be taken to avoid damaging the adjacent vessels, and often a myotomy (a cut in the muscle) is performed to reduce the risk of spasticity to the muscle.

Oesophageal trauma and/or perforation
External trauma can be caused by stab, bullet or crush wounds. Internal trauma can be caused by swallowing foreign bodies, puncture from sharp objects or following an investigative procedure. Examples of these are metallic objects, dentures, fishbones and medical instruments. Other trauma effects can be through the ingestion of poisonous substances, or continuous unrelieved strain caused by vomiting, resulting in mucosal trauma (Mallory–Weiss tear) or full-thickness rupture of the oesophagus.

Intervention   Oesophagoscopy is commonly undertaken with removal of the foreign body or dilatation. In severely traumatized cases a gastrostomy is created for the insertion of a feeding tube to allow the traumatized area of the oesophagus and oedema to subside. Antibiotics may be prescribed following a perforated oesophagus, as there is an increased risk of infection.

Oesophageal achalasia
Oesophageal achalasia is a neuromuscular change that causes benign spasm of the lower oesophageal sphincter, sometimes with marked dilatation of the oesophagus. The lower oesophageal sphincter fails to respond and relax in order to facilitate swallowing. This results in the patient's feeling that food is stuck in the gullet. Food is often regurgitated, and oesophageal

distension occurs. There is a danger of spillover of food from the oesophagus into the trachea, causing respiratory aspiration. Diagnosis is through OGD and barium swallow.

Intervention   The aim would be to dilate the lower oesophageal sphincter using a balloon under pressure, inserted under X-ray or endoscopic guidance. There is a risk of perforation in a small percentage of the procedures. A surgical oesophagomyotomy, i.e. division of the muscle wall, may be performed if dilatation fails.

Oesophageal varices
Oesophageal varices are enlarged, swollen, engorged vessels at the base of the oesophagus that are at risk of rupturing, causing a torrential haemorrhage, which can be life threatening.

Intervention   The aim of treatment is to stop the haemorrhage. This is done endoscopically by injecting the varices with adrenaline (epinephrine) or placing a band around the bleeding vessel. In an emergency situation a Sengstaken–Blakemore tube is inserted to block the gastro-oesophageal junction to stop bleeding.

Oesophageal stricture
Oesophageal stricture may be caused by intensive and prolonged radiotherapy; through external pressure on the oesophagus by an enlarged adjacent organ or tumour; cancer of the oesophagus; and ingestion of caustic substances. The commonest cause of oesophageal stricture, however, is an inflammatory stricture caused by acid reflux (see below). Diagnosis involves a specific comprehensive history of any recent changes in swallowing, and investigations include endoscopy and biopsy.

Intervention   Intervention is by treatment of the underlying cause and may include dilatation of the lumen of the oesophagus and possibly the insertion of a stent.

Oesophagitis
The mucosal lining of the oesophagus becomes inflamed following an acute or chronic episode of infection, e.g. fungal; irritation, which includes malignancy, chemical ingestion or prolonged use of a nasogastric tube; complications following gastric/duodenal surgery; or trauma, caused by repeated vomiting, reflux, bending, coughing, stooping or straining. Investigations include a specific history, oesophagoscopy and/or biopsy (Day, 2003).

Intervention   Intervention is by treatment of the underlying cause and may involve medical treatment or dilatation, oesophagastrostomy, fundoplication, vagotomy and pyloroplasty.

Oesophageal cancer

This is the ninth most common type of cancer in the UK, with nearly 7200 new cases each year. Approximately 5% of the total cancer deaths in the United Kingdom are caused by oesophageal cancer (Cancer Research UK, 2004). It is more common in people over the age of 60, and is twice as common in men as in women. The 5-year survival rate is 7% in men and 8% in women.

There are two main types of oesophageal carcinoma:

- *Squamous cell carcinoma* accounts for half of the diagnosed cases, and develops in the squamous cells which form the lining of the oesophagus.

- *Adenocarcinoma* is cancer that begins in the gland cells. In this case it is the cells that make the mucus in the lining of the oesophagus. It is found in the lower third of the oesophagus. It may infiltrate adjacent structures up and down the oesophagus, is insidious in its onset and does not cause symptoms in the early stages. Symptoms may include involvement of the vocal cords, i.e. hoarseness, dysphagia leading to total blockage in some cases, anorexia with weight loss, pain, regurgitation of undigested food, persistent cough or clearing of the throat, halitosis or foul-smelling breath and haemoptysis. The tumour may eventually invade other adjacent organs, such as the bronchi, trachea, pericardium and great blood vessels, with metastases in the lymph nodes and liver. A patient with Barrett's oesophagus is 50 times more likely to get this type of cancer. It is therefore important that the individual has regular gastroscopies.

These carcinomas are thought to be associated with an increased consumption of alcohol, tobacco, hiatus hernia and Plummer–Vinson syndrome (i.e. cricoid webs causing dysphagia and achalasia). There may be a decreased incidence if an adequate intake of vitamins A and C and the mineral zinc are included in the diet.

Investigations   Investigations include a specific history as outlined in assessment, barium swallow, OGD, biopsy, endoscopic ultrasound and CAT scan. A bronchoscopy may also be performed to rule out any tracheal involvement.

Endoscopic ultrasound   Endoscopic ultrasound has revolutionized the staging of oesophageal cancers. The patient undergoes a gastroscopy, but a fibreoptic tube with an ultrasound crystal is inserted, instead of the camera. The tumour can then be sized, its relation to adjacent structures established and involvement of lymph nodes assessed.

Intervention   Surgical intervention is undertaken if the tumour is considered curative, i.e. partial or total

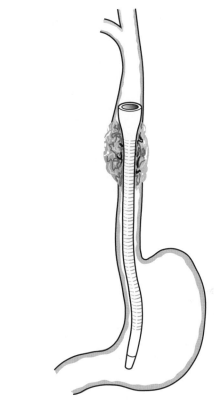

Figure 15.1   Oesophageal stent.

oesophagectomy, or palliative intervention may include the insertion of a self-expanding metallic stent. Treatment may also involve chemotherapy, jejunostomy or laser treatment. Radiotherapy may be effective with an early-stage carcinoma, or as a palliative measure in the advanced stages.

Insertion of a stent   When the carcinoma is severely advanced or involves adjacent organs and tissues, palliative intervention may be the option of choice. An expanding stent is passed to ensure that the oesophagus remains patent (Fig. 15.1), thus allowing a soft diet to be taken enterally by the patient (Bailey, 2004).

Surgical intervention   Surgical intervention is by an oesophagectomy, when part or all of the oesophagus is removed. The surgical approach may be through the thorax and abdomen, abdomen alone or thorax alone, leaving the stomach positioned in the thoracic cavity. Radiotherapy and chemotherapy can also be used in conjunction with an oesophagectomy, either prior to or following surgical intervention. In palliative care, oesophageal stents are widely used in order to provide some symptomatic relief.

Box 15.1 Specific issues related to eating and drinking

- Nutritional deficit – due to alteration in appetite as a result of nausea, anorexia, regurgitation, dysphagia or pain on ingesting food.
- Increased weight loss – following alteration in appetite/pathology.
- Potential risk of malnutrition following decrease in nutritional status/pathology.

Specific objective will be to ensure that adequate nutritional levels are maintained and that the patient is well nourished prior to surgical intervention. Any associated pain and discomfort is relieved or removed.

Nursing intervention and rationale

- Assess the ability of the patient to retain food and fluids. Document food, calorie and fluid intake on the appropriate charts along with weight charts. This will help to monitor nutritional intake and any weight fluctuation, and identify need for further intervention.
- Facilitate passage of food by offering drinks along with food intake; sometimes, soda water will help to clear the blockage and dislodge any food that is trapped. Small, frequent, light meals should be offered that are easy to swallow. All meals should be offered in a conducive environment.
- It may be necessary to give liquidized nutritional intake with vitamin supplements and high-protein fluid drinks, or totally replace enteral nutritional intake with parenteral feeding in order to provide the nutritional requirements.
- It is advisable to involve the dietitian and/or the nutritional specialist nurse to provide additional educational input, thus preventing further complications or problems following the introduction of special diets.
- Initialize appropriate referral to dietitian and possibly gastroenterologists.
- Maintain food chart/nutritional documentation to monitor patients' requirements.

Oesophageal surgery – specific preoperative assessment

Eating and drinking is clearly one of the problems for a patient undergoing an oesophagectomy, and should be discussed in detail as part of the specific preoperative assessment. Questions should be asked and documented in relation to the specific history to identify changes in appetite, increasing dysphagia, substernal pain, regurgitation, vomiting, severe weight loss, increased anxiety, metastatic gland enlargement in the neck, haematemesis and, finally, melaena or anaemia. Examples of questions are: 'How long have you had difficulty in swallowing?' 'Does it affect all foods or just fluids?' 'Do you regurgitate the food?' 'How long does it take you to swallow the food?' 'Where does the food stick?' 'Does it cause pain?' 'If so, whereabouts?' 'Is it getting worse or better?' As a result of the appropriate questions being asked, specific problems are identified, as shown in Box 15.1.

Specific postoperative nursing interventions

Maintaining a safe environment

Immediate assessment is made of the patient's airway, colour, oxygen saturation levels, vital signs and level of consciousness to prevent further complications arising of hypovolaemic shock, postoperative atelectasis and unrelieved pain.

Breathing

Specific postoperative assessment should consider the respiratory needs and possible management of a closed chest drain. This drainage system is positioned in the pleural cavity and may or may not be on suction to ensure that the lungs remain inflated. The water should be deep enough to cover the drainage tube in the drainage bottle and has the function of acting as a valve to prevent air from re-entering the pleural cavity. Circulatory needs require the monitoring of vital signs to identify if the patient is at risk of hypovolaemic shock. Encourage movement by passive and active exercises to prevent thromboemboli complications.

Eating and drinking

It is important that postoperative nutritional and fluid needs are met by a regime of fluid replacement and volume expanders intravenously, including total parenteral nutritional (TPN) replacement and/or supplements. Often, a jejunostomy tube is inserted at operation for postoperative feeding, before the patient is allowed to ingest food some days later when the anastomosis has healed.

Personal cleansing and dressing

There is a high risk of wound infection. Therefore, careful monitoring of the wound for signs of clinical infection, i.e. redness, swelling, heat, pain and exudate, should be undertaken. Comfort needs include assistance with hygiene and creating a safe environment.

Elimination

Monitor for urinary retention, which is related to the neuroendocrine response to stress, anaesthesia and recumbent position.

Additional specific potential complications

These complications include anastomotic leakage, malnutrition, pneumothorax, aspiration pneumonia, wound infection, blocked stent, fistula development, poor prognosis and associated high levels of anxiety.

STOMACH

Anatomy and physiology

The anatomy of the stomach is consistent with the rest of the digestive system tract, but it has the specific function of accommodating and digesting the food following ingestion. This is achieved by its shape and modification to receive food and become a reservoir when full. The contraction and churning of the stomach contents is aided by the muscular lining of smooth oblique, circular and longitudinal muscles. The upper part of the stomach wall is thought to be thinner with little contractile ability, and the pylorus is thicker with an increased contractile function. The passage of food from the oesophagus, stomach and duodenum is controlled by neuromuscular control and sphincter activity.

The mucosa has the ability to secrete enzymes through gastric glands that are present in the columnar epithelium in the mucosa. These cells are known as zymogenic and secrete pepsinogen; parietal cells secrete hydrochloric acid; and mucous cells are responsible for secreting mucus and the intrinsic factor.

Secretion of gastric juices and hydrochloric acid is stimulated by the hormone gastrin from the pyloric mucosa. Gastrin is stimulated by protein foods in the stomach and is released into the bloodstream to reach the gastric glands. Water and glucose are absorbed by the stomach wall along with some drugs and alcohol. The normal pH of the stomach is 2, and is maintained by the secretion of hydrochloric acid (Smith, 2003).

Pathology

Hiatus hernia

There is a herniation of the stomach through an opening in the diaphragm opening into the thoracic cavity. In patients who are symptomatic, gastro-oesophageal reflux is displayed in which the acid contents backflow into the oesophagus, causing inflammation. It is thought to affect 40% of the population. It is more common in females, and the risk increases with age. Muscular weakness and diaphragmatic abnormalities cause the herniation to occur, and these may result from increased intra-abdominal pressure, e.g. because of pregnancy, obesity, malignancy, trauma or persistent coughing/sneezing.

Sliding hiatus hernia Sliding hiatus hernia accounts for 90% of cases. The upper stomach and gastro-oesophageal junction are moved upwards and slide in and out of the thorax. Diagnosis is through radiological studies and fluoroscopy. Clinical manifestations are classically heartburn, regurgitation and dysphagia. The modern surgical management, if the patient is symptomatic, is a laparascopic Nissen fundoplication, although open procedures are still practised by some surgeons.

Para–oesophageal hiatus hernia All or part of the stomach pushes through the diaphragm opening next to the gastro-oesophageal junction. Investigations are the same as for a sliding hiatus hernia. Clinical manifestations often present with fullness after eating, or chest discomfort, haemorrhage, obstruction, and pain as a result of strangulation of the hernia, which is aggravated when lying flat. Reflux does not usually occur, and it is thought that 10% of the patients who have this type of hiatus hernia are asymptomatic.

Surgical intervention Anterior gastropexy can be performed, where the weak portion of the stomach is placed in its normal position and anchored to the abdominal wall.

Gastric dysfunction

This condition is reduced absorption, leading to an accumulation of fluid; reversed peristalsis, causing vomiting; and failure of mucus to act as a barrier.

Peptic ulceration

Peptic ulceration refers to erosion and ulceration of the mucosa of the stomach or duodenum. It is thought that most of these ulcers are due to the infection caused by *Helicobacter pylori*, but, clearly, increased acid secretion is also required. These ulcers, which can be gastric ulcers, duodenal ulcers or stress ulcers, are diagnosed by gastroscopy, barium studies and breath test for *H. pylori*.

Gastric ulceration Peptic ulceration occurs in the pre-pyloric area of the stomach and accounts for approximately 20% of all peptic ulcers. It has the added complication of a higher mortality associated with complications of bleeding. Very few of these ulcers are malignant, and most malignant gastric ulcers occur in the antrum body. The age range most affected is 45–70 years old; however, gastric ulceration particularly affects women over the age of 65. It is particularly associated with a familial tendency, stress, alcohol consumption, smoking and ulcerogenic drugs.

Aspirin, phenylbutazone and other non-steroidal anti-inflammatory drugs (NSAIDs) predispose to gastric peptic ulcers because they inhibit prostaglandin synthesis. Prostaglandins contribute to the protective effect

Table 15.3 Peptic ulceration – conditions and surgical intervention

Condition	Intervention
Gastric ulceration	Partial gastrectomy
	Total gastrectomy
	Oesophagogastrectomy
Duodenal ulceration	Truncal vagotomy
	Highly selective vagotomy
	Antrectomy
	Pyloroplasty

whereby the mucosa resists damage from gastric juices and hydrochloric acid. Steroids and chemotherapy drugs have similar effects. Other factors that have an influence on the mucosal layer, causing damage, are intestinal reflux, and hypersecretion of hydrochloric acid, which produces gastritis.

Clinical manifestations are mainly associated with burning pain in the epigastric region that occurs approximately 45–90 minutes following a meal, and this is often relieved by vomiting. Food does not help and may increase the pain. Other manifestations can include persistent belching, haematemesis, and the patient may appear malnourished.

Intervention   Treatment is by blocking acid secretion by proton pump inhibitors, as well as eradication of H. pylori by combination antibiotics. The vast majority of patients never require surgery, which until 20 years ago was the only treatment available. Surgery is now only required for complications such as bleeding, perforation or cancer (Table 15.3).

Duodenal ulcer   A duodenal ulcer is located in the first 1–2 cm of the duodenum and is the result of excessive gastric acid release and H. pylori. It is often seen in the age range around 50 years old, is more common in males (3:1) and is four times more common than gastric ulcers. There is a high association with blood group O (35% are more susceptible), and it is more common in adults with responsible decision-making jobs. The patient generally appears well nourished.

Clinical manifestations are again associated with pain, which presents in the mid-epigastric region 2–3 hours following the intake of food and often during the early hours of the morning between 1 and 2 a.m. It is often described as back pain, or heartburn. This pain may be relieved by the intake of food, particularly milk or antacids. Duodenal ulcers are rarely malignant, but have for many years been associated with the ingestion of caffeine, stress, alcohol abuse, cirrhosis, chronic pancreatitis, chronic renal failure and smoking. Investigation

and diagnosis is by gastroscopy, blood tests in order to correct any anaemia, and a general physical examination. Gastric function tests, to detect the presence or absence of hydrochloric acid and hypersecretion, are occasionally undertaken.

Intervention   Treatment is again by the use of proton-pump inhibitors such as omeprazole and lansoprazole and other new preparations, which are extremely potent suppressors of acid secretion, as well as combination antibiotics, e.g. amoxicillin, metronidazole or clarithromycin, to eradicate H. pylori. Surgery is reserved for acute complications such as bleeding and perforation, as previously discussed. On very rare occasions when medical treatment fails and there is recurrent symptomatic ulceration despite maximum medical treatment, then elective surgery can be considered (see Table 15.3).

Stress ulcer   Stress ulcer may result following infection, shock, burns or severe trauma, and can occur either in the stomach or duodenum. It is thought to be associated with increased pepsin, acid and ischaemia of the stomach wall. Its onset is rapid, initially within the first 48 hours, and it may be very extensive by the 5th–6th day. As long as the stressful circumstances remain, the ulcers will spread. The patient is generally treated symptomatically with antacids.

Acute complications

- *Haemorrhage* is a common complication of peptic ulceration and occurs most commonly in the distal stomach and proximal duodenum. Haemorrhage is characterized by melaena but is also often life threatening. It must be corrected by replacing lost fluids, giving blood or blood derivatives, e.g. plasma. Adrenaline (epinephrine) or fibrin/thrombin can be injected at endoscopy to stop the bleeding.
  Surgical intervention may be necessary for bleeding that is not responsive to endoscopic treatment or for heavy bleeding.

- *Perforation* and subsequent peritonitis has a sudden onset, sometimes without prior warning. It is a surgical emergency, and surgery should be performed as soon as the patient's condition allows it. Upper abdominal pain is experienced, which may be referred to the right shoulder. The abdomen is distended and rigid. The patient may rapidly become shocked.
  Surgical intervention is by oversewing of the perforation, with intravenous antibiotic therapy to treat bacterial peritonitis.

- *Obstruction* results when scarring and stenosis occur in the pyloric sphincter. The patient feels full and becomes nauseated and vomits, often leading to

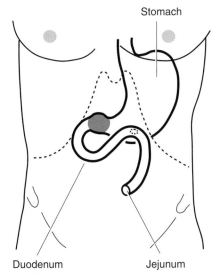

Stomach

Duodenum   Jejunum

Figure 15.2   Gastroenterostomy.

weight loss. Decompression is required and can be achieved by removing the stomach contents via naso-gastric tube aspiration.

Surgical intervention: gastroenterostomy is a pallia-tive operation for pyloric obstruction (Fig. 15.2). Vagotomy and antrectomy involve severing the vagus nerve and removing the antrum of the stomach. This will help to reduce hypersecretion of hydrochloric acid if treatment with proton pump inhibitors fail. These patients may require TPN if severe weight loss has occurred.

Gastric cancer

Gastric or stomach cancer is the fifth most common cancer for men, and the ninth for women, with over 9800 new cases diagnosed each year. It is twice as com-mon in men than women, and more common in the 50–70 years old bracket. Gastric cancer constitutes 4% of cancer deaths and has a mean suvival of 14% (Cancer Research UK, 2004).

There are predisposing factors which include:

- *Dietary*: eating a lot of salted, cured and smoked foods are suggested to increase an individual's risk.
- *Infection*: H. pylori is a common bacterial infection of the stomach. It is diagnosed on gastroscopy and biopsy, and a simple course of antibiotics often eradi-cates it. If left untreated, it increases the individual's risk of developing gastric cancer by up to 5 times.
- *Previous stomach surgery* is suggested to increase the risk of stomach cancer, due to reduced acid production.

- *Pernicious anaemia* is also a predisposing factor, in that the stomach does not produce enough gastric enzymes to take up vitamin B_{12}. However, vitamin B_{12} levels can be topped up with regular 3-monthly injections of hydroxocobalamin.

The prognosis is poor, as many tumours are asymptom-atic and therefore present late, often with metastases. Those situated in the lesser curvature do not cause gas-tric function disorder, while some tumours that occur in the cardiac or pyloric orifice display symptoms caused by disturbed gastric motility. Up to 80% of cases on presentation are too advanced for surgical intervention (Ellis and Cunningham, 1994). Because of the asymp-tomatic nature of the disease in its early stage, there has been speculation as to the advantage of a screening programme for all patients over 40 years old who present with dyspepsia. However, dyspepsia is a very common disorder and affects a large proportion of the general population, whereas gastric cancer is relatively uncommon.

Clinical presentation includes dyspepsia over 4 weeks, anorexia, nausea, vomiting or haematemesis, hoarseness, epigastric discomfort, abdominal disten-sion, pain, weight loss, blood in stool and iron deficiency anaemia.

Diagnosis can be made through investigating occult bloods, while OGD/gastroscopy is the gold standard investigation which allows biopsies and histological confirmation. CT scan and occasionally laparoscopy are carried out to stage the disease and determine resectability.

Intervention   A partial or total gastrectomy may be performed (Figs 15.3 and 15.4). Total gastrectomy is often associated with a high morbidity and mortality. It is often ineffective, although it may improve palli-ation, and long-term trials are being undertaken to address this both preoperatively and postoperatively (Cancer Research UK, 2004).

Pre- and postoperative care of patients with gastric cancer

Specific preoperative assessment

Patients with gastric cancer may have many problems that require nursing intervention. Anxiety related to the impending surgical procedure is common in most surgical patients, but is made more threatening by the possible diagnosis of cancer and poor prognosis. Other specific problems associated with gastric cancer are nutritional deficiency related to anorexia; subsequent weight loss; and pain. The management of pain pre-and postoperatively in gastric cancer surgery is para-mount, and questions should be focused on the nature

Figure 15.3
Gastroduodenostomy –
Bilroth I.

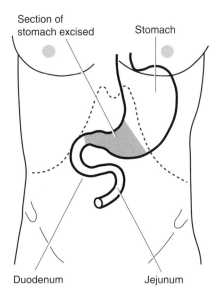

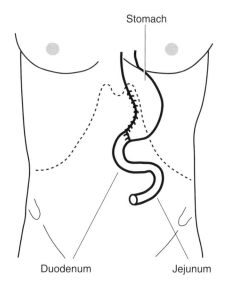

Figure 15.4   Polya
partial gastrectomy –
Bilroth II.

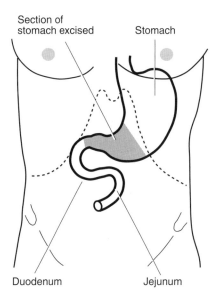

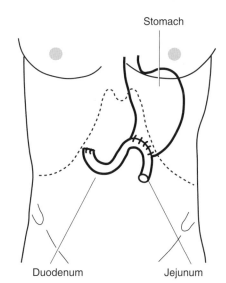

of the pain, location, pattern, duration, intensity and reaction to the pain, in order to plan nursing care effectively (Box 15.2).

Specific postoperative nursing interventions
Maintaining a safe environment   Immediately, postoperatively, the patient should be placed in the semirecumbent position for comfort and to help with breathing.

Breathing and communicating   To avoid pulmonary complications, analgesics should be given which will

encourage deep breathing and productive coughing. This will result in increased oxygen and carbon dioxide interchange, therefore providing adequate oxygen content for circulation. Adequate analgesics will prevent shallow breathing and allow for physiotherapy.

Eating and drinking   A nasogastric or nasojejunal tube may be in situ. Irritation or bleeding from the position of the nasogastric tube on the mucosa should be avoided, by observing and checking the position of the tube and giving nose and mouth care. Drainage contents should also be monitored. Oral fluids are often

---

Box 15.2   Specific issues related to pain

- Pain related to abnormal presence of epithelial cells in tumour formation, sometimes causing pressure on nerves and other organs.
- Pain related to presence of metastases or ascites.

Specific objective will be to ensure that pain is relieved and aim for the optimum state of being pain free.

Nursing intervention and rationale

- Use a pain assessment chart to monitor for the possible indicators of pain: e.g. restlessness, irritability, verbalization and withdrawal. Verbal reports may not always be accurate, because of the effects of the disease process and medication.
- Analyse the information on the assessment chart to indicate pain characteristics. This will aid in the differential diagnosis of pain, therefore ensuring that the appropriate intervention is implemented.
- Discuss with the patient the purpose of pain control and that the aim is to strive for a pain-free state. This will ensure that patients understand why they should report any increase in pain sensation before the pain becomes severe.

- Use a variety of non-pharmacological strategies to relieve the pain: positioning, cutaneous stimulation and massage with oils. Due to the multiple factors that cause and exacerbate pain, a combination of methods of relieving pain may be more effective than a single approach.
- Behavioural pain-relieving strategies may include distraction, relaxation and imagery. These strategies enable patients to divert their attention from the pain and may stimulate endorphin release through having a sense of control and relaxed muscles.
- Liaise with the medical staff to discuss and determine an effective method and dose of analgesics. These may include opioids, non-opioids and adjunctives.
- Discuss impending surgery and the method of controlling pain postoperatively. Ensure that patients have time to ask questions related to the surgery and post-operative management. This will provide patients with as much information as they require to ensure that they understand what is expected of them.
- Initiate appropriate referral to the specialist pain service/nurse specialist for monitoring and advice.

---

withheld, in order to protect the anastomosis. There may be a risk of dehydration; therefore, fluid intake will need to be monitored and replaced by an intravenous infusion. This will compensate for loss in drainage and vomit, as well as maintaining normal hydration needs. Accurate recording is required, and the nasogastric tube is removed once it is felt that the anastomosis has healed. Often a contrast X-ray is performed prior to removal of the nasogastric or nasojejunal tube. Oral fluids are gradually increased as tolerated, but again strict observation should be made for signs of abdominal distension and pain.

There is also an increased risk of malnutrition and/or starvation. Once eating is re-established, dietary needs should be met by offering small bland and frequent meals and drinks. It may also be necessary to replace vitamin B_{12}, and give vitamin supplements, since following resection of the stomach it is possible that the absorption of vitamins will be affected, including the production of intrinsic factor, which is important for the absorption of cyanocobalamin (vitamin B_{12}). The patient should be observed for any evidence of regurgitation that may be caused by eating too much, eating too fast or as a result of oedema along the anastomosis.

Occasionally, when there is prolonged ileus or complications, it may be necessary to commence parenteral feeding support for 5–6 days postoperatively, commencing normal eating when bowel function returns and the patient feels hungry.

Mobilizing   The patient may have limited mobility because of the disease process, the surgery, pain on movement and effects of anaesthesia. Mobility should be encouraged by giving sufficient analgesics, and monitoring for the side-effects of low blood pressure and dizziness. The goal is to increase mobility daily as the individual is able.

Personal cleansing and dressing   There may be a risk of wound infection, so it is important to observe for signs of wound infection. The amount and type of wound drainage should be monitored. The dressing should be changed as necessary. The dressing may be removed and the wound left exposed around the third day. Sutures/staples are removed after approximately 7–10 days.

Additional specific complications

These may include shock, haemorrhage, pulmonary complications and the following.

Steatorrhoea   Unabsorbed fat in the stools results from rapid gastric emptying, where the pancreatic and biliary secretions have not had the opportunity to break down and digest the gastric contents.

Dumping syndrome Dumping syndrome is where vasomotor and gastric symptoms occur after meals, usually after about 10–90 minutes. If the stomach has been anastomosed to the jejunum, the contents may pass through too quickly; therefore, full absorption may not occur. This has implications for the absorption of carbohydrates and electrolytes, as they need to be diluted before absorption can occur. If fluids are taken at meal times, this will also encourage the stomach to empty too quickly, giving rise to the symptoms of dizziness, faintness, weakness, sweating, pain and fullness. These symptoms occur as a result of rapid distension of the jejunal loop anastomosed to the stomach, caused by the hypertonic solution of intestinal contents drawing the extracellular fluid into the intestinal contents for dilution.

Gastritis Because of the removal of the pylorus, its function as a barrier to reflux of duodenal contents is impaired; likewise, the same for the oesophagus when the cardiac sphincter is involved. Vitamin B_{12} deficiency, leading to anaemia, can occur on occasions.

Education and discharge planning

For the patient who is undergoing surgery for an upper gastrointestinal disorder, it is important that the condition is fully addressed and that the patient is fully informed of all procedures and investigations that they are expected to undergo. The procedures and results should be explained in appropriate language that facilitates the asking of questions. The adjustment period is very important for the patient, who is required to alter their lifestyle as a result of surgical intervention or palliative management. A multidisciplinary approach that involves health professionals, the patient, close family and friends will assist in the planning of aftercare and rehabilitation. If the disorder has not been cured, it may be necessary for the patient to have nutritional advice on how to adjust their diet to meet altered nutritional needs; information so as to identify any complications; appropriate contact numbers for specialist support; advice on how to control and manage their pain; and how to manage specialized equipment, i.e. gastrostomy tube or parenteral feeding. In advanced disease, early referral to the palliative care team is a prerequisite before the patient is discharged back into the community. This ensures that adequate care and support is in place, which can help prevent and/or anticipate some of the distressing symptoms produced by advanced gastric cancer.

GALL BLADDER

Anatomy and physiology

The gall bladder, a small muscular pouch or sac, is tucked underneath the liver, and is attached to the liver by connective tissue and to the common bile duct via the cystic duct. Its inner walls are similar in construction to the mucous membrane of the stomach. Bile is secreted from the liver into the hepatic duct continuously, but the majority of bile is concentrated and stored in the gall bladder. Bile is then secreted into the duodenum in response to the ingestion of food under neuroendocrine control. Concentrated bile may become saturated with cholesterol and form crystals which mark the beginning of gallstones.

Bile flow is stimulated by vagus nerve activity. When foods are released into the duodenum, the sensory receptors are stimulated, causing reflex activity in the vagus. Acetylcholine is released and the gall bladder muscle contracts. At the same time the duodenal mucosa produces the hormone cholecystokinin, which stimulates the gall bladder to contract and eject the stored bile into the digestive system in order to assist with the emulsification of fats.

Bile consists of water, conjugated bile salts – i.e. sodium glycocholate, sodium glycochenodeoxycholate, sodium taurocholate and sodium taurochenodeoxycholate – derived from cholesterol, bile pigments – i.e. bilirubin and biliverdin – and a number of lipids. It is a dark yellow/green substance that has a bitter taste. It has a pH of 7.6–8.6 and approximately 800–1000 mL is secreted daily. It also has the dual function of aiding digestion of fats by emulsifying them, and aids excretion through stimulating peristalsis. When erythrocytes are broken down, iron, globin and bilirubin are released. The iron and globin are recycled, but some of the bilirubin is excreted into the bile ducts. It is eventually broken down in the small intestine, giving colour to the faeces, and assisting in the synthesis of vitamin K.

Incidence of gall bladder disease

Suggested predisposing factors for developing gall bladder disease are female, taking the contraceptive pill, aged between 40 and 60 years old, and obesity; also, having a high blood cholesterol level may increase the risk (Royal College of Surgeons of Edinburgh, 2004).

Clinical presentation

Many patients have a history of biliary discomfort, colic and intolerance to fatty foods, but have not sought medical advice. Gall bladder disease can induce symptoms ranging from mild discomfort following a fatty

Box 15.3   Gall bladder disease

- *Cholelithiasis*

  presence of gallstones in the gall bladder or common bile duct.
  Intervention:
  dissolution of stones, ERCP, with or without sphincterotomy, cholecystectomy, choledocholithotomy, exploration of common bile duct, and percutaneous removal of gallstones

- *Cholecystolithiasis*

  gallstones in the gall bladder.
  Intervention:
  open cholecystectomy, or laparoscopic cholecystectomy

- *Choledocholithiasis*

  gallstones in the common bile duct.
  Intervention:
  dissolution of stones, ERCP, choledocholithotomy, cholecystectomy with exploration of common bile duct

- *Cholangitis*

  inflammation of bile ducts.
  Intervention:
  conservative and symptomatic management

- *Cholecystitis*

  inflammation of the gall bladder.
  Intervention:
  conservative and symptomatic management, or surgery

meal, to the patient who presents to their doctor with acute nausea, vomiting and severe pain. The pain is situated in the right hypochondrium, often radiating to the right shoulder. It is severe and intense and can be spasmodic, easing when stones have been passed from the gall bladder to the common bile duct. If the pain remains untreated and persistent vomiting occurs, shock can ensue. Pyrexia may be present due to infection. Jaundice can be present as a result of the gallstones obstructing the common bile duct (Box 15.3).

Conservative and symptomatic management

Many patients in this acute stage are admitted to the surgical ward for symptomatic control prior to surgical intervention. Until recently it has been common practice to avoid surgery until the inflammation has subsided, often for a period of up to 6 weeks.

However, because there is a risk that the patient may present with another attack prior to surgery, modern trends in management are to perform surgery within a week of the initial attack. The rationale for this is that, with antibiotic cover, the risk of complications is reduced (Alexander et al, 2000).

Nursing issues   The patient is given regular analgesics for the severe pain. There is a risk of peritonitis following perforation of the gall bladder; therefore, pain levels and vital signs are monitored and appropriate interventions implemented. Patients are allowed fluids but may be prevented from eating solids, particularly if nauseated and vomiting. A nasogastric tube may be passed for persistent vomiting. Fluids are replaced by intravenous infusion, and fluid and electrolyte balance is carefully monitored. Antibiotic therapy is commenced to reduce the inflammation of the gall bladder associated with the infection.

Investigations include abdominal X-rays, ultrasound examination, and ERCP or endoscopic ultrasound if there is jaundice or cholangitis.

Laparoscopic cholecystectomy

A laparoscope is introduced into the abdomen under general anaesthetic. Carbon dioxide is used to inflate the abdomen to give clear vision. Three more small incisions are made to facilitate the manipulation of instruments. The gall bladder is then dissected, and removed via the umbilicus. There are a number of advantages to this procedure. The patient is able to mobilize more fully at an earlier stage in their recovery, thus preventing the possibility of complications. Surgical disfiguration is limited, and any drains are removed within 24 hours. This procedure is less painful; therefore, there is a reduced need for opioid analgesics, although there is some discomfort experienced following the introduction of carbon dioxide. However, in up to 5–10% of cases the procedure is not possible laparoscopically and an open choleycystectomy is performed.

It is very important that surgeons performing this type of surgery have undertaken a specialized training programme to avoid bile duct injury, which is a catastrophic complication (Guilbeau et al, 1990).

Specific postoperative management

Nursing management is consistent with normal recovery from a general anaesthetic. Analgesics are required for any discomfort associated with the procedure and inflation with carbon dioxide. Oral fluids can be commenced when fully recovered from the anaesthetic and diet taken usually the following day. Normal discharge is within 24 hours, although increasingly the procedure

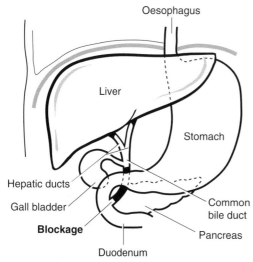

Figure 15.5   Cholecystoduodenostomy.

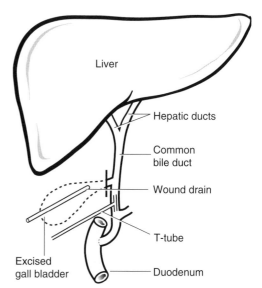

Figure 15.6   Cholecystectomy (exploration of common bile duct).

is being carried out as a day case. Sutures will then need to be removed after a week by the practice nurse.

Surgical interventions (invasive)

Cholecystoduodenostomy

This is a surgical procedure for obstructive jaundice, arising from a stricture of the bile duct caused by congenital factors, inflammation, previous surgery or inoperable tumours of the pancreas or local lymph nodes. The gall bladder is anastomosed to the duodenum, bypassing the common bile duct, ampulla of Vater and sphincter of Oddi (Fig. 15.5). This allows the bile to flow directly into the duodenum.

Choledochostomy (exploration of the common bile duct)

This technique allows the removal of stones from the bile duct, and insertion of a T-tube to allow drainage from the bile duct and a precautionary wound drain to the gall bladder bed (Fig. 15.6).

Cholecystectomy

This is the removal of the gall bladder and occasional insertion of a precautionary wound drain to the gall bladder bed, through a subcostal incision rather than laparoscopically (see Fig. 15.6).

Cholecystectomy and exploration of the common bile duct

This is the removal of the gall bladder followed by an explorative procedure in the common bile duct, and is usually performed to remove gallstones. A T-tube

drain is inserted to ensure the common bile duct remains patent for the safe passage of bile (see Fig. 15.6). This tube is then removed approximately 2 weeks postoperatively, following a postoperative cholangiogram. A precautionary wound drain is often inserted to the gall bladder bed. This procedure can be performed laparoscopically or as an open procedure.

Cholecystojejunostomy

This is a palliative surgical procedure for obstructive jaundice due to a tumour of the pancreas. The gall bladder is anastomosed to the jejunum, bypassing the common bile duct, ampulla of Vater and sphincter of Oddi (Fig. 15.7). A precautionary drain may be inserted to the area of anastomosis.

Pancreatectomy (Whipple's operation)

This procedure is for carcinoma of the head of pancreas. The duodenum and part of the pancreas are resected, and the common bile duct and pancreatic ducts are joined to the jejunum (Fig. 15.8). There are many variations of this procedure.

Principles of a T-tube   During the operation, a cholangiogram is performed to detect gallstones in the common bile duct. If stones are identified, then the surgeon will usually explore the common bile duct and remove the stones or gravel. Following this procedure, the common bile duct is susceptible to leakage, inflammation and oedema; therefore, a T-tube is inserted to maintain the patency of the duct. The function of this

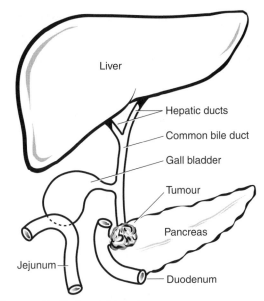

Figure 15.7 Cholecystojejunostomy.

T-tube is to allow safe drainage of bile, approximately 300–450 mL during the first day, which gradually decreases as the oedema subsides.

A postoperative cholangiogram is performed approximately 8–10 days following the cholecystectomy. Depending on the surgeon, some T-tubes are clamped prior to the postoperative cholangiogram. Particular attention should be paid to any complaints of pain associated with the clamping of the tube. If this arises, then the clamp should be removed immediately and the surgical team informed.

The results are viewed by the surgeon, and if they indicate that the oedema has subsided and there are no stones present and no leakage of bile, then the T-tube is removed by the nursing staff. It is usual to give the patient analgesics at least 30 minutes prior to the removal of the T-tube. After removal it is important to monitor the patient for a sudden drop in blood pressure, or rise in pulse, and for evidence of pain, as this may indicate that the patient has developed biliary peritonitis caused by seepage of bile into the peritoneal space.

Pre- and postoperative care of patients undergoing biliary surgery

Specific preoperative assessment
The patient who requires surgery for biliary dysfunction has many problems that require nursing intervention. The specific problems are associated with the risk of peritonitis due to possible perforation of the gall

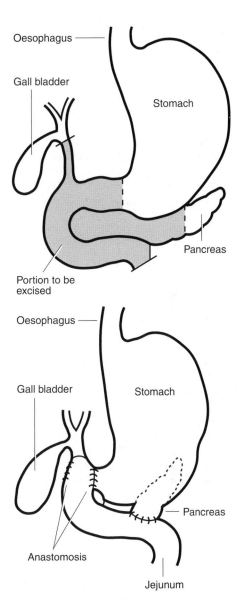

Figure 15.8 Pancreatectomy (Whipple's operation).

bladder; haemorrhage associated with reduced vitamin K production and absorption, following obstructive jaundice; wound infection following the obstruction or dislodgement of the T-tube; and postoperative chest infection due to the pain associated with the high abdominal incision. However, with the advent of laparoscopic cholecystectomy, more that 90% of these operations are being carried out using minimally invasive techniques, which therefore reduces the need for a subcostal incision. The specific problems associated with breathing are detailed in Box 15.4.

Box 15.4   Specific issues related to breathing

- Inadequate air exchange – due to reduced ventilation of the lungs.
- Reduced ventilation of the lungs – due to frequent, shallow respirations.
- Shallow respirations – due to the risk of associated pain when expanding the lungs.
- Potential risk of chest infection – due to the difficulty in expectorating sputum and limited mobility.
- Difficulty in expectorating sputum – due to the tenacity of the lung secretions and a lack of strength to expectorate.

Specific objective will be to maintain optimal air exchange (lung expansion) and prevent chest infection.

Nursing intervention and rationale

- Accurate recordings and monitoring should be carried out postoperatively to establish the depth and frequency of respirations.
- Deep breathing (diaphragmatic) should be taught to the patient prior to surgery and encouraged postoperatively. This will allow full lung expansion and prevent consolidation of lung secretions. Involve the physiotherapist, especially if the patient has had respiratory problems identified prior to surgery.
- Ensure the patient's pain is assessed and analgesics are administered prior to intensive deep breathing exercises or physiotherapy and mobilization.
- Instruct the patient in supporting their abdominal wound prior to coughing and expectorating sputum, thereby reducing any stress or pulling on the incision line.
- Encourage a good fluid intake, which will have the effect of reducing the tenacity of the lung secretions and facilitating expectoration of sputum.
- Mobilize as soon as the patient's condition allows, as this encourages deeper respirations, therefore ensuring that the lungs are adequately ventilated.
- Initiate appropriate referral to physiotherapist, for mobility and check.

Specific postoperative nursing interventions

Maintaining a safe environment   It is important to monitor vital signs for possible shock; the abdomen for signs of distension; and level of pain, including location and character. These all indicate the possibility of peritonitis, perforation and/or haemorrhage. Early detection will ensure that immediate action can be implemented, i.e. fluid replacement and/or emergency surgery.

Communication   Pain has already been mentioned in detail in the section on gastric surgery and in relation to breathing following biliary surgery. However, the management of pain also has important implications for mobilization and the prevention of deep vein thrombosis.

Eating and drinking   Eating and drinking can usually be commenced immediately postoperatively following a laparoscopic cholecystectomy, and up 24 hours following an open procedure.

Personal cleansing and dressing   Wound management has been discussed in previous nursing interventions, although there is a risk of infection associated with the T-tube drain. Any signs of clinical infection, redness, swelling, heat, pain, purulent drainage or odour should be documented and reported, as this will ensure that systemic antibiotic therapy is introduced if required.

Signs of T-tube obstruction should be observed for, by noting any change in skin colour (jaundice), pale stools, dark yellow urine, nausea and vomiting, and reduced amount of drainage in the bile bag. Any of these signs can indicate that the passage of bile is obstructed, causing pressure within the common bile duct and sometimes the liver and portal system. The skin surrounding the T-tube should be observed for any redness and excoriation, and protected with a small keyhole dressing, as bile contents, when leaking around the tube, can cause skin irritation and pain.

Additional specific complications

It should be remembered that the elderly have an increased risk of morbidity and mortality when undergoing surgery of the biliary tract in an emergency, due to increased risk of complications associated with the cardiovascular system. It is estimated that 70% of people over 75 years old have long-standing illness and are therefore at greater risk when undergoing surgical intervention (Office of Health Economics, 1992).

Education and discharge planning

As previously stated in this chapter, it is important that the patient who undergoes surgery should be fully educated and aware of the implications of the surgery. The patient who has had a cholecystectomy may have symptoms that are associated with the free passage of bile. The gall bladder is no longer there to be used as a reservoir, so the bile will be continually secreted. This may mean that when fatty foods are eaten the patient may feel nauseated, and may develop post-cholecystectomy diarrhoea. The patient should also be aware of the need to report any further pain, nausea or change in skin colour, as this may indicate further biliary obstruction.

LOWER GASTROINTESTINAL DISORDERS

SMALL INTESTINE

Anatomy and physiology

The small intestine is a long, muscular, tubular organ which runs from the pylorus through to the caecum, terminating at the ileocaecal valve. It consists of the same layers throughout the intestinal canal, which have been described in detail in the section related to the oesophagus. However, the submucosa and mucosa differ, as their main function is to absorb and assist in the final stages of digestion. The small intestine is divided into three main sections – the duodenum, jejunum and ileum – and is approximately 2.5 cm in diameter, and approximately 3–8 m in length.

The mucosal layer has an increased surface area created by folds and villi that help in the absorption of the intestinal contents. In between the villi are small pits lined with glandular epithelium, referred to as glands or crypts (crypts of Lieberkühn), their main function being the secretion of intestinal digestive enzymes.

These digestive enzymes leave the intestinal walls vulnerable to enzymatic action. Therefore, the walls of the small intestine are protected by alkaline secretions from Brunner's glands in the duodenum, and mucus throughout the small intestine, which have the effect of neutralizing the acid and enzymes.

Normal function

Food is propelled along the small intestine by peristalsis. This action involves muscular activity by rhythmic, relaxing and propulsive movement. These actions allow the food to be mixed and broken down for absorption and move the chyme through the small intestine. Intestinal juices are secreted to assist in the digestion of carbohydrates and proteins. Fats are converted into fatty acids and monoglycerides by the action of pancreatic lipase. Bile salts then assist in converting them into a water-soluble form, for absorption by the villi. The small intestine is responsible for absorbing approximately 90% of the nutrients through the villi by a variety of processes. This is facilitated by the secretion of enzymes, particularly the pancreatic enzymes, amylase and protease, that chemically assist the breakdown of food into smaller molecules.

Abnormal function

Increased peristalsis may cause colic and diarrhoea, which can result in the malabsorption of nutrients. Sometimes, abdominal surgery causes a paralytic ileus, thereby preventing the passage of food and reducing the absorption of nutrients.

Small bowel obstruction

Intestinal obstruction refers to the blockage or slowing down of the normal flow of intestinal contents and may be partial or complete (Table 15.4). The intestine above the blockage becomes dilated, and secretions accumulate, causing stagnation of the contents or even reverse flow. The involved area collapses and loses its function. The intestinal contents build up as the bowel dilates and can cause vomiting, often feculent in nature. Over half of small bowel obstructions are said to be caused by adhesions. Other causes are hernias, diverticular disease and cancer of the large intestine.

Clinical manifestations

Clinical manifestations depend on the degree of obstruction and portion involved, but, in acute small bowel obstruction, present as sudden onset, associated with severe symptoms of colicky pain, nausea, vomiting and dehydration, resulting in loss of electrolytes. Often the blockage can be complicated by interference with the blood supply, which may result in ischaemia, tissue necrosis and the threat of perforation. This type of obstruction requires immediate surgical intervention. Clinical manifestations of chronic or subacute small bowel obstruction present with a slower onset, as the lumen gradually obstructs. Symptoms progressively become worse as the condition develops. This type of obstruction will require surgery, but is less urgent in nature.

Small bowel obstruction is often referred to as either mechanical or paralytic and may be diagnosed by observing for clinical manifestations, particularly the vomiting of faeculent fluid, absence of faeces, colicky pain and abdominal distension.

Diagnosis

A detailed history, abdominal examination and abdominal X-rays are often all that is required.

Mechanical obstruction

Mechanical obstruction can occur anywhere in the small intestine and may be simple in nature or complicated by strangulation. This type of obstruction arises from either an internal blockage that occludes the lumen, or external pressure to the lumen of the bowel.

Foreign body   This type of obstruction is rare and can be due to gallstones or a food bolus that has not been digested and remains lodged in the small intestine, causing a blockage. Intervention is by surgical laparotomy to deal with the underlying cause.

Table 15.4 Small bowel obstruction – causes and surgical interventions

Cause	Intervention
Mechanical – blockage of the lumen	
Foreign body	Laparotomy, excision and removal, repair
Mechanical – lumen wall altered by disease	
Crohn's disease – strictures	Small bowel resection or strictureplasty
Intussusception	Reduction or resection and anastomosis
Meckel's diverticulum	Reduction, repair or resection
Volvulus	Small bowel resection
Neoplasms	Resection, excision of tumour and end-to-end anastomosis
Mechanical – occurring outside the lumen	
Strangulated hernia	Reduction and repair or resection
Adhesions	Division of adhesions
Neoplasm	Resection, excision of tumour and end-to-end anastomosis
Paralytic	
Previous surgery	Decompression by nasogastric intubation
Infection	Withhold all food and fluid; antibiotics
Mesenteric ischaemia	Surgical resection and anastomosis

Crohn's disease strictures The formation of scar tissue as a result of frequent exacerbation of the disease results in the narrowing of the lumen of the small intestine. Intervention is by small bowel resection, strictureplasty or, if accessible, by endoscopic dilatation.

Intussusception Intussusception is caused by telescoping of the intestine, often very close to the ileocaecal valve, and occurs frequently in young infants. One portion of the bowel prolapses into the lumen of another portion. Specific clinical manifestations include those already described, but it may also present with blood in the stools. Diagnostic investigations include barium enema. Intervention is by reduction, resection and anastomosis of the bowel.

Meckel's diverticulum Meckel's diverticulum is a congenital condition where there is incomplete closure of the yellow stalk, a duct that links the yellow sac with the midgut of the embryo, leaving a sac which protrudes from the wall of the ileum. Its length can vary from 2 to 50 cm, and it is susceptible to inflammation. It is often asymptomatic, but it may present similarly to appendicitis, or intestinal obstruction. Intervention is by surgical resection of the affected part of the bowel.

Volvulus Volvulus is a twisting of the small bowel occurring more commonly in the ileum, but it can also occur in the caecum or sigmoid colon. It can lead to ischaemia, necrosis, perforation and peritonitis if not corrected. Specific clinical manifestations include nausea, vomiting, severe colicky pain and the absence of bowel sounds. The abdomen is distended and rigid by the accumulation of gas and fluid that has become trapped. Diagnosis is by abdominal X-ray. Intervention is usually by surgery but endoscopic decompression may be enough for a caecal or sigmoid volvulus.

Neoplasms New growth of tissue (tumour) may be benign or malignant. Diagnosis may be by barium radiological studies, colonoscopy, sigmoidoscopy, proctoscopy and stool specimens for occult blood. Intervention is by resection, excision of the tumour and anastomosis of the bowel, with or without a stoma. Further treatment may be necessary with radiotherapy and/or chemotherapy.

Strangulated hernia Strangulated hernia is a weakness in the muscle wall which allows peritoneum and bowel to protrude. It is irreducible and becomes constricted, therefore reducing the blood supply and causing ischaemia, necrosis and gangrene of the contained omentum or loop of bowel. Clinical manifestations also include colicky pain and increased swelling of the herniation. Diagnosis is by abdominal examination and X-ray. Intervention is by reduction and repair or resection of bowel.

Adhesions Adhesions result from formation of scar tissue within the peritoneal cavity. This usually occurs during the inflammatory response of healing, when tissue becomes attached to part of the intestine. It is associated with previous surgery, presence of infection, inflammation or injury. Clinical manifestations result when the intestine becomes twisted or kinked; they depend on the degree of obstruction but generally include nausea, vomiting, abdominal cramp pain and distension. Diagnosis is by abdominal X-ray. Intervention is by dividing the adhesions to free the intestine if the obstruction does not settle with conservative management.

Paralytic obstruction (paralytic ileus)

This condition is an absence or decrease in peristaltic action, which results in the bowel contents not flowing efficiently through the small intestine. Although not strictly a specific complication, it is appropriate to mention it at this point. The condition is associated with abdominal surgery, infection or mesenteric ischaemia. Clinical manifestations include those already addressed but may be complicated by fever, dehydration, electrolyte imbalance and respiratory distress. Diagnosis is by abdominal examination and abdominal X-ray. Intervention includes symptomatic management.

Nursing intervention

Many patients who are admitted with small bowel obstruction are treated as surgical emergencies, therefore time to improve nutritional and fluid levels is restricted. Fluids lost through vomiting or diarrhoea should be replaced and electrolytes corrected by intravenous infusion. The patient should be encouraged to rest and abstain from taking food or fluids orally until bowel function returns. A nasogastric tube on continuous drainage and intermittent suction is usually inserted to allow decompression of the bowel. Vital signs are monitored and pain control management evaluated.

Occasionally, surgical intervention, e.g. laporotomy with or without resection, and with either anastomosis or stoma, is required if the paralytic ileus results in a complication such as ischaemia or perforation.

Inflammatory bowel disease

Inflammatory bowel disease usually refers to two disorders – Crohn's disease and ulcerative colitis – although there are other forms.

Crohn's disease

Otherwise known as regional ileitis or granulomatous enteritis, this subacute and chronic inflammatory disorder was identified in 1932 by the American physician Burrill B. Crohn. The disease is often considered together with ulcerative colitis; however, it has a different aetiology and clinically presents differently. It can affect any part of the digestive system, but is common in the small intestine, particularly the terminal ileum. The diseased segments are often separated by normal bowel segments and can appear as isolated 'skip' lesions in other parts of the intestine. The inflammation may cause excessive production of fibroblasts and angiogenesis, i.e. new capillary buds, and is histologically distinguishable by the formation of a granuloma.

Clinically, there is a thickening of the bowel wall and the mucosal lining, giving the cobblestone appearance at the advanced stage. There is also a danger of the affected section of bowel forming abscesses that may rupture, or narrowing of the lumen through fibrosis and transmural damage, causing fistulas or sinuses (Cuschieri et al, 2002).

Crohn's disease is particularly common in young adults, although it can occur at any age and in both sexes equally, and in developed countries, with higher frequency in whites and the Jewish population. The incidence is thought to be higher than recorded, because many people remain undiagnosed (Harrison, 1984). There is still much speculation as to the cause of the disease, but, like many other disorders, it is multifactorial, with genetic and environmental factors. Many genes have been identified and it can be associated with autoimmune disorders, food additives, allergens and individual response to stress (Cuschieri et al, 2002).

Clinical manifestations Clinical symptoms of the disease are insidious and often well advanced before the patient seeks help. The patient may present to the doctor complaining of tiredness associated with lethargy and sometimes a persistent elevated temperature.

Other specific symptoms include abdominal pain that is often described as similar to cramp, particularly after meals. This is the result of peristalsis following the intake of food, and the inability of the contents to flow through the narrowed lumen. Some patients will complain of chronic mild pain which is persistent in nature, occurring between the cramping spasms, and some may have a painful and an ineffective desire to empty the rectum (tenesmus). Chronic inflammation of parts of the intestine and oedema may result in diarrhoea. The patient will often admit to having lost weight as a result of withholding food to avoid the cramping pain. This may lead to malnutrition and anaemia, as the patient may already be malnourished due to the malabsorption of nutrients through the small intestine. Diagnosis is through patient history, physical examination, barium and radiological studies, colonoscopy and ileoscopy, blood (leucocytosis), erythrocyte sedimentation rate (ESR), haemoglobin, C reactive protein (CRP), and stool specimens for infective organisms, fat content and occult blood.

Complications Complications may arise due to obstruction, perforation, malabsorption, melaena due to bleeding ulceration, and the formation of abscesses. Other effects of the disease may present as skin ulceration and infection, iritis, arthropathy and perianal sepsis in the form of anal fistulae.

Intervention   The vast majority of patients are treated medically, long term, with 5-ASA (5-aminosalicylic acid) compounds, steroids and immunosuppressants, such as azathioprine. Up to 70% of patients will, however, at some point in their life require surgical intervention. This may include segmental resection of the small bowel, subtotal colectomy, or total colectomy with formation of ileostomy, or surgery for perianal disease. Patients may require surgery on many separate occasions (often more than 50% in an attempt to ease the symptoms of the disease).

Ulcerative colitis

This is the term used to describe diffuse inflammation and multiple ulcerations of the superficial mucosa and occasionally the submucosa of the large intestine and rectum. The mucosa becomes oedematous and reddened with bleeding, and eventually becomes ulcerated. This ulceration results in the large intestine developing numerous continuous lesions that eventually cause muscular hypertrophy, which will shorten, narrow and thicken the bowel. The patient will have periods of exacerbation and remission. There is a danger of toxic dilatation, especially in the transverse colon in severe acute disease, that may result in perforation (Donnelly, 2003).

Aetiology and incidence   This is generally unknown but is similar to Crohn's disease. Some personality traits may influence the progression of ulcerative colitis. Individuals often present as passive and dependent personalities who are anxious to please (Whitehead and Schuster, 1985). Consequently, they find it more difficult to cope and may become psychologically, physically and emotionally stressed. Stress and emotional disturbance may influence the blood supply to the colon, which may result in eventual ulceration. Ulcerative colitis has also been associated with an immunological response to antigens (Mahilda, 1987).

As in Crohn's disease, ulcerative colitis has a familial tendency (Mahilda, 1987), and commonly affects young adults to the middle aged (Morson et al, 1979; Goligher et al, 1980; Day, 2003). Other conditions such as arthritis, ankylosing spondylitis, pyoderma gangrenosum and hepatitis may be associated with ulcerative colitis (Kelly, 1994).

Clinical manifestations   These are similar to those as described in Crohn's disease but histologically crypt abscesses are seen, which can become necrotic and ulcerated. There is intermittent tenesmus with urgency and cramping pain. Loose bowel action may occur, often 10–20 times daily. Rectal bleeding may be present, sometimes with anaemia. Eventually, the debilitating progression of the disease may extend to

Table 15.5   Inflammatory bowel disorders – causes and surgical interventions

Cause	Intervention
Crohn's disease	Segmental resection
	Subtotal colectomy
	Total colectomy
	Strictureplasty
Ulcerative colitis	Kock's pouch
	Parks' pouch
	Proctocolectomy
	Total colectomy

such a degree that it affects normal activities of daily living and social interactions. It can also be so advanced that fistulas and abscesses may be present.

Diagnosis is by barium radiological studies and blood tests, which may identify a high white blood count (WBC), platelets and ESR. Colonoscopy is the diagnostic tool of choice; however, there are some reservations on performing the procedure on patients who have active colitis due to the increased risk of perforating the bowel (Hardman et al, 1995).

Intervention   If medical intervention and control with 5-ASA compounds and steroids does not bring about remission, or the disease has been active for the most part of 20 years, the patient may have an increased risk of developing adenocarcinoma of the colon and rectum, and surgery is then advisable. Emergency life-threatening complications usually require surgical intervention.

Surgical intervention may include subtotal colectomy and ileostomy, or, either proctocolectomy with formation of ileostomy or ileal-pouch–anal anastomosis (Table 15.5). The pioneer in this field was Sir Alan Parks, who developed the Parks' pouch procedure in the late 1970s (Parks and Percy, 1982). The main types of pouch are the J pouch, where the ileum is folded once into a 'J'-shaped reservoir, then sutured directly to the anal canal, and the W pouch, which has four sections similarly joined to make a pouch and then sutured to the anal canal (Cuschieri et al, 2002) (Figs 15.9 and 15.10).

With increasing specialization in recent years, this type of surgical intervention has become more favoured over the traditional procedure of proctocolectomy and formation of an ileostomy. The purpose of ileal-pouch–anal anastomosis is to restore the continuity of the gastrointestinal tract and to promote acceptability, especially in younger patients, by preserving the sphincter control and promoting continence (Wiltz et al, 1991). The implications of the

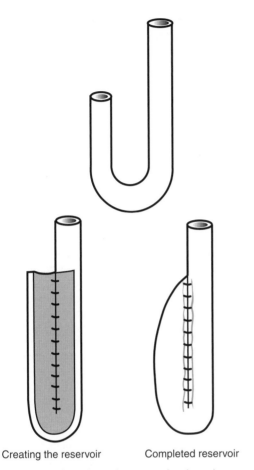

Creating the reservoir   Completed reservoir

Figure 15.9 Ileal-pouch–anal anastomosis – J pouch (two sections of small bowel to form the pouch).

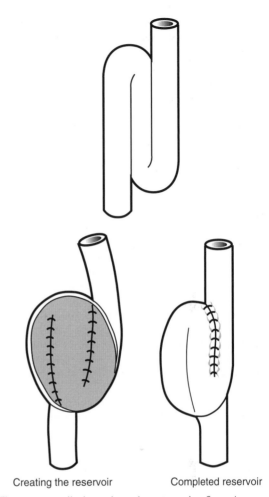

Creating the reservoir   Completed reservoir

Figure 15.10 Ileal-pouch–anal anastomosis – S pouch (three sections of small bowel to form the pouch).

formation of an ileostomy are well documented, especially the psychological aspects associated with an altered body image (Black, 2000). An attempt is made to preserve the anal sphincter and provide an ileal–anal reservoir by resecting the colon and most of the rectum. The remaining rectum has the mucosa excised, leaving the sphincter muscles around the anus intact. A reservoir or pouch is constructed by using the lower part of the small bowel and is joined to the anus. Alternatively, a double-stapled pouch is formed and stapled to the upper anus without excising the mucosa. The bowel contents are usually diverted from the newly constructed reservoir by an ileostomy, until it is healed. Approximately 2 months after the operation, healing is checked by a water-soluble contrast enema (pouchogram) and an examination under general anaesthetic. If healing is satisfactory and the anal sphincter muscles are sufficiently strong, the ileostomy is closed.

This whole procedure may be performed in three stages:

- *Stage 1* includes the colectomy, preservation of the rectum and anal sphincter and formation of the ileostomy.
- *Stage 2* includes the formation of the reservoir and loop ileostomy. This may be easily closed when the reservoir or pouch has healed. Stages 1 and 2 can be performed in one operation for elective cases.
- *Stage 3* is closure of the loop ileostomy.

Ileostomy

In this operation, ileum is brought through an opening to the abdomen. It is usually performed following pan-proctocolectomy or total colectomy, when the diseased or inflamed bowel has been removed, e.g. in ulcerative colitis or Crohn's disease. The opening is higher up the bowel (the ileum); therefore, the bowel contents are more fluid, as the water has not been absorbed via the large colon.

Pre- and postoperative care of patients with inflammatory bowel disease

Specific preoperative assessment

If the patient has been in a period of exacerbation for some weeks, they may already be dehydrated and malnourished. Therefore, nursing intervention should include the replacement of fluids and blood, and a nutritional support programme undertaken prior to surgical intervention; this may include total parenteral nutrition. If the patient is not in a state of exacerbation, then a low-residue diet is encouraged with small portions several times a day. When steroid therapy has been a part of the previous management regime, this is continued and sometimes larger doses are given at the time of surgery, then slowly reduced over a period of time following surgery. Antibiotics are often prescribed as a prophylactic measure. In both types of surgery involving the formation of an ileostomy and ileal-pouch–anal anastomosis, psychological preparation and support from the stomatherapist should be an integral component of care planning.

The stomatherapist will also be involved in marking the site for the ileostomy, i.e. in siting it appropriately for the patient in terms of clothing, previous surgery and body fat distribution. Assessing the patient's needs and matching these with the types of ileostomy appliances available is also important. A vital part of preparation for this type of surgery includes providing education and knowledge of the disease and surgical interventions in a language that the patient will understand and respond to by asking appropriate questions. There are many patient information leaflets available from such organizations as the Ileostomy Association of Great Britain and Ireland, and the British Colostomy Association, as well as the manufacturers of stoma products.

One of the problems that may arise with this type of surgery and formation of ileostomy is the anxiety of the patient who feels that they may have lost control over faecal elimination, therefore increasing the risk of body image disturbance (Box 15.5).

Specific postoperative interventions

Eating and drinking   In the immediate postoperative period the patient may have a nasogastric tube in position, which will be on continuous drainage and may be aspirated every 4 hours. This will ensure that there is no retention of gastric fluid, which will cause distension of the abdomen. Fluid loss will be from the stoma drainage, so fluids will need to be replaced by intravenous infusion. This method of replacing fluids will be necessary until there is evidence of bowel activity following surgery. Fluids are often given orally in small amounts and gradually increased if there is no abdominal distension, discomfort or vomiting. If distension and intolerance to fluids does occur, then the patient is restricted from taking oral fluids until the distension subsides. If this is not resolved, the patient may require intravenous nutrition support or occasionally further surgical intervention, as the bowel may be obstructed. Diet is commenced once oral fluids are tolerated and this may initially be a low-residue, high-calorie diet, until the patient has become adjusted to his altered digestive function.

Elimination   The management of an ileostomy involves observation of the stoma for any signs of stoma necrosis, oedema and/or retraction. The colour should remain a healthy pink; if the stoma changes to a bluish/black colour, then it may indicate ischaemia, and that the stoma is at risk of developing tissue necrosis. If tissue necrosis does occur, then surgery is required to remove the ischaemic bowel. Sometimes the tissue surrounding the stoma becomes oedematous, and this can cause the skin to stretch the blood vessels, resulting in occlusion of the blood supply to the stoma. The bag size should be checked, when the oedema subsides, for a correctly fitting appliance. It is important that all fluid loss is measured and documented in order to calculate the patient's fluid replacement requirements for every 24 hours.

The stoma should also be observed for any signs of retraction. This can be caused by poor healing of the suture line, through poor nutrition, or due to technical problems with formation of the stoma. The patient may have been on steroid drugs for some time, and therefore will be more susceptible to wound and suture line breakdown (Anstead, 1998).

Personal cleansing and dressing   The integrity of the skin is very important for patients with an ileostomy. The skin surrounding the stoma is vulnerable to excoriation if the stoma bag is not positioned correctly and faeces leak onto the skin surface. This is more likely to occur if the diet is not correct and the faeces are more fluid, containing enzymes and digestive secretions. It is important that the stoma bag is the correct size and fits to the contours of the skin. Sometimes problems can be avoided by using a drainable bag, skin sealant and/or barrier paste, e.g. Stomahesive.

Sexuality   There is a possibility that the patient may experience some sexual dysfunction following surgery, and this can be associated with damage to the nerves at the time of surgery or from the psychological

Box 15.5 Specific issues related to having a stoma

- Increased anxiety due to the possible presence of odour and flatulence from the ileostomy.
- Increased anxiety associated with possible visibility of the stoma appliance through clothing.
- Anxiety associated with adapting to the ileostomy and ability to apply coping mechanisms.
- Anxiety regarding relationships with partners and expressing sexuality.

Specific objective will be to preserve the patient's body image, and empower the patient in retaining sense of control over bowel function.

Nursing intervention and rationale

- The possibility of odour is one of the problems that causes the patient considerable anxiety, and in order for the patient to control the odour, it is important that they change the bag regularly, and have the knowledge of odourproof bags and deodorants that are available for use when the bag is emptied and changed.

  Advice should be given on which types of food can be eaten that will reduce odour, e.g. orange juice and yogurt. Some foods should be avoided, such as cabbage, onions, beans and garlic, in order to avoid associated embarrassment of flatulence.
- The patient should be educated as to what foods may cause an increase in flatulence, and period of time between ingestion and the production of flatus. If flatus is difficult to control, it can lead to increased social embarrassment.

The patient should also be taught to anticipate the need for the correct bag and deodorant filters to be attached, therefore minimizing the effects of flatus by releasing the flatus through the deodorized filter.
- The patient should be educated as to how to conceal the bag underneath a stretchy layer of clothing. This will hold the bag next to the skin surface, thereby reducing the bulk. This will have the effect of enhancing the body image by enabling the patient to dress acceptably in clothes that they already have.
- Discussion should be encouraged with the patient and family of the normal emotional response to the ileostomy. This gives the opportunity for negative feelings to be explored and accepted. Coping strategies should be addressed with the patient and their family, as these may need to be altered, adapted or new methods adopted.
- Specialist advice and information on other specialist organizations should be offered, as contact with others in a similar situation will reduce some of the isolation that the patient may be feeling. It will also increase the patient's awareness of the condition being manageable.
- Specialist advice should also be provided on how to manage the ileostomy in normal occupation, social and sexual activities. This will enable the patient to consider coping strategies for these activities, therefore helping to ensure successful outcomes.
- Ensure patients have the contact details of their local stomatherapist for advice and follow-up.

impact of an altered body image. It is important, therefore, that opportunities are given to the patient and the family for full, open and honest discussion of their ability to adapt to the ileostomy, and adopt measures to disguise the ileostomy during sexual activity.

Wound Particular attention should be paid to the sutures around the stoma, ensuring that they are not pulling the wound, nor are they too tight, causing wound breakdown or infection.

Additional specific complications

Other complications include stoma necrosis, oedema and retraction, as previously described. Sometimes, acute obstruction can occur as a result of paralytic ileus or oedema.

Skin excoriation can occur as a result of diarrhoea and poor wound healing, or wound breakdown due to long-term malnutrition. If the patient and the family have a knowledge deficit regarding the condition and the after-care, it is possible that there may be adverse psychological implications with respect to both the acceptance of the ileostomy and alteration of body image.

Education and discharge planning

Prior to discharge, the documentation should indicate that the patient does not have fever or any condition that would delay recovery, and that they will be able to progress satisfactorily in their own home. This should reduce the risk of readmission. Education and advice should also be given on how to manage the stoma. A routine should be established for changing the bag, with all equipment ready prepared. The surrounding skin should be cleaned with warm water. The used bag should be sealed in a plastic bag and disposed of in the dustbin, not flushed down the toilet. Supportive literature highlighting these points and contact numbers may also be given.

There are no restrictions on diet, but the patient should be advised to avoid any food that produces wind or discomfort. There are no problems with travel, but the patient should make certain that they have all the equipment for changing the bag to hand. It is usual to return to work 6–8 weeks after the final operation. Patients who have a pouch formation may return to work in between operations, depending on how they feel.

A full explanation should be provided to patients of how to use community facilities, special organizations and support groups, and how to seek advice or contact appropriate health professionals for support if they are worried about their progress.

LARGE INTESTINE

Anatomy and physiology

The colon has a serous peritoneal lining forming a mesentery in parts. Its muscular component consists of circular and longitudinal muscle that together help to propel and mix the bowel content. It is approximately 1.5 m long and divided into sections. Its mucosa contains no villi, but has goblet cells that secret mucus to aid the passage of intestinal residue, which may stay in the colon for several days depending on the amount of dietary fibre content.

Normal function

Absorption of water from the end products of digestion is approximately 1 L in 24 hours. Faeces are propelled along the colon by the action of peristalsis. Whenever food enters the stomach, a reflex action occurs that opens the ileocaecal valve. This action causes the food to be passed along the small intestine and into the colon. Peristaltic movements occur four to five times daily.

An additional function of the large intestine is to synthesize vitamin K in the presence of stercobilinogen and bacteria. Vitamin K is absorbed through the gut wall into the bloodstream and has an important function in clotting.

Abnormal function

Peristalsis may be dormant, causing the water to be absorbed from the colon, resulting in constipation; or quickened, resulting in diarrhoea, altering the bowel elimination pattern.

Constipation

The stool becomes very hard and may become impacted, causing infrequent bowel actions and, depending on the cause, may result in complete absence of defecation. Other terms used to describe constipation include

Table 15.6 Diarrhoea and constipation – causes and interventions

Cause	Intervention
Diarrhoea	
Infection	Antibiotics
Diet	Avoid hot spicy foods and alcohol
Irritable bowel syndrome	Avoid stress, coffee and alcohol
Ulcerative colitis	Steroids, surgery, ileostomy
Crohn's disease	Steroids, surgery
Carcinoma	Surgery
Metabolic disorders	Medication
Malabsorption	Avoid certain food, e.g. fats
Medications	Identify causative drug
Constipation	
Diet	High-fibre diet, education
Medication	Avoid drugs that affect gut motility
Nerve damage	Surgery
Obstruction/carcinoma	Surgery
Iron supplements	Alternative iron replacement therapy

feeling bloated or full, and experiencing difficulty or the inability to pass a hard stool (Ross, 1993).

Causes of constipation Constipation may be due to poor dietary fibre intake, poor mobility, some types of medication (particularly, strong analgesic preparations, antidepressants, hypotensives and iron), carcinoma and damage or abnormality of the nerve supply (Table 15.6).

Diarrhoea

Sometimes malfunction occurs as a result of excessive bowel movement, resulting in diarrhoea. Other terms used to describe this condition include passing a liquid stool, and urgency associated with abdominal cramps (Ross, 1993). This condition should be recognized as potentially harmful, and consideration should be given to the loss of water and electrolytes. Potassium depletion and dehydration, if not replaced adequately, can have very serious consequences, especially for small children and the elderly.

Causes of diarrhoea Diarrhoea may be due to infection (viral or bacterial), hot spicy foods, irritable bowel syndrome, diverticular disease, ulcerative colitis, Crohn's disease, carcinoma, radiation, overactive thyroid gland, malabsorption, or side-effects from medication, e.g. antibiotics and NSAIDs (see Table 15.6).

Elderly patients are particularly vulnerable to alteration in bowel elimination pattern (McShane and McLane, 1985; Read and Timms, 1986; Bruckstein, 1988;

Ross, 1993), especially when in hospital. These are thought to be linked to the changes in lifestyle imposed through the hospital environment: e.g. different eating patterns and diet, reduced or limited mobility, increased anxiety and inability to cope with stress (Meek, 2000).

Pathology

Diverticular disease

Diverticula commonly occur in the sigmoid colon and are caused by pouch-like herniations of mucosa through the muscular layer of the colon. They are thought to be associated with a low-residue diet, constipation and excessive use of aperients, causing changes in the colonic pressure. They are commonly asymptomatic, but those patients who are affected often present with bleeding and complain of cramp-type pain over the sigmoid colon in the left iliac fossa. Barium investigations and colonoscopy for rectal bleeding identify diverticular disease. Diverticulitis results when the area becomes infected and inflamed and there may be abscesses forming. An increased diet of fibre, e.g. fruit, vegetables and bran, will assist in the movement of faeces through the colon, thus preventing aggravation and obstruction (Hyde, 2003).

Surgical intervention   Resection of the affected colon may be carried out, and the two ends anastomosed together. Sometimes, depending on the condition of the patient, a resection is performed initially and the anastomosis undertaken at a later stage. This is commonly referred to as a Hartmann's excision (Box 15.6). This procedure includes the formation of a colostomy, which may be temporary or permanent.

Appendicitis

Appendicitis is acute inflammation of the appendix. The appendix, a tubular projection approximately 5–10 cm long, is attached to the caecum. Its function originally was to digest cellulose, in herbivores, but this function diminished when the consumption of meat was increased in the diet (Alexander et al, 2000). However, it does fill with faeces and empties on a regular basis. Problems occur when the faeces or foreign bodies become lodged in the tubular lumen and cause obstruction; the lumen then becomes inflamed and painful. Appendicitis may first appear chronic and mild or grumbling, often changing to become acute and severe, and can lead to a strangulated appendix, which becomes gangrenous and has an increased risk of perforation.

Clinical manifestations   The main symptoms of acute inflammation include nausea, vomiting, anorexia, pyrexia and tachycardia, and blood tests will show a

---

> **Box 15.6   Large bowel disorders**
>
> *Diverticular disease*
> - *Indication for surgery*: haemorrhage, perforation, peritonitis, abscess formation, fistula formation, obstruction
> - *Types of surgery*: Hartmann's procedure
>
> *Large bowel obstruction*
> - *Indication for surgery*: cancer, diverticular disease, inflammatory bowel disease, benign tumours
> - *Types of surgery*: segmental resection of colon, abdominoperineal resection, colostomy formation, Hartmann's procedure, bypass surgery (palliative)

---

rise in leucocytes. The pain and tenderness initially presents in the upper central section of the abdomen, but gradually radiates to become severe in the lower right quadrant. Age range is usually older children, teenagers and young adults, and it is more common in males than females.

Investigation and diagnosis   This is based on a thorough general history and clinical examination, although occasionally ultrasound may be performed if diagnosis is unconfirmed.

Intervention   The main objective is to reduce the associated pain and infection by giving appropriate antibiotics and analgesics, and to replace fluid loss prior to surgery.

Surgical intervention   Appendicectomy is the management of an inflamed or infected appendix, because of the high risk of perforation leading to peritonitis. It can be life threatening and constitutes a surgical emergency.

Peritonitis (inflammation of the peritoneum)

The peritoneal cavity is a potentially sterile environment that, once contaminated by infected pus and bacteria, faecal fluid and products of digestion, becomes inflamed and irritated, producing copious amounts of serous fluid. This serous fluid and leakage from the rupture or perforation has the potential of spreading throughout the peritoneal cavity, and, if bacteria are present, the resulting toxins will be absorbed through the peritoneum.

Clinical manifestations   The pain associated with peritonitis can be very severe and immediate, although somewhat diffused at first. It is quickly followed by the symptoms of shock with associated nausea, vomiting and loss of fluids and electrolytes. Body temperature is elevated, and the patient is extremely lethargic and weak. Initial increased motility of the gastrointestinal

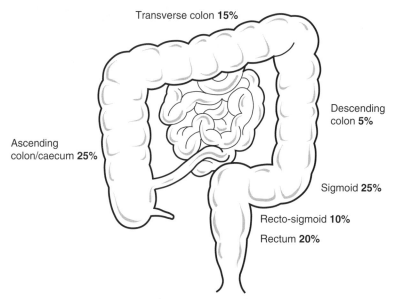

Figure 15.11   Distribution of cancers of the large bowel. (From Butcher, 2003.)

tract is evident, but this is followed by decreased activity known as paralytic ileus, a temporary loss of smooth muscle tone resulting in the abdomen becoming rigid and tender.

Investigations and diagnosis   This is through X-ray examination, which will identify any air or fluid levels present. They may also give an indication of the site of perforation or evidence of abdominal obstruction.

Surgical intervention   Peritonitis constitutes a surgical emergency, along with appropriate antibiotic therapy, fluid and electrolyte replacement. A laparotomy is performed and the perforation or other underlying cause is repaired, excised or resected, and the cavity drained of the leaked contents. As there is a risk of septicaemia, intravenous antibiotics are commenced at an early stage.

Colorectal carcinoma
Cancer of the bowel is the second most common cause of death from cancer in the UK. In 2002 the deaths attributed to cancer of the bowel in the UK were approximately 16 220 (Cancer Research UK, 2004).

Aetiology and incidence   Colorectal carcinoma is commonest in people over the age of 60 years and has a slightly higher incidence in men (Cancer Research UK, 2004). Generally, adenocarcinoma accounts for 90–94% of cases, and the theory is that a substantial number of colorectal cancers arise from adenomatous polyps, i.e. benign tumours that develop from the normal colonic mucosa (Cuschieri et al, 2002).

Cancer of the large bowel is due to genetic factors and may be familial. It can also be influenced by environmental factors: e.g. lack of exercise (Ballard-Barbash et al, 1990; Little et al, 1993); diet that is low in fibre and has a high fat content (Burkitt, 1971); a high intake of beer, which is associated with a high incidence of rectal cancers (Faivre, 1992). High levels of calcium are thought to protect against colorectal cancers, but not sufficiently to recommend a dietary increase (Buset et al, 1986). Similarly, there is evidence to suggest that inhibition of malignant transformation may occur as a result of vitamins acting as antioxidants (Paraskeva and Logan, 1993).

Some families have a genetic predisposition to developing colorectal cancer (Kinzler et al, 1991; Peltomaki et al, 1993). These predispositions relate to two conditions: the first accounts for approximately 1% of colorectal cases in the Western world, and is called familial adenomatous polyposis (FAP), i.e. thousands of polyps that line the entire large intestine; the second accounts for 4–13% of colorectal cancers in industrialized nations and is referred to as hereditary non-polyposis colorectal cancer (HNPCC). Other conditions that are thought to predispose to cancer are long-standing inflammatory bowel disorders, particularly ulcerative colitis (Paraskeva and Logan, 1993). The general percentage distribution of the cancers within the large bowel is shown in Figure 15.11. It can be seen that rectal cancers account for approximately 38% of cases reported, followed by 28% in the sigmoid colon (Butcher, 2003).

Box 15.7   TNM classification of stages of colorectal tumours (from Taylor et al, 2002)

Primary tumour (T)

Pathological staging

TX   Primary tumour cannot be assessed

T0   No evidence of primary tumour

Tis   Carcinoma in situ: intraepithelial or invasion of lamina propria

T1   Tumour invades submucosa

T2   Tumour invades muscularis propria

T3   Tumour invades through the muscularis propria into the subserosa, or into non-peritonealized pericolic or perirectal tissues

T4   Tumour directly invades other organs or structures and/or perforates the peritoneum

Ultrasound staging (u)

uT0   Benign tumour

uT1   Invasion into but not through the submucosa

uT2   Invasion into but not through the muscularis propria

uT3   Invasion into perirectal fat

uT4   Invasion into adjacent organs

Regional lymph nodes (N)

NX   Regional lymph nodes cannot be assessed

N0   No regional lymph node metastasis

N1   Metastases in 1–3 regional lymph nodes

N2   Metastases in 4 or more regional lymph nodes

uN0   No metastatic perirectal node

uN1   Metastatic perirectal nodes

Distant metastases (M)

MX   Distant metastases cannot be assessed

M0   No distant metastases

M1   Distant metastases

Stage grouping

AJCC/UICC[1]				Dukes[2]
Stage 0	Tis	N0	M0	–
Stage 1	T1	N0	M0	A
	T2	N0	M0	–
Stage 2	T3	N0	M0	B
	T4	N0	M0	–
Stage 3	Any T	N1	M0	C
	Any T	N2	M0	–
Stage 4	Any T	Any N	M1	D

[1]American Joint Committee on Cancer /International Union Against Cancer.
[2]Dukes B is a composite of better (T3/N0/M0) and worse (T4/N0/M0) prognostic groups, as is Dukes C (Any T/N1/M0 and Any T/ N2/M0).

Colorectal cancers are classified by using the TNM staging system. This system provides a more accurate description of the tumour itself and its relation to other organs than the older Dukes' classification system. The tumours are classified into four stages, as shown in Box 15.7.

Clinical manifestations   Symptoms are often insidious, and the tumours very often are quite advanced by the time the patient seeks help from the doctor. The main presenting manifestation is an altered bowel pattern. This may be either constipation, diarrhoea or both. Rectal bleeding may also be evident, and on further investigation the patient may present with anaemia. Some abdominal discomfort may occur, especially if the tumour is large and causing pressure on soft tissue and nerves, although this is not one of the main clinical manifestations.

Investigations   These include digital rectal examination, abdominal examination and X-rays to establish evidence of a palpable mass, faecal occult bloods, proctoscopy, sigmoidoscopy, colonoscopy, barium enema, and diagnostic investigation if metastases are suspected, such as a staging CT scan.

Surgical intervention   Surgery includes right or left hemicolectomy, transverse colectomy, anterior resection and abdominoperineal excision of colon, depending on the position of the tumour (Figs 15.12–15.15).

Screening   Survival rates may improve if early diagnosis of colorectal cancer is made. There is currently ongoing research investigating the use of flexible sigmoidoscopy, with or without faecal occult blood screening as a one-off for people aged 55–60 years old (Atkin, 1999; Wardle et al, 1999). Dr W Atkin and team at the Cancer Research UK, Colorectal Centre in London, are currently investigating if screening for bowel cancer will prevent further deaths, due to earlier diagnosis and treatment.

Pre- and postoperative care of patients undergoing colonic surgery

Specific preoperative assessment

Treatment of choice for colonic cancer is surgery. The tumour is removed along with the surrounding margin of tissue. If early diagnosis and intervention occurs, patients with TNM stages 1 and 2 have a good prognosis, and do not require further treatment. It is

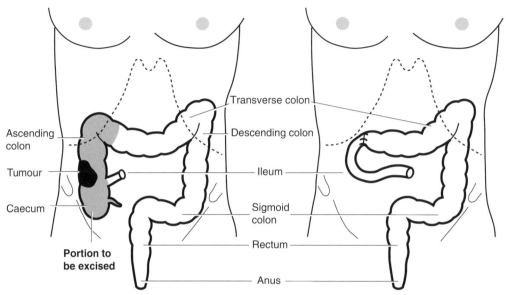

Figure 15.12 Hemicolectomy (right).

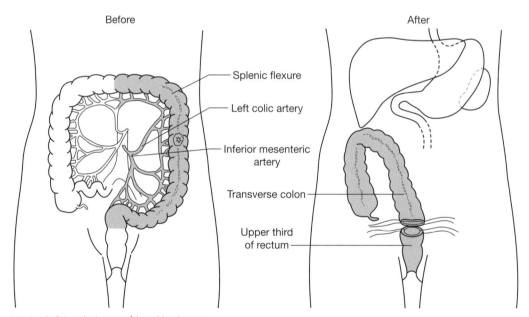

Figure 15.13 Left hemicolectomy/sigmoid colectomy.

also important to remember that the skills of the surgeon are important in the prognosis of the disease (McArdle and Hole, 1991). Increasingly, multidisplinary teams are involved in providing the best care for patients.

The nurse has an important role in facilitating and documenting the provision of information, teaching activities, physical examination, laboratory tests or diagnostic procedures, informed consent, psychological preparation, physical preparation of the gastrointestinal tract and skin and administration of medications. These are important areas that enable the patient to proceed safely through surgery.

Bowel preparation may be indicated to prevent infection and remove faecal matter. This is achieved by

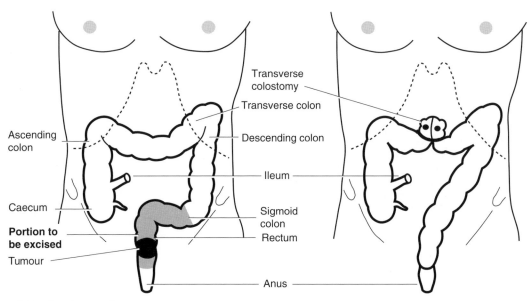

Figure 15.14   Anterior resection.

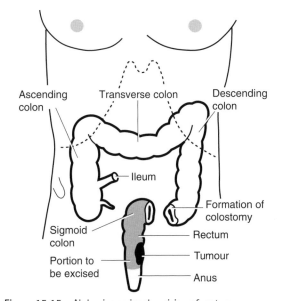

Figure 15.15   Abdominoperineal excision of rectum.

administering an enema/colonic irrigation, or prescribed bowel preparation (polyethylene glycol, sodium pico-sulphate or phosphate solutions), and antibiotics may be given orally (Solla and Rothenberger, 1990). During these procedures some patients may need careful monitoring, due to possible unpleasant side-effects and fluid loss (Box 15.8).

Stoma formation and management
Stoma is the Greek term used to describe a mouth or opening – in this context an opening in the abdominal wall through which the contents of the bowel are evacuated.

Colostomy   A healthy piece of colon is brought through an opening onto the abdomen. It may be referred to as single-barrel, double-barrel or loop colostomy that is supported by a rod, and can be temporary or permanent. A temporary colostomy is performed to give time for the colon to recover and heal prior to resuming its functions. A permanent colostomy is usually performed following the removal of part of the bowel, particularly following the removal of a malignant tumour. The position of the colostomy can vary according to the area of colon that is affected.

Nursing issues   Optimum management is that all patients who are to undergo bowel surgery and have the formation of a stoma, have the condition and implications discussed with them and their family. However, in some emergency situations, this is not possible. In most hospitals a specialist nurse in stomatherapy is available for education and counselling purposes. Specialist advice may be given, and the patient is informed of the self-help or support organizations. The stomatherapist may also advise on the most appropriate position for the formation of the stoma. Consideration should be given to the position of the incision line, bones, scars, skin creases, activities and type of clothes the patient wears.

Box 15.8 Specific issues related to preoperative bowel preparation

- Potential risk of infection if the bowel is not adequately cleansed/operation cancelled due to inadequate preparation.
- Potential loss of fluid and electrolytes due to the physical preparation/dehydration from the cleaning solutions.
- Potential risk of abdominal pain caused by the physical preparation.

Specific objective will be to ensure that the bowel is clean prior to surgery and to minimize the side-effects of vomiting and abdominal pain.

Nursing intervention and rationale
- Ensure the physical cleansing preparation procedure is correctly carried out and the instructions for any laxatives or irrigation carefully followed and monitored. The result of the preparation should be fully documented, and any difficulty in carrying out the procedure should be reported to the surgeon who is performing the surgery.
- All fluid loss associated with diarrhoea and vomiting should be recorded on the appropriate documentation, thereby ensuring that fluid and electrolytes can be replaced by intravenous infusion. Antiemetics may be used to relieve excessive nausea and vomiting.
- Identify the characteristics of the abdominal pain, e.g. location, duration and intensity, and provide appropriate analgesics, ensuring the effectiveness is evaluated. Any associated discomfort through diarrhoea is relieved by ensuring the anal area is clean and dry following the bowel action and by providing anaesthetic creams and protective barrier creams.

All patients who have a stoma formed should receive the appropriate educational material, which will enable them to understand what changes have occurred to their body, what activities they may safely pursue and how to deal with minor complications.

Specific postoperative nursing interventions

Eating and drinking Oral fluids are initially restricted but should return to normal as soon as possible following the surgery. A good indication to commence oral fluids and diet is when the patient has bowel sounds and passes flatus. It is important, therefore, that the patient receives intravenous fluids to replace the loss of fluid and electrolytes. There is also a potential risk of paralytic ileus resulting from the handling of the bowel during surgery. This may be managed by resting the bowel. If the patient has resumed oral fluids, these will be withheld and intravenous fluids recommenced until bowel sounds again return.

The advice for patients with a colostomy is similar to that already described for patients with an ileostomy. However, depending on the stage of the disease and extent of surgery, some patients may need further nutritional supplements of protein, calories and carbohydrates.

Elimination Particular management of the stoma has already been discussed in the section referring to the formation of an ileostomy. However, it is important that the patient is educated and given the option to choose which appliance to use, and how to remove and change the appliance. Supervision and education are usually provided by the stomatherapist or nurses working in specialized colorectal surgical wards.

Change of body image and sexual activity The major area of concern relates to the patient's accepting the colostomy from an early stage. Some patients may wish to discuss the aspect of sexual rehabilitation. Common fears are those of impotence and appearing mutilated, and the consequent effect on their sexuality. Examples have previously been given and highlighted in Box 15.5.

Skin care The risk to skin integrity around the stoma has already been discussed under the management of an ileostomy. However, if the patient has a perineal suture line, there is an increased risk of wound infection or necrosis. This area is also very painful for the patient, due to the presence of sutures and drains; therefore, along with appropriate analgesics, a specialized cushion should be used, e.g. a Valley cushion.

Additional specific complications Other complications include the risk of pulmonary complications, paralytic ileus, wound infection, stoma necrosis and breakdown of the anastomosis/suture site.

Education and discharge planning
Educational advice is similar to that given for inflammatory bowel disease, especially if there has been the formation of a colostomy. Instruction should be given as to how and when to change the bag, irrigate the stoma if necessary and clean the surrounding skin. Used bags are disposed of by placing them in a sealed plastic bag for refuse collection.

Dietary advice is important so that the patient can control the intake of certain foods that may give rise to excessive wind, constipation or loose bowel action.

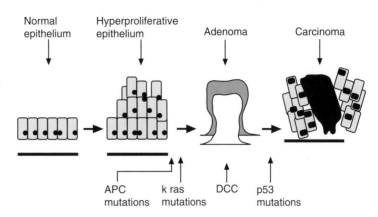

Figure 15.16 Polyp cancer sequence. Proposed adenoma to carcinoma sequence in colorectal cancer. Adenomatous polyposis coli (APC) gene mutations and hypermethylation occur early, followed by k ras mutations. Deleted in colon cancer (DCC) and p53 gene mutations occur later in the sequence, although the exact order may vary. (Printed with permission from BMJ Books.)

Supportive literature and contact numbers may also be given for use in case of an emergency or if the client is worried about their condition.

Rectal surgery

Polyps

Polyps occur from the mucous membrane and are small benign tumour-like growth projections that are more common in the large intestine, i.e. sigmoid and rectum. They are often benign; however, they can be the precursor in the development of malignant polyps and cancer of the bowel. Figure 15.16 illustrates the sequence of a benign polyp becoming malignant. There is a condition known as familial adenomatous polyposis (FAP), when large numbers of polyps occur in the large intestine, and it is thought to be precancerous; therefore, the aim of management is to remove the colon surgically. This is thought to account for only 1–3% of all bowel cancers. However, hereditary non-polyposis colorectal cancer (HNPCC) accounts for between 5 and 10% of bowel cancers. This inherited condition requires surveillance by colonoscopy and possible surgery.

Clinical manifestations Polyps are often asymptomatic, although they may bleed, and so the patient presents with rectal bleeding. Symptoms are determined by the number of polyps, position and size.

Investigations These include rectal examination, proctoscopy, sigmoidoscopy, colonoscopy and occasionally barium enema.

Surgical interventions Surgery includes excision of polyps, often endoscopically. However, surgical intervention such as total colectomy and ileo-anal anastomosis may be required for those patients with familial polyposis.

Abscess

An abscess is formed as a result of localized infections, resulting in a cavity in the pararectal spaces, which contains pus and is surrounded by inflamed tissue.

Clinical manifestations These include a very painful site, raised temperature and oedema. There may be an associated malodorous discharge from the rectum. Abscesses may result from perianal fistulae.

Intervention This requires antibiotic therapy and excision and drainage of the abscess. If a fistula has developed, this may require surgery at a later date where the fistula is laid open and healing occurs through secondary intention. Antibiotics are rarely required, except where there is significant cellulitis and induration despite following adequate surgical drainage.

Fistula

A fistula is an abnormal opening between two epithelial surfaces, but commonly in this condition it is an opening at the cutaneous surface near the anus (Fig. 15.17). It is common in Crohn's disease, but most are caused by a local crypt abscess.

Clinical manifestations These include a rise in temperature and associated pain with a presenting abscess. Sometimes a rectal discharge is present, which often causes excoriation of the surrounding skin and pruritus.

Surgical intervention This will often take the form of incision and drainage if there is an abscess, and excision or laying open of the fistulae tract to allow healing by secondary intention. The insertion of a seton, or suture material threaded through the fistula tract, allows the tract to drain and can then be laid open surgically. The insertion of a cutting seton cuts through the sphincter muscle, rather like a cheese wire, preventing

Figure 15.17 Anal sphincters showing anal fistula positions.

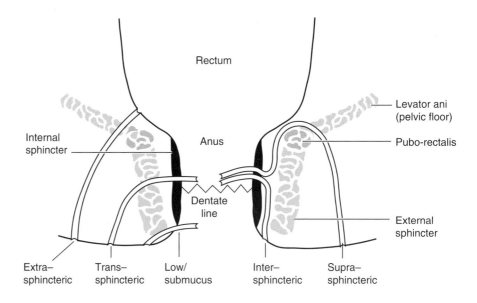

it from retracting while it heals (Hibberts and Carapeti, 2003).

Fissure

A fissure is a tear or crack in the lining of the anus. It is often due to straining on defecation and having a very hard stool.

Clinical manifestation There is extremely sharp pain on evacuation of faeces. It may be managed by the local application of anaesthetic creams/gels, the administration of a mild laxative and increased consumption of water to prevent constipation.

Surgical intervention This may sometimes be required, e.g. sphincterotomy, although many fissures resolve themselves. The operation involves cutting a section in one of the anal sphincter muscles. The implications of undergoing this type of surgery must be discussed with the patient, as temporary or permanent faecal and flatus incontinence may result.

Haemorrhoids (piles)

These are cushions of spongy connective tissue and blood vessels in the anus which, with prolonged straining and hard stools, can descend down the anal canal and cause bleeding. Sometimes they become large enough to protrude from the anus and may become constricted and painful. This condition arises from years of constipation, whereby straining to pass a stool increases the intra-abdominal pressure, resulting in their prolapse. They can also be strangulated and thombosed, which requires urgent attention.

Clinical manifestations There may be evidence of fresh blood and increased pain when opening the bowels. This is thought to be due to the constipation and straining that is associated with this condition.

Investigations These include digital rectal examination, proctoscopy and sigmoidoscopy.

Intervention Many patients manage the condition themselves by the use of local applications of topical medication to lubricate, anaesthetize and shrink the haemorrhoids. If medical advice is sought, this would include health promotion of a high-fibre intake and possibly a bulk laxative.

Surgical interventions Surgery includes injecting the haemorrhoidal veins, which initiates fibrosis and atrophy; ligation, which causes the vessels to shrink through prolonged constriction; and excision and ligation of the haemorrhoid, e.g. haemorrhoidectomy.

Nursing implications Nurses must be aware that straining to defecate and constipation contribute to the development of haemorrhoids. Pregnant women should be encouraged to remain free from constipation.

Complications Haemorrhoids may rupture or thrombose, but most of these resolve spontaneously and conservative treatment is all that is required.

Pilonidal sinus

Pilonidal sinus is a blind ending subcutaneous cavity communicating with the skin and may contain hair. It is most frequently situated over or close to the tip of the coccyx. Abscess formation is common following irritation and subsequent infection.

Clinical manifestations   These include pain and discharge associated with the abscess formation, and often affect males during adolescence.

Intervention   This includes a course of appropriate antibiotics and analgesics, if there is no abscess present and only the presence of cellulitis. Abscesses should be drained surgically and the wound allowed to heal by secondary intention. Aims of elective surgery for pilonidal sinus are excision of the sinus and achievement of skin closure. Many techniques have been described from simple laying open to primary suture, to various plastic flap techniques. Recurrence is common after surgery, and the more complex techniques, although more demanding, seem to result in a better outcome long term.

Education and discharge planning

Following rectal surgery, patients should be given advice on how to prevent further complications arising. It is important that they recognize that straining and constipation should be avoided; therefore, they must pay particular attention and defecate in response to the initial sensation. The risk of constipation will be lessened by increasing the fibre intake in their diet, and by taking exercise and medications to soften the stool. Patients should observe for any bleeding or signs of inflammation, which they should report to their doctor.

It is of particular importance that personal hygiene to the anal area is attended to frequently in order to avoid the risk of infection. Washing the area with warm water is soothing and cleansing, and taking warm baths will reduce pain and keep the anal area clean.

Organizations providing patient information leaflets

British Colostomy Association
15 Station Road
Reading
RG1 1LG
Tel: 0118 939 1537
http://www.bcass.org.uk (accessed 4th July 2004)

The Ileostomy Association
Peverill House
1–5 Mill Road
Ballyclare
Co. Antrim
BT39 9DR
info@the-ia.org.uk
http://www.the-ia.org.uk (accessed 4th July 2004)

National Association for Crohns and Colitis (NACC)
4 Beaumont House
Sutton Road
St Albans
Herts
AL1 5HH
http://www.nacc.org.uk (accessed 4th July 2004)

Summary of key points

■ This chapter has described the pathophysiology of the organs of the upper and lower gastrointestinal tract. Diagrams have been used to facilitate understanding, and the dysfunction of the organs and surgical interventions have also been discussed. Aetiology and epidemiological data, where appropriate, have been included but it must be remembered that, as medical intervention progresses and research is undertaken, these statistics may alter. Some guidance has been offered to assist the nurse to use a problem-solving approach in assessment, planning care, setting goals and initiating intervention for those patients who undergo surgery for a variety of disorders of the gastrointestinal tract.

■ Finally, patient education and preparation for discharge has been highlighted, suggesting that it is necessary to focus on the importance of health promotion. Patient education plays an important part in preventing complications from arising, and in dealing with the implications of failed surgery that may require further intervention.

References

Alexander, M. F., Fawcett, J. N. & Runciman, P. J. (2000) *Nursing Practice: Hospital and Home: The Adult*, 2nd edn. Edinburgh: Churchill Livingstone.

Anstead, G. M. (1998) Steroids, retinoids and wound healing. *Advances in Wound Care* 11(6): 277–285.

Atkin, G. (1999) Implementing screening for colorectal cancer. *British Medical Journal* 319(7219): 1212–1213.

Ballard-Barbash, R., Schatzkin, A., Albanes, D., et al (1990) Physical activity and risk of large bowel cancer in the Framingham study. *Cancer Research* 50(12): 3610–3613.

Bailey, K. (2004) Management of dysphagia in patients with advanced oesophageal cancer. *Gastrointestinal Nursing* 2(2): 18–22.

Black, P. K. (2000) *Holistic Stoma Care*. London: Baillière Tindall.

Bruckstein, A. H. (1988) Acute diarrhoea. *American Family Practitioner* 38(4): 217–228.

Burkitt, D. P. (1971) Epidemiology of cancer of the colon and rectum. *Cancer* 28(1): 3–13.

Buset, M., Lipkin, M., Swaroop, F. & Friedman, E. (1986) Inhibition of human colonic epithelial cell proliferation in vivo and in vitro by calcium. *Cancer Research* 46(10): 5426–5430.

Butcher, G. P. (2003) *Gastroenterology*. Edinburgh: Churchill Livingstone.

Cancer Research UK (2004) Statistics. [Online] Available at http://www.cancerresearchuk.org/about cancer/statistics (accessed on 29 May 2004).

Cuschieri, A., Steele, R. J. C. & Moossa, A. R. (2002) *Essential Surgical Practice: Basic Surgical Training*, 4th edn. London: Arnold Press.

Day, H. (2003) The role of HCl and the gastric mucosa in gastric and duodenal ulceration. *Gastrointestinal Nursing* 1(10): 28–32.

Department of Health (2001) HSC 2001/023 *Good practice in consent: achieving the NHS plan's commitment to patient centred consent practice*. London: HMSO.

Donnelly, L. (2003) Biophysical persepectives in ulcerative colitis. *Gastrointestinal Nursing* 1(1): 27–30.

Ellis, P. & Cunningham, D. (1994) Management of carcinomas of the upper gastrointestinal tract. Current Issues in Cancer. *British Medical Journal* 308(26): 834–838.

Faivre, J. (1992) Diet and colorectal cancer. In: Benito, E., Giacosa, A. & Hill, M. J. (eds) *Public Education on Diet and Cancer*. Dordrecht: Kluwer.

Goligher, J., Duthie, H. & Nixon, H. (1980) *Surgery of the Anus, Rectum and Colon*, 4th edn. London: Baillière Tindall.

Guilbeau, A. M., Young, L. S. & Kirshenbaum, G. (1990) Laser laparoscopic cholecystectomy: laying the groundwork. *AORN Journal* 52(4): 780–789.

Hardman, K. A., Manjunath, S. & Trash, D. B. (1995) Safety of colonoscopy. *Journal of the Royal College of Physicians of London* 29(5): 338–340.

Harrison, R. J. (1984) *Textbook of Medicine*. London: Hodder and Stoughton.

Hibberts, F. & Barnes, E. (2003) The use of ERCP. *Nursing Times* 99(05): 28–30.

Hibberts, F. & Carapeti, E. A. (2003) Caring for the patient with an anal fistula. *Gastrointestinal Nursing* 1(9): 26–28.

Holland, K., Jenkins, J., Soloman, J. & Whittam, S. (2004) *Applying the Roper–Logan–Tierney Model in Practice*. Edinburgh: Churchill Livingstone.

Holloway, N. M. (1993) *Medical Surgical Care Planning*, 2nd edn. Pennsylvania: Springhouse Corporation.

Hyde, C. (2003) Diverticular disease. *Gastrointestinal Nursing* 1(5): 34–38.

Kelly, M. P. (1994) *Colitis*, 2nd edn. London: Tavistock/Routledge.

Kinzler, K. W., Nilbert, M. C., Su, L. K., et al (1991) Identification of FAP locus genes from chromosome 5q21. *Science* 253(5020): 661–665.

Little, J., Logan, R. F., Hawtin, P. G., et al (1993) Colorectal adenomas and energy intake, body size and physical activity: a case control study of subjects participating in the Nottingham faecal occult blood screening programme. *British Journal of Cancer* 67(1): 172–176.

McArdle, C. S. & Hole, D. (1991) Impact of variability among surgeons on post-operative morbidity and mortality and ultimate survival. *British Medical Journal* 302(6791): 1501–1505.

McShane, R. E. & McLane, A. M. (1985) Constipation: consensual and empirical validation. *Nursing Clinics of North America* 20(4): 801–808.

Mahilda, Y. R. (1987) Aetiopathogenesis of ulcerative colitis. In: Jewell, D. & Mahilda, Y. (eds) *Topics in Gastroenterology*, Vol. 15. Oxford: Blackwell.

Meek, R. (2000) Surgery in the older person. In: Manley, K. & Bellman, L. (eds) *Surgical Nursing: Advancing Practice*. Edinburgh: Churchill Livingstone.

Morson, B., Dawson, I. & Spriggs, A. (1979) *Gastrointestinal Pathology*, 2nd edn. Oxford: Blackwell.

Office of Health Economics (1992) *Compendium of Health Care Statistics*. London: HMSO.

Paraskeva, C. & Logan, R. F. A. (1993) Cancer Research Campaign. *Factsheet* 18.1–18.4.

Parks, A. G. & Percy, J. P. (1982) Resection and sutured colo-anal anastomosis for rectal carcinoma. *British Journal of Surgery* 69(6): 301–304.

Peltomaki, P., Aaltonen, L. A., Sistonen, P., et al (1993) Genetic mapping of a locus predisposing to human colorectal cancer. *Science* 260(5109): 810–812.

Read, N. W. & Timms, J. M. (1986) Defecation and the pathophysiology of constipation. *Clinics of Gerontology* 15(4): 937–965.

Ross, D. G. (1993) Subjective data related to altered bowel elimination patterns among hospitalized elder and middle-aged persons. *Orthopaedic Nursing* 12(5): 25–32.

Royal College of Surgeons of Edinburgh (2004) Surgical Knowledge of Skills Website. Management of gall stones. [Online] Available at http://www.edu.rcsed.ac.uk (accessed on 29 May 2004).

Rutishauser, S. (1994) *Physiology and Anatomy: A Basis for Nursing and Health Care*. London: Churchill Livingstone.

Smith, G. (2003) Gastro-oesphageal reflux disease. *Gastrointestinal Nursing* 1(4): 32–38.

Solla, J. A. & Rothenberger, D. A. (1990) Preoperative bowel preparation: a survey of colon and rectal surgeons. *Diseases of the Colon and Rectum* 33(2): 154–159.

Taylor, I., Garcia-Agular, J. & Goldberg, S. (2002) *Colorectal Cancer – Fast Facts*, 2nd edn. Health Press.

Wardle, J., Taylor, T., Sutton, S. & Atkin, W. (1999) Does publicity about cancer screening raise the fear of cancer? Randomised trial of the psychological effect of information about cancer screening. *British Medical Journal* 319(7216): 1037–1038.

Whitehead, W. & Schuster, M. (1985) *Gastrointestinal Disorders: Behavioral and Physiological Basis for Treatment*. Orlando, Florida: Academic Press.

Wiltz, O., Hashmi, H. F., Schoetz, D. J., et al (1991) Carcinoma and the ileal pouch–anal anastomosis. *Diseases of the Colon and Rectum* 34(9): 805–809.

Further reading

Hind, M. & Wicker, P. (2000) *Principles of Perioperative Practice*. Edinburgh: Churchill Livingstone.

Hyde, C. (2003) Diverticular disease. *Gastrointestinal Nursing* 1(5): 23–25.

Platt, V. (2003) Malignant bowel obstruction. *Gastrointestinal Nursing* 1(1): 33–38.

Porock, D. & Palmer, D. (2003) *Cancer of the Gastrointestinal Tract: A Handbook for Nurse Practitioners*. London: Whurr.

Porrett, T. & Daniel, N. (1999) *Essential Coloproctology for Nurses*. London: Whurr.

Smith, G. (2003) Gastro-esophageal reflux disease. *Gastrointestinal Nursing* 1(4): 32–38.

Swan, E. (2004) *Colorectal Cancer for Nurses*. London: Whurr.

Chapter **16**

Patients requiring surgery on the renal and urinary tract

Martin Beynon

Key objectives of the chapter

After reading the chapter the reader should be able to:

- give an overview of the anatomy and physiology of the kidney and lower urinary tract

- list the functions of the kidney

- discuss renal and urological investigations and the preparation required by the patient

- describe the pre- and postoperative care for individuals undergoing surgery on the kidney and lower urinary tract

- discuss discharge advice that would be given to individuals following surgery on the kidney and urinary tract.

INTRODUCTION

During the last 20 years the field of urology has undergone extensive growth as a surgical specialty. As technological advancement has occurred, surgical intervention has moved away from conventional open procedures to minimally invasive and non-invasive surgery for a variety of nephro-urological conditions. The use of improved screening and diagnostic tools has, however, seen surgery for certain conditions become more radical, with an overall improved prognostic outcome. This chapter addresses the management and treatment of individuals with specific renal and urological conditions and explores the nursing interventions and care.

ANATOMY AND PHYSIOLOGY OF THE URINARY TRACT

The urinary tract consists of:

- two kidneys
- two ureters
- the urinary bladder
- the urethra.

THE KIDNEYS

The kidneys play a vital role in regulating homeostasis. Their main functions are:

- maintenance of fluid, electrolyte and acid–base balance
- excretion of nitrogenous waste products of metabolism
- excretion of drugs and poisons
- regulation of blood pressure through the maintenance of fluid volume
- erythropoiesis
- metabolism of vitamin D

(McLaren, 1996).

The kidneys are situated on the posterior abdominal wall on either side of the vertebral column, between the twelfth thoracic and third lumbar vertebrae. The right kidney is normally slightly lower than the left due to displacement by the liver. The kidney is approximately 14 cm long, 6 cm wide and 3 cm thick, and weighs between 135 g and 150 g in adults. The adrenal glands are situated immediately above each kidney.

Each of the kidneys is surrounded by a protective capsule made up of fibrous connective tissue, along with an additional layer of perinephric fat; these layers help to cushion and protect the organ against direct trauma. The renal arteries, renal veins, lymphatic supply and the nerves both enter and leave the kidney at the renal hilum, which is recognized as an indentation on the medial, concave border of the kidney. The funnel-shaped upper end of the ureter also enters at the hilum and expands to become the renal pelvis.

Two distinct areas lie beneath the capsule of the kidney: the outer cortex and the inner medulla body making up the renal parenchyma. Within the medulla there are 8–18 wedge-shaped structures evident, called the medullary pyramids. These drain into minor and then major calyces, which are hollow protrusions of the renal pelvis. The calyces distend as the urine collects within them, leading to peristaltic contraction of the smooth muscle in the walls of the calyces and renal pelvis. The urine is then projected forward from the renal pelvis into the ureter.

The nephron

The nephron is the functional unit of the kidney and each kidney contains approximately 1 million nephrons. The nephron consists of a 'tuft' of capillaries called the glomerulus and the renal tubule. The renal tubule can be subdivided into five distinct regions:

- The *Bowmans capsule* forms the spherical, dilated upper end of the tubule which surrounds or invaginates the glomerulus. The glomeruli lie in the cortex of the kidney and originate from an afferent arteriole; once filtered, the blood then leaves the glomerulus via the efferent arteriole. The efferent arteriole, in turn, branches into a thick capillary network which surrounds the renal tubule and is involved in the reabsorption process. The entire structure is 150 mm in diameter with a vast glomerular capillary surface area of approximately 5000–15 000 cm^2 per 100 g of tissue. It is suggested that the glomerular capillaries are far more permeable to water and solutes than the extra-renal capillaries. The capillary endothelium lies on a basement membrane, and on the other side of the membrane rests the epithelium which lines the Bowman's capsule. The glomerular epithelium has foot-like structures projecting from it known as pedicles; they lie on the basement membrane and are separated by filtration slits. Selective filtration is achieved within the first part of the nephron. In total, 170–180 L of plasma in 24 hours is filtered by the glomerulus at a rate of 125 mL/min; thus, the filtrate within the Bowman's capsule is an ultrafiltrate of plasma. The glomerular membrane is permeable to water and other small molecules but is not permeable to blood cells or to proteins, which are only filtered if the kidney is diseased. The glomerular filtrate has approximately the same pH, osmolarity and solute concentrations as plasma.

- The *proximal convoluted tubule* extends from the Bowman's capsule for a length of 12–14 mm and is lined throughout its length by columnar epithelial cells. These cells are adapted on the inner surface to create a border of microvilli (finger-like projections), which increases the surface area inside the proximal tubule, where most of the solute reabsorption takes place. The volume of glomerular filtrate is reduced by 75–80% in the proximal tubule, and active reabsorption of glucose, sodium, phosphate, chloride, potassium and bicarbonate occurs.

- The *loop of Henle* extends from the proximal convoluted tubule, dips down as the descending limb into the medullary region of the renal parenchyma, and forms a U-shape before coursing back up into the cortex via the ascending limb. The columnar cells within the loop of Henle are flatter and have fewer microvilli on the internal surfaces. Passive reabsorption of water, sodium and chloride takes place in the loop of Henle.

- The *distal convoluted tubule* extends from the ascending limb of the loop of Henle and is 4–8 mm in length. Reabsorption of water is controlled here by antidiuretic hormone, a secretion from the posterior lobe of the pituitary gland. The reabsorption of sodium is controlled by the secretion of aldosterone, a hormone secreted by the adrenal cortex.

- The *collecting tubule* – the distal convoluted tubule leads into the collecting ducts which pass through the renal medulla. Antidiuretic hormone secretion regulates reabsorption of water from the collecting tubules and is independent of sodium reabsorption.

The result of this complex process of filtration, selective reabsorption and secretion is the production of urine.

THE URETERS

The two ureters are hollow muscular tubes which extend from the renal pelvis to the posterior wall of the bladder, entering the bladder at its base. Each ureter is approximately 30 cm long, 6 mm in diameter and lies behind the peritoneum.

The wall of the ureter is composed of three layers:

- inner layer of transitional epithelium
- middle layer of thick muscle
- outer layer of connective tissue.

Peristaltic contractions in the muscle layer of the ureter propels urine forward which has drained from the calyces into the renal pelvis and down the ureter into the bladder. The ureters enter the bladder at an oblique angle, thus preventing reflux of urine back along the ureter and into the kidney.

THE BLADDER

The bladder is a hollow, collapsible muscular organ which lies in the anterior pelvis when empty and expands upwards and forwards in the abdominal cavity during filling. The bladder is bordered in front by the pubic bone and laterally by the walls of the pelvis.

The bladder is lined with transitional cell epithelium which acts as a protective barrier and allows a stretch facility as it fills with urine. The second submucosal layer is constructed of connective tissue and is known as the lamina propria. The third layer consists of smooth muscle bundles, known as the detrusor muscle. The detrusor muscle contains both longitudinal and circular fibres, which are thought to be distributed throughout the bladder wall rather than arranged in one layer (Bullock et al, 1994). The detrusor muscle has a unique function, as it facilitates stretch during the filling phase of the bladder with little or no change in internal pressure (Berne and Levy, 1999); there is also a voluntary component in controlling the storage and emptying ability of this muscle. The superior surface of the bladder is covered by the peritoneum when empty, but during the filling phase the peritoneum lifts upwards and backwards and is therefore not a 'true' layer of the bladder.

At the base of the bladder is a triangular area known as the trigone, which represents the area between the ureteric orifices and the internal urethral meatus. Smooth muscle fibres at the apex of the trigone help to form the bladder neck mechanism. The trigone is very sensitive to stretch and is irritated by the presence of foreign bodies, e.g. indwelling urethral catheters.

The bladder and the urethra function together as a complex unit for the storage and expulsion of urine. The bladder neck differs in males and females and its role in the maintenance of continence is not clearly understood; however, it might have some impact on maintaining closure pressure while the bladder fills with urine.

THE URETHRA – FEMALE

The function of the urethra is to convey urine from the bladder to the exterior. The female urethra is approximately 3–5 cm in length and lies anterior to the vagina. The external urethral meatus opens between the clitoris and vaginal orifice. The urethra is lined with transitional epithelium and with squamous epithelium nearer the external meatus. The external sphincter mechanism is made up of musculature within the urethra in conjunction with the levator ani muscle of the pelvic floor; these combined structures are paramount in the mechanical maintenance of urinary continence. The integral urethral muscle maintains urethral closure, and the pelvic floor muscle increases that closure capacity during a raise in intra-abdominal pressure, e.g. on coughing, laughing, jumping. It is important to note that urine is only found in the urethra during micturition and during the filling phase of the cycle it remains empty and closed.

The male urethra will be discussed in Chapter 17.

The complex process of urine storage and micturition is controlled by the coordinated activity of parasympathetic, sympathetic and somatic nerves, with control by higher centres in the brain (Blandy, 1998).

RENAL AND UROLOGICAL INVESTIGATIONS

URINALYSIS

Simple urinalysis is a non-invasive test using a chemically impregnated strip to measure the urine pH and to detect the presence of blood, glucose, protein, bilirubin, urobilinogen, ketones, leucocytes and nitrites (Beynon and Nicholls, 2004). It is important to use a clean container to collect a fresh specimen of urine for testing, so avoiding contamination of the specimen. The colour, consistency and smell of the urine should also be noted during routine analysis, and the findings documented. Some things to observe for are a cloudy appearance, an offensive or 'fishy' smell, blood and possibly mucose like strands, which may all be indicative of a urinary tract infection.

URINE SPECIMENS FOR CULTURE

If a urinary tract infection is suspected, the collection of urine for culture to identify the offending organisms is indicated. Ideally, a specimen should be obtained before antibiotic therapy is commenced. Urine specimens for culture are usually either a midstream specimen of urine (MSU) or a catheter specimen of urine (CSU) and should be collected in a way that avoids contamination of the specimen with new bacteria.

Midstream specimen of urine

The procedure should be explained to the patient to gain consent and to provide reassurance. The patient is asked to void into a jug or the toilet and to collect the middle part of the voided urine into a sterile container. Urine passed normally may be contaminated by organisms around the urethral meatus and that is why the midstream urine is required for examination. Many nurses still advocate cleansing of the vulva in the female and the glans in the male, prior to collection of the specimen, but there is no statistical evidence to support its continued use and the practice has been deemed unnecessary by some (Brown et al, 1991).

The urine should be sent to the laboratory as soon as possible, with the specimen labelled correctly and accompanied by the appropriate investigation request form. Rapid growth of microorganisms will occur at room temperature and lead to an invalid culture; therefore, specimens should be kept refrigerated at 4°C if transport is delayed.

Catheter specimen of urine

A specimen of urine is obtained by withdrawing approximately 2 mL of urine via the 'sampling port', usually found in the tubing of the catheter drainage bag. The equipment used must be sterile and in most instances a needle and syringe is required. A clamp should be applied below the sampling port to allow collection of the urine. Once the sample is obtained, the clamp should be released and the specimen transferred into a sterile universal container and transported to the laboratory (Mallett and Dougherty, 2000).

Early morning urine

The first urine voided in the morning is collected for three consecutive days. Early morning urine (EMU) is more concentrated and therefore provides a better medium to locate specific types of cells, e.g. tuberculosis or malignant cells.

24-HOUR URINE COLLECTION

This is the collection of the total volume of urine voided in a 24-hour period and is of value in the diagnosis of a number of renal and urological conditions, e.g. renal calculi/stone disease and impaired renal function. The patient is asked to void, the time is noted and this first specimen is discarded. All urine voided for the next 24 hours is collected in a large specimen container. The patient is asked to void at the end of the 24 hours, and this specimen is included in the collection. Care should be taken not to spill any preservative present in some of the containers, as it may be corrosive.

It is essential that 'all' the urine collected in this time frame is kept, as the overall results will be invalid if an incomplete picture is presented. It is important that the nurse and patient have a full understanding of the procedure.

URINARY FLOW RATE

This measures the rate and volume of urine voided in millilitres per second and is an important investigation in the individual with urinary outflow problems (Schafer et al, 2002). Various types of equipment can be used to measure the flow rate, e.g. rotating disc or dipstick, and all entail the individual voiding into the funnel of a monitoring machine.

Preparation of the patient involves:

- full explanation of what the procedure entails
- ensuring a comfortably full bladder, but avoiding overdistension, and consumption of large volumes of fluid prior to the investigation

Table 16.1   Blood tests

Blood test	Rationale
Haemoglobin	Reduced in anaemia, which may occur as a result of urinary tract bleeding, e.g. in bladder or kidney cancer
White blood cells	Raised in infection, e.g. urinary tract infection
Urea, creatinine and electrolyte estimation	Relates to renal function: e.g. creatinine is raised in renal impairment or failure
Prostatic specific antigen	Raised in prostate cancer
Liver function tests	Performed in suspected liver metastases
Calcium	Raised levels may correlate with stone formation
Blood group	Blood transfusion may be required before, during or after surgery
Clotting screen	Particularly important if taking anticoagulants

- instructing the patient to void into the flow rate machine
- maintaining privacy while the patient voids.

A more accurate assessment will be obtained if a series of three successive flow rates is recorded (Welford, 1994).

BLOOD TESTS

Blood analysis is an important part of the investigation of the individual requiring surgery for a renal or urological condition. Blood tests commonly performed are shown in Table 16.1.

RENAL FUNCTION STUDIES

Evaluation of renal function includes measurement of plasma urea and creatinine. Renal damage may occur before plasma urea and creatinine levels rise; therefore, creatinine clearance (normally 125 mL/min), which closely correlates to the glomerular filtration rate (GFR), is a more reliable indicator of renal function. This is calculated from measurement of urine volume, plasma creatinine and urine creatinine. Twenty-four hour urine collection and a blood sample are required.

RADIOLOGICAL INVESTIGATIONS

Plain abdominal X-ray of kidneys, ureters and bladder

A plain abdominal X-ray is taken to include the kidneys, ureters and bladder (KUB). This is particularly useful for detecting urinary calculi (90% are radio-opaque). It is also useful immediately prior to surgery for stone removal to check on stone location.

Intravenous urogram

An intravenous urogram (IVU) is a commonly performed urological investigation. It is an important investigation for the individual with renal stones, haematuria, urinary tract infection and urinary tract tumours. Following a plain abdominal film, contrast medium containing iodine is injected intravenously and a series of films taken as the contrast medium is excreted by the kidneys and through the urinary tract.

The preparation of the individual varies between departments. It is also dependent on the individual's general health and whether other medical conditions are present, e.g. diabetes, impaired renal function. A full explanation of the procedure must be given and time taken to answer any queries. Patients are normally fasted for 4–6 hours and the bowel should be clear of faecal matter to avoid obscuring the film with air and colon content. If bowel preparation is required, the method employed should follow individual patient assessment and local policy/protocol.

An allergic reaction to iodine in the contrast medium can be severe and may result in cardiac arrest. X-ray departments must be fully equipped for cardiac/respiratory resuscitation. Ninety per cent of severe reactions occur within 5–15 minutes of injection (Doyle et al, 1989) and over 20% of patients do experience some reaction, such as nausea or skin irritation, to the contrast medium. It is therefore vital that any history of allergy is highlighted before the procedure is undertaken.

Renal scanning (renogram)

In this procedure, radioisotope-labelled substances which are known to be selectively taken up and excreted by the kidney are injected intravenously. The compound used is then detected and measured by a gamma camera, and information regarding kidney function is obtained, e.g. structure and function of the kidneys and differential kidney function.

The patient should be given adequate information and support prior to undergoing the procedure, and instructions regarding disposal of urine following the scan must be made clear to the patient and ward/departmental staff. Most nuclear medicine departments will provide instructions on the appropriate disposal of urine.

Computerized tomography

In computerized tomography (CT) scanning, specific areas of the body are X-rayed at different angles using high-resolution imaging. Two-dimensional cross-sectional images are reconstructed by computer. In urology it is a particularly useful investigation when planning management/treatment of renal, prostate, testicular and bladder tumours.

Patient information prior to the procedure is of the utmost importance. The machinery used can be very claustrophobic due to the confined space, and many patients find this distressing.

Ultrasound scan

High-frequency sound waves are transduced through a probe over the area being investigated, e.g. kidney, bladder. The reflected image is analysed by computer and displayed on a monitor.

Ultrasound scanning is a very useful and valuable diagnostic investigation; it can differentiate between solid and cystic masses and is used to assess urinary tract obstruction, e.g. hydronephrosis, urinary outflow obstruction.

Patient preparation for ultrasound is minimal. An explanation of the procedure, which is non-invasive in most instances, must be given. When undertaking bladder ultrasonography, it should be noted that the bladder lies low in the pelvis when empty and expands upwards and forwards in the abdomen when it fills; a full bladder is therefore important in order for the sound waves to be transmitted. If the patient has a urinary catheter in situ, it should be clamped for approximately 1 hour prior to the investigation and the patient asked to drink moderate volumes of fluid to aid the bladder-filling process.

Retrograde pyelography

This procedure is usually performed under general anaesthetic following cystoscopy. A small-bore catheter is passed up the ureter to the renal pelvis, contrast medium is injected into the upper renal tract and X-rays taken of the renal pelvis and pelviureteric junction (Beynon and Nicholls, 2004).

Retrograde pyelography is a useful investigation in the management of patients with a suspected obstruction within the upper urinary tracts. It may also be used to obtain urine samples from each kidney, e.g. for cytological analysis in patients with suspected renal carcinoma.

Preparation of the patient is as for a general anaesthetic. Following the procedure, the patient should be observed for any signs or symptoms of urinary tract infection, which can occur as a result of instrumentation of the urinary tract: i.e. loin pain, pyrexia and pain on voiding. Allergic reaction to the contrast medium also needs to be observed for.

Antegrade urography

Antegrade urography is performed when an obstructed ureter has been diagnosed or is suspected. Ultrasound is used to locate the renal pelvis. A fine-bore needle is inserted into the renal pelvis and a cannula passed over the needle to allow contrast medium to be injected and X-rays taken. If an obstruction is diagnosed, a nephrostomy tube can be placed to allow drainage of urine from the renal pelvis. The procedure is usually performed under sedation (Bullock et al, 1994).

Renal arteriography

Renal arteriography involves injection of contrast medium through a fine catheter which is inserted into the femoral artery and passed via the abdominal aorta to the renal artery. A series of X-rays can then be taken. The films give an outline of the renal blood supply and are useful in the diagnosis of renal artery stenosis and renal tumours.

Although the procedure is performed under local anaesthetic with sedation, it is highly invasive. If complications arise, further intervention may be necessary; therefore, the patient is fasted for 4–6 hours. A full explanation of what to expect is given to the patient and informed consent obtained. Following the procedure, bedrest is maintained for up to 12 hours, as there is a risk of haemorrhage from the puncture site. If leakage occurs at the femoral artery puncture site, a longer period of bedrest may be necessary. Pedal pulses in the foot are checked to evaluate peripheral blood supply, and blood pressure, pulse, puncture site and capillary return are monitored 1/2 hourly initially until stable (Beynon and Nicholls, 2004).

Renal biopsy

Renal biopsy is an important investigation in the assessment of the individual with renal disease. The procedure can be performed under X-ray control, ultrasound or CT scanning, and a local anaesthetic is used to anaesthetize the area down to the kidney capsule. Preparation of the patient involves obtaining informed consent following a full explanation of the procedure.

Blood specimens pre-procedure are obtained for:

- full blood count
- clotting screen
- blood group and save serum for cross-match.

In some centres it is advocated that bedrest is maintained for 24 hours following the procedure. Blood pressure and pulse are recorded 1/2 hourly initially and at reduced intervals thereafter if within the patient's normal parameters. A good fluid intake should be encouraged following the procedure (if not medically contraindicated) and observations made of urine output, noting any haematuria. The patient may experience pain after undergoing a renal biopsy and therefore appropriate analgesics should be administered as prescribed (Gower, 1991).

Cystoscopy

Cystoscopy involves direct visualization of the bladder and urethra and is an important investigation in the individual with a urological problem: e.g. haematuria, lower tract obstruction, or follow-up check cystoscopy for bladder cancer. A rigid or flexible cystoscope is used, and the procedure is performed under either a local or general anaesthetic. The bladder is examined and, if abnormal, biopsies are taken for histological examination. Preparation of the patient involves obtaining informed consent following a full explanation of the procedure. The patient is prepared for either a general or local anaesthetic. Following the procedure, patients might experience urethral discomfort and voiding difficulties. The patient is encouraged to drink 2–3 L in 24 hours (unless medically contraindicated), and the urine should be examined for evidence of haematuria. Any pre-existing urinary tract infection is treated with prophylactic antibiotics.

Specific investigations relating to surgical interventions are summarized in Table 16.2.

Table 16.2 Specific investigations related to surgical interventions on the kidneys or urinary tract

Surgical intervention	Investigation
Pyeloplasty	Intravenous urogram – this will confirm diagnosis by demonstrating hydronephrosis on the affected side Renogram – this will measure overall contribution of the obstructed kidney to renal function Urea and electrolyte estimation – to determine renal function Full blood count – to exclude anaemia and treat infection prior to surgery Group and cross-match – blood will be available if required
Nephrectomy	Blood – group and cross-match 2–4 units – urea and electrolyte estimation – full blood count – clotting screen Midstream specimen of urine Intravenous urogram Ultrasound Renogram Computerized tomography (CT scan)
Laparoscopic nephrectomy	Blood – group and cross-match 2 units – urea and electrolyte estimation – full blood count – clotting screen Intravenous urogram Ultrasound Midstream specimen of urine ECG
Percutaneous nephrolithotomy	Urea and electrolyte estimation – to assess renal function Full blood count – to exclude anaemia Clotting screen – it is important to establish prior to the procedure that the patient does not have a clotting disorder nor is taking aspirin regularly (nor other anticoagulants) Group and cross-match 2 units of blood – blood will be available should the patient require transfusion Midstream specimen of urine – if a urinary tract infection is present, the appropriate antibiotics can be prescribed

(Continued)

Table 16.2 (*Continued*)

Surgical intervention	Investigation
	Intravenous urogram – this will demonstrate the location and size of the stone and whether it is causing an obstruction
	Plain abdominal X-ray – this is done prior to the procedure to show location of the stone
Extracorporeal lithotripsy	Blood clotting screen, urea, creatinine and electrolyte estimation
	Midstream specimen of urine
	Blood pressure recorded
	Kidney, ureter and bladder X-ray to locate current position of stone
Cystectomy and ileal conduit urinary diversion	Blood
	– urea and electrolyte estimation
	– liver function tests
	– full blood count
	– group and cross match 6 units
	– blood glucose
	– clotting screen
	Urine
	– midstream specimen of urine
	– cytology
	Chest X-ray
	ECG
	Ultrasound of kidneys/bladder or intravenous urogram
	CT scan

NURSING ASSESSMENT OF INDIVIDUAL REQUIRING SURGERY FOR A UROLOGICAL CONDITION

The initial patient assessment provides an ideal opportunity for the nurse to establish the nurse–patient relationship. The way in which the patient is approached when the patient attends the preadmission clinic or on admission to the ward is extremely important. The patient interview and collection of pertinent information should be done in an environment that provides privacy and maintains confidentiality. A friendly, relaxed, informal atmosphere should be aimed for, with a two-way exchange of information taking place between the nurse and the patient (Rungapadiachy, 1999).

An assessment should explore the patient as a 'whole' being, addressing physical, psychological, emotional, social and cultural needs; the impact of the patient's urological condition on these needs should then be established. Patient assessment is usually performed using a 'model of nursing' and various assessment frameworks which are relevant to the patient experience and/or need.

The assessment undertaken will gather information which includes:

- Recording of baseline observations:
  - temperature
  - pulse
  - respirations
  - blood pressure
  - urinalysis
  - weight.
- Relevant personal details, including past medical and surgical history.
- Current health status: how well does the patient feel?
- Breathing: does the individual have any respiratory problems? How much exertion causes breathlessness?
- Eating/drinking: is the patient overweight/underweight? What is their usual fluid intake in 24 hours, and what type of fluid do they normally drink? Fluid intake is particularly important for the individual experiencing urinary frequency and urgency, or those with renal stones and/or recurrent urinary tract infections.
- Level of independence/dependence and home circumstances: it is very important to establish whether help will be required during the convalescent period after surgery, so that the best possible arrangements can be organized.
- Is the urological condition causing/contributing to mobility problems? The individual with carcinoma of the prostate might have metastatic bone disease causing pain and often restricted mobility.

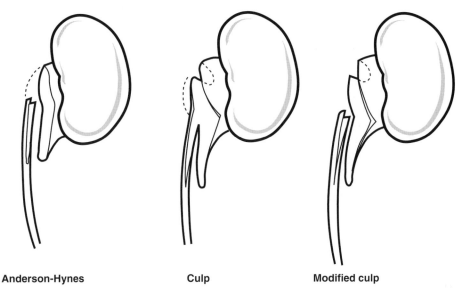

| Anderson-Hynes | Culp | Modified culp |

Figure 16.1   Types of pyeloplasty. (Reproduced from Blandy (1991) by courtesy of Blackwell Science Ltd.)

ELIMINATION

For many patients this is a very sensitive and often embarrassing subject to discuss, but one very much impacted upon by urological disease. A voiding history should be undertaken, which includes information on patients' experiences of urinary frequency, urgency, hesitancy, dysuria, nocturia and haematuria. Patients should be asked to describe their urinary stream when voiding; is the stream strong, do they have to strain to void, do they feel empty on completion? Is urinary leakage or urinary incontinence a problem? Many patients find this a disturbing disease symptom, as it remains a stigmatized problem within society (Shaw, 2001). Patients often need support, empathy, clear guidance and good clinical advice when tackling this urinary symptom. Signs and symptoms of urinary tract infection also need to be observed for, e.g. pyrexia, dysuria and offensive smelling urine. Bowel habits/function should also be assessed, as constipation can be a major contributing cause of urinary symptoms.

SLEEPING

Sleep is often affected in some groups of patients experiencing urinary tract disease. It is important that in the initial assessment it is established if sleeping is interrupted by the need to void, and, if so, how many times does the patient need to get up at night?

BODY IMAGE/EXPRESSING SEXUALITY

Urological disease can have an impact on the physical and psychological needs of the patient, and this can affect individuals' perception of their body image and sexual function (Price, 1995). A great deal of sensitivity is required when exploring this issue, although it is paramount that the nurse addresses and guides the patient through this care activity and does not take the easy route of avoidance. It is important to establish if the patient is sexually active, as some minor and intermediate urological procedures can have a direct impact on sexual function. Retrograde ejaculation is often experienced following transurethral resection of the prostate gland or bladder neck incision, which could render the patient infertile. There is also the risk of impotence/erectile disorder following surgery to combat both bladder and prostatic cancer. Having a urethral catheter in situ following surgery impacts on sexual function, but also might have a more profound effect on the patient's personal body image. Sexual function and activity, and the impact of surgical intervention, are topics that the surgical nurse should be able to tackle with all patients in their care (RCN, 2000).

SURGICAL INTERVENTIONS ON THE KIDNEY

PYELOPLASTY

Pyeloplasty is the operation performed through a loin incision, or via a laparoscopic approach, to relieve an obstruction at the pelviureteric junction often caused by a ring of fibrous tissue (Fig. 16.1). The defect can be a congenital anomaly or the result of repeated infection or injury; this results in dilatation within the renal pelvis due to a narrowed ureter, inhibiting the free flow of urine.

Signs and symptoms of pelviureteric junction obstruction include:

- loin pain, often associated with a large fluid intake
- infection, due to stasis of urine in the renal pelvis
- nausea and vomiting
- impaired renal function.

Specific preoperative nursing care

Psychological/communication

A full explanation is given of what to expect pre- and postoperatively, and time is taken to answer any questions and allay any fears the patient might have.

Controlling body temperature

Any pre-existing urinary tract infection should be treated with an appropriate antibiotic.

Specific postoperative nursing care

Pain control/communication

The surgical approach is a loin incision, and pain control is particularly important if complications due to reduced mobility are to be avoided. A continuous intravenous or subcutaneous opioid infusion or patient-controlled analgesia (PCA) can be an effective choice in pain management (Seymour, 1996). The patient's pain should be assessed and then the patient is assisted into a position in which he feels comfortable. The wound drain, nephrostomy tube (if present) and urethral catheter should be secured to avoid dragging and causing unnecessary pain.

Breathing

It is important that the physiotherapist's teaching of deep breathing exercises is reinforced by nursing staff, because the position of the surgical incision is such that the individual is at risk of developing a chest infection. The patient should be observed for signs of respiratory depression. This is particularly important if an opioid infusion is used to control pain.

Eating and drinking

Intravenous fluid replacement is necessary in the initial postoperative period. Fluids and diet can be gradually reintroduced when bowel sounds are present. An appropriate antiemetic should be prescribed and administered if the patient feels nauseous.

Elimination

An accurate fluid balance is maintained to avoid dehydration/overhydration. The colour and consistency of the urinary output should be observed for blood loss, as a blood transfusion may be necessary if haematuria persists. The patient will have either a nephrostomy tube or a double J stent in situ.

Nephrostomy tube A nephrostomy tube allows external drainage of urine from the renal pelvis. The tube must be kept patent to avoid overdistension of the renal pelvis and the associated potential breakdown of the new surgical anastomosis. Dressings to the site should be performed aseptically with a non-adherent dressing, and then secured to avoid kinking or accidental removal of the nephrostomy tube. Approximately 10–12 days after surgery the tube is clamped for 24 hours, and if the patient does not experience pain or develop a pyrexia, the tube is removed. In some centres a nephrostogram is performed prior to clamping, to ensure healing has taken place and the ureter is patent. Any leakage of urine from the nephrostomy tube site should subside within 24 hours. If urinary leakage persists, a drainage bag, e.g. a urostomy bag, can be applied to the site. The patient is reassured that the drainage will decrease – usually within 48 hours – when a non-adherent dressing can then be applied (Champion and Longhorn, 2004).

Double J stent The double J stent extends from the kidney down the ureter and into the bladder. The stent is normally left in situ for up to 3 months. Following stent insertion, the patient may experience urinary frequency, urgency and haematuria. Suprapubic pain or discomfort can also be a problem. An increased fluid intake is encouraged and oral analgesics given for pain/discomfort. These symptoms should resolve within 48 hours. The patient will attend day surgery for stent removal under a local anaesthetic.

Patient education and advice on discharge will be discussed following the section on nephrectomy.

NEPHRECTOMY

Nephrectomy is the surgical removal of the kidney, and is performed through either a loin incision, abdominal incision or laparoscopic route.

Indications for nephrectomy include:

- Renal cancer – this accounts for around 9% of all urothelial cancers and includes disease of the renal parenchyma and the urothelium. Within the renal parenchyma, adenocarcenoma accounts for around 80% of disease, with nephroblastoma (Wilms' tumour) making up another 15%. Within the urothelium of the renal pelvis and the ureter, transitional cell carcinoma accounts for the highest percentage of disease. Surgery in all cases may be radical and involve removal of the kidney, adrenal gland, perinephric fat, lymph nodes, ureter and removal of tumour from the inferior vena cava.

- Non-functioning kidney – this may be as a result of a chronic infection that has destroyed renal tissue.
- Renal injury, causing haemorrhage.
- Live donor renal transplant.

Specific preoperative nursing care

Psychological/communication

The prospect of losing a kidney is extremely worrying for most individuals, as they are concerned about what will happen if the other kidney becomes diseased or injured. Time must be taken to address these psychological concerns, and provide the patient with appropriate and accurate information in the process of gaining informed and evidence-based consent.

Specific postoperative nursing care

Maintaining a safe environment

There is a potential risk of haemorrhage due to the highly vascular nature of the kidney. The wound dressing and wound drain(s) should be observed for blood loss. The amount of wound drainage is measured and recorded. The wound drain is removed, when 24-hour drainage is less than 50 mL. Blood pressure and pulse are recorded 1/4 to 1/2 hourly initially and the frequency reduced as the patient's condition dictates.

Pain control/communication

Pain control after nephrectomy is crucial, as the open surgical approach leaves the patient with a large incision/wound that causes problems associated with effective breathing and mobility (Carr and Goudas, 1999). To avoid the patient experiencing severe pain and discomfort, pain assessment and management must be effective. A continuous intravenous, subcutaneous or epidural opioid infusion can be most useful in controlling pain. Patient-controlled analgesia gives patients independence and involvement in their pain management. However, if PCA is to be successful, adequate preoperative teaching regarding the use of the device must be given (Rowbotham, 1992).

Breathing

The loin incision, below the level of the twelfth rib, is in close proximity to the diaphragm, pleura and the muscles involved in respiration. This contributes to the potential risk of respiratory problems in the postoperative period. The respiratory rate and effort must be observed and recorded, and any problems seen acted upon quickly. It is important to reinforce the physiotherapist's teaching of deep breathing exercise

and to encourage the patient to cough; good positioning and effective analgesia are important in achieving this. As soon as their general condition allows, patients should be nursed in an upright position to further aid chest expansion. Pneumothorax is a complication associated with this surgery, and therefore regular respiratory monitoring is an essential component of the nurse's observation of the patient.

Elimination

An accurate fluid balance must be maintained to provide an early indication of dehydration or fluid overload. Hourly urine volumes are measured initially, and if output falls below 30 mL/h, medical staff should be informed. The presence of a urethral catheter allows accurate measurement of urinary output, and is necessary for bladder healing to take place at the area where the ureter has been incised if a radical procedure has been performed. The urethral catheter will normally remain in situ for between 48 and 72 hours.

Eating and drinking

Intravenous fluid replacement is necessary in the initial postoperative period. Fluids and diet can be gradually reintroduced when bowel sounds are present, normally on the second or third postoperative day. An appropriate antiemetic should be prescribed for nausea and vomiting.

Complications

Complications of nephrectomy include:

- *Haemorrhage/shock*: this is caused by reduction in circulating blood volume.

- *Pneumothorax*: the pleura may be damaged during the procedure, resulting in a pneumothorax. This can occur when the procedure has been difficult. On return to the ward the patient will have an underwater seal chest drain in situ (Collins, 2004).

- *Chest infection*: this is often as a result of poor chest expansion after surgery and may be a consequence of inadequate pain management.

- *Wound infection*: this may result if a pre-existing infection has not been treated appropriately, or if bacteria are introduced during changing of the wound dressing.

- *Urinary tract infection*: the presence of a urethral catheter increases the incidence of urinary tract infection.

- *Deep vein thrombosis*: this may be as a result of reduced mobility. The wearing of thrombo-embolytic deterrent (TED) stockings (Mallett and Dougherty, 2000), and prophylactic anticoagulant administration, can help to reduce the risk of a thrombosis occurring.

LAPAROSCOPIC NEPHRECTOMY

Laparoscopic nephrectomy is a recent innovation in urology. The first laparoscopic nephrectomy in a human was performed in 1990. Patients suitable for this method are those with a small and non-malignant kidney. It is not considered in those patients who are overweight. The procedure is performed under a general anaesthetic and involves the kidney being dissected laparoscopically in the peritoneal cavity and placed in an impermeable bag. The kidney is morcellated within the bag. The substance is then removed via a mini incision in the abdomen (Clayman et al, 1991; Coptcoat, 1992).

Open nephrectomy has inherent operative and postoperative complications. The main advantages of laparoscopic nephrectomy are claimed to be less pain, a shorter hospital stay (3–4 days) and a quicker return to normal activities and work (Gill, 1998). However, the procedure is still in its infancy within many urological centres and therefore not without risk for the patient – not least the prolonged operative time of between 3 and 4 hours.

SPECIFIC PATIENT EDUCATION AND ADVICE ON DISCHARGE FOLLOWING NEPHRECTOMY/PYELOPLASTY

Written information should be available, which is given in addition to individual verbal advice by nursing and medical staff. Understanding should be evaluated and information reinforced as necessary.

Advice is given regarding the following:

- *Rest and activity*: The patient may feel weak and tired after surgery and should be aware that this is expected. As their strength returns, activity should be increased, with the aim of returning to a normal routine within 3–4 weeks.

- *Wound healing*: before discharge the patient will be informed whether the sutures are dissolvable or will need to be removed. If sutures are to be removed, an appointment should be made with the practice nurse at the GP's surgery or with the district nursing service. The patient is instructed regarding the need to observe the wound for signs of infection, e.g. redness, discharge. Appropriate dressings are provided if required.

- *Elimination*: the patient is advised to drink 2 L in 24 hours (unless medically contraindicated). If signs of urinary tract infection occur, e.g. pain/burning when voiding, urinary frequency or pyrexia, then the GP should be consulted and an appropriate antibiotic prescribed if indicated.

- *Return to work*: this will depend on the type of work in which the patient is employed. The difference in physical demands requires that a manual worker has a longer period of convalescence than a sedentary worker.

- *Sexual activity*: this can be resumed when the individual feels adequately recovered from surgery.

- *Driving*: driving insurance policies have restrictions following surgery; therefore, individual policies should be referred to. It is advisable not to drive for approximately 3–4 weeks or until one is able to perform an effective emergency stop.

- *Follow-up*: a follow-up appointment is given for 4–6 weeks after surgery. This is to ensure that recovery has taken place and to arrange any further investigations which may be necessary.

URINARY TRACT CALCULI

The incidence of urinary tract calculi is estimated at 2–5% of the UK population and is more common in men than in women. Around 20–40% of those affected will require hospitalization due to pain, obstruction or infection (Lingeman et al, 1989). Calculi or stones can occur at any point within the urinary tract (Bullock et al, 1994).

Factors predisposing to calculi formation include:

- metabolic causes, e.g. an increased excretion of calcium, urate and cystine in the urine
- urinary infection
- hyperparathyroidism.

Signs and symptoms include:

- Renal pain/colic – this can be severe pain of sudden onset which radiates from the loin to groin. The pain causes distress and is often accompanied by nausea and sweating.
- Urinary tract infection – may be recurrent.
- Haematuria.

Conservative management of renal colic

It is important that the patient's pain is relieved by adequate analgesics, and an antiemetic drug prescribed to control any nausea. A high fluid intake of 2–3 L in 24 hours is recommended, to try to flush out the stone (i.e. a stone small enough to pass through the renal tract). All urine voided is strained and, if the stone is passed, it can be collected and sent for biochemical analysis. Urinary infection should be treated with an appropriate antibiotic.

Indications for surgery include:

- the stone is too large to pass through the urinary tract, therefore constituting a potential risk of obstruction
- recurrent urinary tract infection, which is difficult to treat while the stone acts as a nucleus for micro-organisms
- recurrent renal colic.

Surgical management of urinary tract calculi

Surgical management depends on the size and location of the stone within the urinary tract. In recent years, as technology has progressed, methods of stone removal have moved towards minimally invasive surgery, i.e. percutaneous nephrolithotomy (PCNL), and non-invasive management, i.e. lithotripsy. For some patients it may be appropriate to combine methods. For example, for an individual with a large staghorn calculus, the initial treatment is a PCNL followed by lithotripsy at a later date to deal with the remaining stone fragments.

Conventional open surgery, e.g. nephrolithotomy, is now a relatively rare procedure. If a kidney stone has caused obstruction, and renal function in that kidney is less than 10% of overall renal function (both kidneys), then nephrectomy is considered, provided that the other kidney is present and has normal function (Bullock et al, 1994).

Percutaneous nephrolithotomy

This procedure involves removal of the calculus under direct X-ray vision and is usually performed under a general anaesthetic. A percutaneous nephrostomy tract is established and enlarged using graduated dilators. This allows a nephroscope to be passed. Stones are removed using grasping forceps passed down the nephroscope. If the stone is too large, it can be fragmented using ultrasonic lithotripsy or electrohydrolic lithotripsy. Following the procedure, it is usual for a nephrostomy tube to be left in situ to allow drainage of blood and urine. The nephrostomy tube is clamped on the first postoperative day and removed on the second postoperative day if the patient is pain free at the site and there is no leakage around the nephrostomy tube (Champion and Longhorn, 2004).

For pre- and postoperative nursing care, see care plans illustrated in Tables 16.3 and 16.4.

Complications of percutaneous nephrolithotomy
- *Haemorrhage*: bleeding occurs in all cases, but the risks are increased with longer operation time and

multiple stone retrieval. A blood transfusion may be necessary depending on the preoperative haemoglobin and estimated blood loss. Regular monitoring of the nephrostomy tube drainage and site should occur in the first 24 hours postoperatively.

- *Infection*: pre-existing infective stones can result in bacteraemia once disturbed. It is important that appropriate antibiotics are commenced prior to the procedure and continued postoperatively.

- *Pneumothorax*: the risk of pneumothorax increases if the puncture to the kidney during the procedure is above the level of the 12th rib (Kekre et al, 2001). An underwater seal chest drain may have to be inserted to draw air from the pleural space.

Patient education and advice on discharge following percutaneous nephrolithotomy

If written information is available, this should be given to the patient on admission (or before) to ensure they are prepared for the postoperative 'journey'; this is provided in addition to any verbal advice given by the nursing and medical staff. Time must be taken to evaluate the individual's understanding and to reinforce the information as required.

Advice is given regarding the following:

- *Wound healing*: the patient is given instruction on observing the nephrostomy tube site for signs of infection, e.g. redness, discharge and pain. The area should be kept covered with a non-adherent dressing until a scab forms. Appropriate dressings should be provided by the nursing staff for the patient to take home.

- *Elimination*: there may still be blood present in the urine in the initial days following surgery; this is normal, but it should noticeably decrease in the first 3–5 days. The patient should be aware of the signs and symptoms of urinary tract infection, e.g. urgency, frequency and pain on voiding. If an infection is suspected, the GP should be consulted, as a course of antibiotics may be necessary.

- *Fluids and diet*: a fluid intake of 2–3 L in 24 hours is recommended to maintain an increased urinary output, which in turn will flush out any blood or stone fragments that might be present. Long-term maintenance of this level of fluid intake might be beneficial in the prevention of future stone formation.

- *Return to work*: this will depend on the occupation of the patient. Manual workers will require longer than the individual with a more sedentary occupation.

Table 16.3 Preoperative nursing care plan for an individual undergoing percutaneous nephrolithotomy

Patient problem	Expected outcome	Action/rationale
Communicating		
Potential anxiety due to admission to hospital and impending surgery	Patient is able to express fears and anxieties and will feel safe and informed regarding surgery	Discuss preoperative and anticipated postoperative care Give the patient the opportunity to express any anxieties and fears and provide a relaxed non-threatening environment Provide information – use diagrams if indicated (Hayward, 1975) Ensure that consent is informed
Breathing, eating/drinking		
Potential respiratory problems due to inhalation of gastric contents while unconscious, or underlying respiratory disease	Gastric contents will not be be inhaled Respiratory problems will not be exacerbated	Reinforce deep breathing exercises taught by the physiotherapist Fast for 6 hours (diet), 2 hours (fluid) prior to general anaesthetic (Phillips et al, 1993)
Controlling body temperature		
Potential postoperative infection, e.g. urine	Temperature will be between 35.5 and 37.5°C Early detection and treatment should infection occur	Record temperature preoperatively and report if outside normal parameters Perform urinalysis – obtain MSU if nitrates present (Laker, 1994) Administer prophylactic antibiotics as prescribed Bath/shower to be taken prior to theatre
Mobility		
Decreased mobility postoperatively could lead to circulatory problems and potential risk of pressure ulcer occurrence	Patient will remain as mobile as condition permits and risk of pressure ulcer occurrence will be minimized	Assess pressure ulcer risk using an appropriate assessment tool Encourage mobility and foot and leg exercises to aid venous return Measure and fit with TED stockings (Mallett and Dougherty, 2000)
Elimination		
Potential risk of incontinence due to loss of voluntary muscle control while unconscious	Patient will remain continent	Give patient the opportunity to void prior to administration of premedication/transfer to theatre Ensure the patient has had a bowel action within 24 hours of theatre
Maintaining a safe environment		
Inability to maintain own safety while sedated/unconscious	Safety of the patient will not be compromised	Ensure the following: - Correctly labelled identity bands are worn - Patient's consent form is signed - Wedding ring is covered with tape - Prostheses are removed, e.g. dentures, contact lenses - Baseline observations and weight are recorded - Any allergies are recorded - Patient's medical notes, blood results, X-rays and nursing documentation are available - Patient is positioned correctly on canvas

- *Sexual activity*: this can be resumed when the individual wishes and feels recovered from surgery.

- *Driving*: individual driving policies should be referred to, as there may be restrictions following a general anaesthetic and surgery.

Extracorporeal lithotripsy

Lithotripsy involves focusing shockwaves which travel through water, onto the stone, under X-ray or ultrasound control. The shockwaves cause the stone to disintegrate into fragments small enough to pass down the ureter (Tolley and Segura, 2002).

Table 16.4   Postoperative nursing care plan for an individual following percutaneous nephrolithotomy

Patient problem	Expected outcome	Action/rationale
Breathing		
Potential problems with breathing following anaesthetic and surgical intervention	Patient's airway will remain clear Early detection should problems occur	Patient to be positioned ensuring clear airway is maintained Observe and record respiratory rate $\frac{1}{4}$–$\frac{1}{2}$ hourly initially and decrease frequency as patient's condition dictates Administer oxygen therapy as prescribed Encourage deep breathing exercises to aid lung expansion
Maintaining a safe environment		
Inability to maintain own safety after surgery and potential risk of shock, e.g. due to blood loss	Early detection and treatment if shock occurs	Observe and record patient's pulse and blood pressure $\frac{1}{4}$, $\frac{1}{2}$, and 1 hourly and decrease frequency as condition dictates Report to nurse in charge/doctor if blood pressure and pulse are outside normal parameters Report changes in patient's peripheral colour and responsiveness Monitor colour/consistency of urine drainage from nephrostomy tube to estimate blood loss Administer blood transfusion if prescribed Follow local protocol regarding blood transfusion
Communicating		
Potential risk of pain/discomfort following surgical intervention and presence of nephrostomy tube	Pain/discomfort will be controlled to level acceptable by the patient	Assess degree of pain/discomfort using verbal and non-verbal communication (McCaffery, 1983) Give analgesics as prescribed and evaluate effectiveness Position patient as feels comfortable, ensuring nephrostomy tube is well secured to avoid traction
Controlling body temperature		
Potential infection following surgical intervention and presence of nephrostomy tube	Temperature will be between 35.5 and 37.5°C Early detection and treatment should infection occur	Monitor temperature 1–4 hourly Report to nurse in charge if outside normal parameters Observe urine, nephrostomy tube site and IV site for signs of infection Note colour, consistency, smell of urine Note redness, discharge at nephrostomy and IV site Give antibiotics as prescribed
Eating/drinking		
Potential nausea/vomiting/dehydration following anaesthetic and surgery	Patient will not feel nauseated or vomit Patient will feel adequately hydrated	Observe patient for signs of nausea Provide vomit bowl, tissues, mouthwash and ensure privacy Administer antiemetic as prescribed and evaluate effectiveness Maintain intravenous fluids as prescribed, discontinue when normal diet and fluids have been resumed Encourage 2–3 L oral fluids in 24 hours
Elimination		
Potential inability to void following surgery Potential blockage of nephrostomy tube due to clots/debris	Patient will void urine within 12 hours of surgery Nephrostomy tube will remain patent and will be removed 48 hours following surgery	Maintain an accurate fluid balance chart Encourage fluid intake of 2–3 L in 24 hours (intravenous fluids and oral fluids initially) Observe colour and consistency of urine Clamp nephrostomy tube on the first postoperative day, on doctor's instructions, following abdominal X-ray Remove nephrostomy tube on second postoperative day if pain has not been experienced since clamping and there is no leakage of urine around the tube Apply non-adherent dressing to drain site Observe for excessive leakage
Personal cleansing		
Potential problem meeting personal hygiene needs following surgery	Hygiene needs will be met	Assist the patient as necessary, maintaining dignity and promoting independence

Since its inception in the early 1980s, there have been great technological advances in the method of delivery of the shockwave system and the efficiency of stone treatment has also improved. The first-generation lithotripter used extracorporeal shockwaves to break up the stones. The patient would be positioned on a chair in a water bath with repeated shockwaves delivered through the water. A general or epidural anaesthetic is required for this procedure, as it can be painful and the treatment might take rather a long period of time (Champion and Longhorn, 2004).

The second-generation lithotripter 'extracorporeal piezolithotripsy', fragments the stone using shockwaves generated across small ceramic piezoelectric crystals. The patient is positioned so that the affected area is in contact with water, which is integral to the lithotripsy machine. Ultrasound is used to locate the stone. The shockwaves emitted are weaker and the focus area for the treatment to the stone is smaller; this results in a less painful and better tolerated treatment which does not require a general anaesthetic to be administered in most patients. Many of the newer-generation systems work in a similar way to the piezoelectric lithotripter using electromagnetic energy to break up the stone. Each system has its own advantages and disadvantages, and there are no clear indications to suggest that one system outweighs the other significantly enough at present in its effectiveness and overall safety (Whitfield, 1998).

Large stones require repeated treatments (e.g. up to five treatments) to break up the stone into small fragments, which will then pass through the urinary system. The treatments are usually carried out on an outpatient basis, each treatment lasting approximately 45–60 minutes unless contraindicated, e.g. in patients with impaired renal function or those who have a solitary kidney.

Preparation for the procedure is minimal. Prior to the procedure, a full explanation of what to expect is essential. Preparation for the procedure involves the patient attending a preassessment clinic where a full clinical history is undertaken.

Many patients who have previously undergone painful procedures or operations for stone removal are understandably very cautious and anxious. For some patients it will be necessary to position a double J stent prior to lithotripsy, to avoid ureteric obstruction caused by stone fragments at the lower end of the ureter. The stent is inserted under a general anaesthetic and is positioned between the kidney and bladder on the affected side. On completion of lithotripsy treatment, admission is then arranged for the removal of the stent.

Patient education and advice following lithotripsy

- *Pain*: following the procedure, some pain may be experienced as the stone fragments pass down the ureter, causing colic-like discomfort. Analgesics are prescribed for the patient to take home.

- *Risk of infection*: prophylactic antibiotics are given, as most stones have a bacterial component and shattering these can result in urinary tract infection and possibly septicaemia. The importance of completing the course of antibiotics is stressed. The GP should be consulted if a pyrexia develops and increased pain is experienced.

- *Elimination*: the patient is advised to drink 2–3 L in 24 hours to help flush out stone fragments and clear any blood in the urine.

- *Activity*: normal activity can be resumed the next day, with a return to work within a few days.

SURGICAL MANAGEMENT OF BLADDER CANCER

Bladder cancer is one of the most common urological malignancies and is found in around 20 per 100 000 of the UK population, accounting for around 8000 new cases per year (Fenwick, 2004). There is an overall higher incidence of bladder cancers within industrialized societies, with a peak age occurrence at around 65 years of age. Men have a higher risk factor than women, but in recent years the incidence in women has increased. The most common form of carcinoma diagnosed is transitional cell carcinoma (TCC), accounting for around 90% of all malignancies, and these tumours are often papillary in nature.

Some of the presenting problems associated with bladder cancer are:

- painless haematuria
- cystitis and urine infection
- outflow obstruction – causing problems with voiding urine
- ureteric obstruction – causing back pressure within the kidney
- non-specific problems; weight loss, anorexia, anaemia, pyrexia.

Surgical management of bladder cancer can take several routes depending on the stage and grade of the diagnosed tumour. However, all patients diagnosed with the disease need support and reassurance throughout their 'journey', and the ability to provide effective and honest information is essential.

TRANSURETHRAL RESECTION OF THE BLADDER

In superficial disease, tumours are managed by transurethral resection using diathermy to remove the diseased tissue, and cautery to stem the bleeding vessels under a general or spinal anaesthetic. Patients will normally return to the ward with a urethral catheter in situ along with a bladder irrigation which flushes out any excess bleeding and maintains catheter patency. The irrigation is normally in place for up to 24 hours and the catheter remains in situ for the initial 24–48 hours.

Complications of transurethral resection of bladder tumours

It is extremely important that nurses are aware of the complications of this procedure, as frequently it is the prompt action of the nurse which prevents these occurring.

Complications include:

- *Postoperative haemorrhage*: this can be moderate if a diathermied blood vessel in the bladder mucosa is not cauterized during surgery. A blood transfusion might be required if bleeding is prolonged.

- *Clot retention of urine*: the patient will have a distended bladder and severe suprapubic pain caused by clots obstructing the urethral catheter. 'Milking' the drainage bag tubing is often successful in dislodging clots. A bladder washout may be necessary to dislodge and evacuate the clots, and must be performed using an aseptic technique.

- *Urinary tract infection*: it is important that appropriate antibiotics are prescribed preoperatively if the patient is known to have infected urine, therefore reducing the risk of postoperative bacteraemia or septicaemia. Principles of risk reduction should also be enforced when managing the urethral catheter and irrigation systems.

Patient education and discharge planning following transurethral resection of a bladder tumour

Discharge planning begins prior to admission if possible. It is important that the patient's home situation and social circumstances are known so that appropriate arrangements for discharge can be organized.

Information booklets should be available and provided to the patient in the outpatients department, at the preassessment clinic prior to admission or in the ward. It must be stressed that any written information must not be a substitute for verbal advice and discussion, as time must be taken to evaluate understanding and to make sure that the patient is well informed and aware of the operative procedure and the required follow-up care and management of the disease.

Advice is given regarding the following:

- *Activity*: it is important to remember that this surgery is not a minor procedure and this is a fact that many patients and healthcare professionals find difficult to understand because there is no visible operative wound. A gradual return to normal activity over a period of 1–2 weeks is recommended. If the patient still works, and depending on whether it is manual or sedentary work, a further 2–3 weeks convalescence may be required.

- *Fluids and diet*: a fluid intake of 2–3 L in 24 hours (provided there are no medical contraindications) should be continued for up to 2 weeks after discharge. A diet high in fibre is advised to avoid becoming constipated and to avoid straining; this could result in episodes of fresh bleeding in the bladder for up to 2 weeks after surgery.

- *Sexual activity*: this can be resumed 2 weeks following surgery if the patient feels comfortable.

- *Return to driving*: individual insurance policies should be consulted, as some may require a longer period of abstinence than the 2 weeks advised.

Patients should be advised to consult their GP should there be any unexpected blood loss in the urine or a burning sensation when voiding, as both are symptoms of a urinary tract infection which might require antibiotic therapy.

The patient will be given an outpatients appointment, usually at 2 weeks, for histological results. Check cystoscopy is normally undertaken at 3 months following initial resection to monitor tumour recurrence, and a course of intravesical chemotherapy might also be administered to reduce tumour recurrence.

For more advanced bladder cancer, the surgical treatment options are:

- cystectomy and formation of a neobladder
- cystectomy and formation of an ileal conduit urinary diversion.

Both types of surgery are indicated for multiple superficial bladder tumours which are not kept under control by intravesical chemotherapy or transurethral resection, and for T2 or T3 staged bladder tumours following radiotherapy (Blandy, 1998). Total cystectomy is a radical procedure and involves removing the bladder, lower ureters, prostate and urethra in men. In women the bladder, lower ureters, urethra and reproductive organs are removed. Radical pelvic node dissection may also be indicated.

CYSTECTOMY AND FORMATION OF A NEOBLADDER

Formation of a neobladder for treatment of bladder cancer involves removal of the native bladder and replacement with a new bladder constructed from bowel. This is classified as major surgery and the outcome criteria need to be discussed with the patient before proceeding. There are postoperative problems associated with this surgery, e.g. high pressures within the neobladder causing ureteric reflux and renal tissue damage, urinary incontinence, and the need to perform intermittent catheterization. Overall outcomes in both men and women have proved to be satisfactory (Mills and Struder, 2000), although numbers performed are not large, and most success appears to have been achieved in the larger specialist urological centres. This form of reconstructive surgery is currently used more often in the UK for patients requiring intervention for congenital anomalies and for those with intractable incontinence.

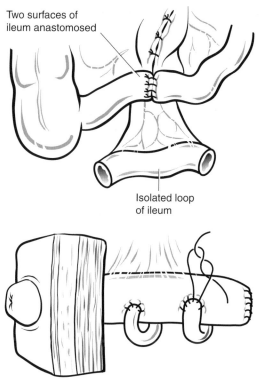

Figure 16.2   Formation of ileal conduit.

CYSTECTOMY AND FORMATION OF AN ILEAL CONDUIT URINARY DIVERSION

This is the main form of diversional surgery offered to patients requiring cystectomy, and therefore greater focus is given to the nursing care and management of this patient group. There are around 2000 'urostomies' formed annually (Fillingham and Fell, 2004), and following their surgery patients will be required to wear a stoma appliance to collect the urinary output from the ileal conduit.

The native bladder is removed, as discussed above, and the ileal conduit is formed by anastomosing the ureters to an isolated loop of the ileum. The other end of the loop is brought onto the abdominal surface to form the urinary stoma (Fig. 16.2).

Management of the patient undergoing such radical surgery involves the ward nursing team working closely with the multidisciplinary team, particularly the stomatherapist.

It should be clear from the outset to the patient that, due to the nature of this surgery, pelvic nerve damage can result in erectile dysfunction for many men, and both men and women may experience a reduced libido and have difficulty in reaching orgasm following surgery (Jones et al, 1980).

Specific preoperative nursing care

Ideally, admission to hospital should be 2–3 days prior to the procedure, so that the patient can be safely prepared for such extensive surgery.

Psychological/communication

If possible, patients should be admitted to an area where they are familiar with the clinical staff. It is important that the nurses involved in the patient's care are knowledgeable regarding the impending surgery and inherent implications, and are able to communicate honestly and openly with the patient. The patient's significant family/friends should be included in preoperative discussions, if the patient agrees, so that any fears they may have are allayed, so allowing them to offer support and understanding in the recovery period and beyond.

Stoma formation can have a major impact on an individual's life both physically and psychologically. Difficulty may be experienced in coming to terms with an altered body image and changes relating to sexuality and sexual function. Many healthcare professionals might feel unable to discuss aspects of care relating to altered body image and sexuality, and this may be due to a lack of knowledge, embarrassment and the possible perceived embarrassment of the patient (Salter, 1996). Input from the stomatherapist is vital in managing this aspect of the patient's care and management.

Maintaining a safe environment

If the patient has had persistent haematuria prior to surgery, this might result in a significant blood loss and consequent anaemia. A preoperative blood transfusion may therefore be necessary.

Breathing

Because of the nature of the surgery, the operating time may be 3–4 hours or longer. Recovery from the anaesthetic and surgery is often influenced by the general health of the patient. The anaesthetist and physiotherapist will be made aware of any pre-existing respiratory problems during their preoperative assessments. Elective mechanical ventilation may be indicated in the immediate postoperative period. If the patient smokes, this should be actively discouraged prior to surgery.

Elimination

Preoperative bowel preparation is necessary as a section of the ileum is resected during the procedure. In many units the method chosen is dependent on the 'surgeon's preference':

- 2 days preoperatively – low-residue diet
- 1 day preoperatively – clear fluids only
- 2 sachets of Picolax.

Whichever method is chosen, it is vital that the patient is adequately hydrated. Ideally, individual assessment should occur, and bowel preparation should be tailored to meet individual needs.

Eating/drinking

A low-residue diet is begun 2 days preoperatively, and clear fluids only are given on the preoperative day. An intravenous infusion should be commenced 12 hours prior to surgery to avoid dehydration.

The role of the stoma care nurse

The stomatherapist will be involved with the patient and family as soon as the decision for surgery is made, so early referral is essential. Areas covered within the stomatherapist's role include giving preoperative information about appropriate appliances, patch testing for these appliances and siting of the stoma. RCN 'Standards of Care' (1992) state that siting should be undertaken by nurses who have taken a relevant academic and clinically assessed stoma course.

Counselling skills are important to enable the nurse to build a rapport with the patient, partner and other family members. Altered body image can have a profound effect on the patient's mental and physical well-being, and it is essential that the stomatherapist is equipped to discuss these issues (Salter, 1996).

Specific postoperative nursing care

Postoperatively, if their general condition allows, the patient is returned to the ward, where one-to-one nursing care should be undertaken for the first 24 hours. The patient will have an assortment of tubes and drains in situ. These include:

- triple lumen line for central venous pressure readings/total parenteral nutrition feeding
- peripheral intravenous infusion
- epidural/intravenous opioid infusion
- nasogastric tube/gastrostomy tube
- ureteric stents
- wound drains
- oxygen therapy.

Breathing

The patient should be observed for signs of respiratory depression. This is particularly important if an opioid infusion is used to control pain. Oxygen therapy is administered as prescribed.

Maintaining a safe environment

Blood pressure, pulse and central venous pressure recordings are monitored as frequently as the patient's condition dictates. The amount of drainage from the wound drains is measured and recorded, and the wound dressings observed for evidence of oozing. Wound drains are removed when drainage is minimal. A blood transfusion may be necessary, and this will depend on blood loss and the patient's preoperative haemoglobin level.

Pain control/communication

A return to independence in activities of daily living is realistic only if pain is controlled to a level acceptable to the patient. Epidural analgesia, an opioid intravenous infusion or PCA is most effective in the initial postoperative period.

Elimination

Two ureteric stents will be in situ, and their function is to splint the ureteric–ileal anastomosis and allow healing to take place. The stents protrude through the end of the stoma and are observed in the stoma bag. The stents are sutured in position (dissolvable sutures) and remain in situ for approximately 10 days. An accurate recording of urine output is maintained with hourly measurements initially. Ureteric stents should not be flushed unless indicated by the stomatherapist or the consultant urologist.

The stoma is checked for viability. This should include:

- *colour*: the stoma may be bruised initially but should look red in colour within the first 48 hours after surgery
- *temperature*: the stoma should be warm, moist and soft to touch.

The patient should be involved in the care of the stoma as soon as this appears to be appropriate, i.e. the patient is emotionally and physically prepared. Further information on stoma care can be found in Chapter 15.

Eating/drinking

A nasogastric tube or a gastrostomy tube is in situ to allow aspiration of stomach contents. Nasogastric tubes can be uncomfortable and inhibit the patient undertaking deep breathing exercises and coughing; therefore the preferable option for the patient is often a gastrostomy tube, but this decision is usually reliant on medical preference.

The patient is kept nil by mouth until bowel sounds return – normally between 5 and 7 days postoperatively. Patients are then allowed restricted amounts of fluid, which are gradually increased before commencing a light diet. If the patient has a prolonged ileus or is in a poor nutritional state, parenteral nutrition may be prescribed.

Controlling body temperature

Prophylactic intravenous antibiotics should be given at induction of the anaesthetic and a course continued postoperatively, to reduce the risk of infection.

Complications

Complications after cystectomy and ileal conduit diversion can be divided into those associated with major abdominal surgery and those associated with ileal conduit surgery.

Complications associated with major abdominal surgery

Complications associated with major abdominal surgery include:

- chest infection
- haemorrhage
- wound infection
- prolonged ileus
- anastomosis leak
- wound dehiscence
- intestinal obstruction
- deep vein thrombosis

- septicaemia
- pulmonary embolism.

Complications associated with ileal conduit surgery

Complications associated with ileal conduit surgery include:

- *Stoma necrosis*: postoperatively, a dark purple stoma suggests a poor blood supply, and urgent medical attention should be sought. Surgery may be necessary to remove a pregangrenous section of bowel.

- *Prolapse*: surgical intervention to refashion the stoma may be necessary if it is not possible to manage the prolapse by manual reduction and use of a firm abdominal support.

- *Retraction*: this can result in unmanageable leakage problems, and refashioning of the stoma is often necessary.

- *Stenosis*: constriction of the outlet of the stoma can lead to reabsorption of urine, infection and dilatation of the upper urinary tract. It may be possible to dilate the stoma using a finger or a catheter but often surgery is necessary.

- *Skin excoriation*: this may be caused by a reaction to the bag adhesive or skin protective agent, or repeated contact with urine, and patients should be aware of the need to seek advice before problems become more difficult to resolve.

Specific patient education and advice on discharge following cystectomy and ileal conduit urinary diversion

Discharge is usually 10–14 days following surgery. However, for some patients, recovery may take longer if complications have arisen. It is vital that discharge planning commences on admission or before, if the best possible arrangements are to be made for the individual's convalescence.

Patient education and advice on discharge are given, as for major abdominal surgery. Specific information is necessary regarding further management of the urinary stoma. This information is normally given by the stomatherapist, who will continue to care for the patient or arrange continuing care in the community. It is important that nurses in the ward are able to reinforce information and answer any questions the patient may have.

Advice is given regarding the following:

- *Skin care*: maintenance of skin integrity around the stoma is extremely important. If the appliance is ill fitting, urine will be in constant contact with the skin, resulting in excoriation. To prevent this happening,

- the size of the appliance opening should be appropriate to the size of the stoma.

- *Stoma equipment*: the patient is given information on how to obtain further supplies of stoma equipment, and prescription details are passed on to the GP.

- *Urinary output*: if blood is seen in the urine, or urinary output decreases or stops, then medical attention must be sought immediately. Mucus is naturally produced from the stoma, and a fluid intake of 2–3 L per day, including two glasses of cranberry juice, can help to reduce the amount of mucus (Leaver, 1996). Individuals who are diabetic should be aware that urine from the stoma is not suitable for testing, as sugar is absorbed into the conduit (Elcoat, 1986).

- *Activity*: return to normal activity should be gradual over a period of several weeks. If patients wish to continue a strenuous job or sporting activity, they should be assessed on an individual basis. There are no restrictions on activities such as swimming.

- *Driving*: if seat belts are uncomfortable, aids are available from car accessory shops. These can relieve pressure.

- *Altered body image/sexual activity*: erectile disorders/impotence, loss of libido and problems associated with body image may cause significant distress. The patient will require ongoing counselling and referral to appropriate agencies if necessary.

- *Follow-up:* the patient will be seen in the outpatients department between 4 and 6 weeks after surgery and at 3-monthly intervals for a year after.

CONCLUSION

Urology as a specialist area of practice has evolved in the last 20 years, and nurses have played a major role in the development and delivery of appropriate care and management programmes. Patient outcomes have improved with the advent of technological advances in diagnostic screening, minimally invasive techniques and in some cases radical treatment options. Ongoing advancement in specialist nursing practice within the field of urology will see the role of the nurse developing in new practice areas in the next decade, giving even more focus on specialist care to those experiencing urological disease.

Summary of key points

- An understanding of the anatomy and physiology of the kidney and lower urinary tract is essential before the most appropriate investigations can be performed, diagnosis is obtained and relevant surgery undertaken.

- This chapter includes both invasive and non-invasive treatments for urological

conditions, encompassing new technology and techniques.

- Sensitive nursing care is required, particularly when dealing with the profound change in body image and sexual function experienced with surgery such as cystectomy.

References

Berne, M. R. & Levy, M. N. (1999) *Principles of Physiology*, 3rd edn. St Louis: Mosby.

Beynon, M. R. & Nicholls, C. (2004) Urological investigations. In: Fillingham, S. & Douglas, J. (eds) *Urological Nursing*, 3rd edn. Edinburgh: Baillière Tindall.

Blandy, J.P. (1991) *Lecture Notes on Urology*, 4th edn. Oxford: Blackwell Scientific.

Blandy, J. P. (1998) *Lecture Notes on Urology*, 5th edn. Oxford: Blackwell Scientific.

Brown, J., Meikle, J. & Webb, C. (1991) Collecting midstream specimens of urine: the research base. *Nursing Times* 87(13): 49–52.

Bullock, N., Sibley, G. & Whitaker, R. (1994) *Essential Urology*, 2nd edn. Edinburgh: Churchill Livingstone.

Carr, D. B. & Goudas, L. C. (1999) Acute pain. *Lancet* 353: 2051–2058.

Champion, J. & Longhorn, S. (2004) Urinary tract stones. In: Fillingham, S. & Douglas, J. (eds) *Urological Nursing*, 3rd edn. Edinburgh: Baillière Tindall.

Clayman, R. V., Kavoussi, L. R., Soper, N. J., et al (1991) Laparoscopic nephrectomy: initial case report. *Journal of Urology* 146(2): 278–282.

Collins, P. (2004) Reconstructive surgery for urinary tract defect.: In: Fillingham, S. & Douglas, J. (eds) *Urological Nursing*, 3rd edn. Edinburgh: Baillière Tindall.

Coptcoat, M. J. (1992) Laparoscopy in urology: perspectives and practice. *British Journal of Urology* 69(6): 561–567.

Doyle, T., Hare, W. S. C., Thomas, K. & Tress, B. (1989) *Procedures in Diagnostic Radiology*. Edinburgh: Churchill Livingstone.

Elcoat, C. (1986) *Stoma Care Nursing*. London: Baillière Tindall.

Fenwick, E. (2004) Urological cancers. In: Fillingham, S. & Douglas, J. (eds) *Urological Nursing*, 3rd edn. Edinburgh: Baillière Tindall.

Fillingham, S. & Fell, S. (2004) Urological stomas. In: Fillingham, S. & Douglas, J. (eds) *Urological Nursing*, 3rd edn. Edinburgh: Baillière Tindall.

Gill, I. S. (1998) Retroperitoneal laparoscopic nephrectomy. *Urology Clinics of North America*. 25(2): 343–360.

Gower, P. E. (1991) *Handbook of Nephrology*. London: Blackwell Scientific.

Hayward, J. (1975) Information – a prescription against pain. *RCN Study of Nursing Care Series*. London: Royal College of Nursing.

Jones, M. A., Breckman, B. & Henry, W. (1980) Life with an ileal conduit: result of questionnaire surveys of patients and urological surgeons. *British Journal of Urology* 52(1): 21–25.

Kekre, N. S., Gopalakrishnan, G. G., Gupta, G. G., et al (2001) Supracostal approach in percutaneous nephrolithotomy: experience with 102 cases. *Journal of Endourology* 15(8): 789–791.

Laker, C. (1994) *Urological Nursing*. London: Scutari Press.

Leaver, R. (1996) Cranberry juice. *Professional Nurse* 11(8): 525–526.

Lingeman, J. E., Smith, L. H., Woods, J. R. & Newman, D. M. (1989*) Urinary Calculi*. Philadelphia: Lea & Febiger.

McCaffery, M. (1983) *Nursing the Patient in Pain*. Adapted for the UK by Beatrice Sofaer. Lippincott Nursing Series, London: Harper & Row.

McLaren, S. M. (1996) Renal function. In: Hinchcliff, S. M., Montague, S. E. & Watson, R. (eds) *Physiology for Nursing Practice*, 2nd edn. London: Baillière Tindall.

Mallett, J. & Dougherty, L. (eds) (2000) *The Royal Marsden Hospital Manual of Clinical Nursing Procedures*, 5th edn. Oxford: Blackwell Science.

Mills, R. D. & Struder, U. E. (2000). Female orthotopic bladder substitution: a good operation in the right circumstances. *Journal of Urology* 163 (5): 1501–1504.

Phillips, S., Hutchinson, S. & Davidson, T. (1993) Preoperative drinking does not affect gastric contents. *British Journal of Anaesthesia* 70(1): 6–9.

Price, B. (1995) Assessing altered body image. *Journal of Psychiatry and Mental Health Nursing* 2(3): 169–175.

RCN (1992) *Standards of Care*. London: Royal College of Nursing.

RCN (2000) *Sexuality and Sexual Health in Nursing Practice*. London: Royal College of Nursing.

Rowbotham, D. J. (1992) The development of safe use of patient controlled anaesthesia. *British Journal of Anaesthesia* 68(4): 331–332.

Rungapadiachy, D. M. (1999) *Interpersonal Communications and Psychology for Health Care Professionals*. Oxford: Butterworth-Heinemann.

Salter, M. (1996) Sexuality and the stoma patient. In: Myers, C. (ed.) *Stoma Care Nursing*. London: Arnold.

Schafer, W., Abrams, P., Liao, L., et al (2002) Good urodynamic practices: uroflowmetry, filling cystometry and pressure-flow studies. *Neurourology and Urodynamics* 21(3): 261–274.

Seymour, J. (1996) Analgesia – under patient control. *Nursing Times* 92(1): 42–44.

Shaw, C. (2001) A review of the psychosocial predictors of help-seeking behaviour and impact on quality of life in people with urinary incontinence. *Journal of Clinical Nursing* 10(1): 15–24.

Tolley, D. A. & Segura, J. W. (2002) *Fast Facts – Urinary Stones*. Oxford: Health Press.

Welford, K. (1994) Urodynamics. In: Laker, C. (ed.) *Urological Nursing*. London: Scutari Press.

Whitfield, H. N. (1998) Surgical management of renal stones. In: Whitfield, H. N., Hendry, W. F., Kirby, R. S. & Duckett, J. W. (eds) *Textbook of Genitourinary Surgery*, 2nd edn. Oxford: Blackwell Science.

Further reading and useful websites

Blandy, J. P. (1998) *Lecture Notes on Urology*, 5th edn. Oxford: Blackwell Scientific.

Fillingham, S. & Douglas, J. (eds) *Urological Nursing*, 3rd edn. Edinburgh: Baillière Tindall.

Karlowicz, K. (1995) *Urologic Nursing, Principles and Practice*. Philadelphia: W. B. Saunders.

http://www.baun.co.uk British Association of Urological Nurses (accessed on 27 May 2004).

http://www.cancerbacup.org.uk Cancer Bacup. Helping people with cancer. (accessed on 27 May 2004).

http://www.cancerhelp.org.uk Cancer Reasearch UK (accessed on 27 May 2004).

http://www.continence-foundation.org.uk The Continence Foundation (accessed on 27 May 2004).

http://www.impotence.org.uk Sexual Dysfunction Association (accessed on 27 May 2004).

http://www.incontact.org UK organization for people affected by bowel and bladder problems (accessed on 27 May 2004).

http://www.malehealth.co.uk Mens Health Forum (accessed on 27 May 2004).

http://www.orchid-cancer.org.uk Orchid Cancer Appeal (accessed on 27 May 2004)

http://www.prostate-cancer.org.uk The Prostate Cancer charity (accessed on 27 May 2004)

http://www.urohealth.org Information for primary care in erectile dysfunction. (accessed on 27 May 2004).

Chapter 17

Patients requiring surgery on the male reproductive system

Martin Beynon

Key objectives of the chapter

After reading the chapter the reader should be able to:

■ give an overview of the anatomy and physiology of the male reproductive system

■ describe the pre- and postoperative nursing care for individuals undergoing surgery on the prostate gland

■ explain discharge advice that would be given following surgery on the prostate gland

■ describe the pre- and postoperative nursing care for individuals undergoing surgery for penile and scrotal conditions

■ explain discharge advice that would be given following penile and scrotal surgery.

INTRODUCTION

This chapter addresses the management and treatment of men with specific conditions of the genitourinary tract. Nursing care related to these specific conditions will be discussed, including the psychological needs of the patient when addressing sexuality and altered body image, and the need for sensitive and empathetic management of this client group. Where necessary, cross references are made to Chapter 16 with regard to investigations and nursing assessment of the individual requiring surgery.

ANATOMY AND PHYSIOLOGY OF THE MALE REPRODUCTIVE SYSTEM

The main structures of the male genitourinary system are:

- the testes and associated ducts
- the accessory glands, e.g. the prostate gland
- the penis.

THE TESTES AND ASSOCIATED DUCTS

The testes are the primary sex organs of the male. They have two functions:

- to produce androgens, which are the male sex hormone (testosterone)
- production of the male reproductive cell (spermatozoa).

The paired testicles sit within the scrotum and a mid-line septum divides the two compartments. The testicles are suspended in the scrotum by the spermatic cord; the blood and nerve supply and lymphatic drainage run through this structure. Arterial blood supply is via the testicular artery and drainage via the testicular vein. The testes are surrounded by two layers of connective tissue, the tunica albuginea and the tunica vaginalis: they help protect the testicle against injury and also cushion the structures during movement.

There are two distinct cell types within the testicle:

- the Sertoli cells, which are responsible for the production of spermatozoa and are found within the seminiferous tubules of the testes
- the Leydig cells, which are found in the interstitial tissue between the seminiferous tubules and are responsible for the production of testosterone.

The tubules and ducts from each testis converge at the posterior aspect of the gland and form the epididymis, where the sperm is stored and matures. The epididymis is a coiled tube approximately 6 m in length and is divided into the head, body and tail. The head of the epididymis receives sperm from the testis and storage occurs within the body and tail regions. The epididymis expands near its tail to become the vas deferens.

The vas deferens is a small muscular tube approximately 45 cm long that begins in the scrotum, travels a course through the inguinal canal into the pelvic cavity and ends where it joins with the duct of the seminal vesicle to form the ejaculatory duct. The ejaculatory ducts open into the urethra on either side of the verumontanum, which is a raised structure found on the posterior wall of the prostatic urethra. The two seminal vesicles are located behind the prostate gland beneath the bladder base and are approximately 5–7 cm in length. Seminal fluid, secreted by the seminal vesicles is viscous, alkaline, yellowish in colour and contains nutrients and enzymes. The fluid is thought to aid sperm motility and makes up around 60% of the ejaculatory volume.

THE PROSTATE GLAND

The prostate gland surrounds the urethra at the bladder neck. The size of the prostate varies considerably – it increases in size at puberty, and in the adult is approximately 15 g in weight. It is likened to a chestnut in shape and has a diameter of approximately 3 cm. At around 55 years of age the prostate gland often undergoes benign hyperplastic change which can result in urinary outflow obstruction. The outer zone of the prostate (the lateral and posterior portions) consists of glandular tissue, and the inner zone (the middle of the gland) is made up of mucosal glands. The prostate is surrounded and encased by an outer fibrous capsule.

The gland produces milky, slightly acidic secretions which contain enzymes (e.g. acid phosphatase) and many additional components (e.g. citrate and calcium). The fluid makes up approximately 10–20% of the ejaculate and is thought to help neutralize the acidity of the vagina and to stimulate the mobility of the sperm (Blandy, 1998); it is also thought to be responsible for the characteristic smell of semen. The prostate gland is reliant on the levels of circulating testosterone for it to function effectively.

The arterial blood supply to the prostate gland arises from the inferior vesical artery. Venous drainage is to a plexus of veins which drain into the internal iliac vein.

THE PENIS

The penis is an elongated organ consisting of three spongy cylindrical bodies – two dorsal corpora cavernosa and one corpus spongiosum – which surrounds the urethra. The corpora act as storage reservoirs for blood and are surrounded by the Buck's fascia, a tough connective tissue layer. The enlarged head of the penis is known as the glans penis and the urethra opens at its end. The glans penis is covered by the prepuce or foreskin, which is removed during the procedure of circumcision.

Penile erection occurs when there is an increased activity of the sacral parasympathetic nerves, causing vasodilatation of the arterioles and constriction of the dorsal veins of the penis. The corpora cavernosa and spongiosum fill with blood, and the penis becomes erect. At ejaculation detumescence occurs and the penis returns to the flaccid state.

All of the above structures are key to the production and transportation of viable sperm. At ejaculation, approximately 3 mL of semen is produced, which contains around 200 million sperm. The whole process of sperm production from inception to completion takes around 74 days.

For investigations and nursing assessment of the individual with a urological problem requiring surgery,

refer to Chapter 16. Specific preoperative investigations are outlined in Table 17.1.

SURGERY ON THE PROSTATE GLAND

Almost every man over the age of 40 years old has some degree of benign prostate hyperplasia (BPH), but only 1 in 10 will get outflow obstruction requiring surgery. The incidence of BPH varies from race to race,

Table 17.1   Specific investigations related to surgical interventions on the male reproductive system

Surgical intervention	Investigation
Transurethral resection of the prostate gland (TURP)	Blood – group and cross-match 2 units – urea and electrolyte estimation – full blood count – prostatic specific antigen Urinary flow rate Midstream specimen of urine ECG Chest X-ray Ultrasound of urinary tract
Retropubic prostatectomy	As above
Laser prostatectomy	Blood – group and save serum – urea and electrolyte estimation – full blood count – prostatic specific antigen Urinary flow rate Ultrasound of urinary tract ECG
Urethroplasty	Blood for: – full blood count to detect anaemia – urea, creatinine and electrolytes to assess renal function – cross-match so that blood will be available for transfusion if required Urethroplasty – urinary flow rate, cystourethroscopy Urethrogram – to determine site and length of stricture Midstream specimen of urine – to detect and treat urinary infection
Penile surgery for impotence	Blood tests – blood glucose estimation – hormone levels: testosterone, follicle-stimulating hormone, luteinizing hormone Doppler ultrasound Cavernosogram
Scrotal surgery – vasectomy – vasovasectomy	Semen analysis
Exploration for suspected torsion of testes	Scrotal ultrasound if indicated

	Not at all	Less than 1 time in 5	Less than half the time	About half the time	More than half the time	Almost always	Patient score
1 Incomplete emptying Over the past month, how often have you had a sensation of not emptying your bladder completely after you finished urinating?	0	1	2	3	4	5	
2 Frequency Over the past month, how often have you had to urinate again less than 2 hours after you finished urinating?	0	1	2	3	4	5	
3 Intermittency Over the past month, how often have you found you stopped and started again several times when you urinated?	0	1	2	3	4	5	
4 Urgency Over the past month, how often have you found it difficult to postpone urination?	0	1	2	3	4	5	
5 Weak stream Over the past month, how often have you had a weak urinary stream?	0	1	2	3	4	5	
6 Straining Over the past month, how often have you had to push or strain to begin urination?	0	1	2	3	4	5	
7 Nocturia Over the past month, how many times did you most typically get up to urinate from the time you went to bed at night until the time you got up in the morning?	0	1	2	3	4	5+	
Total IPSS							

	Delighted	Pleased	Mostly satisfied	Mixed	Mostly dissatisfied	Unhappy	Terrible
Quality of life due to urinary symptoms If you were to spend the rest of your life with your urinary condition the way it is now, how would you feel about it?	0	1	2	3	4	5	6

Figure 17.1 Chart for recording the International Prostate Symptom Score.

being more common in caucasian and black men, while rare in Chinese and Japanese men (Kirby et al, 1995).

Signs and symptoms of prostate outflow obstruction are:

- *urinary frequency*: needing to void often, usually more than 10 times daily
- *nocturia*: waking at night to void, usually more than twice
- *urgency*: sudden and strong desire to void
- *poor urinary stream*: often worse early morning and may need to strain
- *hesitancy*: experiences a delay in voiding although desire is present
- *urinary tract infection*: residual urine caused by bladder obstruction increases risk of infection
- *dysuria*: pain on voiding, which may be caused by infection
- *urinary incontinence*: occurs as a result of overdistension, with overflow incontinence as a result
- *acute retention of urine*.

The severity of symptoms can be assessed and evaluated using the International Prostate Symptom Score (IPSS), which consists of seven questions related to the severity of symptoms (Fig. 17.1). A separate question is asked regarding the bothersomeness of symptoms. Thirty-five is the maximum possible score; a score above 20 is regarded as severe. Digital rectal examination of the prostate gland will provide useful information regarding the size, consistency and anatomical limits of the prostate gland. Examination of the abdomen should also be undertaken to detect a palpable bladder that might indicate chronic retention of urine.

During the investigative stage it is important to rule out carcinoma of the prostate gland. The combined results of a digital rectal examination and prostate-specific antigen (PSA) blood screen will aid in the diagnosis.

In recent years there has been an increased trend to use medications to treat and manage benign prostatic hyperplasia. Alpha-1 adrenoceptor blockers, 5-alpha reductase inhibitors and occasionally hormone manipulation have had varying degrees of success, depending on the outcome measurement tools used (Kirby et al, 1995). However, surgical management remains the most successful option in terms of symptom and outcome improvement. Surgical treatment is indicated if there is upper tract obstruction with renal function impairment, and for acute or chronic retention of urine. Surgical intervention is not indicated, however, for symptoms of frequency alone, unless it interferes with the individual's normal lifestyle (Blandy, 1998).

Surgical procedures include:

- transurethral resection of the prostate gland (TURP)
- retropubic prostatectomy
- laser prostatectomy
- insertion of prostatic stents.

TRANSURETHRAL RESECTION OF THE PROSTATE GLAND

Transurethral resection of the prostate is the operation of choice for 80–90% of men who require surgery, and remains the 'gold standard' treatment for benign prostatic hyperplasia (Blandy, 1998). The operation is performed under a general or spinal anaesthetic, and a cystoscopy is undertaken prior to transurethral resection to allow direct visualization of the bladder and to detect any abnormalities. A resectoscope is then passed along the urethra and the obstructing part of the prostate gland is removed using a cutting loop; diathermy is also used to control bleeding. The bladder neck is excised during the procedure (resulting in retrograde ejaculation), but the prostatic capsule and tissue below the verumontanum remain intact.

Transurethral resection of the prostate gland can be a difficult procedure to perform but, in the hands of a skilled and competent urologist, is generally considered safe. Controversy exists as to whether a transurethral resection or an open procedure should be performed on large prostate glands, i.e. 50 g and over (Lewis et al, 1992).

The pre- and postoperative nursing care for individuals undergoing TURP is outlined in the care plans in Tables 17.2 and 17.3.

Complications of transurethral resection of the prostate gland

It is extremely important that nurses are aware of the complications of TURP, as frequently it is the prompt action of the nurse which prevents more serious and even life-threatening situations arising.

Complications include:

- *Postoperative haemorrhage:* this can be severe as the prostate gland is very vascular. It is vital that blood for transfusion is readily available.

- *Clot retention of urine:* the patient will have a distended bladder and severe suprapubic pain. 'Milking' the drainage bag tubing is often successful in dislodging any clots. Irrigation should be stopped and a bladder washout may be necessary using an aseptic technique (Forristal and Maxfield, 2004).

Table 17.2 Preoperative nursing care plan for an individual undergoing transurethral resection of the prostate gland

Problem	Expected outcome	Action/rationale
Communication		
Potential anxiety due to hospitalization and impending surgery	Patient is able to express anxieties and fears and will feel safe and informed about his operation	Discuss preoperative and anticipated postoperative care Provide a non-threatening relaxed environment in which the patient will feel able to express his anxieties and ask questions Provide information, using diagrams if necessary (Hayward, 1975) Ensure that informed consent is obtained before administration of a premedication Provide environment conducive to restful sleep
Breathing, eating/drinking		
Potential respiratory problems due to: – inhalation of gastric contents while unconscious – underlying respiratory disease	Gastric contents will not be inhaled Respiratory problems will not be exacerbated	Report any breathing problems the patient may be experiencing Reinforce deep breathing exercises taught by the physiotherapist Fast for 6 hours (diet), 2 hours (fluid) prior to general anaesthetic (Philips et al, 1993)
Mobility		
Decreased mobility could lead to circulatory problems and increase risk of pressure ulcer occurrence	The patient will remain as mobile as condition permits, and risk of deep vein thrombosis and pressure ulcer occurrence will be minimized	Perform pressure ulcer risk assessment Perform mobility risk assessment as per local policy Encourage mobility during preoperative period Reinforce physiotherapist's teaching of leg exercises Measure and fit with anti-embolic stockings (Mallett and Dougherty, 2000)
Controlling body temperature		
Potential postoperative infection, e.g. urine	Temperature will be between 35.5 and 37.5°C Early detection and treatment if infection occurs	Record temperature preoperatively and report if outside normal parameters Perform urinalysis – obtain MSU if nitrates present on dipstick (Laker, 1994) Prophylactic antibiotics to be given as prescribed Bath or shower to be taken prior to theatre Clean theatre gown/bed linen to be provided
Elimination		
Potential risk of incontinence due to loss of voluntary muscle control while unconscious	Patient will remain continent during anaesthetic	Ensure patient has had a bowel action within 24 hours of theatre Give patient the opportunity to void prior to administration of premedication/transfer to theatre
Maintaining a safe environment		
Inability to maintain own safety while sedated/unconscious	The safety of the patient will not be compromised	Correctly labelled identity band is in place Patient's consent form is signed Wedding ring is taped Prostheses are removed, e.g. dentures, contact lenses Baseline observations and weight are recorded Any allergies are documented Patient's medical notes, blood results, X-rays and nursing documentation are available Patient is positioned correctly on canvas

- *Transurethral resection syndrome:* also called dilutional hyponatraemia, it occurs as a result of excessive absorption of the irrigation fluid into the bloodstream, causing haemodilution and circulatory overload. If undetected, it can lead to respiratory/cardiac arrest (Bullock et al, 1994).

- *Urinary tract infection:* prophylactic antibiotics are essential preoperatively if the patient is known to have infected urine; this will help reduce the risk of postoperative bacteraemia or septicaemia.

- *Deep vein thrombosis and pulmonary embolism:* these are potential complications following pelvic surgery,

Table 17.3   Postoperative nursing care plan for an individual undergoing transurethral resection of the prostate gland

Problem	Expected outcome	Action/rationale
Breathing		
Potential risk of problems with breathing due to anaesthetic/surgical intervention	Patient's airway will remain clear Early detection of hypoventilation	Position patient ensuring clear airway is maintained Observe and record respiratory rate $\frac{1}{4}$ – $\frac{1}{2}$ –1 hourly initially and decrease as patient's condition dictates Administer oxygen therapy as prescribed Follow anaesthetist's instructions regarding position if patient has had a spinal anaesthetic, i.e. length of time patient is to lie flat Encourage deep breathing exercises
Maintaining a safe environment		
Inability to maintain own safety after surgery Potential risk of shock and haemorrhage, e.g. due to blood loss	Patient's safety will be maintained Early detection of signs of shock/ haemorrhage	Observe and record pulse and blood pressure $\frac{1}{4}$ – $\frac{1}{2}$ –1 hourly and decrease as patient's condition dictates Report to nurse in charge/doctor if blood pressure and pulse are outside normal parameters Monitor colour, consistency of urine for blood loss or blood clots Administer blood transfusion if prescribed and follow local protocol Report changes in patient's peripheral colour and responsiveness
Communicating		
Potential risk of pain/ discomfort due to surgical intervention and presence of urethral catheter	Pain/discomfort will be controlled to a level acceptable to the patient	Assess degree of discomfort/pain experienced by use of verbal/non-verbal communication Position patient as he feels comfortable Ensure catheter is patent – observe urinary drainage Secure urethral catheter to avoid traction Give analgesics as prescribed and evaluate effectiveness
Controlling body temperature		
Potential difficulty in maintaining body temperature in immediate postoperative period Potential infection following surgical intervention and presence of urethral catheter	Temperature will be between 35.5 and 37.5°C Early detection and treatment should infection occur	Monitor temperature 1 hourly, and decrease as condition dictates Observe urine for signs of infection, i.e. note colour, consistency and odour Inspect IV cannula site for signs of infection; note any discomfort, redness, discharge Instruct patient regarding catheter toilet using soap and water; to be performed twice daily Give antibiotics as prescribed
Eating and drinking		
Potential risk of nausea/vomiting due to anaesthetic Potential risk of dehydration following surgery	Patient will not feel nauseated, will not vomit	Observe patient for signs of nausea Administer antiemetic as prescribed and evaluate effectiveness Monitor IV fluids as prescribed Commence oral fluids when fully awake (if general condition allows) and increase as tolerated Discontinue IV fluids when oral intake is 2–3 L in 24 hours and diet is tolerated
Elimination		
Potential risk of clot retention following surgery Potential inability to void following removal of urethral catheter Potential inability to eliminate faeces normally	Urethral catheter will remain patent Patient will void urine within 12 hours of catheter removal Patient will eliminate faeces normally before removal of urethral catheter	Maintain an accurate fluid balance chart Maintain bladder irrigation – rate to correspond to colour of urine Discontinue bladder irrigation on the 1st postoperative day if blood loss in the urine is decreasing Observe colour and consistency of urine – if clot retention occurs, perform bladder washout using an aseptic technique, following local protocol Ensure patient does not strain to have his bowels open Administer aperient as prescribed and evaluate effectiveness Remove urethral catheter as directed by doctor at midnight on the 2nd postoperative day (Chillington, 1992) or the morning of the 3rd postoperative day

(Continued)

Table 17.3 (*Continued*)

Problem	Expected outcome	Action/rationale
		Instruct patient to use a urinal when he voids and maintain an accurate record of urinary output
Personal cleansing Potential problem performing hygiene needs	Hygiene needs will be met at a level acceptable to the patient	Assist as necessary, maintaining dignity and promoting independence Instruct patient regarding how to perform catheter toilet using disposable wipes, soap and water
Mobility Potential complication of reduced mobility following surgery: e.g. pressure ulcers, chest infection and deep vein thrombosis	Independence in mobility will be achieved at a level acceptable to the patient	Assess pressure ulcer risk using recognized assessment tool Use aids as necessary Assist in promoting independence Anti-embolism stockings to be supplied and worn Reinforce deep breathing exercises as taught by the physiotherapist

but are often overlooked in patients undergoing TURP.

- *Infertility:* as a result of bladder neck resection, there is retrograde ejaculation of semen into the bladder instead of down through the distal urethra. Following surgery, patients will experience a dry orgasm.

- *Incontinence:* this occurs due to damage of the external sphincter and if severe may require additional surgical intervention.

Patient education and discharge planning

Discharge planning should ideally begin prior to admission, but this is not always possible, especially in those who experience acute retention. It is important that the patient's home situation and social circumstances are discussed if the best possible discharge planning arrangements are to be made.

In most surgical wards and departments, information booklets are made available to patients requiring TURP before they have their surgery. It must be stressed that any written information should be provided in addition to verbal advice and discussion, as time must be taken to evaluate understanding and to make sure that informed consent is gained.

Advice should be provided on the following:

- *Activity:* it is important to remember that TURP is a major surgical intervention, a fact that patients and sometimes healthcare professionals often find difficult to understand because they cannot see a wound. A gradual return to normal activity over a period of 2–3 weeks is recommended. If the patient still

works, and depending on whether it is manual or sedentary work, a further 2–3 weeks' convalescence may be required.

- *Fluids and diet:* a fluid intake of 2–3 L in 24 hours (provided there are no medical contraindications) should be continued for up to 3 weeks after discharge. This will help the raw area in the prostatic bed to heal and will also clear any blood still present in the urine. A diet high in fibre is advised to avoid constipation and straining at stool, as this may contribute to fresh bleeding from the prostatic bed.

- *Pelvic floor exercises:* instruction should be given in the different types of exercise which will help to strengthen the pelvic floor musculature. Advice sheets should be made available within wards and departments, and are often available from relevant charities, e.g the Continence Foundation, and patient support groups, e.g Incontact.

- *Sexual activity:* this can be resumed 2 weeks following surgery. It should be stressed that retrograde ejaculation should not be seen as a reliable form of contraception, and an alternative method should be used if necessary. It should also be noted that this surgery carries a 4–30% risk of erectile dysfunction/impotence (Tanagho and McAninch, 1992) and this should be discussed with the patient preoperatively.

- *Return to driving:* individual insurance policies should be consulted, as some may require a longer period of abstinence than the 2 weeks advised.

The patient should be advised to consult his GP should there be any unexpected episode of haematuria, or burning/dysuria on voiding, as both might indicate a urinary tract infection which may require intervention with antibiotic therapy. An outpatients appointment for 6 weeks is usually provided and at this follow-up the patient will be required to perform a urinary flow rate to evaluate the effectiveness of the surgery on the patient's urinary flow. Histological information is also provided, and if the prostate chips retrieved from the surgery contain foci of carcinoma the required interventional and management options are explored and discussed with the patient. It is estimated that around 5% of patients will need to undergo a repeat procedure within 5 years due to regrowth of the gland (Tanagho and McAninch, 1992).

RETROPUBIC PROSTATECTOMY

This surgical operation was used to manage BPH before the advent of the transurethral approach. It is usually the surgery of choice in patients with a prostate gland above 60 g in weight, as a transurethral approach in this group would involve a longer operative period, increasing the risk of perioperative haemorrhage and transurethral resection syndrome. A Pfannenstiel incision is made, the prostate capsule cut transversely and a finger used to 'scoop' out the gland.

Nursing care

In addition to the pre- and postoperative nursing care required for TURP (see Tables 17.2 and 17.3), the patient will have an abdominal wound and will require regular effective analgesics to avoid problems arising due to reduced mobility. The wound is observed for signs of infection, i.e. redness, inflammation, or discharge – and the wound drain removed when drainage over a 24-hour period is minimal. Fluids and diet are reintroduced on the first postoperative day. The hospital stay for open surgery is often twice as long as for TURP.

LASER PROSTATECTOMY

Laser prostatectomy is a relatively new technique which involves the insertion of a specially designed laser fibre through an endoscope to the prostate. The laser beam is directed through the fibre into the prostate gland and literally 'burns' it. Laser treatment causes little or no bleeding (Kirby et al, 1995), and patients are able to go home on the evening of surgery or the following morning, usually with a urethral catheter in situ. Before discharge, time must be taken to teach the patient how to manage his catheter and drainage system. The patient returns for trial without the

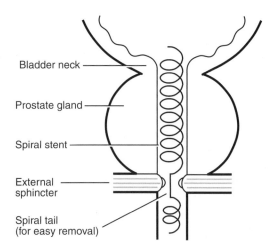

Figure 17.2 Prostatic stent.

catheter 5–7 days after surgery. It is important to emphasize that an improvement in symptoms will take 6–12 weeks. During this time the dead tissue fragments will be passed and the prostate gland will gradually get smaller (Anson et al, 1994).

PROSTATIC STENTS

Prostatic stents are implantable devices which hold open the prostatic urethra from the verumontanum to the bladder neck (Fig. 17.2). They are intended for use in men either as a temporary or permanent treatment to relieve urinary obstruction secondary to BPH. Stents have been most commonly used for patients who are not fit enough to undergo more invasive surgery, but their popularity in recent years has diminished with the introduction of improved medical and other minimally invasive management options.

Types of stent include the following:

- *Macroporous tubular mesh*: the urothelium grows over the mesh, which becomes incorporated within the urethral wall over a period of 6–8 months. The stent is permanent and is inserted transurethrally using a local anaesthetic.

- *Prostatic spirals*: normally used for temporary relief of prostatic obstruction prior to admission for prostatectomy. Cystoscopy and transrectal ultrasound are used under a local anaesthetic to place the stent, which can be removed at a later date (Chapple et al, 1990).

Following insertion of the stent, prophylactic antibiotics are given to reduce the risk of infection. Should the patient experience difficulty in voiding, it is necessary to insert a suprapubic catheter, because of the possibility of displacing the stent if a urethral catheter is used. Patients should be told to expect mild discomfort, haematuria and urgency in the first few weeks following placement of the stent. These symptoms usually resolve spontaneously. It is possible for the stent to move, e.g. into the bladder, and if this occurs the stent will need to be removed by cystoscopy under local/general anaesthetic.

CARCINOMA OF THE PROSTATE GLAND

Prostate cancer has become a major men's health issue over the last decade as a result of improved screening and diagnostic tools, and the introduction of new treatment and management modalities. Kirby et al (1995) estimate that the risk of developing microscopic disease stands at 30%; however, clinical disease is only evident in 10% of men. The risk factors proposed include ageing, race, a genetic predisposition, androgen activity, saturated fat intake and possible environmental factors. Diagnosis may result as a consequence of routine health screening, or following presentation with lower urinary tract symptoms similar to those seen in men with benign prostatic disease.

For organ-confined prostate cancer there are several potential curative treatment options available; radical prostatectomy is the only surgical intervention and the procedure is generally only undertaken in major urological units. External beam radiotherapy and radioactive seed implantation (brachytherapy) are the other treatments used. Much of the nursing management of patients undergoing radical prostatectomy involves a similar plan of care provided to those undergoing a retropubic prostatectomy. However, clear instruction on the time the catheter will stay in situ should be sought and reflected in local policy, as it differs in some units. Emotional support is paramount in both the pre- and postoperative phases, and involvement of specialist nurses can have a significant impact on long-term patient outcomes.

PENILE CONDITIONS AND SURGERY

PHIMOSIS

This is the term given to the inability to retract the foreskin over the glans penis. The condition is often not detected until the individual is sexually active and complains of painful erections. The individual may also present with balanitis, i.e. inflammation of the foreskin, which is often a result of inadequate hygiene.

PARAPHIMOSIS

In this condition the foreskin is retracted over the glans penis and cannot be pulled forward again, resulting in a swollen glans penis and foreskin. The condition occurs following sexual intercourse, masturbation, catheterization or surgical instrumentation (e.g. cystoscopy or TURP). Nurses and the patient should be aware of this potential problem in the postoperative period and ensure that the foreskin is maintained in the forward position.

If an early diagnosis of paraphimosis is made, then often it can be treated conservatively with gentle compression to reduce the oedema and manipulation of the foreskin using an anaesthetic gel. If this fails, then surgical intervention will be necessary and usually a circumcision is performed.

CIRCUMCISION

This is surgical removal of the foreskin and is indicated as treatment for balanitis, phimosis and paraphimosis (Fig. 17.3). It is also commonly performed in male infants for religious and ritual beliefs (Fuller and Toon, 1988).

Specific complications are:

- *Haemorrhage:* bleeding can be brisk following circumcision, because of the close proximity of the dorsal vein and frenular artery.
- *Pain:* erections in the postoperative period can cause increased pain. Administration of prescribed analgesics will be of assistance.
- *Oedema:* supportive underwear should be encouraged.

PEYRONIE'S DISEASE

In this disease, plaques of fibrous tissue are found in the sheath of the corpora cavernosa of the penis, which adhere to the overlying Buck's fascia (Blandy, 1998). This results in penile curvature on erection, and the patient may experience pain and difficulty achieving penetration during sexual intercourse.

Aetiology of the condition is unknown, although it can be associated with retroperitoneal fibrosis and Dupuytren's contracture (Bullock et al, 1994). Surgical treatment for this condition is usually the Nesbit's procedure and is indicated if penile deformity on erection is such that sexual intercourse is impossible or if the patient is impotent. The operation involves making an incision in the Buck's fascia, in the opposite side to the curvature, leaving the fibrotic plaque intact (Fig. 17.4). Circumcision is often performed at the same time. The procedure results in a shortening in the length of the

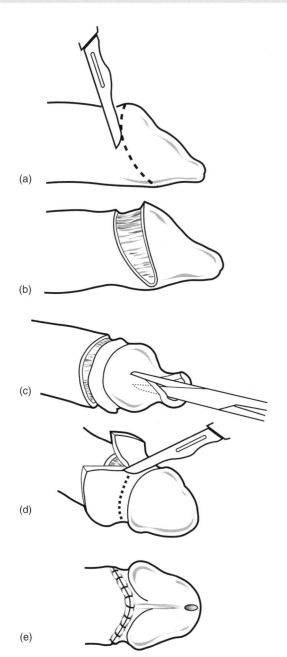

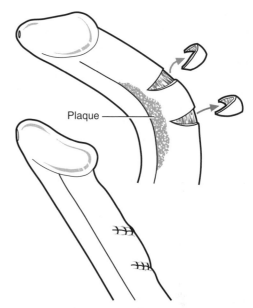

Figure 17.4 Nesbit's procedure. (Reproduced from Blandy (1991) by courtesy of Blackwell Science Ltd.)

PRIAPISM

Priapism is defined as 'a persistent painful erection which is not associated with an appropriate sexual desire' (Bullock et al, 1994). The corpora cavernosa become engorged as a result of venous congestion, and the glans penis and the corpus spongiosum remain flaccid. The condition is often extremely painful and frightening for the patient. Priapism should be seen as a urological emergency, as a delay in treatment increases the risk of erectile dysfunction/impotence.

In many cases the cause of priapism is unknown, but there are some predisposing causes:

- sickle cell trait
- leukaemia
- malignant tumour spread to the penis, causing obstruction
- drugs, e.g. marijuana, antihypertensives and anticoagulants
- injection into the corpora cavernosa used in the treatment of erectile dysfunction

(Fillingham and Douglas, 2004).

Management of priapism initially involves the insertion of a large-bore cannula into the corpora cavernosa under sedation, with an attempt made to wash out the blood clots with saline. If this is unsuccessful, vasoconstrictors are used along with aspiration. If these fail, then surgical intervention is necessary (Blandy, 1998).

Figure 17.3 Circumcision. (Reproduced from Blandy (1991) by courtesy of Blackwell Science Ltd.)

penis, and the patient must be fully informed of this prior to surgery.

The Lue procedure is an alternative surgical intervention and involves the division of the fibrous plaque with inlaying of saphenous vein in the created space. The advantage of this surgical approach is that there is no shortening of the penis.

Surgery involves the urologist performing a 'shunt' procedure to create a venous bypass for the blood to escape through. The long saphenous vein is divided and anastomosed to the corpus cavernosum. The patient must be fully informed of the complications associated with this surgery, i.e. permenant erectile dysfunction.

ERECTILE DYSFUNCTION/IMPOTENCE

Erectile dysfunction or impotence can be defined as the persistent or recurrent inability to achieve or maintain an erection sufficient for satisfactory sexual activity (American Psychiatric Association, 2000). It is estimated that the incidence of erectile dysfunction may be 1 in 10 men across all age groups (Frank et al, 1987). Most men experience erectile dysfunction on at least one occasion, but when it occurs on a more regular basis it becomes significant (Stedman, 1994).

Causes of impotence include:

- diabetes mellitus
- vascular disease, e.g. venous leaks
- pelvic surgery, e.g. cystectomy
- drugs, e.g. alcohol, antihypertensives
- psychogenic.

It is important to distinguish through clinical assessment and investigation whether the problem has a physical or psychogenic basis, although many patients will show a mixed picture.

Investigations

- *Nocturnal penile tumescence studies*: penile strain gauges are attached to the penis and linked to a computer to monitor night-time erections, which occur naturally during periods of rapid eye movement sleep. Interpretation of the graph can distinguish organic dysfunction from psychogenic dysfunction. This investigation requires overnight admission to hospital for 1–3 nights (Bullock et al, 1994).

- *Blood tests*: these include measurement of testosterone, follicle-stimulating hormone and luteinizing hormone levels to exclude hormonal imbalances. Blood glucose estimation is also undertaken to exclude diabetes mellitus.

- *Doppler ultrasound*: measures penile blood flow and can exclude vasculogenic impotence.

- *Cavernosogram*: this involves the injection of a radio-opaque substance into the corpora cavernosa and is useful in identifying impotence caused by erectile deformity (Bullock et al, 1994).

Management of impotence

Once the cause of impotence is established, then treatment can be discussed with the patient. If the impotence is psychogenic in origin, then the individual and his partner may be referred for psychosexual counselling; however, medical interventions can also be used in conjunction with counselling to assist in the treatment programme.

In the last 5 years oral agents for the treatment of erectile dysfunction have revolutionized the management of this condition/disorder. They have become the first-line treatment and are more acceptable to the patient and their partner (Lawless and Cree, 1998). Sildenafil citrate (Viagra) promotes cavernosal muscle relaxation, which results in the promotion of an erection in the presence of sexual stimulation. In the last 12–18 months, similar oral agents have become available that offer an additional treatment option in this management portfolio, e.g. tadalafil (Cialis) and vardenafil (Levitra).

Prior to the advent of oral agents, intracavernosal injections were often used in the treatment of patients with diabetic neuropathy, spinal cord injuries or other neurological causes of erectile dysfunction. This method has been used since 1974 and is still the best treatment option in some patient groups. Alprostadil is the most commonly used drug causing smooth muscle relaxation and increased cavernosal blood flow. The patient (or his partner) is taught to self-inject the penis with the amount of drug needed to produce an erection, which will last between 40 minutes and 4 hours. However, prolonged erection, which may lead to priapism, is a complication of this method. Some men also find it difficult to self-inject and will discontinue treatment.

External vacuum devices also have a part to play in the management of erectile dysfunction and are popular with some patients who do not want medical or surgical intervention. An erection is artificially created using a vacuum pump and a constriction ring is applied to the base of the penis maintaining penile engorgement. The ring should only be left on for up to 30 minutes at a time and then removed to allow sufficient blood flow back into the penis. This is a very successful method of management as there are very few side-effects or complications.

Surgical management

Surgical treatment for erectile dysfunction does not make up a large proportion of the work of most urologists; however, there are several operations available to those for whom non-surgical interventions have not been successful.

Penile revascularization surgery

This is indicated for arterial exclusion and involves microsurgery, which is often very difficult to perform.

Venous leak repair

Identified veins can be ligated to improve erections.

Insertion of penile prosthesis

An implantable penile prosthesis can be used in patients with neuropathic impotence and for those with organic disease unresponsive to medical intervention. The operation involves the insertion of a prosthesis into each corpus cavernosum (Bullock et al, 1994).

There are three main groups of prosthesis:

- Semi-rigid malleable rods.
- Cylinders with fluid-filled reservoirs.
- Inflatable penile implants; they consist of two inflatable silicone cylinders, a fluid reservoir and a pump. This prosthesis gives the best functional and most realistic result; however, cost may be an inhibitory factor.

A common complication following insertion of a penile prosthesis is infection; therefore, prophylactic antibiotic therapy should commence preoperatively.

SCROTAL CONDITIONS AND SURGERY

VASECTOMY

This is the operation for sterilization of the male and is commonly performed under a local anaesthetic. An incision is made in the scrotum, the vas deferens are located and approximately 1 cm removed from the epididymal end; this is then turned back on itself and ligated. This last stage should prevent the tube from rejoining.

It is important that both partners fully understand the implications of having a vasectomy and that it is seen as a permanent form of contraception. Most health authorities and trusts require both partners to sign consent for surgery. Advice is given regarding alternative contraception for 6–8 weeks following vasectomy, as spermatozoa within the genital tract may remain viable for this time period (Rous, 1996). The use of contraception will be necessary until semen analysis confirms azoospermia.

VASOVASOSTOMY

This operation is performed to reverse a vasectomy and is usually done under a general anaesthetic. An incision is made in the scrotum or lower abdomen. The ends of the vas are located and reanastomosed. Vasectomy reversal is most commonly requested when the male has a new partner, there has been the tragic death of a child or a couple have improved financial circumstances.

The incidence of pregnancy following vasectomy reversal is 40–70% (Bullock et al, 1994); however, better results are obtained from improved microsurgical techniques and success also depends on the time interval from the original surgery.

Due to financial constraints within the National Health Service, surgery may not be available in some areas unless the couple are able to pay.

VARICOCELE

A varicocele is often described as feeling like a 'bag of worms' in the scrotum. It is formed when the veins of the pampiniform plexus, which drain the testes, become varicosed and distended. It is most commonly found in the left side and is possibly due to an incompetent or absent valve mechanism at the end of the left testicular vein (Nieschlag and Behre, 1997). A varicocele can also be formed as a result of venous obstruction due to a renal or retroperitoneal tumour. Men undergoing investigation for infertility will need to have the presence of a varicocele excluded, as there are indications that an increase in scrotal temperature might affect spermatogenesis (Bullock et al, 1994).

Signs and symptoms include:

- 'dragging' discomfort or ache in the scrotum
- scrotal swelling
- 'bag of worms' felt on examination when the patient is standing.

Treatment is indicated only if the varicocele is causing symptoms. Surgery is by ligation of the varicocele, which is performed under either a local or general anaesthetic, and involves ligation of all veins except one in the inguinal canal.

HYDROCELE

A hydrocele is a collection of fluid in the tunica vaginalis, the outer covering of the testes. In many cases the cause is unknown, although it can occur secondary to trauma, infection or tumour. In most cases the patient is asymptomatic, but for some patients the hydrocele may be so large that it causes a dragging pain and discomfort in the scrotum. The size of the swelling can also cause the patient much embarrassment.

Treatment is initially by aspiration of the fluid, using a trocar and cannula. This can be performed on an outpatient basis. Unfortunately, the fluid usually reaccumulates and surgery is necessary. Surgery is performed through a scrotal incision and involves excision and plication of the hydrocele sac.

TORSION OF THE TESTIS

Torsion of the testis can occur at any age, but is predominantly seen before the age of 20–30 years old (Marcozzi and Suner, 2001). It is caused by excessive mobility of the testis, allowing it to twist on its mesentery and interfere with the blood supply. If misdiagnosed or untreated, this can lead to infarction of the testicle. Torsion should be assumed until proven otherwise.

Signs and symptoms include:

- sudden acute pain in the scrotum
- referred pain to the lower abdomen/groin
- testis is tender to touch
- red swollen oedematous scrotum.

Treatment

Surgical exploration of the torsion is performed through a scrotal incision. The viability of the testis is assessed and if infarcted it is removed. If the testis is viable, an orchidopexy is performed. This is fixing of the testis by suturing it to the inner wall of the scrotum. During the procedure the other testis should be examined and orchidopexy performed if it is thought that torsion may occur in the future.

ORCHIDECTOMY

This is the operation for the removal of the testis and is indicated in the following:

- *Torsion of the testis* (if infarcted).
- *Advanced prostatic cancer*: bilateral subcapsular orchidectomy is performed to try and delay progression of the disease.
- *Testicular tumour*: this is the commonest neoplasm in young men between 25 and 34 years old (Foley et al, 1995). Most tumours are prone to metastatic spread; therefore, additional treatment will be required, e.g. chemotherapy or radiotherapy.

NURSING CARE FOR PENILE AND SCROTAL SURGERY

SPECIFIC PREOPERATIVE CARE

Psychological care

Patients and their partners are often very frightened, embarrassed and anxious about hospitalization and the impending surgery. It is very important that patients are allowed to express any fears and anxieties they may have. It is within the nurse's role to provide a relaxed and supportive environment and give emotional and psychological support (Wilson-Barnett and Batehup, 1988).

Patients often have to come to terms with an altered body image (e.g. following orchidectomy, vasectomy, insertion of penile implants). If the nurse is unable to fulfil the role of counsellor, then they should be able to recognize their limitations, and an appropriate referral should be made.

It is the doctor's responsibility to gain informed consent. Information must be given in sufficient detail to enable the patient to give consent. The nurse must allow time to ensure that the patient fully understands the implications and outcome of surgery and that consent is truly informed.

Potential risk of infection after surgery

The penile and scrotal area is in close proximity to the end products of elimination and therefore is an ideal environment for the multiplication of bacteria. Antibiotic therapy is indicated if a pre-existing infection is known, e.g. urinary tract infection. If the operative site needs to be cleared of hair prior to surgery, this should be performed in the operating theatre, so as to further reduce the risk of infection and also save the patient unnecessary embarrassment (Seropian and Reynolds, 1971).

SPECIFIC POSTOPERATIVE CARE

Pain control

It is unacceptable for patients to suffer pain in the postoperative period. Pain should be assessed and controlled with the administration of adequate analgesics. It is the nurse's responsibility to evaluate the effectiveness of analgesics through verbal and non-verbal communication.

The scrotum and penis should be supported with a correctly fitting scrotal support (it is a good idea to take note of the patient's waist size before surgery) or, if unavailable, net elastic pants and a wound dressing pad will work as well. This will help to relieve pain and enable the patient to mobilize with greater ease. Wound drains in situ should be well secured to avoid pulling. Penile and scrotal pain is often accompanied by nausea and, if present, an appropriate antiemetic should be prescribed.

Wound care

Dressings should be left intact for 24–48 hours unless they require changing, e.g. if excessive oozing or wound infection is suspected. The wound is left exposed or redressed with a non-adherent dressing, depending on the patient's preference. Signs of infection should be observed for, including redness, inflammation and discharge; they might also be accompanied by a pyrexia. A swab of the wound should be obtained for culture and sensitivity if infection is suspected and the appropriate antibiotics can be administered as prescribed. The importance of thorough hand washing in reducing the incidence of infection should be emphasized, and correct hand-washing technique should be taught if necessary. If a wound drain is in situ, it is removed when drainage is minimal.

The patient should be warned that extensive bruising is a possible outcome of surgical intervention in this area and its appearance should not cause undue distress. Sutures will be dissolvable; therefore, a shower is recommended rather than a bath for at least 4 days postoperatively.

Elimination

It is expected that patients will pass urine within 12 hours after surgery; this, however, will obviously be dependent on whether there has been an adequate fluid intake. Some patients experience anxiety about voiding after surgery for fear of pain and discomfort. If the patient feels the need to void but is unable to, the nurse can assist by:

- ensuring the patient is pain free
- assisting the patient into a position in which he feels comfortable
- removing restricting dressings and support
- ensuring privacy (with nurse call bell at hand).

Voiding for the first time after surgery and having to stand or sit up may cause the patient to feel faint. To maintain safety, the nurse should remain in close proximity to the patient, in case assistance is needed.

It is important that the patient does not strain when defecating, but fear of 'bursting stitches' can lead to constipation. Reassurance is needed that this should not happen and it may be necessary to administer a mild aperient or suppositories.

COMPLICATIONS AFTER PENILE AND SCROTAL SURGERY

Haemorrhage

Because of the vasculature of the area, bleeding can be brisk. Observation of the wound site should be made and, if excessive bleeding occurs, firm pressure applied and medical attention sought. A large haematoma can

occur, which will require evacuation in the operating theatre.

Retention of urine

The provision of privacy, assistance with removing dressings and adequate pain control are often necessary if urinary retention is to be avoided. Insertion of an intermittent urethral catheter to drain the bladder may be necessary if the above measures fail.

Infection

If an infection is present, an appropriate antibiotic should be prescribed. The patient should not be discharged home with an untreated pyrexia; this is especially important in patients who have had insertion of penile implants. In this instance infection can result in the prosthesis eroding through the end of the penis and may also cause damage to the urethra. In extreme situations, penile and/or scrotal necrosis might occur.

Urethral damage during surgery

If the urethra is damaged during surgery, urinary drainage will be required and either a urethral or suprapubic catheter is inserted. The catheter is left in situ for approximately 1 week, although the length of time will depend on the extent of the urethral damage.

Psychological disturbances

Expectations of surgery are not realized for some patients, and this can lead to considerable psychological trauma. Referral to an appropriate professional should be made, e.g. a psychosexual counsellor.

PATIENT EDUCATION AND DISCHARGE ADVICE

If written information is available, this should be given to the patient on admission (or before). Time must be taken to evaluate the patient's understanding of the surgery and to reinforce appropriate information as necessary. Following penile and scrotal surgery, discharge can be on the same day (e.g. for vasectomy) or within 72 hours of surgery.

Advice is given regarding the following:

Wound care

Instruction is given regarding the need to observe the wound for signs of infection, e.g. redness, swelling or discharge. If an infection is suspected, the GP should be consulted, as a course of antibiotics may be required. The patient should be aware that it can take up to 3 weeks for sutures to dissolve. A scrotal support or supportive pants should be worn for 2 weeks or longer, as it often takes this time for bruising to subside. Wound dressings should not be necessary.

Hygiene

A shower is recommended for the first few days. A bath may then be taken if preferred, but 'soaking in the bath' should be avoided until the suture line has healed.

Pain control

Advice is given on the frequency with which prescribed analgesics should be taken. The GP should be contacted if pain is not controlled.

Activity

The patient should be aware of his own limitations, and a gradual return to normal activity is recommended. Contact sports, e.g. football or rugby, should be avoided for at least 2 weeks and up to 4 weeks following vasectomy reversal.

Sexual activity

Sexual intercourse can be resumed 1–2 weeks following discharge for most procedures. Following insertion of penile implants, abstinence is advised until the patient is reviewed at the 6-week outpatient appointment. The patient may be advised to attempt intercourse before the review so that he can report on the outcome.

Return to work

This very much depends on the type of work in which the patient is employed. For example, if he is a manual worker and this involves heavy lifting, then he will require longer than an individual with less strenuous employment.

Driving

Individual driving insurance policies should be referred to. Driving is discouraged until an emergency stop can be performed without straining.

SURGERY ON THE MALE URETHRA

URETHRAL STRICTURES

A stricture is a narrowing of the lumen of the urethra, usually as a result of scar tissue formation.

Causes of urethral strictures include:

- *trauma to the urethra*: following pelvic injury, straddle injury, passage of a stone
- *iatrogenic*: due to instrumentation, catheterization
- *infection*: sexually transmitted infection, non-specific urethritis.

Signs and symptoms of urethral strictures include:

- poor urinary stream, which may be thin, forked and forceful
- difficulty in initiating voiding
- postmicturition dribbling
- feeling of incomplete bladder emptying
- repeated urinary tract infections
- urinary retention.

Treatment

Treatment of urethral strictures is by one of the following procedures:

- dilatation of the urethra
- urethrotomy
- self-dilatation
- meatomy, meatoplasty
- urethroplasty

Dilatation of the urethra

This procedure, which involves regular dilatation of the urethra using graduated steel or plastic bougies, is often the treatment of choice for elderly gentlemen who may be unsuitable for alternative management. It is normally performed on an outpatient basis. Local anaesthetic gel is used to anaesthetize the urethra prior to insertion of the dilators using an aseptic technique. If the patient is known to have a pre-existing urinary tract infection, an appropriate antibiotic should be prescribed.

Urethrotomy

Urethrotomy is used in the initial and the long-term management of urethral strictures. An endoscopic knife (optical urethrotome) is used under vision to cut the stricture along its length (Albers et al, 1996). The procedure is usually performed under a general anaesthetic (Blandy, 1998).

Postoperatively, the patient will have a urethral catheter in situ for approximately 48 hours, although the length of time will depend on the surgeon's instructions. Haemorrhage and urinary tract infection are potential complications. The patient should be reassured that it is normal for the urine to be blood-stained initially and that this will improve with an increased fluid intake.

The patient may experience discomfort or pain on voiding following removal of the catheter; this is due to contact of the urine with the healing tissue in the urethra.

Urethrotomy generally gives short-term relief of symptoms and often has to be repeated. However, the introduction of self-dilatation following urethrotomy has improved the management of strictures for many patients (Harriss et al, 1994).

Self-dilatation

In this procedure the patient is taught to self-dilate the urethra using a lubricated disposable catheter. The technique is simple to learn and should cause minimum discomfort. However, the success of the procedure is dependent on a well-motivated patient, taught by a skilled, knowledgeable and supportive nurse.

The patient normally performs self-dilatation twice weekly for a month, then at weekly intervals. A urinary flow rate is performed in the outpatient department at regular intervals, e.g. 3-monthly, to evaluate progress.

Meatomy/meatoplasty

Strictures of the external urethral meatus can be treated by:

- *meatomy*: incision of the meatus
- *meatoplasty*: surgical reconstruction of the urethral meatus.

Postoperatively, a catheter remains in situ in the urethra for at least 24 hours after both procedures. Following removal of the catheter, the patient is taught to self-dilate the urethral meatus by introducing a lubricated meatal dilator, on a weekly or twice-weekly basis.

Urethroplasty

Urethroplasty is an open operation to reconstruct the urethra. The surgical technique employed will depend on the length, severity and location of the stricture (Collins, 2004). If the stricture is short, i.e. 1.5 cm or less, the area can be excised and an end-to-end anastomosis of the urethra performed.

A 'substitution' urethroplasty is performed for strictures longer than 1.5 cm. A perineal incision is used to expose the affected area, which is excised and substituted with grafted skin, e.g. buccal mucosa from inside the mouth, skin from behind the ear or skin from the penis or scrotum. The procedure can be performed in one or two stages, depending on the difficulty of the surgery and the type of skin used for the graft.

Specific preoperative nursing care

- *Psychological care*: the patient must be given time and the opportunity to express any anxieties they might have regarding the impending surgery and expected outcome.

- *Skin preparation*: the perineal area should be cleansed prior to surgery. In some areas the use of antiseptic preparations in the preoperative bath may be prescribed. The area should not be shaved; however, if shaving is necessary, it should be done in the operating theatre.

- *Elimination*: the patient's normal bowel habits should be understood before surgery. If constipation is a problem, then bowel preparation may be necessary to avoid postoperative straining and possible damage to the surgical wound.

- *Infection*: there is an increased risk of postoperative wound infection due to the close proximity of the perineum and the anus. Prophylactic antibiotics should be prescribed preoperatively.

Specific postoperative nursing care

- *Pain and discomfort*: the combination of an opioid infusion and a non-steroidal anti-inflammatory drug (NSAID) is often most effective in managing the patient's pain.

- *Potential haemorrhage/haematoma*: the area is highly vascular and therefore must be observed for any undue swelling or bleeding. A foam compression dressing is often used and is generally most effective in helping to reduce swelling for penile urethroplasty. The amount and type of drainage in the wound drain should be recorded. The wound drain used is either a vacuum or a corrugated drain.

- *Wound care*: the wound dressing is left intact for 3 days if possible. The wound drain is removed when drainage is minimal. The wound is examined each day and healing evaluated. A bath should be taken daily from the fourth day postoperatively and a fresh supportive dressing applied. The patient is instructed regarding the correct hand-washing technique and the importance of perineal cleansing following a bowel motion, to avoid contamination of the wound.

- *Elimination*: a urethral and, in some cases, a suprapubic catheter will be in situ and remain in for up to 3 weeks. The urethral catheter must be secured to avoid damage to the urethra caused by pulling. It is important that the catheters remain patent; therefore, a fluid intake of 3 L in 24 hours should be encouraged. A urethrogram is performed prior to removal of the urethral catheter, to exclude a 'fistula' in the new urethra. If the urethrogram is satisfactory, the urethral catheter is removed and, if present, the suprapubic catheter clamped. Once a voiding pattern is established, the suprapubic catheter is removed. A urinary flow rate should be performed.

- *Mobility*: to reduce the risk of damaging the urethra, mobility is minimal for the first few days postoperatively. Instruction is given regarding leg and deep breathing exercises, and anti-embolism stockings should be worn and subcutaneous heparin prescribed, to reduce the risk of a deep vein thrombosis occurring.

Patient education and discharge advice

This is the same as for penile and scrotal surgery, with the addition of the following information:

- To avoid damaging the new graft, sexual intercourse should not resume until at least 6 weeks

after surgery. Sitting for any length of time should be avoided, as should driving long distances.

- If any problems are encountered with voiding, e.g. retention of urine, a suprapubic catheter should be inserted and the patient seen by the operating urologist as soon as possible.

CONCLUSION

The field of urological nursing is a progressive and expanding specialty. As nurse involvement in specific urological procedures increases, it is essential that as a profession nurses have a sound knowledge base of the genitourinary tract and the disease processes which may require surgery. It is hoped that this and the previous chapter will provide such information to the reader.

Summary of key points

- An understanding of the anatomy and physiology of the kidney and lower urinary tract is essential before the most appropriate investigations can be performed, diagnosis is obtained and relevant surgery undertaken.

- Benign prostatic hyperplasia is one of the more common diseases to affect men beyond middle age.

- The symptoms experienced by this condition often greatly affect the individual's quality of life.

- A number of treatment options are available for benign prostatic hyperplasia.

- Penile and scrotal conditions and the ensuing surgery can be very frightening and embarrassing for the individual patient.

- Psychological preparation and support for men undergoing penile or scrotal surgery is paramount.

References

Albers, P., Fitchner, J., Bruhl, P. & Muller, S. C. (1996) Long term results of internal urethrotomy. *Journal of Urology* 156(5): 1611.

American Psychiatric Association. (2000) *Diagnostic and Statistical Manual of Mental Disorders*, 4th edn. Washington DC: American Psychiatric Association.

Anson, K., Seenivasagam, K., Miller, R. & Watson, G. (1994) The role of lasers in urology. *British Journal of Urology* 73(3): 225–230.

Blandy, J. P. (1991) *Lecture Notes on Urology*, 4th edn. London: Blackwell Scientific.

Blandy, J. P. (1998) *Lecture Notes on Urology*, 5th edn. London: Blackwell Scientific.

Bullock, N., Sibley, G. & Whitaker, R. (1994) *Essential Urology*, 2nd edn. Edinburgh: Churchill Livingstone.

Chapple, C. R., Milroy, J. G. & Rickards, D. (1990) Permanently implanted urethral stent for prostatic obstruction in the unfit patient. *British Journal of Urology* 66(1): 58–65.

Chillington, B. (1992) Early removal advances discharge home. *Professional Nurse* 8(2): 84–89.

Collins, P. (2004) Reconstructive surgery for urinary tract defects. In: Fillingham, S. & Douglas, J. (eds) *Urological Nursing*, 3rd edn. Edinburgh: Baillière Tindall.

Fillingham, S. & Douglas, J. (2004) Penile disorders. In: Fillingham, S. & Douglas, J. (eds) *Urological Nursing*, 3rd edn. Edinburgh: Baillière Tindall.

Foley, S., Middleton, S., Stitson, D. & Malhoney, M. (1995) The incidence of testicular cancer in Royal Air Force personnel. *British Journal of Urology* 76(4): 495–496.

Forristal, H. & Maxfield, J. (2004) Prostatic problems. In: Fillingham, S. & Douglas, J. (eds) *Urological Nursing*, 3rd edn. Edinburgh: Baillière Tindall.

Frank, E., Anderson, C. & Rubenstein, D. (1987) Frequency of sexual dysfunction in 'normal' couples. *New England Journal of Medicine* 299(3): 111–115

Fuller, J. H. S. & Toon, P. D. (1988) *Nursing Practice in a Multicultural Society*. Oxford: Heinemann.

Harriss, D. R., Beckingham, I. J., Lemberger, R. J. & Lawrence, W. T. (1994) Long term results of intermittent self catheterisation in patients with recurrent urethral strictures. *British Journal of Urology* 74(6): 790–792.

Hayward, J. (1975) Information – a prescription against pain. *RCN Study of Nursing Care Series*. London: Royal College of Nursing.

Kirby, M., Kirby, R. S., Fitzpatrick, A. & Fitzpatrick, J. (1995) *Shared Care for Prostatic Disease*. Oxford: ISIS Medical Media.

Laker, C. (1994) *Urological Nursing*. London: Scutari Press.

Lawless, C. & Cree, J. (1998) Oral medications in the management of erectile dysfunction. *Journal of the American Board of Family Practice* 11(4): 307–314.

Lewis, D. C., Burgess, N. A., Hudd, C. & Mathews, P. N. (1992) Open or transurethral surgery for the large prostate gland. *British Journal of Urology* 69(6): 598–602.

Mallett, J. & Dougherty, L. (eds) (2000) *The Royal Marsden Hospital Manual of Clinical Nursing Procedures*, 5th edn. Oxford: Blackwell Scientific.

Marcozzi, D. & Suner, S. (2001). The nontraumatic acute scrotum. *Emergency Medicine Clinics of North America* 19(3): 547–552.

Nieschlag, E. & Behre, H. M. (1997) *Male Reproductive Health and Dysfunction*. Berlin: Springer Verlag; 138–140.

Phillips, S., Hutchinson, S. & Davidson, T. (1993) Preoperative drinking does not affect gastric contents. *British Journal of Anaesthesia* 70(1): 6–9.

Rous, S. N. (1996). *Urology: A Core Textbook*. Massachusetts: Blackwell Science; 333–345.

Seropian, R. & Reynolds, B. (1971) Wound infections after preoperative depilatory versus razor preparation. *American Journal of Surgery* 121(3): 251–254.

Stedman, Y. (1994) Common psychosexual problems in males. *British Journal of Sexual Medicine* 21(4): 6–10.

Tanagho, E. A. & McAninch, J. W. (eds) (1992) *Smith's General Urology*, 12th edn. London: Prentice Hall.

Wilson-Barnett, J. & Batehup, L. (1988) *Patient Problems: A Research Base for Nursing Care*. London: Scutari Press.

Further reading and useful websites

Allison, M. (1996) Discharge planning for the person with a stoma. In: Myers, C. (ed.) *Stoma Care Nursing: A Patient Centred Approach*, London: Arnold.

Blandy, J. P. (1998) *Lecture Notes on Urology*, 5th edn. Oxford: Blackwell Scientific.

Fillingham, S. & Douglas, J. (eds) (2004) *Urological Nursing*, 3rd edn. London: Baillière Tindall.

Karlowicz, K. A. (1995) *Urologic Nursing, Principles and Practice*. Philadelphia: W. B. Saunders.

Kirby, R. S. & McConnell, J. D. (1995) *Fast Facts: Benign Prostatic Hyperplasia*. Oxford: Health Press.

Kirby, R. S., Oesterling, J. E. & Denis, L. J. (1996) *Fast Facts: Prostate Cancer*. Oxford: Health Press.

Shah, J. (1997) *Fast Facts: Urology Highlights 1996*. Oxford: Health Press.

See Chapter 16 for useful website addresses.

Chapter **18**

Patients requiring gynaecological surgery

Jacky Cotton

CHAPTER CONTENTS

Key objectives of the chapter

After reading this chapter the reader will understand:

■ the relevant anatomy and physiology of the female reproductive system

■ specific investigations that may be required by a woman undergoing gynaecological surgery

■ different types of gynaecological surgery

■ what women will experience in hospital and during recovery at home

■ discharge advice for specific operations

■ sexual aspects of gynaecological surgery.

INTRODUCTION

Surgery on any part of the body is likely to cause anxiety, but gynaecological surgery is a particularly sensitive area. Outpatient appointments and admission to hospital often involve vaginal examinations – the most personal of all medical examinations, and a cause of anxiety to many women. It is crucial to gain a woman's confidence and provide a relaxed environment where her dignity and privacy are maintained.

Gynaecological surgery may also pose a threat to a woman's concept of her body image, her role as a woman and as a mother, her sexuality, her relationship with her partner (Lee and Rider, 2001) and having to undergo intimate procedures (Nelson, 2001).

A major area of concern to many women is their femininity, and often fertility following surgery, and this is a subject often forgotten by nurses. Webb (1985) stresses that the more knowledge people have about human sexuality, the more open and flexible they are likely to be towards their own and others' behaviour.

The aim of this chapter is to promote awareness of the wider issues of the psychological effects and related sexuality surrounding gynaecological surgery. Nurses will then be better informed to care sensitively for these women.

ANATOMY AND PHYSIOLOGY OF THE REPRODUCTIVE SYSTEM

The female reproductive system consists of the internal genitalia situated in the pelvis – two ovaries, two Fallopian (or uterine) tubes, uterus, cervix, vagina – and the external genitalia, comprising the vulva.

THE OVARIES

The two almond-sized ovaries are the female gonads or sex glands. They lie on either side of the uterus within the pelvic cavity. They measure about 3.5 cm in length, 2 cm in depth and 1 cm in thickness. Each ovary is attached to the broad ligament by a thin mesentery, the mesovarian. The ovaries obtain blood from the ovarian arteries, which arise from the dorsal aorta on the posterior abdominal wall.

The ovaries produce ova or eggs, and secrete the hormones oestrogen, progesterone and small amounts of androgens.

The ovary is composed of a cortex and medulla. It is surrounded by a layer of germinal epithelium.

At birth each ovary contains at least two to three million primordial follicles. Some of these follicles will develop within the ovarian cortex and become mature cystic follicles. These are known as Graafian follicles. The ovum is embedded within the Graafian follicle and, when mature, one will be released each month, at ovulation, ready for fertilization by a sperm.

Ovulation occurs 14 days before the onset of menstruation, midcycle in a 28 day cycle. Some women experience pelvic pain each month when ovulation occurs, known as 'mittelschmerz'. Conception is most likely to occur shortly after ovulation.

The menstrual cycle prepares the uterus for pregnancy. If conception occurs, menstruation does not take place. If the ovaries are removed, menstruation ceases and pregnancy cannot occur.

THE MENSTRUAL CYCLE

The menstrual cycle occurs in most women every 28–39 days, but may vary from 21 to 42 days. It is controlled by ovarian and pituitary hormones.

Follicle-stimulating hormone (FSH) from the anterior pituitary gland causes the follicle to grow and stimulates the granulosa cells in the Graafian follicle to produce oestrogen. As the level of oestrogen rises, it inhibits further production of FSH but stimulates the release of luteinizing hormone (LH), and ovulation occurs.

Accompanying the ovarian and pituitary cycles are a series of changes in the uterine endometrium. When menstruation occurs, the endometrium is shed down to its basal layer and is accompanied by bleeding. Under the influence of oestrogen, regeneration begins and the endometrium grows thicker. This is the proliferation phase and lasts about 10 days.

Following ovulation and the production of progesterone, the endometrium becomes thicker and the glands more tortuous. This is the secretory phase and lasts about 14 more days, after which the lining is shed again.

After the discharge of the ovum from the Graafian follicle, the granulosa cells multiply rapidly and a convoluted, solid greyish body is formed. This is known as the corpus luteum and it functions as an endocrine gland, secreting oestrogen and progesterone. It persists for about 14 days, after which it degenerates if fertilization has not occurred.

When pregnancy occurs, the corpus luteum continues to produce both oestrogens and progesterone for about 12 weeks, after which the placenta takes over the production of these hormones.

The corpus luteum is sustained by human chorionic gonadotrophin (hCG), which is produced by the cells of the trophoblast (embryo) from the time of implantation.

THE FALLOPIAN TUBES

Two Fallopian tubes (also known as uterine tubes) join the uterus just below the fundus, or upper part, of the uterus. Each tube is 10–14 cm long and opens out into a funnel-shaped structure of small, finger-like projections, known as fimbriae, which are positioned close to the ovaries during ovulation.

The tubes are mobile, which enables them to pick up eggs (ova) released from the ovaries and carry sperm upwards to meet them. Fertilization takes place in the tubes, which then carry the fertilized ovum into the uterus, wafted along by the ciliated epithelial cells which line the tubes.

UTERUS

The uterus is a hollow, pear-shaped muscular organ lying between the bladder and the rectum. It is made up of the fundus, body and cervix.

The thick muscular wall of the uterus is called the myometrium, while the body of the uterus is lined with a mucous membrane called the endometrium. This is a very vascular layer which differs in thickness throughout the menstrual cycle and is largely shed during menstruation.

The uterus normally lies in an anteverted position, meaning that the long axis of the uterus is directed forwards. It is held in place by muscular and fibrous supports. The muscle is arranged in a spiral form running from the cornum to the cervix, giving a circular effect around the Fallopian tubes and cervix, and an oblique effect over the body of the uterus. The important muscular supports are the levator ani muscles. The uterine ligaments include:

- anteriorly – the round ligaments
- laterally – the transverse cervical ligaments
- posteriorly – the uterosacral ligaments.

The broad ligaments, although referred to as a ligament, are folds of peritoneum attaching the uterus to the pelvic side walls, helping to hold the uterine fundus in an anteverted position (Tortora and Grabowski, 2003).

The blood supply to the uterus is derived from two pairs of arteries: the uterine and ovarian arteries.

CERVIX

The cervix is the neck of the uterus and extends into the top of the vagina. The cervix is 2–3 cm long and dilates during childbirth to allow the passage of the baby.

The outer surface of the cervix in the vagina is covered with squamous epithelium. Squamous cells begin to grow from beneath the columnar epithelium and gradually replace it. The point at which the squamous cells of the ectocervix (outer cervix) meet the columnar cells of the endocervix (inner cavity) is known as the squamocolumnar junction.

The normal replacement of one type of cell by another is called squamous metaplasia, and where it takes place is called the transformation or transitional zone. The squamocolumnar junction and the transformation zone are the sites where most precancerous changes originate (Hughes, 2001).

During the menstrual cycle the crypts or glands in the cervix respond to rising levels of oestrogen by secreting an abundance of mucus. This mucus becomes increasingly thinner, stretchier, clearer and more watery. It resembles raw egg white and a drop can be stretched between two points to form a thread of up to 15 cm long, known as the spinnbarkeit phenomenon (Govan et al, 1993). The molecules of fertile mucus are arranged as long canals, through which sperm can pass. Obviously, this is most evident at the time of ovulation, and followers of 'natural family planning' or the Billings method (Billings and Westmore, 1980) rely on changes in their cervical mucus to predict their fertile period. This mucus also maintains the life of the sperm by providing nourishment and changing the pH of the vagina. Fertile mucus is alkaline, and this neutralizes the acidic vaginal secretions.

Following ovulation, as the progesterone level rises, the mucus becomes thick and sticky, forming a plug at the cervix and preventing sperm entry.

VAGINA

The vagina is a muscular canal joining the uterus to the external genitalia. It is about 8 cm long, and normally the anterior and posterior walls are in close contact with one another. They lie in folds called rugae, which expand during sexual intercourse and childbirth.

During the reproductive years, Döderlein's bacilli, a form of lactobacilli, appear in the vagina and produce lactic acid by acting on the glycogen in the epithelial cells. This results in a vaginal environment with a pH of 4, which helps prevent infection.

VULVA

The vulva (meaning 'cover' in Latin) is the collective name given to the external female reproductive organs. It extends from the mons pubis to the perineum and is bounded by the labia majora.

SPECIFIC INVESTIGATIONS FOR PATIENTS REQUIRING GYNAECOLOGICAL SURGERY

PELVIC EXAMINATION

Vaginal examination

After a thorough history has been taken from the patient, the gynaecologist will usually wish to perform a vaginal examination. This may be a digital examination, or involve the insertion of a speculum. This is a most intimate procedure, and most women worry about this aspect of a gynaecological outpatient appointment. It is crucial that the nurse acting as a chaperone provides support to the woman, ensures privacy and maintains the woman's dignity at all times. The woman values the support of the nurse in providing an explanation of what occurs during the examination (Duffin and Nash, 2001). The nurse should continually talk to the woman, encouraging her to relax and breathe deeply. Some women prefer to be told exactly what is happening; others like to be distracted by talking about their children or holidays, etc. She should be advised that the more relaxed she is, the less uncomfortable the examination. It is advisable that the woman empties her bladder first, so she is more comfortable, and is allowed to remove her underclothing in private. A blanket should always be available to maintain her dignity during the examination.

Speculum examination

The clinician will often need to use a speculum to view the cervix. The most common type of speculum is a Cusco's or bivalve speculum, which parts the vaginal walls, enabling the cervix to be visualized. A high vaginal swab may be taken if any discharge is present, and in sexually active young women a chlamydia swab may be taken. Chlamydia is a sexually transmitted infection which may be difficult to detect since often women have no symptoms. It can cause pelvic inflammatory disease and infertility (Sutton, 2001).

Another speculum is a Sims' speculum, used when the woman is lying in a modified left lateral position. It is used to detect any prolapse of the uterus or vaginal wall. The woman may be asked to cough to demonstrate any signs of stress incontinence.

Bimanual palpation

Often a woman will be examined both abdominally and vaginally in the outpatient clinic. After the gynaecologist has palpated the abdomen, the woman will be asked to draw her knees up with her ankles together, and asked to relax her knees apart. This is the dorsal position and is most commonly used, since it is convenient for bimanual palpation.

The procedure is carried out with two hands palpating together, one on the woman's abdomen, pressing down on the fundus (top) of the uterus, and one inside the vagina. The size, position and movement of the uterus are determined. Other structures such as the ovaries and Fallopian tubes are located. Any masses, such as a pregnancy, ovarian cyst or tumour are noted.

Cervical smear

Also known as a Pap test, a cervical smear is a screening test undertaken to detect early changes in cells from the cervix, which might lead to squamous cell carcinoma. George N. Papanicolaou (1883–1962) demonstrated changes in the vaginal epithelium at different phases of the menstrual cycle and developed a cytological test for malignant changes in the squamous epithelial cells of the cervix.

The cells are obtained during a speculum examination using a specific wooden spatula and brush. Cells are taken from the squamocolumnar junction of the cervix, and the sample is then smeared across a cytology slide, which is sent to the laboratory for histological examination. All women during their reproductive years should have a smear test every 3 years or more frequently if they have had an abnormal result (Department of Health, 1993).

Sometimes the cervix may appear red. This is a quite normal physiological state and occurs when there is only a single layer of columnar cells covering the connective tissue and blood vessels. In the past this condition has been called an 'erosion', but the name given to the area now is an 'ectropion'.

Any abnormal or dyskaryotic cells are known as cervical intraepithelial neoplasia (CIN), meaning 'new change in the outer layer of the cervix'. There are three stages of cervical intraepithelial neoplasia, as follows:

- *CIN 1* refers to cells which are abnormal, in that they have minor changes in cell structure which are the first signs of precancer. Approximately one-third of CIN 1 cases revert to normal (Hughes, 2001). Repeat smears may be required more frequently, depending on local policy.

- *CIN 2* is the next stage, which usually correlates with moderate dyskaryosis where there are more marked changes. A repeat smear or colposcopy is usually recommended.

- *CIN 3* is the most severe preinvasive abnormality and is also known as carcinoma in situ. There are definite changes of premalignancy, and one in three lesions will progress to invasive cervical cancer unless the abnormal cells are removed. An urgent colposcopy and biopsy are required to determine whether the malignant cells have become invasive.

Colposcopy

The word colposcopy is derived from the Greek word 'colpos' meaning 'bay' or 'bosom-like hollow' and 'scope' meaning to inspect. A colposcopy is the observation of the cervix and its surrounding tissue with binocular magnification. A microscope is used, which allows magnification of up to 10 times.

Colposcopy may be undertaken in a general gynaecology outpatient clinic, specific colposcopy unit or genitourinary department. Increasingly, nurses are undergoing specialist training and performing the role of nurse colposcopist, undertaking both diagnostic colposcopy and treatments. This is often more acceptable to women than being treated by a male doctor. It is advisable to explain to the woman that the large-looking microscope and its attachments will not go inside her. In fact, the procedure is similar to taking a cervical smear, apart from the fact the woman's legs will be in a lithotomy position, i.e. in stirrups. A biopsy may also be taken under a local anaesthetic. In many units, the woman may be given the opportunity to view her cervix on a television screen.

Colposcopy is indicated when there have been changes in the cells of the cervix, noted on the woman's smear test. It enables the position and extent of the CIN to be ascertained, so that the correct management is chosen. Sometimes, treatment may be carried out at colposcopy, using local ablative therapy such as laser, cold coagulation or diathermy loop excision.

Discharge advice following colposcopy

- There may be a bloodstained discharge or it may be watery. A panty liner should be used for sufficient protection. Tampons should not be used for the first period after treatment, to reduce the risk of infection.

- Follow-up is crucial to the ongoing care of women who have had an abnormal smear test. Most women will have a follow-up colposcopy after 6 months and then annual smears for 2 years.

- If the woman has had treatment to the cervix, she should refrain from sexual intercourse for 4–6 weeks to enable the biopsied area of the cervix to heal. Signs of local infection include heavy fresh bleeding or an offensive smelling discharge.

Pelvic ultrasound scan

Ultrasound is used as a means of examining various organs of the body by means of high-frequency sound waves. These form pictures on a screen and enable any abnormalities to be detected. The uterus and ovaries can be identified and any tumour located and measured. During the menstrual cycle, the growth of a Graafian follicle may be observed and the thickness of the endometrium measured, so that the timing of ovulation is confirmed.

A full bladder is necessary as it helps push the uterus and ovaries into a better position for examination. The woman should fill her bladder by drinking 1 litre of fluid (not fizzy drinks) during the 2 hours before the appointment. This can be very uncomfortable for the woman.

The procedure takes between 5 and 10 minutes and is not painful but may be uncomfortable. This is because the radiographer has to press firmly, using cold gel, against the abdomen and full bladder, in order to produce a clear picture.

Transvaginal ultrasound scan

This type of scan facilitates a much clearer view of the abdominal organs than an abdominal scan. It is useful in confirming the presence of an early intrauterine or ectopic pregnancy, and a missing intrauterine contraceptive device may be located.

The tip of a round-edged probe is covered by a disposable condom, then inserted into the vagina. An ultrasound scan cannot harm a pregnancy.

Endometrial biopsy

It is possible to obtain tissue for endometrial biopsy without a general anaesthetic in the outpatient clinic. This may be more suitable for women who do not wish to have a general anaesthetic or for whom a general anaesthetic may be unsuitable, such as very elderly women. In the past this was done using a small suction aspirator (Vabra aspirator). Now, a narrow plastic pipette is introduced into the endometrial cavity and a biopsy taken. The woman should be advised that this can be uncomfortable. However, some gynaecologists believe that a full dilatation and curettage under general anaesthetic should be performed if a larger sample is required. A hysteroscopy must be carried out prior to this procedure, so the gynaecologist has inspected the endometrial cavity before the curettage.

Hysterosalpingogram

A hysterosalpingogram (HSG) is an X-ray examination of the female genital tract and takes about 15–20 minutes. The test must be done during the first 10 days of the cycle, after menstruation has ceased, but before ovulation. It must not take place during the follicular phase, as it could disturb a pregnancy if conception has occurred. An HSG should not take place if there is evidence of active infection, since infected material could enter the tubes.

A speculum is inserted into the vagina, and radio-opaque dye is injected into the cervical canal via a cannula. The dye may cause a warm flush in the abdomen with some abdominal cramping pains. Progress of the dye through the uterus and Fallopian tubes can be followed on a television screen. The dye is harmlessly absorbed into the bloodstream and excreted via the urine.

An HSG is a diagnostic aid and demonstrates internal uterine abnormalities such as fibroids or a bicornuate uterus. The test also illustrates the site of tubal occlusion in cases of infertility. If the Fallopian tubes are patent, radio-opaque dye will spill into the pelvic cavity. However, in many cases of infertility, the usefulness of this procedure has now been superseded by the 'laparoscopy and dye' test, which gives more detail about the nature of the tubal occlusion.

Hysteroscopy

This procedure allows the gynaecologist to view directly inside the uterus and examine the endometrium. A small fibreoptic telescope is passed through the cervix into the uterus. The walls of the uterus are separated with gas or fluid to enable the telescope to view inside the uterus. Some surgeons prefer not to carry out this procedure if the woman is bleeding vaginally, since this can impair the view.

Hysteroscopy may be used to diagnose the cause of postmenopausal bleeding, and in this instance a dilatation and curettage will be carried out simultaneously. Hysteroscopy is increasingly performed as an outpatient procedure, so eliminating the need for a general anaesthetic.

Laparoscopy

This test enables the direct visualization of the pelvic organs using a fibreoptic light and a telescope-like instrument known as a laparoscope. Under general anaesthesia, the woman is catheterized and placed head downwards in the Trendelenburg position to allow the upper abdominal contents to fall away from the pelvic organs. A small incision is made below the umbilicus, and 2–3 L of carbon dioxide is introduced into the abdominal cavity. This produces a pneumoperitoneum, which helps to displace the intestines and allows the pelvic and abdominal organs to be viewed easily via the laparoscope. A second instrument is inserted through a small cut near the upper pubic hairline.

Thorough observation of the pelvic organs can then be undertaken. As an investigation for infertility, methylene blue is injected through the cervix and observed via the laparoscope as it passes from the uterus through the Fallopian tubes and out via the fimbrial ends into the pelvic cavity. The dye illustrates any blockages in the tubes which might prevent the eggs from the ovaries reaching the uterus. If the dye flows through (referred to as 'fill and spill'), the tubes are assumed to be patent, although the state of the cilia in the lining cannot be seen. If the test is performed during the follicular phase of the cycle, developing follicles may be viewed.

The woman should be warned that she may feel bloated and have an aching pain around the shoulders. This is quite normal and is caused by the carbon dioxide in the abdomen irritating the phrenic nerve. Paracetamol and hot peppermint water can give relief. Sometimes the incisions may bleed or ooze a little, but an ordinary plaster should be a sufficient covering. There may be blue staining on her sanitary towel, and urine may appear green or blue as it mixes with dye from the vagina.

URODYNAMIC INVESTIGATIONS

When a woman complains of stress incontinence, it is important to ascertain whether she has genuine stress incontinence, which may be treated surgically, or detrusor instability which does not require surgery.

- *Genuine stress incontinence* is defined as 'the involuntary leakage of urine in the absence of detrusor activity' (Govan et al, 1993:356). There may be displacement of the bladder neck due to pelvic floor weakness, which prevents it responding normally to increases in intra-abdominal pressure such as coughing.

- *Detrusor instability* (also known as unstable bladder) refers to a condition whereby the bladder contracts uninhibitedly during bladder filling. This leads to symptoms of frequency and urgency.

Urodynamic investigations measure changes in bladder pressure with changes in bladder volume. A catheter is inserted into the bladder, and a pressure catheter is placed in the rectum to measure abdominal pressure. This eliminates movement artefacts which may be produced if the intravesical pressure alone is measured. The rectal pressure is subtracted from the intravesical pressure to give the detrusor pressure.

The bladder is filled at a fast rate of 100 mL/min. The woman indicates when she first feels the sensation of filling and when her bladder feels full. The water flow is switched off; she then stands up and is asked to cough to demonstrate any urinary leakage. She then sits on the uroflowmeter (a commode-like lavatory) and empties her bladder in private while the peak flow rate and maximum volume pressure are noted.

Videocystourethrography (VCU) can also be carried out, which allows visualization of the urethral sphincter mechanism and demonstrates any associated bladder pathology.

Cystoscopy

This procedure involves the thorough examination of the bladder under a general anaesthetic. A cystoscope, a fine telescope-like instrument with a light source, is inserted into the urethra and passed into the bladder. This enables the urogynaecologist to view inside the bladder, and a biopsy may be taken.

This operation is carried out to investigate the cause of recurrent urinary tract infections or haematuria (blood in the urine). Small polyps in the bladder or a caruncle (a small fleshy lump) at the urethral entrance can be removed during the procedure.

Occasionally, a woman may have a urethral catheter inserted at the end of the procedure if it is felt that the bladder needs to be rested.

PREGNANCY TESTING

A diagnostic pregnancy test detects human chorionic gonadotrophin, which is excreted in the urine. The level in blood and urine reaches its highest point in normal pregnancy between the 8th and 12th weeks.

Human chorionic gonadotrophin levels in an ectopic pregnancy (i.e. one occurring in a Fallopian tube) are lower than those found at a comparable period of gestation in a normal pregnancy. In instances of suspected ectopic pregnancy, the measurement of serum concentration of the β subunit of human chorionic gonadotrophin (β-hCG) is of great value, especially when used in conjunction with ultrasound scanning.

If the level of β-hCG is above 6000 mlu/L the patient is likely to have a normal intrauterine pregnancy, especially if the level rises rapidly. Absence of β-hCG eliminates pregnancy, but levels below 6000 mlu/L may indicate a tubal pregnancy, a missed abortion or very early intrauterine pregnancy. Repeat blood tests may be required after 48 hours to assess the increase of β-hCG levels. Doubling of this level after 48 hours is suggestive of an ectopic pregnancy, whereas in an intrauterine pregnancy the increase is much larger.

RHESUS STATUS

After a pregnancy loss, whether a miscarriage, termination or an ectopic pregnancy, it is crucial that a woman's rhesus status is checked to prevent haemolytic disease of the newborn.

The rhesus factor is found in the red blood cells of 85% of the population (rhesus positive); the other 15% are rhesus negative (Tortora and Grabowski, 2003). If a woman with rhesus-negative blood becomes pregnant by a man with rhesus-positive blood, the fetus will have rhesus-positive blood. A small amount of fetal blood may pass into the woman's blood, which will then form antibodies. If the woman continues with the pregnancy, there will be no harm to the fetus, but if she becomes pregnant again by a rhesus-positive man, the woman's blood will 'attack' the fetus (Fig. 18.1). This will either cause a miscarriage or the child will be born with haemolytic disease of the newborn and will require a full exchange of blood.

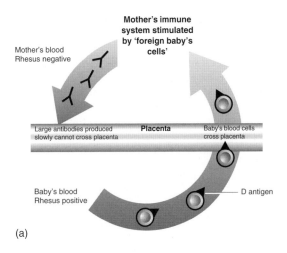

(a)

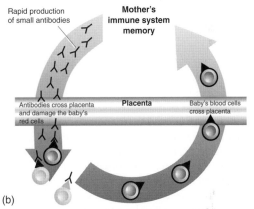

(b)

Figure 18.1   Rhesus disease and (a) first and (b) second pregnancies. (Reproduced with permission from Baxter Healthcare.)

Rhesus disease may be prevented by the injection of immunoglobulin 'Anti-D', which destroys any rhesus-positive cells that have entered a woman's bloodstream. It therefore prevents the woman's body from making the antibodies, but must be given within 72 hours of the placenta separating.

ASSESSMENT OF PATIENT REQUIRING GYNAECOLOGICAL SURGERY

The majority of gynaecological operations are undertaken as planned elective admissions, giving nurses the opportunity to prepare a woman both physically and psychologically for surgery. Gynaecological nursing is a particularly sensitive area, and very often the ward nurse is the first person a woman can talk to openly about her problems and anxieties. Once a diagnosis has been made, finding an empathic listener can be the first step a woman takes in coming to terms with a difficult diagnosis, be it an unwanted pregnancy or a suspected cancer.

Following surgery, women are being discharged back to their families earlier, which reduces postoperative complications and hastens recovery (Taylor et al, 1993). It is important that a full nursing assessment is made as soon as possible after admission and the nurse establishes a rapport quickly so support can be provided for the woman, who may find the situation both distressing and embarrassing (Cotton, 2003).

Many hospitals provide preadmission clinics several weeks before the operation date. The woman will visit the clinic, where a nurse will assess her health status. Ward procedures and the planned surgery will be explained, information leaflets given and any preoperative investigations performed. The National Institute for Clinical Excellence has produced guidelines for routine preoperative tests based on the American Society of Anaesthesiologists' (ASA) grading and grading of surgery booked (NICE, 2003). These may include a full blood count, and group and save for women undergoing major surgery. Here the laboratory saves some of the patient's blood so that it can be cross-matched with appropriate units of blood in case she should haemorrhage during surgery. Electrophoresis is required for those of Afro-Caribbean and Mediterranean origin to exclude sickle cell disease and β thalassaemia. Women aged 60 years old or above often require an electrocardiogram to detect any unknown cardiac problems.

At this stage the nurse may carry out the assessment. This is to establish a baseline assessment from which change and progress may be compared. It is important to obtain a general medical and social background, as well as a specific obstetric and gynaecological history. An obstetric history listing the number of pregnancies, miscarriages and terminations should be obtained, although some women prefer that any terminations revealed are not actually recorded. For women undergoing continence surgery, any babies weighing more than 8 pounds should be noted. The length of labour and type of delivery is also pertinent (Cardozo et al, 1993), since a long labour resulting in a forceps delivery may damage the pelvic floor and urethra. The terms 'gravida' meaning 'pregnancy' and 'para' meaning 'live children' are often used. Thus, a woman described as being G4 P2^{+2TOP} means four pregnancies leading to two live children and two terminations.

A menstrual history is also recorded. Every woman has her own idea of what a 'normal' period is like, and therefore it is helpful to ask specific questions such as how many pads/tampons a day does she use during a period. The length of the period and duration of cycle are important, as is the occurrence of any dysmenorrhoea (period pain) and premenstrual tension. Menstrual cycle is often denoted as, for example, 5/28, meaning 5 days of bleeding every 28 days.

Any contraception being used should be noted. Women using the oral contraceptive pill may be advised to stop taking it before surgery, due to the risk of developing deep vein thrombosis following surgery.

An assessment of bowel and urinary function should also be carried out. Many women suffer constipation following surgery. It is helpful to know if a woman suffers from this, so as to plan her care accordingly. An overview of a woman's bladder dysfunction is particularly crucial if she is undergoing continence surgery. Urinary incontinence has been a 'taboo' subject for many years, and women have often been too ashamed or embarrassed to admit that they leak urine. It may be that the woman has been admitted for an unrelated problem and has never told anyone that she sometimes feels wet. Asking the woman direct questions at an appropriate time will often be a relief to her that the subject has been mentioned. Sometimes, closed questions (questions to which the reply is yes or no) are more useful to elicit information from the woman, than open questions which may be misinterpreted. For example, the question, 'Do you ever leak urine when you sneeze or during exercise?' is very clear.

Sometimes, assessment may take place while casually talking about another topic or when performing a physical task. Selby (2001) refers to the 'moment of truth' when the woman identifies a moment when she is enabled to talk about her inner feelings, where intimacy and touch by the nurse are the releasing factors. This is particularly true of a vaginal examination, which offers a 'moment of truth' for women who have troubled sexualities (Tunnadine, 1992). Many nurses feel out of their depth discussing sexual matters, but often the patient just wants the opportunity to talk about her experiences and feelings.

Webb (1985) recommends that potentially threatening or embarrassing questions can be 'unloaded' by preceding them with a general statement such as, 'Many people feel ... how about you?' Questioning methods like this prevent conveying assumptions about the patient. In this way, for example, when discussing surgery for a woman admitted for a vulvectomy, it may be helpful to ask, 'Many women don't like to feel inside their vagina or look at themselves down below, how do you feel about this?'

Shingleton and Orr (1987) recommend various questions to open up discussion of sexual anxieties following hysterectomy (Box 18.1). They provide an ideal framework to begin discussing any sexual concerns with women and can be adjusted to whichever operation an individual woman is having.

Box 18.1 Questions to open up discussion of sexual anxieties following hysterectomy

- What does your uterus mean to you?
- How will hysterectomy change your life?
- What is the most important function of your uterus?
- What are your thoughts about losing your uterus?

Obviously, not all nurses are trained to perform vaginal examinations, but it is a skill with enormous benefits for the woman and the nurse. It may become a basis for a psychosexual nursing assessment without medical staff being present. Many continence and family planning nurses assess pelvic floor function while performing a vaginal examination, and it makes teaching pelvic floor exercises much easier (see p. 399).

Discharge planning should be commenced at preoperative assessment to determine, prior to admission, the home environment and what care is available from the family. If the woman is single, with no family or carers – particularly for older women who may live alone – plans should be made at the earliest stage for any support services that may be required on discharge from hospital, by involving a social worker in her care.

The preadmission clinic provides an ideal opportunity for all these assessments to be undertaken by nursing staff. Unfortunately, due to the very busy nature and rapid turnover of most gynaecological wards, a nurse may only have 10–15 minutes to admit each patient, so the assessment must be straightforward and relatively quick.

The model of care based on activities of daily living developed by Roper, Logan and Tierney (2000) is frequently used as an assessment framework for planning care, since it is relatively easy to use. Often 'standard' care plans are used where the care required changes rapidly pre- and postoperatively. However, it is important that the psychological care of the individual woman and her family are also considered. Gould (1990) criticizes Roper et al's model, since its contribution towards planning psychological care is somewhat limited. However, it may be used to plan care for discharge, and to identify areas where patient teaching is required.

The primary goal of gynaecological nursing is to help the woman become independent and self-supporting (RCN, 1991). Orem's Self-Care Model (1985) may therefore be more suitable for women with gynaecological conditions, since its central theme is patients taking responsibility for their health needs. The model promotes partnership in care of the woman and her

named nurse, and assumes the woman to be capable of making her own decisions regarding care.

Nurses must provide individualized nursing care, using a problem-solving approach based on an holistic assessment that includes the woman's perception of her own anatomy and physiology, with special attention to body image and sexuality. In many units, integrated care pathways are used as the basis for planning the care and services women admitted for specific procedures will require.

MINOR GYNAECOLOGICAL SURGERY

HYSTEROSCOPY, DILATATION AND CURETTAGE

Hysteroscopy, followed by dilatation of the cervix and curettage of the uterus (D and C), is the most common minor gynaecological procedure undertaken. A telescope is introduced into the endometrial cavity via the cervix, where the size and shape of the uterine cavity and the endometrium can be viewed directly.

This procedure is diagnostic where there has been occurrence of postmenopausal bleeding, postcoital bleeding (after sexual intercourse) or any instance of increased bleeding, both during menstruation and between periods. It may reveal an endometrial polyp, or the pathology of the endometrial curettings may show an endometrial cancer.

Evacuation of retained products of conception

A dilatation and curettage may also be used as a therapeutic intervention to treat heavy bleeding where the cause is retained products of conception following a miscarriage. This procedure is known as evacuation of retained products of conception (ERPC).

A miscarriage may be described as the expulsion of the fetus from the uterus before it is viable, i.e. before it is capable of independent existence. This is considered to be before 24 weeks' gestation. The correct medical term for a miscarriage is spontaneous abortion, but this can cause additional distress to women, so the term miscarriage is preferred.

The cervix is gently dilated and a curette (spoon-like instrument) is used to scrape away the lining of the uterine cavity. The procedure only takes a few minutes, and the cervix closes naturally afterwards.

The language used when caring for women who have miscarried is always important. It is advisable that the procedure is not referred to as a 'scrape', since this can understandably upset mothers. Women are particularly vulnerable at this time and appreciate health professionals' recognizing their loss as significant and as a real baby rather than a fetus.

Women not only need physical and emotional support at this time but they also require information to be given clearly, honestly and in a sensitive manner. Evacuations of retained products of conception are often performed at the end of a booked theatre list, as they are not considered a priority compared with other emergency cases, e.g. trauma, and for this reason women may have to wait several hours for surgery. This can further add to their distress, particularly when they have not been allowed to eat or drink and the nursing staff have no idea when the operation will be performed.

Surgical treatment is now only one of three options the woman should be counselled about, so she can make an informed decision. The other options are conservative or medical treatment:

- *Conservative management* – this should only be offered if the woman is not bleeding heavily. Nature is allowed to take its course and a spontaneous miscarriage occurs. A full explanation must be given of what the woman should expect in terms of pain, bleeding and the expected appearance of the products of conception. She must be given contact phone numbers of the hospital in case the bleeding or pain becomes excessive. A scan is arranged for 1 week later to assess for retained products of conception. This is a natural option and offers women the opportunity of being in control of their bodies with an alternative to medical or surgical treatment. However, some women cannot cope with the psychological effects of carrying a dead baby for possibly several weeks; for these women, one of the other alternatives may be more appropriate.

- *Medical management* – this has developed over recent years and has been shown to be extremely effective. The woman is given a combination of the antiprogesterone mifepristone and prostaglandin E, either orally such as misoprostol or vaginally such as gemeprost (RCOG, 2001). The first dose of mifepristone is usually given to the woman while in the early pregnancy assessment unit, and she returns to the ward for completion using misoprostol 36–48 hours later. The woman must be counselled fully about the effects of the treatment, i.e. that she will have some bleeding and may even miscarry at home. Any products passed must be examined closely for fetus, membranes and placental tissue, to ensure there are no retained products. The woman must be able to return to the hospital at any time should she start to miscarry before the second dose. An advantage of this treatment is that the woman does not require a general anaesthetic, but she will have to experience a process during the expulsion of the products similar to labour.

Termination of pregnancy

A similar procedure is also used to perform an early suction termination of pregnancy (STOP) during the first trimester – up to around 12 weeks' gestation (Campbell and Monga, 2000). The cervical canal is dilated to take the aspiration cannula, the size used depending on how far the pregnancy has advanced. The vacuum is switched on and by moving the cannula within the uterine cavity, the products of conception are dislodged and aspirated. A small curette is then used to check the completeness of the evacuation. The pregnant uterus is obviously enlarged and more vascular, so the risks of uterine perforation or need for a re-evacuation if not all the products of conception are removed should be explained fully. These procedures are usually performed as day cases under general anaesthesia, but some hospitals do offer the option of a local anaesthetic, which reduces waiting times.

Terminations in the second trimester – 13–20 weeks' gestation – can be undertaken by administering mifepristone. This drug causes the embryo to detach, uterine muscles to contract and the cervix to dilate, by blocking the effect of progesterone. The care is similar as that for women undergoing medical management of miscarriage.

LAPAROSCOPIC SURGERY

LAPAROSCOPIC ADHESIOLYSIS OR SALPINGOLYSIS

This operation is performed via the laparoscope and consists of dividing the peritubal adhesions around the upper ends of the Fallopian tubes. If the fimbriae are not damaged and the adhesions are not too extensive, the lining epithelium of the Fallopian tubes is likely to be intact and its function may be restored. Campbell and Monga (2000) state that 30–50% of patients could become pregnant up to 6 months following surgery but that ectopic pregnancy occurs in up to 5% of these patients.

LAPAROSCOPIC TREATMENT FOR ENDOMETRIOSIS

Endometriosis is a condition which occurs in women of reproductive age where endometrial tissue (that usually lines the uterus) is found outside the uterus. If it is confined to the myometrium, it is called adenomyosis. Endometriosis may be found on the ovary, broad ligament, bowel and bladder and occasionally has been seen in the lung. In severe endometriosis the ovaries, Fallopian tubes, uterus and bowel are stuck together by dense adhesions.

The range of symptoms and pain experienced by different women vary considerably. During menstruation the endometrial tissue is subject to the same hormonal changes as the uterus. The blood released has no way of escape and is reabsorbed into the bloodstream. The inflammation caused gives rise to scarring and adhesions. The deposits may be seen as tiny black spots or larger cysts know as 'chocolate cysts' from the appearance of altered blood. This condition can be treated by ablating the tissue either by laser therapy or diathermy.

The word 'laser' refers to **l**ight **a**mplification by **s**timulated **e**mission of **r**adiation. The carbon dioxide (CO_2) laser vaporizes tissue so that malignant or unwanted tissue, such as adhesions or endometriosis, may be removed painlessly and completely under the enhanced vision of the laparoscope. The laser has a sealing effect on the blood vessels, and the risk of bleeding is greatly reduced (Sharp and Jordan, 1986). The Nd:YAG laser is an exceptional coagulator which delivers an invisible beam near to the infrared range of the spectrum. New techniques being developed with diathermy are considerably cheaper than the laser.

LAPAROSCOPIC TREATMENT FOR POLYCYSTIC OVARIAN DISEASE

Laser laparoscopy or diathermy may also be used to treat polycystic ovarian disease. This condition occurs when the ovaries are enlarged and contain numerous cystic follicles. The normal production of oestrogen is affected, resulting in absence of periods (amenorrhoea) or irregular periods (oligomenorrhoea). A woman is considered to have polycystic ovarian syndrome when she has other symptoms in addition to the cysts on the ovaries, such as acne, hirsutism, weight gain, pelvic pain and infertility.

Therapeutic laparoscopy replaces the old-fashioned wedge resection which was often followed by spontaneous ovulation. Cauterization and multiple ovarian biopsy have also been used to mimic a wedge resection, but can cause formation of adhesions and haematomas. Using a laser, multiple holes are made in the ovary, causing drainage of the subcapsular cysts, which contain high levels of androstenedione. This will lead to a rise in FSH secretion and ultimately spontaneous ovulation should occur. Armar et al (1990) report a high success rate, with the hormonal abnormalities

being corrected and subsequent ovulation and conception frequently occurring. Where ovulation does not occur spontaneously, women often respond to clomiphene, even where they were resistant to it before surgery. Although the effect is usually temporary, it allows 'a window of opportunity' for women to attempt conception without having to resort to expensive infertility options.

LAPAROSCOPIC STERILIZATION

Female sterilization involves the blocking or excision of the Fallopian tubes, thereby preventing the ovum from meeting the sperm and fertilization taking place. The various methods of blocking the tubes are shown in Figure 18.2.

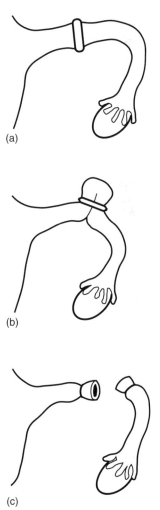

(a)

(b)

(c)

Figure 18.2 Female sterilization techniques: (a) Filshie clip; (b) Fallope ring; (c) tying of ends after the tube has been cut.

In the past it was necessary for women to have a laparotomy (large incision of the abdominal wall). Nowadays, the majority of sterilizations are performed laparoscopically. Occasionally, a mini-laparotomy (8–10 cm scar) may be necessary if access and visualization of the Fallopian tubes is difficult. This may be due to the woman being obese and/or she has had previous pelvic surgery, or she has had infections which have resulted in multiple adhesions. In this instance, a stay in hospital of 1 or 2 days will be recommended and heavy lifting should be avoided for about 3 weeks.

Pregnancy following this operation is rare – 1 in 200 operations (RCOG, 1999) – but if it does occur there is usually a higher risk of an ectopic pregnancy (Campbell and Monga, 2000). The woman must also be warned of the risk during laparoscopy of damage to adjacent organs or vessels, and advice should be given about pelvic and shoulder tip pain that can develop following laparoscopy.

It is not advisable to carry out sterilization at the same time as a termination of pregnancy, because of the vascularity of the tissues involved, or after delivery by caesarean section where the uterus may be large and the tubes high in the abdomen. The woman must consider this operation to be irreversible.

NURSING CARE FOR MINOR GYNAECOLOGICAL AND LAPAROSCOPIC SURGERY

PREOPERATIVE CARE

Preoperative care and information is a vital part of the preparation of a woman to undergo any operation, whether minor or major. This is particularly true of women experiencing a miscarriage or termination. A miscarriage is a problem which occurs suddenly. The woman is admitted to hospital quickly, without time to make plans for the care of any other children. It is important to consider the feelings of both partners and ensure family members have a direct telephone number to the ward.

Most minor gynaecological procedures are carried out as a day case, although increasingly procedures are being undertaken in the outpatient setting. The nurse must ensure the woman feels relaxed and not part of a conveyor belt, by appearing unhurried and focused on the woman. Every woman is entitled to her own Named Nurse in accordance with the RCN's 'Standards of Care. Gynaecological Nursing' (1991).

POSTOPERATIVE CARE

Women usually recover very quickly from minor investigations and operations. Providing their observations are stable and vaginal bleeding is not heavy, they may be escorted to the lavatory to pass urine. Once they have tolerated fluids and a light diet, they may go home, usually a minimum of 4 hours after their anaesthetic.

It is important that a partner or friend collects the woman following day surgery, and a written information leaflet containing discharge advice and a contact telephone number should be given to her.

Discharge advice

- It is common to have some bleeding after the procedure, which may be bright red at first and should gradually decrease to a brownish stain.
- If the bleeding becomes heavier than a normal period, offensive smelling or there is a raised temperature, then the ward should be contacted, since these are indications of an infection.
- The woman should be accompanied home and overnight in case of complications developing.
- Sanitary towels rather than tampons should be used to reduce the risk of infection.
- Mild painkillers such as paracetamol or ibuprofen may be used to help any pain.
- It is advisable for the woman to take a few days off work and resume a normal lifestyle and work when she feels ready.

Specific advice following an evacuation of retained products of conception or a suction termination of pregnancy

The advice for women following these two procedures is similar to that for a dilatation and curettage. Breast tenderness may be a problem, especially if the miscarriage or termination occurred later in the pregnancy. Women should be warned about this since it can be a distressing symptom. A well-supporting bra will help reduce discomfort, but it is not usually necessary to take any medication.

Contraceptive advice

- Following a termination, it is crucial that women are offered comprehensive contraceptive advice. They may begin taking the oral contraceptive pill the evening of the operation or the following morning. They can return to their GP 6 weeks after the operation for a general check-up and further contraceptive prescriptions.

- A follow-up appointment is not usually offered unless the woman has had three consecutive miscarriages, or has a miscarriage in the second trimester of pregnancy.

- The Miscarriage Association and SAFTA (Support after Termination for Abnormality) have a useful range of booklets.

- Some hospitals have their own Miscarriage Group run by the hospital bereavement counsellor, and many have an annual remembrance service for all the babies that have died before or at birth in the previous year.

In Tables 18.1–18.3 a care plan details Roper's Activities of Living for Jean, a 30-year-old woman who has lost her baby through a miscarriage and is to undergo an evacuation of retained products of conception. Jean was 10 weeks pregnant and had recently had her first scan. Last night she began to have mild backache and found she was bleeding from her vagina. Her 5-year-old son David had accompanied her when she had her first scan.

Table 18.1 Assessment of patient who is to undergo an evacuation of retained products of conception, using the Roper, Logan and Tierney model of nursing

Activity of living	Assessment baseline
Maintaining a safe environment	Baseline observations: – Pulse 84 bpm – Respiration 18 rpm – Blood pressure 100/60 mmHg – Weight 64 kg Blood loss per vagina: moderate to heavy No known allergies
Communication	Would like to be known as Jean Very anxious and tearful at present
Breathing	Tendency to hyperventilate when anxious Non-smoker
Eating and drinking	Vegetarian diet
Elimination	Bowels: BO twice daily but tendency to constipation during pregnancy Haemorrhoids during last pregnancy Bladder: – Urinary frequency – Urinalysis NAD
Personal cleansing and dressing	Daily shower
Controlling body temperature	Temperature 37°C
Mobilizing	Fully mobile Plays badminton twice a week Not at risk of pressure ulcer since Jean can move around the bed
Working and playing	Full-time solicitor Nanny employed to look after son Enjoys patchwork making and reading
Expressing sexuality	Married with one son aged 5 Husband accompanied Jean on admission LMP 16.3.03 K–4–5/28–30 Contraception: condom G3, P1 Baby Christopher died aged 2 days in October 2001 Last smear October 1991 Checks breasts when she remembers
Sleeping	Usually 6–7 hours/night

Table 18.2 Preoperative care plan for patient undergoing an evacuation of retained products of conception

Activity of living	Problem	Aim	Nursing care	Rationale	Evaluation
Communicating	Anxiety due to hospitalization	To ensure Jean is as calm and relaxed as is possible	1. Jean has one nurse to look after her as far as possible 2. Approach Jean in a calm friendly manner 3. Explain all nursing care and procedures to Jean 4. Allow Jean to ask questions 5. Encourage Jean to verbalize her anxieties	The woman with a gynaecological condition is able to establish a meaningful relationship with her nurse (Coults, 1985).	Jean is very tearful and particularly worried about her 5 year old son, David. The hospital is reminding her of Christopher's death and all that it entailed
	Pain due to uterine contractions	To ensure Jean is pain free, or feels in control of any pain she may experience	1. Offer analgesics as prescribed 2. Observe for effectiveness 20–30 minutes later 3. Check for non-verbal signs of pain 4. Position comfortably in bed 5. Offer use of heat pad 6. Encourage Jean to tell nurse of any pain she has	It can be very soothing	Jean has refused analgesics. She wants to 'suffer pain for her baby as it has suffered'. Jean states her pain is not unbearable
Maintaining a safe environment	Bleeding due to miscarriage	To detect excessive blood loss	1. Observe Jean's vaginal loss $\frac{1}{2}$ hourly 2. If very heavy (>1 sanitary towel/$\frac{1}{2}$ h), save pads and any tissue passed for doctor 3. Administer ergometrine if prescribed	To monitor uterine haemorrhage	Jean's blood loss is moderate to heavy
	Lack of preparation for theatre	Jean is adequately prepared for theatre	1. Record vital signs, pulse, temperature, respirations, blood pressure 2. Ensure Jean has removed all her make-up and nail varnish 3. Ensure Jean has removed all her jewellery except her wedding ring 4. Check that consent form has been signed	To establish a baseline for postoperative observation Make-up obscures cyanosis, and nail beds are used to ensure adequate tissue perfusion To prevent diathermy burns from static electricity Legal requirement	Pulse 84 bpm Temp 37°C Respiration 18 rpm B/P 100/60 mmHg
Eating and drinking	Lack of preparation for theatre	Jean is fasted for 4–6 hours before surgery	1. Explain to Jean why she cannot eat or drink 2. Place 'nil by mouth' sign above bed 3. Offer mouth washes	To ensure stomach is empty and gastric contents cannot be aspirated into lung	Jean last drank coffee at 8 a.m. this morning
Elimination		To reduce injury or infection of bladder	Ensure Jean has emptied her bladder an hour before surgery	A full bladder may be damaged during procedures	Jean has passed urine before leaving ward
Personal cleansing and dressing		Jean is wearing a theatre gown	Give Jean a clean theatre gown to wear, with no underwear underneath	To reduce risks of postoperative sepsis	Jean has a gown which she will put on shortly before theatre: prefers to keep her nightshirt on at present

Table 18.3   Postoperative care plan for patient after evacuation of retained products of conception

Activity of living	Problem	Aim	Nursing care	Rationale	Evaluation
Maintaining a safe environment	Potential problem of haemorrhage postoperatively	To detect excessive haemorrhage	1. Record vital signs: $\frac{1}{2}$ hourly for 2 h, 1 hourly for 2 h, and then 4 hourly 2. Observe Jean's PV loss $\frac{1}{2}$ hourly. 3. Inform doctor if excessive	To detect signs of hidden blood loss by use of pulse and blood pressure To detect uterine haemorrhage (remember blood pools in vagina while supine)	Pulse 75 bpm: blood pressure stable at 100/60 mmHg Blood loss moderate
	Potential problem of rhesus incompatibility	To protect Jean's future pregnancies	1. Check Jean's rhesus factor 2. Administer anti-D gamma globulin if necessary 3. Explain the reasons for this to Jean and her husband	Haemolytic disease of the new born may develop in the next pregnancy if mother is rhesus negative, and baby that was miscarried was rhesus positive	Jean is rhesus positive
Communication	Pain baseline: Jean is awake able to communicate her needs	To ensure Jean is pain free	1. Offer analgesics as prescribed 2. Observe for effectiveness 20–30 minutes later 3. Check for non-verbal signs of pain 4. Position comfortably in bed 5. Encourage Jean to tell nurse of any pain she has	'Communication is not an optional extra in a feature of the role of the nurse' (Friend, 1981)	Jean is given two Co-dydramol with good effect
Eating and drinking	Inadequate hydration baseline: Jean states she is 'starving'	For Jean to be adequately hydrated and nutritional needs met	1. Offer Jean water, followed by tea and toast/biscuits and resume normal diet as tolerated 2. Order Jean supper if she feels like it	Minor gynaecological patients do not need to be kept nil by mouth following surgery, as long as they do not feel nauseated	Jean enjoyed a cup of tea and some biscuits
Elimination	Potential problem of retention of urine	To promote normal micturition	1. Encourage Jean to pass urine as soon as possible 2. Walk Jean to the bathroom if not feeling faint 3. Undertake bladder scan if not passed urine within 6 hours 4. Pass residual catheter if required 5. Encourage Jean to continue with fluids and mobilize up to toilet	To detect any damage to bladder/ureters and prevent infection caused by urinary stasis To check volume of urine in bladder To empty bladder initially	Jean is unable to pass urine at first attempt, but is reassured that this is normal Passes urine later in evening
Personal cleansing	Jean needs assistance at the moment	To resume normal cleansing and	1. Offer Jean a bowl of water and towel to freshen up	Theatre gowns cause patients to lose their identity	Jean will change into her nightshirt later when she is not so drowsy

(Continued)

Table 18.3 (Continued)

Activity of living	Problem	Aim	Nursing care	Rationale	Evaluation
		dressing activities	2. Change soiled gown if necessary 3. Change sanitary towels as required 4. Offer assistance with mouth wash or cleaning teeth		
Mobility	Reduced mobility	To promote return to mobility following surgery	1. Offer to walk Jean to bathroom when she is ready 2. Ensure adequate pain control	To prevent all complications of bedrest	Jean walks to bathroom, although she feels quite dizzy. She is still anxious to return home
Expressing sexuality	Jean is very upset	To allow Jean to feel able to communicate her innermost feelings to her nurse	1. Spend time talking with Jean about her ability as a mother following death of a second baby. Christopher's death is still fresh in her mind 2. Provide privacy and confidentiality	To provide a non-judgmental acceptance of her sexual attitudes (Shapiro, 1984) using communication skills: active listening, silences, reflection	Jean showed some photographs of Christopher and talked about his short life
Working and playing	Lack of discharge advice	For Jean and her husband to feel confident on discharge	1. Spend time talking with Jean and Michael about the miscarriage, physical and psychological factors 2. Offer miscarriage leaflet and read through it with them, pointing out Miscarriage Association and telephone number of nurse counsellor at the hospital	Every woman should have access to information which will enable her to maintain a healthy lifestyle	Jean is worried about returning to work, as she has not told her colleagues that she is pregnant and 'wants to put it all behind her now'. She is also worried about telling her son David

MARSUPIALIZATION OF A BARTHOLIN'S ABSCESS

The Bartholin's glands, which lubricate the vulva, lie behind the vestibule with a duct which opens at the vaginal introitus. They are susceptible to infection by sexually transmitted diseases and also general micro-organisms such as staphylococci and *Escherichia coli*. If the duct becomes blocked, the mucous secretions which lubricate the original opening during intercourse are unable to drain and a cyst forms. The cyst may resolve or it may become infected, resulting in a painful Bartholin's abscess, which is often initially noticed during sexual intercourse.

The abscess can be extremely painful and appear hot, red and swollen. The woman may have difficulty in walking, be unable to sit down and is reluctant to pass urine. It is preferable not to excise the gland, because it provides lubrication for sexual intercourse. Instead, marsupialization is performed, from the Greek 'marsipos' meaning bag. The abscess is opened to facilitate drainage and the walls of the abscess are sutured to the surrounding skin to leave a large orifice to facilitate drainage of the pus (Fig. 18.3).

A new duct forms as healing occurs. During the operation a swab will be taken for microscopy, culture and sensitivity, and antibiotics may be prescribed. The cavity is loosely filled with ribbon gauze impregnated with a solution such as glycerine or proflavine. This is to keep the skin edges apart so that healing can occur by granulation. If the skin edges heal together before this happens, a sinus can be left under the skin which may harbour recurrent infections.

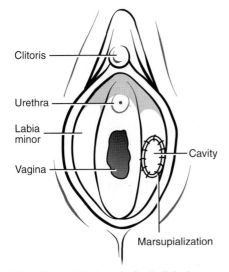

Figure 18.3   Marsupialization of a Bartholin's abscess.

Labels: Clitoris, Urethra, Labia minor, Vagina, Cavity, Marsupialization

Postoperative care

This operation is often performed as an emergency, and women usually go home 24 hours later, once they have passed urine. The vaginal pack will be removed either by the nurse or by the woman herself. This can be helped by sitting in a warm bath. The area should be kept clean and a hair dryer can be used instead of a towel for drying the area. Antibiotics are not given routinely unless infection is proven. It is probably advisable not to have sexual intercourse for 2 weeks following the operation, so as to avoid reinfection and to allow the area to heal.

MYOMECTOMY

A myomectomy is a major operation to remove fibroids from the uterus. A fibroid (also known as a myoma or leiomyoma) begins as a single cell in the endometrium of the uterus, which multiplies to become a mass of muscle and fibrous connective tissue. Most fibroids are no larger than a pea, but they can grow to the size of a grapefruit. Fibroids seem to occur more frequently in West Indian and West African women, although the reason for this is not clear (Campbell and Monga, 2000).

It is not entirely clear why fibroids develop, but they are dependent on oestrogen. Before a myomectomy, the woman may be prescribed Zoladex (goserelin) to suppress the release of oestrogen and cause the fibroids to shrink (Campbell and Monga, 2000).

REASONS FOR MYOMECTOMY

Small fibroids are asymptomatic and treatment is not required. However, where diagnosis of the pelvic mass is in doubt, where the mass is larger than the size of a 16-week pregnancy, or where there are unpleasant symptoms or causing infertility, surgery is required.

Menorrhagia (heavy periods) is a common problem caused by the larger area of endometrium that is shed at menstruation. Large fibroids may press on the bowel, causing constipation, or on the bladder, causing urinary frequency or retention.

A myomectomy involves the 'shelling out' of the fibroids and is preferable for women who still want children. If no further pregnancies are desired, then a hysterectomy may be the operation of choice.

During myomectomy, there is a risk of haemorrhage from the incision of the uterine muscle. Women should always be aware of the risk that, if bleeding cannot be controlled, a hysterectomy will be performed.

The woman may require a blood transfusion, and therefore this operation is not always suitable for women who do not accept blood products, e.g. Jehovah's Witnesses.

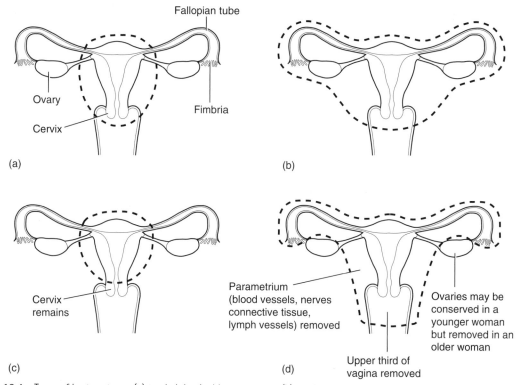

Figure 18.4   Types of hysterectomy: (a) total abdominal hysterectomy; (b) total abdominal hysterectomy and bilateral salpingo-oophorectomy; (c) subtotal hysterectomy; (d) Wertheim's hysterectomy.

The woman will often stay in hospital for 5–7 days, depending on the healing of the wound. Since the development of new techniques in microsurgery, it has been possible to remove certain fibroids either via a hysteroscope or a laparoscope. Since this is minimally invasive surgery, women are able to return to an active life 7–10 days following surgery, and have no scar. This kind of procedure is also advantageous because, following laparotomy, any suture lines may weaken the wall of the uterus and may necessitate a caesarean section at subsequent births.

Some women who have had a myomectomy due to multiple fibroids may have had a 'full feeling' during intercourse. She and her partner may now experience an 'empty sensation' once the fibroids are removed. If a woman wishes to become pregnant following myomectomy, many gynaecologists recommend that she tries to conceive in the first 3–6 months following surgery before the fibroids grow again.

POSTOPERATIVE ADVICE FOLLOWING LAPAROSCOPIC REMOVAL OF FIBROIDS

This operation is usually performed as a day case, so the woman should make sure someone is available to take her home. Advice should be given about risks of damage to adjacent organs and how to treat the pelvic or shoulder tip pain that can occur following any laparoscopy. It normally takes a woman a few days to recover fully from a laparoscopy, and she should resume normal activities and work when she feels ready.

HYSTERECTOMY

Despite a slight decline in numbers in recent years in the United Kingdom (DOH, 2004), hysterectomy is still the most frequently performed major gynaecological operation (Skea et al, 2004). There are various types of hysterectomy (Fig. 18.4), and the type of hysterectomy suggested will depend on the reason for the operation (Box 18.2).

TOTAL ABDOMINAL HYSTERECTOMY

This operation involves the removal of the uterus and cervix through a horizontal cut in the abdomen just above the pubic bone, i.e. Pfannenstiel or 'bikini-line' incision. Some women may require a vertical incision where there is a large abdominal swelling or a previous scar.

Box 18.2   Reasons for hysterectomy

- painful or irregular periods or episodes of unexplained vaginal bleeding
- fibroids, which can cause pain, heavy bleeding and occasionally pressure on other pelvic organs, e.g. the bladder
- uterine prolapse, which may interfere with bladder and bowel function
- chronic pelvic pain caused by pelvic infection
- gynaecological cancers of the vagina, cervix, endometrium, Fallopian tubes or ovaries
- occasionally a hysterectomy is performed in an emergency, e.g. in instances of postpartum haemorrhage or following a gynaecological procedure where haemostasis cannot be maintained

---

Table 18.4   International classification of endometrial carcinoma

Stage/grade	Classification
Stage I	Carcinoma is confined to the corpus
Stage II	The carcinoma has involved the corpus and the cervix but has not extended outside the uterus
Stage III	The carcinoma has extended outside the uterus, but not outside the true pelvis
Stage IV	The carcinoma has extended outside the true pelvis or has obviously involved the mucosa of the bladder or the rectum

Source: taken from Campbell and Monga (2000).

BILATERAL SALPINGO-OOPHORECTOMY

Bilateral salpingo-oophorectomy refers to the removal of both Fallopian tubes and ovaries and is often performed at the same time as a total abdominal hysterectomy, particularly where there is evidence of disease, or if the woman is approaching the menopause, or is already postmenopausal. Oophorectomy obviously prevents ovarian cancer from occurring in the future. For premenopausal women, an attempt is made to conserve the ovaries if they are healthy, so as to avoid a sudden decrease in oestrogen, which could cause severe menopausal symptoms. It has been shown, however, that if the ovaries are conserved, they may have a decreased hormonal function in premenopausal women, possibly because their blood supply may be compromised during surgery. Siddle et al (1987) found that hysterectomy alone, i.e. with conservation of one or both ovaries, has also been shown to bring forward the age of menopause in some women.

SUBTOTAL HYSTERECTOMY

In this procedure the uterus is removed but the cervix is left in situ. Cervical smears are still needed annually to screen for cervical cancer.

RADICAL/WERTHEIM'S HYSTERECTOMY

This operation is an extended hysterectomy where the uterus, ovaries, Fallopian tubes, adjacent pelvic tissue, lymph ducts and the upper third of the vagina are removed. This is necessary in cases of advanced cervical and endometrial cancer. In 1900, Thomas Cullen

of The Johns Hopkins Hospital, Baltimore recommended abdominal hysterectomy with the removal of adnexae as the best treatment for endometrial cancer. Table 18.4 illustrates the stages of endometrial cancer.

Today, total abdominal hysterectomy and bilateral salpingo-oophorectomy is still the treatment of choice for women with low-risk Stage I disease. High-risk Stage I and Stage II cases may also be treated with adjunctant radiation therapy. For Stage III disease a total abdominal hysterectomy, salpingo-oophorectomy and debulking of any pelvic disease is undertaken followed by pelvic irradiation. Stage IV is extremely rare, as women usually present with early symptoms such as postmenopausal bleeding. However, where it is diagnosed, treatment is individualized. Surgery is not usually the first line of treatment (Campbell and Monga, 2000) but usually will include radiotherapy for palliative control and chemotherapy for control of metastatic disease (Martin-Hirsch and Reynolds, 2001). Surgical intervention may then follow.

A radical or Wertheim's hysterectomy is usually carried out for cervical cancer. This kind of surgical treatment is suitable for fit patients with small Stage I, grade 2 tumours and a few patients with disease that involves the cervix and the body of the uterus. Table 18.5 illustrates the International Federation of Gynaecology and Obstetrics (FIGO) classification for staging of cancer of the cervix.

Surgical treatment for women who are diagnosed as having ovarian cancer will depend on the extent of the disease. Unfortunately, because there is an insidious onset of this disease, many women present in advanced stages. Chemotherapy may be the treatment of choice if the disease is too far advanced for surgical treatment. However, if surgery is indicated, laparotomy is performed with a total abdominal hysterectomy, bilateral salpingo-oophorectomy and excision of

Table 18.5   FIGO (International Federation of Gynaecology and Obstetrics) classification of cancer of the cervix

Stage/grade	Classification
0	Pre-invasive disease
I	Cancer confined to cervix
II	Involvement of vagina except the lower third or infiltration of the parametrium. No involvement of side wall
III	Involvement of the lower third of vagina with extension to pelvic side wall
IV	Extension of cancer beyond the reproductive tract

Source: taken from Campbell and Monga (2000).

pelvic lymph nodes. Due to the relatively high morbidity of this disease, oncology nurse specialists are paramount in providing both patients and family with support, and Jefferies (2002) demonstrated the positive impact nurses can have at this time.

VAGINAL HYSTERECTOMY

This operation involves the removal of the uterus through the vagina, leaving no apparent scar. A vaginal hysterectomy is usually performed where there is prolapse of the uterus. Contraindications to vaginal hysterectomy include a bulky uterus (larger in size than a 14-week uterus) and suspected or known malignancy. One of the most recent developments in gynaecological surgery is that of laparoscopic-assisted vaginal hysterectomy, including removal of the ovaries. This procedure is not designed to replace either abdominal or vaginal hysterectomy, but it offers a less-invasive option to women facing abdominal hysterectomy and oophorectomy. The operation can take longer than conventional hysterectomy but the hospital stay is reduced to 2 days. There is little postoperative pain, intraoperative blood loss is reduced significantly and low small incisions replace a large abdominal wound.

PSYCHOLOGICAL ASPECTS OF HYSTERECTOMY

All major surgery has implications for an altered body image, but the removal of a uterus can alter a woman's self-image, her perceived femininity and have a profound effect on her feelings of sexuality. The inability to reproduce, even if the woman did not want to, can mark a major life event. To many women, the suggestion of

having a hysterectomy provokes fear and horror on account of the misconceptions and old wives' tales surrounding this particular operation. The Ancient Greeks believed the uterus (hystero) to be the source of all emotions; hence, the words 'hysteria' and 'hysterectomy'.

The role of the nurse is of utmost importance, to uncover anxieties and fears, to correct any myths and misconceptions, and to give clear, accurate advice. Unfortunately, instead of the detailed information women require, they are often only given brief hints about 'not lifting', and important concerns such as when to resume sexual activity are neglected. Webb (1985), in her study of gynaecology nurses, found that although nurses did talk to their patients and were aware that hysterectomy patients feared 'losing their womanhood', they interpreted this as referring only to patients' sex lives and not to the wider aspects of sexuality, self-concept and self-esteem.

Some women do not realize that they will no longer have periods following a hysterectomy, and others who have suffered from premenstrual syndrome may mistakenly think that the hysterectomy will cure this problem. However, if the ovaries have been conserved, cyclical symptoms will persist, leading to ovarian cycle syndrome as described by Backstrom et al (1981).

NURSING CARE FOR MAJOR GYNAECOLOGICAL SURGERY

PREOPERATIVE CARE

The importance of preoperative care for minor gynaecological cases has already been discussed earlier in the chapter. Obviously, when a more serious operation is taking place it is even more vital that the woman and her family feel adequately prepared. It is in these instances that a preadmission clinic can help allay some of her fears, as she will have had ward procedures explained to her prior to her admission. Some hospitals also organize preadmission hysterectomy groups where women can discuss their concerns with health professionals and other women before admission.

It is a good idea to introduce new patients to one another, particularly if they are having the same operation. Wilson-Barnett (1978) found that patients derive considerable support from one another. It may also be beneficial for a woman who is very scared to meet with a woman who is recovering from a similar operation, providing all went well!

A full admission assessment should be undertaken (see p. 375), and the nurse should explain exactly what will happen. It is also necessary to prepare the woman physically for surgery. She may be given two glycerin suppositories or a small enema to ensure the bowel is empty prior to the operation. A pubic shave may be required, performed by either the woman herself or the nurse, as it allows the surgeon a more accurate view.

There is a risk of deep vein thrombosis following major abdominal and pelvic surgery (RCOG, 1995), so women are measured and fitted for anti-embolism stockings and may be given prophylactic heparin.

Patients undergoing major gynaecological surgery are starved prior to surgery to prevent gastric aspiration. ASA (1999) guidelines recommend a minimum of 6 hours for food and 2 hours for clear fluids. On the morning of the operation, the patient will be advised to have a bath or shower. Some women prefer to have a premedication to help them relax before going to theatre. The anaesthetist will discuss this with the woman if she requests one when they assess the woman for anaesthesia. All patients should be advised to give up smoking for at least 48 hours before surgery.

All women will be required to sign a consent form for the operation after the benefits, and serious and frequently occurring risks have been fully explained to her. These should have been explained fully to her during her original outpatient consultation and at preoperative assessment, to ensure that gaining her consent has been a process and not just signing a form (DOH, 2001).

In teaching hospitals, medical students are likely to be present at all stages of her care pathway. Some women find it intimidating to discuss their personal symptoms in front of an audience, and the nurse must act as the woman's advocate. All women have the right to refuse to participate in the teaching of undergraduates, and if this is the case her wishes should be respected. At some hospitals women may sign a consent form for medical students to perform vaginal examinations while they are in theatre under general anaesthesia. The woman may request a female doctor to examine her and this should be supported where possible. A male doctor should always be chaperoned and it is now recommended that all clinicians, regardless of their gender, should be chaperoned (RCOG, 2002).

See Table 18.6 for a detailed preoperative care plan for a patient undergoing major gynaecological surgery.

POSTOPERATIVE CARE

A detailed postoperative care plan is shown in Table 18.7. Major gynaecological surgery such as hysterectomy, myomectomy or vaginal repair can take from 45 minutes to an hour depending on the specific operation. Oxygen therapy will be required following the general anaesthetic, and this will be continued from recovery onto the ward.

The patient will have an intravenous infusion in progress, which will stay in situ for 24–48 hours, and occasionally a blood transfusion may be required, depending on the estimated blood loss during the operation. A urinary (Foley's) catheter will keep the bladder empty, and a Redivac drain will protrude from a point near one end of the incision site. This drain has a vacuum and drains off excess blood from the operation site to prevent formation of a haematoma. Unless there is particularly heavy oozing from the wound, a light dry dressing will be sufficient covering for the wound for 48 hours. Following a myomectomy, there is an increased risk of the formation of a haematoma, and also adhesions may develop later between the intestines and the suture lines on the uterus. Careful monitoring of temperature is required to detect a haematoma.

Women who have had a vaginal hysterectomy and/or a vaginal repair will have a 'vaginal pack' (a length of ribbon gauze soaked in glycerin) in situ, which is inserted into the vagina rather like a large tampon. This exerts pressure and stops any bleeding from suture points. It may be removed after 24 hours, and this is most comfortably done while the woman sits in a warm bath.

In some cases of vaginal hysterectomy and repair, a suprapubic catheter is inserted via the abdomen, since it is thought to reduce the risk of postoperative urinary tract infections. The other advantage of suprapubic catheters is that they may be clamped temporarily and a system of bladder retraining commenced (Cardozo, 1993).

Strong analgesics will be required for the first 24 hours and morphine sulphate is often administered via an intramuscular injection, or by patient-controlled analgesia (PCA) where the patient can administer the amount required themselves, via a pump. In some units, epidurals are available. Diclofenac sodium suppositories are frequently used for their anti-inflammatory and excellent analgesic properties. Prochlorperazine or metoclopramide may be given for nausea. In addition, acupressure can help and this can be applied to the inner aspect of the wrists using Seabands.

On the day following major surgery the woman will be encouraged to sit out of bed for a short while and a physiotherapist may visit to encourage leg exercises, pelvic rocking, i.e. moving hips from side to side, and deep breathing. These will help prevent common postoperative problems such as deep vein thrombosis and chest infections.

When bowel sounds resume, the woman can start sipping water and gradually progress to a light diet. Her intravenous infusion will be discontinued, in addition to the removal of her urinary catheter. A strict fluid balance chart should be maintained. Some women

Table 18.6 Preoperative care plan for patient undergoing major gynaecological surgery

Universal self-care requisites	Problem	Aim	Patient activity	Nursing activity
Promote normality	Anxiety related to hospital admission	Alleviate anxiety associated with admission and unfamiliar surroundings and people	Patient to familiarize herself with staff, fellow patients and ward layout	Welcome patient to ward. Introduce to staff and identify named nurse to patient
	Unfamiliar surroundings and disturbance in usual life activities	To give adequate information regarding treatment stay and discharge	Patient is able to ask questions and express anxieties and fears	Explain ward layout and toilets, bathrooms and day room. Give patient necessary information about activities, e.g. visiting times, meal times, ward telephone number, etc. Give appropriate explanation of intended treatment and surgery (using information aids if appropriate). Answer questions posed by patient. If unable to, refer to appropriate member of multidisciplinary team
				Be sensitive to patient's anxieties and fears, which may be expressed in speech or in non-verbal behaviour
				React sensitively to these fears and anxieties
				Discuss any family/social problems arising from admission
Prevention of hazards to life, well-being and functioning	Unprepared for surgery	Safe preparation for theatre	Patient understands rationale for fasting. Patient assists in preoperative skin preparation	Full preoperative nursing assessment: measurement of temperature, pulse, respiration and weight and urinalysis. Check consent form is signed and premedication given if required
			Patient has bath/shower Patient assists in bowel preparation procedure Patient empties bladder prior to premedication	Attach ID band Record results of preoperative investigations: – Full blood count – Sickle cell trait – Urea and electrolytes – ECG if required Check shave Ensure bowels have been opened prior to surgery or give suppositories/enema if needed
			Patient wears operating gown and antiembolic stockings	Patient measured for antiembolic stockings Fast patient for 6 hours Escort to theatre

Source: adapted and published with permission from Lisa Stewart.

Table 18.7 Postoperative care plan for a patient following major gynaecological surgery

Universal self-care requisites	Problem	Aim	Patient activity	Nursing activity
Maintain sufficient intake of oxygen	At risk of respiratory insufficiency/infection	Clear airway Independent ventilation	Understands reason for actively performing breathing exercises 4 hourly postoperatively Understands reason for adequate pain relief in order to perform breathing exercises Participates in physiotherapy exercises Understands and uses PCA appropriately	Safe administration of oxygen as per anaesthetist's instructions Observe and record respiratory rate, depth and patient colour Reinforce breathing exercises Offer and assist with mouthcare Monitor patient's pain and administer analgesics as prescribed Observe for side-effects such as respiratory depression
Prevention of hazards of life, well-being and functioning	At risk of postoperative complications	Maintain patient safety: – haemorrhage – hypovolaemia – infection – pain – hygiene		Record pulse, blood pressure, patient's colour, level of consciousness according to individual assessment Observe and record Redivac drainage Report any anomalies to senior nursing and medical staff Record temperature Administer antibiotic therapy Remove dressing around 2nd day after operation Remove sutures according to assessment and instructions Assess level of pain Monitor and administer prescribed analgesics Assist patient to find comfortable position Assist with hygiene needs Maintain patient dignity
Maintain sufficient intake of fluids	Fluid intake affected due to surgery	Adequate hydration and electrolyte balance	Understands reason for IV hydration until bowel sounds return If able, assists in completion of fluid balance chart	Maintain IVI as per prescription Explain rationale for IV hydration to patient Instruct patient to complete fluid chart Check IV patency and cannulation site for signs of infection

(Continued)

Table 18.7 (Continued)

Universal self-care requisites	Problem	Aim	Patient activity	Nursing activity
			Able to drink fluids independently once IV has been discontinued	Offer and assist with mouthcare Monitor patient's record of fluid balance Provide vomit bowls and tissues
Maintain sufficient intake of food	Enforced fasting and temporary anorexia	Balanced diet Adequate calories	Understands reason for being nil by mouth	Keep patient nil by mouth until bowel sounds re-established Observe for signs of paralytic ileus Introduce fluids slowly
			Understands rationale for slow reintroduction of solids once bowel sounds have returned	Offer a light diet progressing to normal diet
			Able to participate in menu choice	Involve dietitian in patient care
			Encourage relatives or friends to bring in own choice of foods	
Care associated with elimination	At risk of urinary retention or incomplete voiding	Passes urine normally once catheter is removed	Understands reason for catheter	Close observation of urinary output and catheter patency
			Understands how to care for and empty: 1. urethral catheter 2. suprapubic catheter, which is used following a bladder repair operation or occasionally a vaginal repair.	Report decrease in urinary output to nursing and medical staff Empty catheter 6 hourly Ensure patient passes urine normally once catheter is removed.
			Is able to assist in completion of fluid chart	Ensure nursing staff complete accurate fluid balance chart
	At risk of constipation	Normal bowel action	Understands rationale to prevent constipation – increased fibre – adequate fluids	Monitor patient's bowel action Instruct patient on how to complete fluid chart
			– to request aperients – increased mobility	Administer aperients prn Advise on measures for avoiding constipation
Maintain balance between activity and rest	Enforced rest and limitation on activity due to surgery and associated fatigue following surgery	For patient to appreciate temporary limitations on activity due to surgery	Understands reason for temporary fatigue	Explain and reinforce limitations on patient
			Understands that usual activities involving abdominal muscles will be altered:	Ensure patient has leaflet and/or advice following major surgery

		To identify discharge facilities and home support	– driving – working – cleaning/lifting – sexual intercourse Patient identifies relative or friend to assist in recuperative period at home Engages in active exercises Patient understands limitations on independence during convalescence and makes appropriate plans for help after discharge	Explore with patient family facilities following discharge Encourage balance between adequate mobilization and adequate rest Encourage patient participation in postoperative exercises Confirm home circumstances following discharge Inform community/social services to implement discharge plan if required
Maintain balance between solitude and social interaction	Alteration in usual communication patterns and privacy	To maintain patient social interaction To express feelings to nursing staff or friend or relative To respect patient privacy and solitude To encourage social activities to limit boredom and seclusion	Patient appreciates alteration in usual patient sociability Involve relative or friend in communication, if appropriate Patient understands rationale for limiting visitors in order to prevent tiring patient	Assist in introduction of fellow patients Allow time for patient to express her feelings (worries, fears, concerns, etc.) To ensure that patient visiting is promoted yet numbers kept within manageable limits
Promote normality	Potential alteration in body image Loss of body part may lead to grieving Temporary physical constraints on sexual functioning related to healing tissues and vaginal discharge Freedom to express spiritual beliefs	Patient feels comfortable' with body image, sexual functioning and spirituality	Patient understands temporary limitations on sexual functioning	Provide the opportunity to express feelings/concerns about temporary restriction in sexual functioning Explore alternative ways of expressing affection if appropriate Involve partner if appropriate Respect patient's spiritual needs

Source: adapted and published with permission from Lisa Stewart.

do contract a urinary tract infection following hysterectomy, and this will be treated with antibiotics. It is important that women empty their bladder fully and squeeze out the last few drops, as this prevents urine being retained in the bladder.

By the second day following surgery, women are usually able to walk to the bathroom and have a shower without too much discomfort. Oral analgesics are now given in conjunction with an anti-inflammatory suppository to control the pain.

Women may worry about 'bursting their stitches' and need reassurance that there are several layers of stitches. They may find it helpful to hold their hand across their abdomen (or hold the sanitary towel in place if they have had a vaginal hysterectomy) when they cough. The sutures or staples are usually removed, without discomfort, on the 4–5th day for a horizontal wound, and on the 7–10th day for a vertical incision. Any vaginal sutures will dissolve or occasionally fall out. Sometimes a tight one may have to be cut, if the wound feels as if it is pulling.

Many women experience griping 'wind' pain after abdominal surgery, which can cause considerable discomfort. Hot peppermint water sipped slowly may help, and some doctors prescribe enteric-coated peppermint oil capsules (Colpermin). Walking around and sitting in a warm bath may also help.

Constipation can be a problem and regular lactulose syrup, Fybogel or Senokot may be prescribed. Glycerin suppositories can be given if the bowels have not been opened by the 3rd day.

It is very common for women to feel 'blue' on the 3rd or 4th day following surgery, and many women find themselves in tears for no apparent reason. They should be reassured that this is a normal reaction and will pass, although some women do experience similar feelings again on leaving hospital. For women who have had a hysterectomy and/or bilateral salpingo-oophorectomy and those who are perimenopausal, hormone replacement therapy will help, but there may be deeper reasons for this feeling of depression.

DISCHARGE ADVICE FOLLOWING MAJOR SURGERY

Women normally stay in hospital for 4–7 days following major gynaecological surgery, and they should be encouraged to go home when they feel ready to do so. Some hospitals have now introduced community gynaecology nurses who visit women at home, providing specialist care. This means that women can be discharged as early as the 3rd day following surgery, which in turn frees hospital beds and reduces waiting lists.

Whatever the situation, it is crucial that the woman, her partner and the rest of her family are aware of what she can and cannot do while she is recovering at home. This should be supported with specific written information, and with an assurance that she can ring the ward for advice at any time. She should also be given the details of any local relevant support networks, e.g. the Hysterectomy Support Group or National Endometriosis Society (see Resources section).

The following issues should be discussed with the woman, her partner and family if appropriate.

Bleeding

There may be a vaginal discharge for up to 4 weeks, which will turn from red to a pale brown colour. If it becomes heavier, brighter in colour, or offensive smelling, medical advice should be sought. Occasional red spotting may occur when the sutures fall out. Sanitary towels rather than tampons should be used, in order to prevent infection for as long as required. If the woman has not had a hysterectomy, this may be until after the next period.

Resting

It is important that the woman should rest sufficiently during the first 2 weeks, and go to bed for a rest when she feels tired. It is common to feel tired for several weeks after discharge. Some women may need iron tablets following surgery if their haemoglobin level is low.

Exercise

Exercise is important, and any exercises taught in hospital should be continued at home, as long as they do not cause undue pain. Some women occasionally feel strange sensations in the abdomen, sometimes described as 'pinging elastic', which is normal. It is advisable to go for short walks, increasing gradually to 45 minutes by 6 weeks after the operation. Swimming may be resumed after about 4 weeks if vaginal bleeding has stopped. Cycling and other light exercises may also be resumed at this stage.

Housework

No housework should be performed for the first 2 weeks by the woman, but, after this, light chores can be safely undertaken. It is very important to avoid lifting anything heavy for the first 4 weeks, and very heavy items, such as shopping, wet laundry, full bin bags or toddlers, should not be lifted for at least 3 months. When anything is lifted, it is important to remind the woman to bend her knees, keep her back straight and hold the object close to her, as this avoids straining her abdomen.

Diet

Many women have heard that they will gain weight or develop a 'middle-aged spread' after a hysterectomy. This is a myth, and any weight gain is due to an increased calorie intake combined with a lack of exercise. It is advisable to eat a variety of foods, including fresh fruit and vegetables to avoid constipation. Some women find prune juice an effective laxative. Other preventative measures such as drinking at least eight glasses of water per day and taking high-fibre foods are also recommended.

Work

Some women feel able to return to work 6–8 weeks following surgery, whereas others may need to take a further 6–8 weeks off work. Obviously, some jobs are more strenuous than others and women should judge for themselves when they feel ready. Some employees may allow women to return on a part-time basis initially, which is an ideal way to readjust to the demands of their job.

Sexual intercourse

Generally speaking, it takes about 6 weeks to feel both physically and emotionally ready to resume sexual intercourse after major gynaecological surgery, and most gynaecologists recommend this time interval before attempting intercourse. It is important to wait until any vaginal bleeding has stopped, to prevent the risk of infection.

The woman's partner should understand the importance of being gentle initially, to avoid undue trauma to the area. Tissue strength is adequate by this time, and the risk of infection is virtually non-existent in the presence of complete healing.

The hormonal effects of oophorectomy, i.e. reduced oestrogen and testosterone, may cause loss of libido, vaginal atrophy and reduction of vaginal lubrication. This may be overcome by hormone replacement therapy or locally applied oestrogen cream. Vaginal dryness may also be helped by using a lubricant such as KY Jelly or Senselle which will reduce chafing and discomfort, and also increase sensitivity.

Hysterectomy usually includes removal of the cervix, which can slightly decrease the length of the vagina, but not to the extent of limiting intercourse. A change in position may be more comfortable initially, such as the female astride or legs together. Some women do report a decreased sexual response after hysterectomy. This may be because the scar tissue at the surgical site within the vagina is not as tactile, and will not engorge and stretch as well as other genital tissues during the excitement and plateau phases of sexual arousal. Sensory nerve pathways to the vagina and perineum may also have been interrupted. While the inner vagina does not contain tactile nerve endings, it has pressure-sensitive nerves that can prompt sexual engorgement. Preoperatively, deep penile thrusting may have been enjoyable because of the pressure it placed on the inner vagina and cervix. Penile thrusting can also produce pleasurable feelings through the movement of internal abdominal organs caused by the motion of the cervix and uterus during intercourse. If this has been part of a woman's enjoyment and arousal pattern, she should be encouraged to focus on other sensations that will assist in building her sexual response.

The character of orgasm for women who have had a hysterectomy may change. This is due to the lack of any uterine contractions, but does not usually affect overall satisfaction.

ENDOMETRIAL ABLATION

Endometrial ablation includes several minimal access procedures that have been developed over recent years (Sutton, 1993). It involves destroying the endometrium, instead of undertaking a hysterectomy, which is a much bigger surgical procedure, with an increase in associated risks and recovery period. The endometrial lining of the uterus is removed while the procedure is observed on a video screen via a hysteroscope. Women have a hysteroscopy prior to the operation, to ensure their suitability for such surgery. A drug such as danazol may be given for 4–6 weeks beforehand to reduce endometrial thickening.

Transcervical resection of the endometrium (TCRE) was one of the first techniques and was initially pioneered in Oxford in 1987. Prior to the development of this procedure, the traditional treatments for heavy menstrual bleeding were drug therapy, a dilatation and curettage, or the option of major surgery in the form of a hysterectomy. Endometrial ablation can be undertaken as a day case and increasingly in outpatient clinics. Consequently, for many women the associated physical, social and psychological implications make it preferable to a hysterectomy.

The advantages and disadvantages of having endometrial ablation compared with a hysterectomy are outlined in Table 18.8. The risk of fluid overload in TCRE is due to the large volume of flushing medium used (Bauman et al, 1993).

Pinion et al (1994) found that women treated by hysteroscopic surgery had a lower morbidity and a significantly shorter recovery period (2–4 weeks) than those treated by hysterectomy (2–3 months). It was

Table 18.8 Comparison between endometrial ablation and hysterectomy

Ablation	Hysterectomy
Disadvantages	
Potential haemorrhage	High risk of haemorrhage
Potential risk of uterine perforation	Potential wound infection
Potential risk of fluid overload (TCRE)	Increased anaesthetic time
Cannot guarantee total cessation of	Postoperative complications:
periods or sterility	– chest infection
Long-term effects unknown	– deep vein thrombosis
May still require hysterectomy for	– constipation
fibroids and ovarian problems	– need for strong analgesics
	Altered body image with change in sexual function
	Large abdominal scar
	Long convalescence required
Advantages	
Can be carried out under sedation	No further periods
and local anaesthetic	Sterility guaranteed
Greatly reduced need for analgesics	No need for further surgery for fibroids, etc.
Rapid recovery and convalescence	
No visible scar	
Short hospital stay, therefore cheaper	
Retains womb, symbol of feminity and fertility	
Quickly resume sexual function	

Box 18.3   Contraindications to endometrial ablation

- Any woman with a vaginal prolapse.
- Endometriosis or fibroids.
- If there is a suspected malignancy, a total abdominal hysterectomy, where biopsies may be taken from other sites in the pelvis, is required.

---

originally felt that an endometrial resection would challenge the hysterectomy as a routine treatment for menorrhagia (Phipps et al, 1990). However, results of long-term studies looking at women after resection indicate that these procedures, while providing alternative treatment, will not replace hysterectomy completely. MacDonald (1993) stated that, in a study undertaken in London, 17% of women required another resection and 10% still required hysterectomy. Endometrial ablation is not an appropriate procedure for all women, and contraindications are listed in Box 18.3.

BALLOON ENDOMETRIAL ABLATION

This relatively new procedure is increasingly undertaken in the outpatient setting, eliminating the need for general anaesthetic. Following hysteroscopy, a special catheter is introduced via the cervix to the endometrial cavity. Water distends the balloon of the catheter so

that it comes into direct contact with the endometrial lining. The water is then superheated to 87°C and left in situ for 8 minutes. The heat produced effectively destroys the endometrium.

LEVONORGESTREL INTRAUTERINE SYSTEM

The levonorgestrel intrauterine system, Mirena, is a T-shaped intrauterine contraceptive device which contains the progesterone levonorgestrel in a sleeve around its stem. Progesterone is released slowly from the core and can be used for both contraceptive purposes and treatment of menorrhagia. It is ideal for older perimenopausal women who require hormone replacement therapy but still need contraception.

If used for women with menorrhagia who do not wish to have surgery, it must be explained thoroughly that the woman may experience erratic, irregular bleeding for the first 3–4 months following insertion. Bleeding then decreases considerably if the woman is able to tolerate this period of uncertainty.

VAGINAL REPAIR SURGERY/ COLPORRHAPHY

Vaginal repair surgery (or colporrhaphy) is carried out to treat uterine or vaginal wall prolapse. Prolapses develop due to lack of support for pelvic organs by either the pelvic floor muscles or ligaments. This can be caused by increased abdominal pressure due to pregnancy and labour, persistent coughing or, more frequently, postmenopausally. The uterus may descend into the vagina and even reach the introitus. In severe cases the uterus extends right outside the vagina and is known as a procidentia. A prolapse is often first discovered when a woman complains of 'something coming down'; she may also have pelvic pain, backache, dyspareunia and urinary symptoms such as stress incontinence. There are several types of uterine prolapse:

- *Cystocele*: prolapse of the bladder and anterior vaginal wall.

- *Cystourethrocele*: the urethra descends as well as the bladder, resulting in urinary problems such as difficulty emptying the bladder, recurrent urinary tract infections and stress incontinence. Stress incontinence may be demonstrated while asking the woman to cough when the bladder is full. A small jet of urine is seen to escape from the urethra while a Sims' speculum parts the vaginal walls.

- *Rectocele*: the rectum prolapses through the adjacent posterior vaginal wall. The woman may have backache or a dragging feeling in the pelvic floor and may have difficulty emptying the bowel.

- *Enterocele*: hernia of the rectovaginal pouch into the upper third of the vagina. It may occur without uterine prolapse and occasionally following hysterectomy where there may be a vault prolapse.

NON-SURGICAL TREATMENT

Many women with a slight prolapse have no discomfort and do not require treatment, apart from being taught pelvic floor exercises. A prolapse which is causing discomfort should be treated by surgery unless the woman plans to have another baby, or if she is too old or frail to undergo an operation. In this instance a polyethylene ring pessary may be inserted into the vagina to support the pelvic organs. The ring pessary needs to be changed every 6–12 months unless there is any bleeding or unusual discharge.

TYPES OF SURGERY

A uterine prolapse is best treated by vaginal hysterectomy combined with a vaginal repair.

Anterior colporrhaphy

This operation is a repair of the anterior vaginal wall and is designed to cure a cystocele or cystourethrocele,

due to urethral sphincter incompetence. The anterior vaginal wall is incised, and a triangular portion of vaginal skin from below the external urethral opening to the front of the cervix is excised. One or two sutures are placed deep around the bladder neck. The edges of the wound are sutured together to provide extra support for the bladder and urethra.

Posterior colporrhaphy

This procedure is used to repair a rectocele, or a rectocele and enterocele. A triangular portion of posterior vaginal wall with its apex at the midvaginal level and its base at the introitus is removed by an inverted T-incision to expose the levator ani muscles. These muscles are brought together with one or two interrupted sutures and closed in a Y-shape to avoid narrowing the entrance to the vagina. The operation also involves the excision of any enterocele and repair of the perineal body (perinorrhaphy).

CONTINENCE SURGERY

There are several different operations that aim to improve continence, and these may be done vaginally or via an abdominal or suprapubic approach.

The aims of continence surgery are to elevate the bladder neck and urethra from the pelvis into the abdomen where intra-abdominal pressure can act as an additional closing cone. Surgery should also support the bladder neck, aligning it to the posterior superior aspect of the pubic symphysis. In some cases this may increase outflow resistance (Cardozo et al, 1993).

It is crucial that prior to surgery a thorough assessment has been made of the woman and her complaint. The first operation for stress incontinence is the one most likely to succeed, so it is important that the most appropriate type of surgery is performed first. Most suprapubic operations in current use produce a subjective cure rate in excess of 85% in patients undergoing their first operation for correctly diagnosed stress incontinence (Cardozo, 1993).

Subsequent surgery may have to be performed on the vagina, which is less mobile and where there is fibrosis of the urethra. In the past, sling operations were performed to elevate the bladder neck and partly to provide support underneath it. Sling material may be organic (rectus sheath fascia) or inorganic (Silastic or Mersilene). The sling may be attached to the rectus sheath or ileoperitoneal ligaments. The amount of tension in the sling will depend upon whether it is being used to obstruct the outflow or to just support the bladder neck.

A procedure known as 'tension free vaginal tape' (TVT) has been developed as a minimally invasive procedure, promoting a quicker recovery than suprapubic surgery. Short-term success rates are approximately 80%, although the long-term success rate is unknown (BSUG, 2003). Two small incisions are made suprapubically and a needle is passed from the vagina upwards to take a length of the tape either side of the bladder and provide a sling to the bladder and urethra. This operation is often undertaken under local or regional anaesthesia, to enable the surgeon to adjust the tape in response to increases in abdominal pressure by asking the woman to cough at certain points of the procedure. Often the woman only requires an overnight stay, and will recover considerably faster than if she had had a suprapubic sling operation.

BURCH COLPOSUSPENSION

This operation is performed through a suprapubic incision. Sutures are inserted on either side of the bladder neck and urethra and passed through the paravaginal fascia, which becomes elevated and is sutured to the ileopecturinal ligaments. As well as raising the urethra and bladder neck to restore the urethrovesicular junction, this procedure elevates the vaginal vault, so any existing anterior vaginal wall prolapse is simultaneously repaired.

The results of this suprapubic operation are better than those for traditional anterior colporrhaphy with bladder neck buttresses, but it requires a longer hospital stay and the use of a suprapubic catheter postoperatively. Women can experience difficulties in voiding urine and so the patient may be discharged home with a suprapubic catheter in situ until urinary function is resumed.

NURSING CARE FOR PATIENTS REQUIRING VAGINAL REPAIR AND CONTINENCE SURGERY

PREOPERATIVE CARE

Preoperative care is very similar to that of women undergoing any major gynaecological surgery. All women will require a full explanation of the proposed surgery, and the chances of success and risks should be honestly discussed so that the woman can make an informed choice before deciding on surgery. Discharge planning should commence at preoperative assessment, since these patients are often elderly.

A midstream urine sample should be sent on admission and antibiotics commenced if necessary. A pubic shave may be required prior to vaginal surgery, as it allows the surgeon a more accurate view.

Even if a woman appears 'elderly' to nurses, it should be ascertained whether she is still sexually active. If so, the gynaecologists should be aware of this when they are suturing near the introitus, to prevent future dyspareunia.

POSTOPERATIVE CARE

These operations usually take about 45 minutes to 1 hour and the care is very similar to that following an abdominal hysterectomy. A vaginal pack will be in situ following a vaginal repair, and if the woman has had bladder surgery, a suprapubic catheter may be in situ. This is a fine plastic tube which is inserted just above the mons pubis and has a plastic disc with four sutures attached to the skin to prevent it from falling out.

Pain can be a particular problem for women who have had a posterior repair. Opioids will be prescribed either via a PCA pump, continuous infusions or by intramuscular injections initially, and diclofenac suppositories are very effective in reducing inflammation and pain. Ice packs can be used, providing they are not used for more than 10 minutes at a time, since they will reduce blood flow to the area where healing needs to occur. Advising the woman to change her position in bed regularly, or maybe by lying prone, can help, in conjunction with advice from the physiotherapist. Women need reassurance following repair surgery, since the pain and discomfort initially may appear to be worsening due to the bruising and the fact that they are probably moving around more than on the day after the operation.

Following a vaginal repair without bladder involvement, the urethral urinary catheter will be removed in the first couple of days. If a suprapubic catheter has been used, it will be left to drain freely for 3–5 days, depending on the urogynaecologist's preference. After this time, a 'suprapubic clamping regime' will commence, to test whether normal bladder function has returned. On the 1st day, the catheter is clamped for an agreed time, e.g. 4 hours, to observe whether the woman can pass urine urethrally. After this time, the clamp is released and the residual that drains into the bag is measured. Initially, the residual may be larger than the amount of urine voided urethrally, but after a few days the residual usually decreases, and when it is less than approximately 100 mL the catheter may be removed. This is a painless procedure, and the small abdominal wound heals quickly without the leakage of urine that women might expect.

The regime used in different hospitals may vary, and initially can appear complicated. Time and patience are required while explaining to the woman about clamping and measuring residuals. Women are usually taught how to clamp their own catheter, empty the drainage bag and record their own fluid balance measurements.

Women often need considerable encouragement, especially when they compare themselves with other patients who may be progressing more rapidly. Occasionally, women are unable to pass urine urethrally due to excessive trauma during surgery, and these women may go home with their suprapubic catheter in situ. They can either leave the catheter on free drainage, or they may continue with the suprapubic clamping regime, where the familiar home environment often produces better results. They are taught how to strap their catheter correctly, how to use a leg bag during the day and how to change to an overnight bag when necessary. Some district nurses will supervise the clamping regime.

Where a urethral catheter has been used, residual amounts of urine can be measured, without further catheterization and its inherent risks of introducing infection, by the use of a bladder scanner. Nurses can be trained to be competent in the use of a small portable scanner, which is far more comfortable for the woman than being catheterized.

In rare instances of women being unable to pass urine urethrally after at least a month following surgery, intermittent self-catheterization will be taught.

Intermittent self-catheterization

This procedure involves introducing a catheter into the bladder intermittently to remove any residual urine. The catheter is then removed until required again. In hospital, this must be done aseptically to prevent cross-infection, but the woman can use a clean technique at home.

Factors such as being well motivated, good cognitive skills, manual dexterity, physical ability and good eyesight are needed for the woman to master the technique (Association for Continence Advice, 2003). Undertaking this procedure is not acceptable to all women and nurses must take this into account.

Gradually the woman may find that she is able to empty her bladder fully, and the residual amount of urine may become less and less when she self-catheterizes. She may well only then need to use the catheter when she wakes in the morning.

Dolman (2001) recommends encouraging the woman to double void: i.e. when she thinks she has emptied her bladder, wait 50 seconds and bear down using the abdominal muscles to try to cause another

bladder contraction. This may prevent residual urine and urinary tract infections.

Many women find that drinking cranberry juice helps prevent cystitis or urinary tract infections developing. As early as the 19th century, Native Americans used crushed cranberries as a herbal remedy for the treatment of urinary infections (Bodel et al, 1959). Many studies have focused on the anti-adherence activity of cranberry juice and its alteration of the urinary pH (Schmidt and Sobota, 1988).

Discharge advice

Women undergoing repair procedures need to be told about their internal sutures since no external wound is visible. They may not understand why precautions about lifting, etc., as discussed on p. 394, are necessary.

Bowel habits
Following any vaginal surgery, care needs to be taken to avoid constipation or straining at stool. Wright (1974) stresses that hospital, with its strange environment and unfamiliar routines, is not the best place to learn new bowel habits. For this reason, health education and discharge advice are crucial. Some women may like to hold a sanitary towel to support the perineum and they should be encouraged to eat plenty of fresh fruit and vegetables and drink plenty of fluids, particularly water.

Pelvic floor exercises
It is crucial that all women having vaginal repair surgery and continence surgery learn how to perform pelvic floor exercises. This increases muscle volume in the pelvic floor. Although originally taught by physiotherapists, this role can be undertaken by nurses. The woman should be instructed to tighten the muscles around the anus as if trying to prevent flatus escaping. The same should then be undertaken around the vagina. Asking the woman to imagine she is on the toilet and trying to stop the flow of urine may help her to visualize just what she should be feeling. Once she can manage this, she should be encouraged to hold these contractions for at least 5 seconds, then repeating 5–10 times for at least 5 times a day. Visual reminders such as stickers on cupboard doors can act as stimuli to remind the woman to do these during the day. Women should be encouraged to do these exercises regularly. All women of all ages should develop a habit of performing pelvic floor exercises every day on a long-term basis in order for it to be effective. They are also especially important after childbirth, and can improve sexual enjoyment.

LAPAROSCOPIC TREATMENT OF ECTOPIC PREGNANCY

This condition is included under major gynaecological surgery because an ectopic pregnancy is potentially life-threatening for the woman.

WHAT IS AN ECTOPIC PREGNANCY?

The word 'ectopic' originates from the Greek *'ektopos'*, meaning 'misplaced', and an ectopic pregnancy occurs when the fertilized ovum implants and develops outside the uterus. In the UK several studies indicate that the incidence is rising. Lewis and O'Drife (2001) reported 11.1 ectopic pregnancies per 1000 pregnancies and Irvine et al (1994) identified the rate as 1 in 60 reported pregnancies. It is often the result of fibrosis or damage to the cilia in the tube following salpingitis (infection or inflammation of the Fallopian tubes). Other contributing factors are shown in Box 18.4.

A woman with a suspected ectopic pregnancy should always be treated as a gynaecological emergency. Despite medical advances in the past decade, there has been no decrease in the number of women dying from an ectopic pregnancy. There were 13 reported pregnancy deaths due to ectopic pregnancy in the 3 years 1997–1999 (Lewis and O'Drife, 2001). This is because there is a high risk of sudden rupture of the Fallopian tubes, which can lead to a massive intraperitoneal haemorrhage. The woman's symptoms vary according to the site of implantation, although most ectopic pregnancies occur in the Fallopian tube. If implantation has occurred within 4–6 weeks of her last period, the woman may not realize that she is pregnant. The first symptoms may include irregular vaginal bleeding and pelvic pain caused by the distension of the tube. Some women arrive at hospital in a state of collapse due to tubal rupture, requiring resuscitation, blood transfusion and immediate surgery by laparoscopy or laparotomy. Symptoms of tubal rupture are listed in Box 18.5.

A diagnosis of ectopic pregnancy can be confirmed using a serum β-hCG pregnancy test, which is accurate 2 weeks after conception, and a pelvic or a transvaginal scan, which will fail to show an intrauterine pregnancy. If the diagnosis remains doubtful, a laparoscopy will be performed. In the past, a laparotomy was required to remove the damaged tube (salpingectomy). However, with the development of minimally invasive surgical techniques, unruptured ectopic pregnancies are now treated laparoscopically.

The commonest technique is to make an incision into the tube and remove the pregnancy. The tube then

---

> **Box 18.4 Factors contributing to ectopic pregnancy**
>
> - tubal surgery, including sterilization
> - post-delivery or post-abortion infection
> - pelvic inflammatory disease
> - endometriosis (where endometrial tissue is deposited outside the uterus)
> - previous ectopic pregnancy

> **Box 18.5 Symptoms of tubal rupture**
>
> - sudden severe pain
> - vaginal bleeding
> - shoulder tip pain, caused by irritation of the diaphragm by blood in the peritoneal cavity
> - pallor and signs of shock and blood loss
> - distended abdomen due to bleeding

---

heals spontaneously. Although laparoscopic treatment is increasingly available, a woman should understand there still remains a risk that a laparotomy may be required.

Another new development in this area has been the use of non-surgical techniques. These include the puncture and aspiration of ectopic sac or the local injection of embryotoxic drugs, such as methotrexate or potassium chloride (Campbell and Monga, 2000). These approaches obviously remove the need for a general anaesthetic with its associated risks but careful follow-up is required to monitor the effects on the woman and the pregnancy.

SPECIFIC PREOPERATIVE CARE

Frequently there is no time to fully admit and prepare a woman for surgery, since she may be rushed to theatre as an emergency. Her partner may arrive on the ward to wait for her postoperatively, and he will need support and information. He may not even realize his partner was pregnant. If a woman does come to the ward initially, she needs to be prepared as if for major surgery, since this is always a possibility. Most importantly, her psychological care is paramount.

Women can be very distressed when an ectopic pregnancy is diagnosed, since they are experiencing a multiple loss, i.e. that of a baby and possibly a Fallopian tube, leading to concerns about their future fertility. They may be very shocked if they were using contraception and had not even realized they were pregnant. On the other hand, a couple may have been trying to conceive for many years, have had a previous ectopic pregnancy or were on an IVF (in vitro fertilization) programme.

POSTOPERATIVE CARE

Postoperative care will depend on whether the woman has had a laparoscopy or laparotomy. Women usually remain in hospital for 24 hours following laparoscopy and for about 3–4 days following laparotomy. It is important that the woman's rhesus status is ascertained before she goes home. Nurses must ensure the woman and her partner are given the appropriate psychological care. This may involve talking about the pregnancy and its outcome or providing the opportunity to meet with a counsellor at a later date. However, the nurse must be aware that women will react differently to this distressing experience and must respect the woman if she does not wish to discuss her feelings at this time.

SPECIFIC DISCHARGE ADVICE

Sexual intercourse may be resumed once any bleeding has stopped. It is probably advisable for the couple to wait until one or two normal periods have occurred before they try for another pregnancy. The couple may also find it useful to contact the Miscarriage Association (see Resources section).

VULVECTOMY

Vulval cancer accounts for approximately 4% of all gynaecological cancers (Hughes and Handscomb, 2001). It is usually seen in elderly women over 70 years old. The most common malignancy of the vulva is squamous cell carcinoma, which accounts for 80% of all vulval cancers (Hughes and Handscomb, 2001). Early signs are pruritus or irritation and in about half of cases a vulval lesion is present. Unfortunately, because it occurs in elderly women there is often a reluctance to seek medical help due to embarrassment. Consequently, although vulval cancer is a slow-growing disease, women often present for diagnosis when it is in an advanced state.

SIMPLE VULVECTOMY

A simple vulvectomy is carried out for chronic vulval dystrophy, intractable pruritus vulvae (vulval itchiness) and vulval intraepithelial neoplasia (VIN) (a precancerous condition with similar histological features to CIN (see p. 372). The skin and subcutaneous tissues of the vulva are removed using a lateral elliptical incision, starting at the mons pubis. The incision runs down the lateral fold of the labia majora and meets the incision at the other side of the vulva at the posterior fourchette. The levator ani muscles between the vagina and the anus are sutured together and the skin closed anteriorly at the mons pubis and posteriorly at the anus. An alternative treatment is a wide local excision of the lesion, which allows full histological examination and may be a definitive treatment that reduces the need for removing the lymph nodes.

RADICAL VULVECTOMY

A radical vulvectomy is performed for invasive cancer of the vulva. In the past the vulval tissue was removed en bloc in one piece, but surgery has developed using the triple-incision technique. This involves the dissection of the invasive lesion, adjoining skin, subcutaneous fat, regional, inguinal and femoral nodes and the vulva. The degree of surgery depends on the location and extent of the primary lesion, and the surgeon will plan to effect treatment but reduce morbidity and postoperative complications. However, if it is necessary to remove a large area of skin, a skin graft may be required from the thigh or abdomen. In the past, removal of larger amounts of tissue led to frequent wound breakdown due to increased tension on the suture lines.

PREOPERATIVE CARE

Preoperative care will be the same as that for any major gynaecological surgery, but it is obviously vital that women and their partners have a full explanation of the operation and its implications. On admission, both ward and specialist nurses must be involved with the woman's care. A full sexual history and assessment should be made. Women may find it difficult to come to terms with the mutilating effects surgery will have, and considerable time will need to be spent preoperatively in discussion with the whole family. There is an excellent BACUP (see Resources section) booklet 'Cancer of the Vulva', which is useful for both women and nurses.

It is probably preferable that women undergoing vulvectomy are nursed in a side-room initially due to the privacy and intensive nursing care required. However, if a woman would rather be with other patients, this should be arranged.

A full 'through' shave will be required before surgery unless there are any open or painful lesions.

Anti-embolism stockings should be measured and fitted, since mobility will be impaired by pain and bulky bandages. These patients are often elderly, and should be taught deep breathing and leg exercises prior to surgery to reduce the risks of deep vein thrombosis. Subcutaneous heparin will also be prescribed, as for all patients undergoing major surgery.

POSTOPERATIVE CARE

The operation will take 2–4 hours. Opioid analgesics will be required postoperatively, either by PCA, infusion pumps or injections, or an epidural may be sited. Intravenous fluid replacement will be required, since fluid loss may be considerable during this complicated operation. After the initial drowsiness and nausea, drinking and eating may be gradually resumed. A low-fibre diet is necessary to avoid bulky stools and straining.

A urethral (Foley) catheter will be in place and it will remain in situ for 1–3 weeks while healing occurs. Although one-third to one-half of the urethra may have been removed, spontaneous voiding is possible. Some women find that urine no longer flows out in a steady stream, so they need to be taught how to squat and sit back slightly to avoid wetting their legs or the floor.

Two Redivac drains are inserted into the groins to prevent haematoma formation and will remain in situ for 7–10 days. Wound care varies between different units and there appears to be very little published research to recommend the best approach. Nursing staff often take the lead in determining the most appropriate wound care, based on the rationale of promoting healing and reducing wound breakdown, which in the past has been associated with this surgery. Following bathing or showering, the area can be dried thoroughly using a hair dryer. However, if there is any infection present, this practice is not appropriate as the hairdryer can blow microorganisms into the atmosphere. In some hospitals women return to theatre for a light anaesthetic before removal of sutures, or inhalational analgesia such as Entonox is used. Surgery involving removal of lymph tissue can result in lymphoedema, whereby lymph is unable to drain properly and so collects in interstitial tissue such as the leg. A specialist nurse can provide advice and help with the treatment and fitting of compression hosiery.

BODY IMAGE ISSUES

All women undergoing vulvectomy require psychologically sensitive nursing care. Women may find it difficult to look at their new altered appearance, and it is advisable they try to do so before going home. If possible, the woman should look with the help of a mirror, in her own time, but with her nurse present if she prefers. Many women in this age group are not used to looking 'down below', so sensitive communication is required. It may be better to wait until the staples or sutures are removed, since they can make the scarring look worse. Many women find it hard to visualize what the scar will look like. Due to the fatty, stretchy nature of vulval skin, the remaining skin can be stretched to leave a very neat scar. Women need to be warned that, because the labia have been removed, the opening of the vagina will be more visible. If the clitoris has been removed the area will now be flat skin, without the usual folds of the vulva. Also, the groin may feel tight at first if lymph nodes have been removed.

DISCHARGE ADVICE

Women usually stay in hospital for 2–4 weeks, and discharge planning from the time of preoperative assessment is essential. Unfortunately, there is no specific support group for vulvectomy patients, but BACUP (see Resources section) is a very helpful organization, and healthcare professionals can network between old and new patients. In general, similar discharge advice should be given, as for patients who have undergone major gynaecological surgery (see p. 394).

SEXUAL ADVICE

It is crucial that, before discharge, there should be discussion about any sexual concerns the couple may have. The psychosexual implications of vulvectomy are of utmost importance, since genitals are intimately associated with a woman's sexuality, body image, gender identity and general quality of life.

Excision of the clitoris is likely to greatly reduce sensation and sexual arousability and orgasm is rare (Wabrek and Gunn, 1984). The scarred tissue at the remaining vaginal opening can be insensitive to penetration, or hypersensitive to friction. Removal of the pelvic lymph nodes can result in oedema of the legs, which can cause embarrassment, and excision of fatty tissue can cause pain on sitting.

A woman who has undergone a vulvectomy should be advised that she may resume intercourse when she feels ready, probably 4–12 weeks following surgery. Couples should be advised to compensate for loss of perineal sensation by exploring other erotic areas, i.e. breasts, buttocks, thighs (Lamb, 1985). It has to be remembered that couples may need explicit advice and information rather than vague generalizations about intercourse, since people's sexual experiences vary enormously. Although such detailed discussion such as alternative recommended positions for love-making may or may not be accomplished by all nurses, depending on their personal expertise and degree of comfort, it is important not to neglect the issue of the patient's altered sexuality, since this will only reinforce the fallacy that her sexual role is over. In such circumstances, specialist oncology nurses should be involved.

TOTAL PELVIC EXENTERATION

Total pelvic exenteration is a very serious operation which may be considered after radiotherapy in a few selected cases of recurrent cervical cancer. It is carried out when the disease has spread into the bladder or rectum, but where clinical evidence of distant metastases is absent.

The surgery involves the removal of the rectum and distal sigmoid colon, the urinary bladder, all reproductive organs and the entire pelvic floor, and necessitates the formation of both a urostomy and a sigmoid colostomy. Vaginal reconstruction can be performed at the time of operation or 12–18 months later, so that total healing can be permitted and early recurrence of cancer detected (Donahue and Knapp, 1977).

Obviously, the chance of a cure entails great sacrifice on the part of the patient. Potential survival involves the loss of reproductive and sexual functions and the formation of a urostomy and sigmoid colostomy, and thus causes drastic alteration to body image, self-respect and sexuality.

Vera (1981) demonstrated that at the time of diagnosis and proposed surgery, sexual function is not an issue of prime consideration. However, as the patient recovers from surgery and the fear of persistent disease lessens, the hope for complete rehabilitation gradually emerges.

Yarborough (1981) devised a teaching plan for patients undergoing total pelvic exenteration, which took a multidisciplinary approach. The teaching objectives of the nurse included education of the patient regarding anatomy and the changes that would occur as a result of surgery. By discussing the outcomes of surgery, the nurse also encourages the patient to voice her feelings about the impending alterations to body image, eliminatory and sexual functions.

McKenzie (1988) stresses the importance of continuing assessment and evaluation of the patient's adjustment after discharge, both at home and in outpatient settings. Follow-up should be continued for as long as the woman feels it to be necessary. If such support is

offered, sexual rehabilitation can become a reality for the couple.

SEXUAL HEALING

All nurses working in specialties where sexuality is a central issue need to realize that patients do have sexual concerns and that nurses can contribute to this crucial aspect of recovery. It is of utmost importance that all gynaecology units maintain a standard for caring for women within a 'sexually aware' environment.

MacElveen-Hoehn (1985) suggests that many nurses are concerned about violating their patients' privacy regarding sexuality and are anxious about raising such issues for fear of being unable to implement helpful nursing interventions. However, nurses working on gynaecology wards do not have to be sexual therapists. They can help their patients by providing information and understanding about self and body, and its relation to sexuality before and after diagnosis and surgery.

It is vital that each woman is treated as an individual and that assumptions about her are not made.

Gynaecology wards usually have a large number of women who are over 60 years old, and it is important that their sexuality is not ignored, but addressed in the same manner as a younger woman's. Older women may be even less likely to initiate discussions about sexual concerns, and therefore the gynaecology nurse must act as a sensitive facilitator. Sexuality in the elderly can be difficult to discuss.

Another common assumption made by health professionals is that everyone is heterosexual. Jones (1988) comments how lesbians may be isolated and deprived of care in hospital and made to feel uncomfortable when their partner visits.

The issue of confidentiality is important for all gynaecology patients, since gynaecology is so intimately related to sexuality, but confidentiality is particularly required by homosexual patients. A patient's sexuality should not be recorded on medical or nursing notes, since its inclusion may leave the patients open to negative attitudes from other staff in the future.

It is also important for nurses to take into account any cultural differences between women they care for. Certain ethnic groups find hysterectomy particularly hard to accept, and nurses should be aware of the impact this operation may have on different cultures and communities. West Indian women view menstruation as a cleansing act, ridding the body of impurities, and so are reluctant to have a hysterectomy. Some also fear they will be 'less of a woman' in the eyes of their men, who may be tempted to look for another 'whole woman'. For this reason they may not wish their partner or family to know exactly what operation they are having, and all staff should respect their right to confidentiality.

The cultural role of modern women is dependent on their fertility; again, it may be difficult for both partners to come to terms with surgery, not only with the patient but also with her partner and other members of the family.

Finally, all nurses should be aware of the Royal College of Nursing Gynaecological Standard Statement for sexuality. It is imperative that a woman experiences a non-judgmental acceptance of her sexual attitude from healthcare professionals caring for her (Shapiro, 1984).

Within gynaecology, the partner can sometimes be forgotten. At the same time as a woman is grieving for losses, whether it is the miscarriage of a much-wanted baby, or losing her uterus by hysterectomy, her partner also grieves. He may be threatened by her loss and, because men have difficulty in revealing their pain and asking for help, he may feel very alone.

Sometimes the partner may feel that he is the cause of the pain. In the case of dyspareunia caused by endometriosis, the partner may well be affected by the fact that he initiates the pain, and this frequently has a harmful effect on the sexual side of the relationship.

In other instances, women and their partners may believe that genital cancer is contagious, and whatever sexual relationship that previously existed may therefore cease. Guilt associated with prior sexual activity and a belief that this may have caused the cancer becomes a deterrent to positive adjustment and recovery. A woman who develops cervical cancer after an abortion, extramarital affair or sexually transmitted disease is likely to interpret her disease as punishment for sin or wrongdoing.

Loss of a pregnancy or baby, for whatever reason, i.e. miscarriage, stillbirth, ectopic pregnancy or even termination of pregnancy, can cause psychological problems for the woman and her partner for some time after the event. Guilt is a common feeling, particularly with women who have undergone a termination, and it may take a sympathetic partner and skilled nursing care to help a woman at this time.

Miscarriage may create problems with a woman's self-concept, inner feelings of failure, loss of faith in her body and other conflicts in the marriage and family relationships.

Touch is a powerful healer. Yet, bereaved parents (former lovers) may be painfully unable to touch each other in sexual intimacy. Sexual contact and simple touching may be experienced as violations. Pregnancy losses have often involved physical invasion (such as an evacuation of retained products, laparotomy or different kinds of termination) of the sexual parts of a woman's body. It may take time and emotional resolution for a woman to feel healed and ready for sexual contact.

Some couples may shy away from lovemaking in order to avoid intercourse and the memory of the dead child's conception. They may also feel guilt, as pleasure or happiness may seem disloyal to the lost pregnancy. Others may be terribly fearful of another pregnancy too soon, and be unwilling to trust contraception. Some women may feel able to receive lovemaking but feel so drained by their grief that there is no energy to give in return.

Hidden agendas – including unexpressed thoughts, feelings or issues – never remain hidden for long in couples who know each other well. They show up in body language and touch, and by discussing fears and needs couples may be released from their tensions, so that physical contact can be fully enjoyed again.

Unfortunately, the psychological impact on fathers has been largely overlooked. Johnson and Puddifoot (1996) examined the psychological impact on the partners of women who had had miscarriages. The duration of the pregnancy and whether the partner had been present at the ultrasound scan confirming the pregnancy were factors related to raised levels of guilt and stress.

A couple who have had a miscarriage should be advised to wait until the woman has had one normal period before trying for another pregnancy. Obviously, this is often the last thing the couple want to do, and it is very crucial that nurses do not assume the attitude, 'Go home and get pregnant again'.

CONCLUSION

Because of constant developments in women's health, it has been impossible to discuss every gynaecological operation. However, it is hoped that this chapter has provided a straightforward overview of gynaecology surgery and insight into the psychological aspects of care. Conflicts can occur on gynaecology wards where some of the women are longing for a pregnancy, while others are terminating them.

Although many of these operations are considered routine by healthcare staff, it should always be remembered that for each individual woman, surgery on an intimate part of the body can be a major life event. The sexual anxieties of women are often forgotten but should be a crucial focus of care. This will enable the woman and her partner to make a full recovery. It is the responsibility of the nurse to ask a woman about her specific anxieties rather than waiting for her to offer them as topics of discussion.

The nurse must ensure that they convey a non-judgmental attitude to all women they care for at all times.

Summary of key points

- Gynaecological surgery is an extremely sensitive area, and this should be taken into consideration when caring for patients, and their partners, who are undergoing any form of gynaecological investigations and/or surgery.

- Nurses need to be aware of the psychological effects and related sexuality surrounding gynaecological surgery.

- A woman's concept of her body image, her role as a woman and mother, her sexuality and her relationship with her partner can be threatened following gynaecological surgery.

- A general medical, social, obstetric and gynaecological history should be obtained during the assessment process.

- The nurse should provide an environment in which the woman and her partner are able to discuss any sexual matters.

- The primary goal of gynaecological nursing is to help the woman become independent and self-supporting following her surgery.

- The nurse must maintain a sensitive, non-judgmental attitude at all times.

Resources

Amarant Trust
11–13 Charterhouse Buildings London, EC1M 7AM
Telephone: 020 7401 3855 Helpline: 01293 413000
Information for women undergoing menopause
http://www.amarantmenopausetrust.org.uk (accessed 15 February 2004)

Association for Continence Advice
102a Astra House, Arklow Road, Newcross, London SE14 6EB
Telephone: 020 8692 4680
http://www.aca.uk.com (accessed 15 February 2004)

BACUP
3 Bath Place, Rivington Street, London, EC2A 3JR
Telephone: 0800 181199 (freephone)
http://www.cancerbacup.org.uk (accessed 15 February 2004)

British Society of Urogynaecology
27 Sussex Place, Regent's Park, London NW1 4RG
Telephone: 0202 7772 6211
http://www.rcog.org.uk/bsug (accessed 15 February 2004)

Continence Foundation
2 Doughty Street, London, WC1N 2PH
http://www.continence-foundation.org.uk (accessed 29 February 2004)

Hysterectomy Support Group
The Venture, Green Lane, Upton, Huntingdon, Cambridgeshire, PE17 5YE

Incontact
United House, North Road, London N7 9DP
Telephone: 0870 770 3246
Fax: 0870 770 3249
Email: info@incontact.org
http://www.incontact.org (accessed 28 February 2004)

Issue (The National Fertility Association)
114 Lichfield Street, Walsall, WS1 1SZ
Telephone: 01922 722 888
Fax: 01922 640 070
http://www.issue.co.uk (accessed 28 February 2004)

Miscarriage Association
c/o Clayton Hospital, Northgate, Wakefield, West Yorkshire, WF1 3JS
Telephone: 019234 200 799
http://www.miscarriageassociation.org.uk (accessed 15 February 2004)

National Association for Premenstrual Syndrome (NAPS)
41 Old Road, East Peckham
Kent, TN12 5AP
Telephone: 0870 777 2178 Helpline: 0870 777 2177
http://www.pms.org.uk (accessed 15 February 2004)

National Endometriosis Society
Suite 50, Westminster Palace Gardens, 1–7 Artillery Row, London, SW1P 1RL
Telephone: 020 7222 2781 Helpline: 020 7222 2776
http://www.endo.org.uk (accessed 15 February 2004)

National Osteoporosis Society
http://www.nos.org.uk (accessed 15 February 2004)

Royal College of Obstetricians and Gynaecologists
27 Sussex Place, Regent's Park, London NW1 4RG
Telephone: 020 7772 6200
http://www.rcog.org.uk (accessed 15 February 2004)

Sands (Stillbirth and Neonatal Death Society)
28 Portland Place, London, W1N 4DE
Telephone: 020 7436 7940 Helpline: 020 7436 5881
http://www.uk-sands.org (accessed 15 February 2004)

SATFA (Support after Termination for Abnormality)
The Hospital for Women, 29–30 Soho Square, London, W1N 6JB
Helpline: 020 7631 0285

The Pre-menstrual Society (PREM SOC)
P.O. Box 429, Alddlestone, Surrey, KT15 1DZ
Telephone: 01932 872560

Well Being
27 Sussex Place, Regent's Park, London NW1 2SP
Research charity of RCOG. Funds research into women's
health

Women's Health
52 Featherstone Street, London, EC1Y 8RT
Telephone: 020 7251 6333 Helpline: 0845 125 5254
http://www.womenshealthlondon.org.uk (accessed 15
February 2004)

References

American Society of Anesthesiologists (1999) Practice guidelines for preoperative fasting and the use of pharmacological agents to reduce the risk of pulmonary aspiration: application to healthy patients undergoing elective surgery. *Anaesthiology* 90(3): 896–905.

Armar, N. A., McGarrigle, H.H. G., Honour, J., et al (1990) Laparoscopic ovarian diathermy in the management of anovulatory infertility in women with polycystic ovaries: endocrine changes and clinical outcome. *Fertility and Sterility* 53(1): 45–49.

Association for Continence Advice (2003) *Notes on Good Practice*. London: ACA.

Backstrom, C.T., Boyle, H. & Baird, D.T. (1981) Persistence of symptoms of pre-menstrual tension in hysterectomised women. *British Journal of Obstetrics and Gynaecology* 88(5): 530–536.

Bauman, R., Magas, A. L. & Kay, J.B. S. (1993) Absorption of glycine irrigation solution during transcervical resection of the endometrium. *British Medical Journal* 300: 305–315.

Billings, E. & Westmore, A. (1980) *The Billings Method*. Harmondsworth: Penguin.

Bodel, P. T., Cotran, R. & Kass, E. (1959) Cranberry juice and the antibacterial action of hippuric acid. *Journal of Clinical Medicine* 56(4): 881–887.

British Society of Urogynaecology (2003) *BSUG Newsletter*, November. London: RCOG.

Campbell, S. & Monga, A. (eds) (2000) *Gynaecology by Ten Teachers*, 17th edn. London: Edward Arnold.

Cardozo, L. D. (1993) Objective and subjective assessment of 184 colposuspensions performed at King's College Hospital (1991–1992). Unpublished data. From: Kelleher, C. J. & Cardozo, L. D. (1993) Treatment options in urinary incontinence. *Review of Contemporary Pharmacotherapeutics* 5: 163–177.

Cardozo, L., Cutner, A. & Wise, B. (1993) *Basic Urogynaecology*. Oxford: Oxford Medical Publications.

Cotton, J. A. (2003) Nursing patients with sexual health and reproductive problems. In: Brooker, C. & Nicol, N. (ed.) *Nursing Adults. The Practice of Caring*. Edinburgh: Mosby.

Coults, L. C. (1985) *Teaching for Health – The Nurse as a Health Educator*. Edinburgh: Churchill Livingstone.

Department of Health (1993) *HSG (93) 41*. London: DoH.

Department of Health (2001) *Good Practice in Consent Implementation: Consent to Examination or Treatment*. London: DoH.

Department of Health (2004) *Hospital Episode Statistics 1999–2002*. [Online] Available at http://www.doh.uk (accessed 28 February 2004).

Dolman, M. (2001) Continence issues. In: Andrews, G. (ed.) *Women's Sexual Health*, 2nd edn. London: Baillière Tindall.

Donahue, V. C. & Knapp, R. C. (1977) Sexual rehabilitation of gynaecological cancer patients. *Obstetrics and Gynaecology* 49(1): 118–121.

Duffin, A. & Nash, J. (2001) Sexual health and sexually acquired infection. In: Andrews, G. (ed.) *Women's Sexual Health*, 2nd edn. London: Baillière Tindall.

Friend, P. (1981) Foreword. In: Bridge, W. & Macleod-Clark (eds) *Communication in Nursing Care*. London: HM&M.

Gould, D. (1990) *Nursing Care of Women*. Herts: Prentice-Hall.

Govan, A. D. T., Hart, D. & Callendar, R. (1993) *Gynaecology Illustrated*, 4th edn. Edinburgh: Churchill Livingstone.

Hughes, C. (2001) Cancer of the uterine cervix. In: Gangar, E. (ed.) *Gynaecological Nursing: A Practical Guide*. Edinburgh: Churchill Livingstone.

Hughes, C. & Handscomb, K. (2001) Cancer of vulva. In: Gangar, E. (ed.) *Gynaecological Nursing: A Practical Guide*. Edinburgh: Churchill Livingstone.

Irvine, L., Hicks, J. L., Blair-Bell, S. & Setchell, M. E. (1994) The incidence of ectopic pregnancy in the City and Hackney Health District of London 1990–91. *Journal of Obstetrics and Gynaecology* 14(1): 29–34.

Jefferies, H. (2002) Ovarian cancer patients: are their informational and emotional needs being met? *Journal of Clinical Nursing* 11(1): 41–47.

Johnson, M. P. & Puddifoot, J. E. (1996) The grief response in the partners of women who miscarry. *British Journal of Medical Psychology* 69(4): 313–327.

Jones, R. (1988) With respect to lesbians. *Nursing Times* 84(20): 48–49.

Lamb, M. (1985) Sexual dysfunction in the gynaecological oncology patient. *Seminars in Oncology Nursing* 1(1): 9–17.

Lee, L. & Rider, I. (2001) Gynaecological investigations and surgery. In: Andrews, G. (ed.) *Women's Sexual Health*, 2nd edn. London: Baillière Tindall.

Lewis, G. & O'Drife, J. (eds) (2001) *Why Mothers Die 1997–1999. Fifth Report of the Confidential Enquiries into Maternal Deaths in the United Kingdom*. London: HMSO.

MacDonald, R. (1993) Audit applied to endometrial ablation. In: Sutton C. J. G (ed.) *New Surgical Techniques in Gynaecology*. Carnforth: Parthenon Publishing Group.

MacElveen-Hoehn, P. (1985) Sexual assessment and counselling. *Seminars in Oncology Nursing* 1(1): 9–17.

McKenzie, F. (1988) Sexuality after total pelvic exenteration. *Nursing Times* 84(20): 27–29.

Martin-Hirsch, P. & Reynolds, K. (2001) Endometrial cancer. In: Shafi, M., Luesley, D. & Jordan, J.(eds) *Gynaecological Oncology*. London: Churchill Livingstone.

National Institute of Clinical Excellence (2003) *Preoperative Tests. The Use of Routine Preoperative Tests for Elective Surgery*. London: NICE.

Nelson, S. (2001) Womens' sexuality. In: Andrews, G. (ed.) *Women's Sexual Health*, 2nd edn. London: Baillière Tindall.

Orem, D. (1985) *Nursing: Concepts of Practice*, 3rd edn. New York: McGraw-Hill.

Phipps, J. H., Lewis, B. V. & Prior, M. V. (1990) Experimental and clinical studies with radio-frequency induced thermal endometrial ablation for function menorrhagia. *Obstetrics and Gynaecology* 76(5): 876–882.

Pinion, S. B., Parking, D. E., Abramovich, D. R., et al (1994) Randomised trial of hysterectomy, endometrial laser ablation and transcervical endometrial resection for dysfunctional uterine bleeding. *British Medical Journal* 309(6960): 979–983.

Roper, N., Logan, W. W. & Tierney, A. J. (2000) *The Roper–Logan–Tierney Model of Nursing*. Edinburgh: Churchill Livingstone.

Royal College of Nursing (1991) *Standards of Care. Gynaecological Nursing*. London: Royal College of Nursing.

Royal College of Obstetricians & Gynaecologists (1995) *Report of RCOG Working Party on Prophylaxis against Thromboembolism in Gynaecology and Obstetrics*. London: Chameleon.

Royal College of Obstetricians and Gynaecologists (1999) *National Evidence Based Guidelines: Sterilisation – Males and Females*. London: RCOG.

Royal College of Obstetricians and Gynaecologists (2001) *Management of Early Pregnancy Loss*. London: RCOG.

Royal College of Obstetricians and Gynaecologists (2002) *Clinical Standards Advice Planning the Service in Obstetrics and Gynaecology*. London: RCOG.

Schmidt, R. D. & Sobota, A. E. (1988) An examination of the anti-adherence activity of cranberry juice on urinary and nonurinary bacterial isolates. *Microbios* 52(224–225): 173–181.

Selby, J. (2001) Psychosocial and emotional care. In: Andrews, G. (ed.) *Women's Sexual Health*, 2nd edn. London: Baillière Tindall.

Shapiro, R. (1984) Putting the sex back into contraception. *Nursing Times: Community Outlook* 80(9): 123–131.

Sharp, F. & Jordan, J. A. (eds) (1986) *Gynaecological Laser Surgery*. New York: Perinatology Press.

Shingleton, M. M. & Orr, J. W. (1987) *Cancer of the Cervix – Diagnosis and Treatment*. Edinburgh: Churchill Livingstone.

Siddle, N., Sarrel, P. & Whitehead, M. L. (1987) The effect of hysterectomy on the age of ovarian failure: identification of a sub group of women with premature loss of ovarian function. *Fertility and Sterility* 47(1): 94.

Skea, Z., Harry, V., Bhattacharya, S., et al (2004) Women's perceptions of decision-making about hysterectomy. *British Journal of Obstetrics and Gynaecology* 111(2): 133–142.

Sutton, A. (2001) Chlamydia and pelvic inflammatory disease. In: Gangar, E. (ed.) *Gynaecological Nursing: A Practical Guide*. Edinburgh: Churchill Livingstone.

Sutton, C. J. G. (1993) *New Surgical Techniques in Gynaecology*. Carnforth: Parthenon Publishing Group.

Taylor, J., Goodman, M. & Luesley, D. (1993) Is home best? *Nursing Times* 89(37): 31–33.

Tortora, G. J. & Grabowski, S. R. (2003) *Principles of Anatomy and Physiology*, 10th edn. New York: John Wiley & Sons.

Tunnadine, P. (1992) *Insights into Troubled Sexuality. A Case Profile Anthology*, revised edn. London: Chapman and Hall.

Vera, M. L. (1981) Quality of life following pelvic exenteration. *Gynaecologic Oncology* 12(3): 355–366.

Wabrek, A. J. & Gunn, J. L. (1984) Sexual and psychological implication of gynaecological malignancies. *Journal of Gynaecological and Neonatal Nursing* 13(6): 371–375.

Webb, C. (1985) *Sex, Nursing and Health*. Chichester: Wiley.

Wilson-Barnett, J. (1978) Factors affecting patients' response to hospitalisation. *Journal of Advanced Nursing* 3(3): 221–228.

Wright, L. (1974) *Bowel Function in Hospital*. London: RCN.

Yarborough, B. (1981) Teaching plan for patients undergoing total pelvic exenteration. *Oncology Nursing Forum* 8(2): 36–40.

Further reading

Andrews, G. (ed.) (2001) *Women's Sexual Health*, 2nd edn. London: Baillière Tindall.

Brooker, C. & Nicol, M. (eds) (2003) *Nursing Adults. The Practice of Caring*. Edinburgh: Mosby.

Campbell, S. & Monga, A. (2000) *Gynaecology by Ten Teachers*, 17th edn. London: Edward Arnold.

Clark, J. (1993) *Hysterectomy and the Alternatives*. London: Virago.

Friday, N. (1976) *My Secret Garden*. London: Quartet.

Gangar, E. A. (ed.) (2001) *Gynaecological Nursing: A Practical Guide*. Edinburgh: Churchill Livingstone.

Gould, D. (1990) *Nursing Care of Women*. Herts: Prentice-Hall.

Govan, A. D. T., Hart, D. & Callendar, R. (1993) *Gynaecology Illustrated*, 4th edn. Edinburgh: Churchill Livingstone.

Haslett, S. & Jennings, M. (1992) *Having Gynaecological Surgery*. Beaconsfield: Beaconsfield Publishers.

Hunter, M. (1994) *Counselling in Obstetrics and Gynaecology*. Leicester: BPS Books.

Jenkins, J. E. (1987) *Caring for Women's Health*. London: Women's Health Concern.

Johnson, J. E. (1987) *Intimacy. Living as a Woman after Cancer*. Toronto: NC Press.

Jolly, J. (1987) *Missed Beginnings. Death before Life has been Established*. Reading: Austen Cornish.

Lambert, H. E. & Blake, P. E. (1992) *Gynaecological Oncology*. Oxford: Oxford University Press.

Llewellyn-Jones, D. (1990) *Fundamentals of obstetrics and gynaecology, Vol 2: Gynaecology*, 5th edn. London. Faber and Faber.

Luesley, D. (ed.) (1997) *Common Conditions in Gynaecology.* London: Chapman Hall.

Moulder, C. (1990) *Miscarriage: Women's Experiences and Needs.* London: Pandora.

Oakley, A., McPherson, A. & Roberts, H. (1984) *Miscarriage.* London: Fontana.

Older, J. (1984) *Endometriosis.* New York: Schribner.

Smith, J. R. & Barron, B. A (1999) *Gynaecological Oncology.* Oxford: Health Press.

Thomas, J. (1992) *Supporting Parents when a Baby Dies. Before or Soon After Birth,* 2nd edn. (Available from J Brown, 1 Millside, Riversdale, Bourne End, Bucks, SL8 5EB, UK.)

Walton, I. (1994) *Sexuality and Motherhood.* Cheshire: Books for Midwives.

Chapter 19

Patients requiring breast surgery

Elisabeth Grimsey

Key objectives of the chapter

At the end of the chapter the reader should be
able to:

- describe the basic knowledge of anatomy and
  physiology of the breast

- demonstrate a basic knowledge and understanding of the investigations used in breast disease

- understand the conditions requiring breast
  surgery and the reasons for it

- assess the needs of patients undergoing breast
  surgery, using a model of nursing care

- plan and implement pre- and postoperative
  nursing care, taking into account current
  research

- plan a discharge from hospital

- give appropriate advice, information and education to the patient.

INTRODUCTION

Breast disease is a common occurrence in women, so it
is likely that most nurses will find themselves caring
for women with breast disease at some point in their
career. It is therefore important to have a good knowledge base and understanding from which to work.

One in ten breast lumps is malignant (Hughes et al, 1989) but, for the woman herself, finding a breast lump instils a fear of cancer. It is essential that the woman is cared for in a caring and sensitive manner and a diagnosis is made quickly.

This chapter looks at both benign and malignant breast disease, the different types of surgery and the nursing care of a patient undergoing breast surgery.

ANATOMY AND PHYSIOLOGY

The breasts, also known as mammary glands, exist in both males and females, and are the accessory organ of reproduction. The breasts are situated on either side of the sternum between the second and sixth rib and overlying the pectoralis major muscle. They are stabilized by a suspensory ligament known as Cooper's ligament, named after Sir Astley Cooper.

The shape of the breast is hemispherical, with a tail of tissue extending towards the axilla. The size varies with the stage of development as well as with age. Size also varies between individuals, and often one breast is larger than the other.

GROSS STRUCTURE

The axillary tail, also known as the tail of Spence, extends towards the axilla.

The areola is the pigmented circular area approximately 2.5 cm in diameter situated at the centre of each breast. The colour varies from a pale pink in fair-skinned women, to a dark brown in dark-skinned women. The colour darkens during pregnancy. There are approximately 20 sebaceous glands called Montgomery's tubercles on the areola that lubricate the nipple.

The nipple lies in the centre of the areola and is approximately 6 mm in length. It is composed of erectile tissue and is highly sensitive. The surface is perforated by the openings of the lactiferous ducts.

MICROSCOPIC STRUCTURE

The breast is made up of three types of tissue – fibrous, glandular and fatty – and is covered by skin.

Fibrous bands divide the glandular tissue into approximately 16–20 lobes. Within each lobe is the milk-producing system. The alveoli are the milk-secreting cells (also known as acini). The alveoli are connected by lactiferous tubules, which then connect to the main lactiferous ducts. The lactiferous ducts are lined with epithelial cells. The lactiferous duct then widens to form the ampulla, which acts as a reservoir for the milk to be stored. The lactiferous duct then continues on from the ampulla and opens onto the nipple.

The glandular tissue of the breast is surrounded by fat. If weight is gained or lost, the shape and size of the breast will vary.

BLOOD SUPPLY

The blood supply to the breast comes from the axillary artery and the internal mammary artery. The venous drainage is through the corresponding vessels into the internal mammary and axillary veins.

NERVE SUPPLY

The nerve supply to the breast is mainly by the somatic sensory nerves and autonomic nerves accompanying the blood vessels. The nipple, being the most sensitive part of the breast, is supplied by somatic sensory nerves, whereas the rest of the breast tissue is mainly supplied by the autonomic nerves.

The medial aspect of the breast is served by the thoracic intercostal nerve, which penetrates the pectoralis major to reach the skin. The upper outer quadrant is served by the intercostal brachial nerve, which comes via the axilla.

LYMPHATIC SYSTEM

The lymph fluid from the outer quadrants of the breast flows into the axillary lymph nodes and eventually into the nodes in the neck. Lymph fluid in the inner quadrant drains towards the sternum via the infra-mammary nodes.

The major lymphatic drainage of the breast is to the axilla, and the axillary nodes are divided into three levels:

- Level I – the nodes lie lateral to the lateral border of the pectoralis minor muscle
- Level II – the nodes lie behind the pectoralis minor muscle
- Level III – the nodes are located medial to the medial border of the pectoralis minor muscle.

PHYSIOLOGY OF THE BREAST

The breast is influenced by two main hormones: oestrogen and progesterone. Oestrogen stimulates the growth of the breast once a girl has reached puberty. Progesterone has a secondary function in the maturation of the glandular tissue.

The breasts undergo cyclical changes with the menstrual cycle, due to the changing levels of the hormone prolactin, which controls the secretion of the ovarian hormones, oestrogen and progesterone. These hormones cause the breast tissue and ducts to enlarge. The breast may change in size and consistency and become tender, swollen and nodular, usually 10–14 days prior to menstruation.

When ovarian activity ceases at the menopause, causing a fall in the level of circulating oestrogen and progesterone, the glandular tissue in the breasts starts to involute and atrophy. The glandular tissue then becomes replaced by fat.

ASSESSMENT AND INVESTIGATIONS

Women will initially present to their general practitioner with a breast symptom. The GP will assess her and decide whether a referral to a breast specialist is appropriate. Following guidelines produced by the Cancer Relief Macmillan Fund (1994) and also those by the Breast Surgeons Group of the British Association of Surgical Oncology (1995), it is advisable that a woman should be referred to a specialist breast unit as opposed to a general surgeon, so she can receive optimum care.

METHODS OF ASSESSMENT

History taking

Prior to a clinical assessment, a detailed history should be obtained from the woman. This not only gives the clinician the information required to help make a diagnosis and assess her risk factors for developing breast cancer but also helps to relax the woman.

The details obtained should include:

- patient's age
- past medical history
- family history of breast cancer
- age at menarche
- age at menopause
- date of last menstrual period (LMP)
- use of hormone replacement therapy
- use of the combined contraceptive pill
- number of pregnancies
- age at first pregnancy
- whether she breast-fed her babies.

It is also very important to note the woman's presenting symptom, noting the duration of the symptom and whether it is cyclical in nature.

Clinical examination

The environment in which the woman is examined is very important. A gown should be provided to ensure the woman's dignity and the door should be locked to ensure privacy. If the examiner is a male, a chaperone should be present.

The clinical examination is divided into two parts:

- palpation
- inspection.

Palpation

The woman is first examined lying supine on the couch, with her arms above her head. This flattens out the breast tissue so it is easier to feel. The examiner, having washed and warmed their hands, uses the flats of the fingers to palpate the whole of the breast tissue with a steady, medium-to-light pressure. This can be done in a variety of different ways: for example, using one hand or both hands; the examiner must find the most suitable method for them. Any lesion found is then examined with the fingertips to assess mobility and fixation. It is important to examine both breasts for comparison. The breast is also palpated when the patient is in the sitting position.

The axillary nodes are then examined either lying down or sitting up, depending on the examiner's preference. The patient's arm is supported to relax the muscles. Nodes are easily missed in a fatty axilla, and correlation between clinical and pathological staging is poor (Dixon and Sainsbury, 1993).

When the patient is sitting up, the supraclavicular area is examined for any enlarged supraclavicular nodes. The hands are then swept down both sides of the chest towards the breasts to assess for any enlarged inframammary nodes.

The Royal College of Nursing (1995) has recommended that nurses do not undertake the practice of breast palpation. However, it acknowledges that a small number of nurses with specialist training, working within a specialist unit, can practise breast palpation.

Inspection

The breasts are inspected with the patient in three positions:

- hands relaxed by the side
- hands in the air
- hands on the hips.

The different positions are important, as changes are sometimes noticed in only one of the positions. Putting the hands on the hips contracts the pectoralis major muscle behind the breast. When this is done, a dimple in the breast may be noted, which has previously not been seen in the relaxed position with the hands by the side.

The size and contour of the breasts are noted, and the breasts are inspected for any skin changes, such as skin dimpling, increased vascularity and skin lesions.

The nipple is inspected for any eczematous changes, discharge, crusting and recent inversion. However, some women will have always had inverted nipples and this is normal for them. Also, in older women, nipple inversion can be due to hypertrophy of the ducts, but this should be investigated to exclude malignancy.

BREAST AWARENESS

Breast awareness has been a topic for much debate over the last few years. In 1991 the chief medical officer, Sir Donald Acheson, made a statement regarding breast screening in his final annual report. He stated that unless breast examination was done correctly, it could either promote a sense of false security or, conversely, a sense of acute anxiety in women. This was said to encourage women to attend for mammographic screening but got misinterpreted by the media, causing a lot of confusion and anger (Burton, 1995).

The Department of Health then tried to clarify this situation. The following chief medical officer, Kenneth Calman, recommended that women should become 'breast aware' by getting to know their breasts. The term 'breast self-examination' was then replaced with 'breast awareness'. In 1991 a pamphlet 'Be Breast Aware' was published by the Department of Health, encouraging women to get to know their own breasts.

It is known that approximately 90% of breast lumps are found by the women themselves or their partners (Cancer Research UK, 2003), so breast awareness may be a better means for picking up early changes than examination by a doctor. However, no trial has been able to prove breast awareness has any effect on reducing breast cancer mortality (Baum et al, 1994).

The nurse plays a role in advising women about breast awareness. There is a breast awareness 5 point code:

- Know what is normal for you
- Know what to look and feel for
- Look and feel
- Report any changes to your GP without delay
- Attend for routine breast screening if you are aged 50 or over.

INVESTIGATIONS

A woman may undergo one or several of the following investigations, depending on her age.

Mammography

A mammogram is a low-dose X-ray of the breast tissue. With modern techniques a dose of less than 1 mGy is used.

A full explanation should be given to the woman prior to the procedure. To obtain the mammogram, the breast has to be compressed between two plates while the exposure is made, which may be uncomfortable. Two views are normally obtained. The oblique view is taken across the breast lengthways, and the craniocaudal is looking at the breast from head to toe.

In women under 35 years old, the breast is relatively radiodense, so a mammogram is rarely indicated in women in this age group. If a woman over 35 years old has a palpable lump, a mammogram may be performed.

For routine breast screening on the NHS Breast Screening Programme, the age range is 50–64 years old (Austoker, 1990), extending to 70 years old from 2004.

Ultrasound

Ultrasound is a painless technique which uses high-frequency sound waves. The reflections are detected and turned into an image. A conductive jelly is placed on the breast, and a probe is used to scan the breast. Ultrasound is used if there is a palpable lump in a woman under the age of 35 years. It is also used as an aid to mammography, as it can differentiate between a cystic and a solid lesion.

Other radiological imaging

Magnetic resonance imaging (MRI) scans and scintimammography are other radiological imaging procedures that can be used in addition to mammography. These are not routine investigations and are usually advised by the consultant radiologist.

Fine-needle aspiration

This test is performed in the outpatient department. If there is a palpable lump, the clinician is able to perform a fine-needle aspiration (FNA). A full explanation is given to the patient prior to the test. The skin is cleaned and a fine needle (21G or 23G) attached to a 10 ml syringe is introduced into the skin. Suction is applied by withdrawing the plunger of the syringe. Several passes are made in to the lump in different directions, to ensure a good sample is obtained from the lump. The plunger is then released and the needle is withdrawn. The material is then spread thinly onto slides and left to air dry, or is fixed with an alcohol fixative (depending on the cytologist's preference). The cytologist then examines the slides under the microscope and a cytological diagnosis can be made.

Results are usually given a numerical scoring (Table 19.1). The advantage of FNA is that, if a cancer is diagnosed, the woman and her family know prior to

Table 19.1   Cytology grading

Grading	Explanation
C1	Inadequate
C2	Benign
C3	Atypical, probably benign
C4	Suspicious, probably malignant
C5	Malignant

Source: from Wells et al (1994).

surgery what they are dealing with, and can make an informed choice.

Core biopsy

If the cytology from the fine-needle aspiration is not conclusive, or if a histological diagnosis is required, a core biopsy can be taken.

This procedure can be performed in the outpatient department. A full explanation should be given to the patient prior to the procedure. If a biopsy gun is used, the patient should hear the sound made as it can cause her to jump if she is not prepared. Local anaesthetic is injected into the breast, and once this has taken effect a small puncture is made by a scalpel blade over the site of the lump. The trocar is inserted through the puncture until the tip touches the tumour, and the central trocar is advanced into the mass. A core of tissue is obtained, inserted into a pot of formalin and sent to the histology department.

Pressure should be applied to the breast to help to prevent bruising, and a pressure dressing should be applied. Extra caution should be taken with patients on warfarin, as their INR needs to be checked prior to the procedure and extra pressure exerted afterwards.

Staging investigations

If a breast cancer is diagnosed, the woman will need to have some further investigations to assess if there has been any metastatic spread. These tests are usually performed as an outpatient at the time of diagnosis, and the appropriate treatment can then be planned. The following blood tests are usually performed:

- full blood count
- ESR (erythrocyte sedimentation rate)
- urea and electrolytes
- albumin
- bilirubin
- alanine aminotransferase
- alkaline phosphatase

- gamma-glutamyl transferase
- calcium
- phosphate.

If any of the above tests is abnormal, the following investigations can be arranged if appropriate.

Bone scan
The procedure involves an intravenous injection of a harmless radioactive isotope, and then, approximately 3 hours later, an X-ray of the whole body is taken. The films are examined by a consultant radiologist to assess for any metastatic spread to the bones.

Liver ultrasound
Liver ultrasound uses the same technique as with the breast ultrasound, but is used to assess if there has been any metastatic spread to the liver.

Chest X-ray
A chest X-ray is also performed to assess for any lung disease.

If there are any neurological symptoms suggestive of metastatic brain disease, a computerized tomography (CT) scan can also be arranged.

BREAST SURGERY

Breast surgery is performed for both benign and malignant breast disease. The two areas will be looked at separately.

BREAST SURGERY FOR BENIGN BREAST DISEASE

Not all benign breast conditions will require surgery: e.g. cysts can be aspirated in the outpatient department. Each breast unit will have its own local policy, so variations may be found.

The informational needs for women with benign breast disease can be met by information leaflets produced by Breast Cancer Care (see Useful addresses section).

The following operations may be performed for benign breast conditions.

Removal of a benign breast lump

The most common breast lump to be surgically removed is a fibroadenoma, which is a benign fibrous lump. They are most commonly found in women in the 15–30-year-old age group, and they account for approximately 13% of all palpable breast lumps (Dixon and Mansel, 2000).

Presentation

Fibroadenomas usually present as a palpable lump, although some may be impalpable and are only detected on mammographic screening. They tend to be smooth, well-circumscribed, firm and mobile lumps. They have been nicknamed 'Breast Mice' as they are so mobile.

Management

Policies for removal of a fibroadenoma may vary between units. In general, the following policy applies:

- *Observation.* If the clinical examination, ultrasound and fine-needle aspiration (known as the triple assessment) confirm this lump to be a benign fibroadenoma and the woman is under the age of 35 years old, the lump can be left in situ and reassessed with clinical examination and repeat FNA in 6–8 weeks' time. Most women, if given the choice, will opt to leave the lump in situ as opposed to having surgery resulting in a scar.
- *Excision.* If the fibroadenoma measures over 4 cm, if there's any clinical suspicion, if the woman is over 35 years of age or if the woman wishes to have the lump removed, then excision is advised.

The reason why women over the age of 35 years old are advised to have the fibroadenoma removed is that the risk of breast cancer increases with age, and there is fear of missing a breast cancer (Wilkinson and Forrest, 1985).

Surgical treatment

Most fibroadenomas are removed as a day case, if the woman meets the criteria set out for day surgery. A small incision is made over the site of the palpable lump, and the fibroadenoma is shelled out. The wound is then sutured, usually with a subcutaneous dissolvable suture to give the best cosmetic appearance possible. If the lump is near the areola, a subareola incision is made, which gives a very good cosmetic result.

Specific nursing care

The general nursing care is the same as that for any patient undergoing surgery. Advice should be given regarding wound care, pain control, bathing, etc. The patient should be advised to wear a supportive non-wired bra, to give support to the breast, so preventing pulling on the scar. She should be reassured and given a contact number should she experience any problems.

An outpatient appointment should be made for 7–10 days postoperatively, for the wound to be checked and for the histology result. If the histology is benign, the woman can be reassured that it is not a cancer and that it does not increase the risk of breast cancer.

The same management and nursing care as described above applies to women having the following removed:

- lipoma (fatty lump)
- discrete nodularity (thickening of the breast tissue).

Excision of fat necrosis

Fat necrosis is usually caused by trauma to the breast, which causes fat cells to burst open. The body does not recognize these altered fat cells, and so reacts to it as if it were a foreign body. Intense scarring occurs, which feels like a firm irregular lump. The scar tissue then contracts, pulling on the Cooper's ligament, causing skin dimpling. Thus, it mimics a cancer (Dixon and Sainsbury, 1993).

Management

A careful history needs to be taken with special regards to trauma. A mammogram and fine-needle aspiration should have been performed in the outpatient department. If there is still bruising present on the breast, it may be appropriate to reassess the woman in a few months' time. If there is any suspicion, excision is advisable.

Surgical treatment

Surgical treatment is as for removal of a benign breast lump.

Specific nursing care

Specific nursing care is as for removal of a benign breast lump.

Microdochectomy

A microdochectomy (excision of a duct) is performed to excise an intraduct papilloma. Duct papillomas are 'warty'-like growths within a duct. They can either be single or multiple. There is a very low malignant potential, if any (Dixon and Mansel, 2000). Microdochectomies are also performed to investigate a bloodstained discharge and to cure a chronic serous discharge.

Presentation

The most common symptom is a spontaneous serous or bloodstained nipple discharge, usually from a single duct.

Management

A mammogram will have been performed in the outpatient department if the woman is over 35 years old, and slides from the discharge will have been taken to send for cytology assessment.

Surgical treatment

A microdochectomy is performed using a small sub-areola incision. The duct containing the papilloma is isolated and removed. The wound is then sutured with either a subcutaneous dissolvable suture or an interrupted Prolene suture. This can be performed as a day case if the woman meets the day surgery criteria.

Specific nursing care

Specific nursing care is as for removal of a benign lump.

Incision and drainage of a breast abscess

Breast abscesses can occur in the non-lactational or lactational breast.

Non-lactational abscess

These abscesses can occur either in the periareolar region or peripherally.

There are several causative factors:

- duct ectasia (a benign condition within the duct, commonly linked with smoking)
- diabetes
- steroid treatment
- trauma
- infected sebaceous cyst

(Dixon, 2000).

Lactational abscess

The incidence of puerperal mastitis and lactational breast abscesses has reduced in recent years due to improvement in maternal and infant hygiene, a change in feeding patterns and the introduction of early treatment with antibiotics (Dixon, 2000). The organism most commonly responsible is *Staphylococcus aureus* or *Staphylococcus epidermidis*. Infection starts usually via a break in the skin, e.g. cracked nipple, and then enters via the nipple.

Presentation

The most common time for presentation is within the first month after delivery. The woman presents with a red, swollen, hot and painful breast. In the later stages there may be a fluctuant mass. The woman may feel unwell with a pyrexia and tachycardia.

Management

Most breast abscesses can be managed conservatively, but some will still require incision and drainage.

Conservative management   Antibiotics, if given in time, can prevent abscess formation. If there is a fluctuant mass, a fine-needle aspiration can be performed to aspirate some pus, which can be sent for macroscopy, culture and sensitivity (MC&S), and antibiotic treatment is continued. The woman is encouraged to continue breast-feeding from both breasts, as this helps to promote drainage.

Surgical treatment   Occasionally, incision and drainage is necessary if the breast abscess is not resolving with the use of antibiotics. This is usually done under a light general anaesthetic. It is now more common practice for women to be allowed to continue breast-feeding provided the incision is away from the baby's mouth. Feeding can continue as normal from the unaffected side (Baum et al, 1994).

Specific nursing care

Postoperatively, the wound will be left open and a daily dressing will be required to lightly fill the cavity to promote healing. Antibiotic therapy is given if there is widespread cellulitis; otherwise, it is unnecessary (Hughes et al, 1989). Adequate pain control should be given, and a supportive bra should be worn.

These women will require the use of a single room, as the baby will usually accompany them. This reduces the risk of hospital-acquired infection for the baby, gives the mother privacy and causes less disturbance to the other patients.

Psychological support may be necessary, as this can be a difficult and emotional time. Practical support with babycare may be necessary if there's no family support, and referral to a health visitor or social worker may be appropriate.

BREAST CANCER

Breast cancer is the most common form of cancer among women. In the UK in 1999, 41 000 women were newly diagnosed with breast cancer. Although the incidence of breast cancer in the UK is slowly rising, the survival rate has improved significantly. In the 1970s the survival rate was around 54%; in the latest figures from 1991–1993 it is quoted to be 74%. Over the last 10 years (1992–2001) the number of female deaths has fallen from 15 200 to 13 000. In the UK, for a woman, the lifetime risk of developing breast cancer is 1 in 9 (Cancer Research UK, 2003). It is important to state that this is a lifetime risk. The risk for a woman up to the age of 25 years old is 1 in 15 000, whereas a woman between the ages of 80 and 85 years old has a 1 in 10 risk.

It is also important to remember that men can also get breast cancer. Approximately 300 men are diagnosed with the disease in the UK each year (Cancer Research UK, 2003).

TYPES OF BREAST CANCER

There are several types of breast cancer:

- invasive ductal
- invasive lobular
- ductal carcinoma in situ (DCIS)
- lobular carcinoma in situ (LCIS)
- Paget's disease of the nipple
- other rare forms

(Baum et al, 1994).

Invasive ductal carcinoma

This is the most common type of breast cancer, usually presenting as a palpable lump. It originates from the epithelial cells lining the ducts within the breast. It breaks out of the duct and into the surrounding breast tissue. As the cancer grows, it can invert the nipple, cause skin dimpling and, in the advanced stage, cause peau d'orange, where the skin looks like the skin of an orange, and eventually leading to ulceration and possible fungation. It has the potential to metastasize. If detected early, the prognosis is improved.

Invasive lobular carcinoma

This cancer is less common than ductal carcinoma, only accounting for 8% of all breast cancers (Baum et al, 1994). The cancer originates from the lobules of the breast, and behaves the same way as ductal carcinomas, but has the tendency to be bilateral and multifocal.

Ductal carcinoma in situ and lobular carcinoma in situ

These cancers are pre-invasive conditions. The cancer cells are contained within the ducts or the lobules and have not broken out into the surrounding breast tissue. They do not have the ability to metastasize. They usually do not present as lumps but are picked up on mammographic screening, by the appearance of a cluster of microcalcifications.

Paget's disease of the nipple

This condition presents as an eczema-type rash on the nipple and areola complex, which progresses to ulceration. Itching, tingling, burning and bleeding are often common accompanying symptoms. If there is any doubt, a biopsy should be performed. On histology, malignant Paget cells are found in the epidermis.

Other rare forms

Cancers arising from connective tissue can also be found in the breast. These are known as sarcomas. The

Table 19.2 Staging of breast cancers

Stage	Explanation
Stage I	Confined to the breast alone, with or without minor skin dimpling or nipple inversion
Stage II	As above, but with involvement of the regional lymph nodes
Stage III	Locally advanced breast cancer where either the breast tumour or the nodes have infiltrated the skin or have become fixed to the muscle or other structures
Stage IV	Obvious metastatic spread

Source: from Baum et al (1994).

breast can also be a site for secondary carcinomas, e.g. malignant melanomas, although this is rare.

STAGING

It is known that the smaller and the less advanced the tumour is at the time of diagnosis, the better the prognosis. There are many different systems of staging breast cancer, and each breast unit will adopt the most appropriate system for their practice. One simple system involves dividing breast cancer into four stages (Table 19.2).

METASTATIC SPREAD

Cells from the breast cancer can spread via the bloodstream and lymphatic system to other organs in the body. The most common sites for breast cancer metastases are in the axillary, supraclavicular and inframammary nodes, the liver, bones, lungs and brain.

SURGERY FOR BREAST CANCER

There are several types of surgery used in the treatment of breast cancer, which will be discussed below. This is often accompanied by axillary surgery, which will be discussed as a separate issue.

The type of surgery performed depends on:

- patient choice
- size of the tumour in comparison to the size of the breast
- location of the tumour
- age of the patient.

There has been a debate as to the timing of breast cancer surgery in relation to the menstrual period. Badwe et al (1991) found that premenopausal women operated on 3–12 days after their last menstrual period had a greatly reduced overall and recurrence-free survival compared with those who underwent surgery on days

0–2 or 13–32. There have not been any other significant data to date, to fully support this.

The different types of surgery will now be discussed.

Breast-conserving surgery (wide local excision)

This surgery involves removal of the palpable lump and some of the surrounding healthy breast tissue to ensure excision of the tumour is complete (Sainsbury et al, 2000). If the tumour is large, a quadrantectomy may have to be performed, which involves removal of a whole quadrant of the breast. This may involve a significant loss of breast tissue, causing an alteration in breast shape. A Redivac drain is inserted into the cavity to prevent a fluid collection.

Needle–localization biopsy

This surgery is performed when there is an abnormality on the mammogram, such as a cluster of microcalcifications, which cannot be felt. To ensure the surgeon removes the correct area, a fine wire has to be inserted into the abnormal area in the breast. On admission, the woman goes to the X-ray department where she is given a local anaesthetic. Under mammographic control, a fine wire is inserted into the abnormal area. There is a small hook on the end of the wire to prevent it moving. The wire is then taped securely to the breast. At the time of surgery the surgeon makes an incision and follows the wire down to the tip and excises an area of tissue around it. The specimen is then X-rayed while the woman is still asleep, to ensure the mammographic abnormality has been completely removed (Blamey et al, 2000).

Mastectomy

Mastectomy is usually performed if the lump is too big to be able to conserve the breast, if the disease is multifocal, or if this is a recurrent breast cancer in the same breast. Some patients will also choose mastectomy, as opposed to breast-conserving surgery, for a variety of reasons, e.g. fear of local recurrence.

There are several types of mastectomy (Table 19.3). The decision regarding the type of mastectomy is usually dependent on the extent of the disease and the position of the cancer. Figure 19.1 shows a mastectomy scar.

Breast reconstruction

Following a mastectomy, breast reconstruction can be performed either at the time of surgery or at later date. There are several types of breast reconstruction:

- silicone implants
- tissue expander

Table 19.3 Types of mastectomy

Type of mastectomy	Explanation
Total mastectomy	Removal of the breast tissue with some of the overlying skin, including the nipple
Subcutaneous mastectomy	Removal of the breast tissue, keeping the nipple
Radical mastectomy	Removal of the breast tissue, including the pectoralis muscle and axillary contents
Modified radical mastectomy	Removal of the breast tissue, leaving the pectoralis major muscle intact but dividing the pectoralis muscle – so allowing the axilla to be cleared
Salvage mastectomy	Removal of the breast tissue for an ulcerating or fungating lesion in advanced breast cancer, with the aim of improving the quality of life and the relief of distressing symptoms

- myocutaneous flaps
- nipple reconstruction.

The type of reconstruction depends on the patient's choice, type of mastectomy performed, condition of the skin on the chest wall and the condition of the muscle.

Silicone implant

This procedure involves insertion of a silicone implant under the pectoralis muscle at the time of mastectomy. This method is only suitable for small-breasted women and is not suitable if a radical mastectomy has been performed or if radiotherapy has been given to the breast in the past.

In the 1990s there was much debate regarding the safety of silicone and the possible harmful effects it may have on the body in the long term. In 1992, the American Food and Drug Administration (FDA) suspended the sale of silicone implants pending investigation. The Department of Health set up an Independent Review Group (IRG 1998) to review the safety of silicone and it has found them to be safe.

Tissue expander

This procedure involves the insertion of a silicone sac under the pectoralis muscle. A commonly used tissue expander is the Becker Tissue Expander. The sac has a port and valve attached. Saline is injected into the sac via the valve at the time of surgery. Postoperatively, the woman attends the outpatient department to have more saline inserted on a weekly or fortnightly basis to achieve the required size.

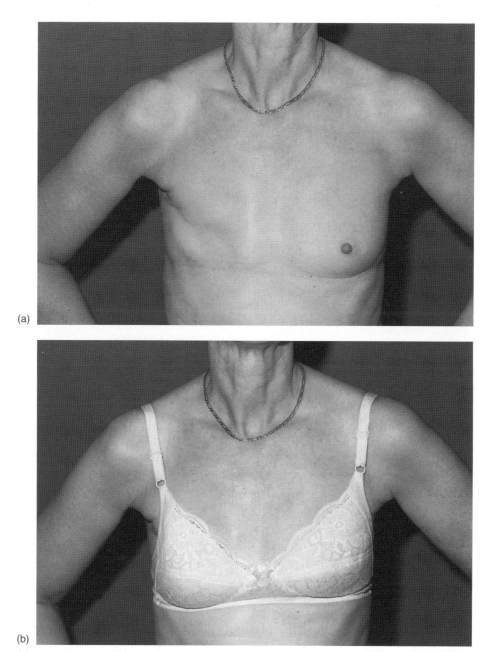

(a)

(b)

Figure 19.1 (a) A mastectomy scar. (b) Same woman wearing bra with prosthesis.

Once the required size is achieved, more fluid is inserted. This overexpansion is done for two purposes. First, when the port and valve are removed, some saline is removed at the same time to match the breast size and to obtain the natural droop of the breast. Secondly, the stretching of the tissues is thought to decrease the incidence of capsule formation (Dixon and Sainsbury, 1993). The port and valve can be removed as a day case.

This method of breast reconstruction is used when the skin is of good quality. It is not suitable following a radical mastectomy unless a myocutaneous flap is used. It is not usually advisable following radiotherapy, as the skin and muscle can be fibrosed.

Myocutaneous flaps

This procedure is used to reconstruct the breast when the skin is damaged by radiotherapy or the breast is large. This technique involves taking a flap of skin and muscle, still attached to its blood supply, from another part of the body to reconstruct the breast. An implant can be inserted underneath this flap, if required, but if the breast is small the flap alone may be sufficient to form a breast mound.

There are two types of myocutaneous flaps used in breast reconstruction: the latissimus dorsi flap (LD flap) and the transverse rectus abdominus myocutaneous flap (TRAM flap).

Latissimus dorsi flap   This procedure involves dissecting the latissimus dorsi muscle from the back, keeping it attached to its own blood supply, rotating it on a pedicle and tunnelling it under the skin of the axilla to cover the deficit from the mastectomy site. The donor site can be taken horizontally so the scar can be hidden by a bra strap, or vertically if low-backed dresses are worn (Berger and Bostwick, 1994). This is the most commonly used myocutaneous flap.

Transverse rectus abdominus myocutaneous flap   This procedure involves dissecting the rectus abdominus muscle, which runs from the pubis to the costal cartilages of the fifth, sixth and seventh rib. Again, it is kept attached to its own blood supply and tunnelled under the skin to cover the deficit. The abdominal scar is transverse and so is well hidden, and a mesh is inserted to prevent herniation. It has the added benefit of giving a 'tummy tuck' at the same time!

Despite the advantages of this flap in being able to take a large area of tissue and the reduced need of an additional implant, it is not as popular as the latissimus dorsi flap. This is because a longer stay in hospital is required and it has a lower success rate. It is not a suitable technique for anyone where the microcirculation is diminished, e.g. diabetics, heavy smokers or in an obese patient (Lerberg and Prin, 1991; Harden and Girard, 1994). It must also be remembered that if the woman has stretch marks on her abdomen, these will then be visible on her reconstructed breast.

Nipple reconstruction

There are several techniques that can be used to reconstruct the nipple. This is usually performed several months following the initial reconstruction.

The most common method is to use the skin and fat from the reconstructed breast to form the nipple, and a skin graft is taken from the inner thigh to form the areola. The graft can be tattooed to obtain the correct colour if necessary. In the past the graft used to be taken from the labia but, for obvious reasons, this was not popular with the women.

There is the potential risk of the graft failing and becoming necrotic. This risk should be explained to the woman prior to surgery. Other techniques have been developed where the areolar complex is tattooed onto the reconstruction and a nipple bud is created from this skin. Further tattooing may be necessary to reshape the areola.

Many women will not opt for nipple reconstruction, preferring to use an adhesive silicone nipple instead when wearing tight-fitting clothes.

(See Chapter 22 for specific nursing care regarding reconstructive surgery.)

Management of the axilla

The management of the axilla is a very controversial issue. There is some debate as to the extent of axillary surgery that is necessary, or if it is necessary at all (Sacks et al, 1994).

Axillary surgery is undertaken for two main reasons:

- for staging and prognostic information, so that adjuvant therapy can be planned – if any of the glands are positive, then adjuvant chemotherapy may be required
- for local control.

If axillary surgery is not performed, radiotherapy may be given to the axilla.

Several complications can arise from axillary surgery or radiotherapy. The possible complications include seromas (fluid collection), reduced arm movement, nerve damage and lymphoedema, the most significant being the development of lymphoedema (Kissin et al, 1986).

Axillary surgery

Each breast unit will have its own policy regarding axillary surgery, which will vary between axillary node sampling (removal of approximately four nodes) and axillary clearance up to Level III. A separate incision is made in the axilla to remove the nodes, and a single suction drain is inserted to prevent a fluid collection. The drain will need to stay in place until the drainage is less than 50 mL over 24 hours (this takes approximately 5–6 days).

The use of sentinel node biopsy is currently undergoing clinical trials, in the hope that it may reduce the need for axillary dissection and all its potential complications. An injection of a blue dye and/or a radioisotope is given several hours before surgery. The theory is that, once injected, the dye and radioactive material will be drawn through the breast to the lymph nodes. The first node it reaches is called the sentinel node. The surgeon excises this node and sends it to pathology for a frozen section. If this node is positive, the surgeon will proceed with an axillary dissection, but if it is negative no further surgery to the axilla will be required. At the time of writing, this procedure is not yet standard care and its use should be restricted to centres involved in relevant clinical trials of the technique. Clinicians using this technique should be adequately trained and be able to demonstrate a false-negative rate below 10% (Sainsbury, 2002).

ADJUVANT TREATMENTS

Adjuvant treatment is decided upon once the histology report is available and will depend on:

- patient choice
- the size and grade of the tumour
- the nodal status
- age and menopausal status
- excision margins
- previous treatment
- oestrogen receptor (ER) status.

The adjuvant treatments to prevent local and distal disease may include all or a combination of the following.

- *Radiotherapy*: this is a high-dose X-ray treatment which kills any residual cancer cells that might be remaining in the breast tissue or chest wall. It is a localized treatment which is given to help prevent local recurrence. It is most commonly given following breast-conserving surgery, but is occasionally given to the chest wall following mastectomy. It is commenced once the wound has healed and full arm movement is achieved; this is usually 4–6 weeks postoperatively (Baum et al, 1994).

- *Chemotherapy*: this simply means 'treatment with drugs'. It is a systemic treatment, so, unlike radiotherapy, it treats the whole of the body. A combination of different cytotoxic drugs is used which kills cells that are dividing rapidly. It is given to women with poor prognostic features, such as involved nodes (Baum et al, 1994).

- *Endocrine therapy*: the most common endocrine treatment is tamoxifen, which is anti-oestrogenic. It competes with oestrogen to lock on to the oestrogen receptor site, preventing growth stimulation. Benefits are greatest in women with tumours that are sensitive to oestrogen, but some benefit is gained

in women with tumours that are less sensitive to oestrogen (Baum et al, 1994). The role of aromatase inhibitors is currently being investigated for the use in the adjuvant setting for postmenopausal women. Once the menopause has passed, the majority of naturally circulating oestrogen has gone. However, oestrogen is still produced, mainly from fat, under the control of the adrenal gland. The enzyme aromatase converts the androgen androstenedione in the fat into oestrogen. The most commonly known aromatase inhibitor is Arimidex (anastrozole). The results of a clinical trial comparing the use of Arimidex against tamoxifen, and also in combination, are currently awaited. Preliminary findings indicate that Arimidex may be superior to tamoxifen and that there are no benefits of using them together. However, further long-term data need to be accrued prior to changing current clinical practice.

NURSING CARE OF A PATIENT UNDERGOING SURGERY FOR BREAST CANCER

The general nursing care for patients undergoing breast surgery is the same as for any surgery, e.g. wound care, but there are specific issues that the nurse needs to be aware of in planning the nursing care. (See Table 19.4 for a case study of a woman undergoing a mastectomy).

PREOPERATIVE INFORMATION

Ideally, the woman should have been seen by a Breast Care Nurse at diagnosis, who will have explained what to expect, but, if not, the ward nurse should be able to provide this information. Written information should also be provided.

The woman should be given an idea about the possible cosmetic outcome of the surgery. The use of a photo album to illustrate the outcomes of different operations may be of help, but it should be stressed that every person is an individual, so outcomes may differ.

If axillary surgery is planned, the woman should be warned that she may lose the sensation under her arm and along the underside of the upper arm. This can be quite an uncomfortable feeling. Sensation may return in a few months postoperatively, but it may never be fully regained. The woman should also be informed about the use of surgical drains postoperatively. Often two Redivacs are inserted, one in the breast and one in the axilla, to prevent a haematoma or a seroma (fluid collection). These are normally left in situ until the drainage is less than 50 mL in a 24-hour period.

A seroma may occur after the axillary drain is removed. The fluid that was previously drained away in the Redivac bottle may collect in the cavity, causing a swelling in the axilla. This causes some discomfort and the feeling of having an orange under the arm. It can simply be drained by inserting a needle into the area and drawing off the fluid. This should be performed by a doctor or the Breast Care Nurse, who has been trained to drain seromas. The woman should be warned that this may reoccur, so that she is not alarmed.

THE POTENTIAL RISK OF LYMPHOEDEMA

Lymphoedema is defined as tissue swelling due to failure of lymph drainage (Mortimer, 1990), and can result from axillary surgery. In a study by Kissin et al (1986) it was found that the incidence of lymphoedema following either surgery or radiotherapy treatment for breast cancer was 25.5%.

Following axillary surgery or radiation to the axilla, the lymphatic channels become obliterated or obstructed. Lymph vessels are able to regenerate and develop collateral vessels, but this can be greatly impaired if there is extensive scar tissue (Mortimer, 1990). Lymphoedema, therefore, occurs when the lymph load exceeds the lymph drainage capacity and swelling occurs.

The woman should be given information regarding skin care to prevent the occurrence of lymphoedema. The skin care advice for the affected arm is of great importance (Box 19.1).

Box 19.1   Skin care advice for the affected arm following surgery

- Gently wash skin, avoiding harsh soaps, and dry thoroughly.
- Apply moisturizer daily.
- Take care cutting nails.
- Avoid getting the arm sunburnt.
- Avoid insect bites (use a repellent).
- Use an electric razor to shave under the arm instead of an open blade.
- Avoid injections and venepuncture.
- Avoid blood pressure recordings.
- Use gloves for washing up and gardening.
- Encourage normal use of the arm, but avoid heavy lifting and housework.
- Treat cuts promptly with an antiseptic ointment.
- See GP for antibiotic treatment if there is any sign of infection.

Source: from Badger (1996).

POTENTIAL IMMOBILITY OF THE AFFECTED ARM

The woman should be seen by a physiotherapist, to be shown some arm exercises so as to prevent a frozen shoulder and also to help prevent lymphoedema. These should be encouraged twice daily (Fig. 19.2).

ANXIETY

When a woman is given a diagnosis of breast cancer, it completely changes her life. It raises many fears and anxieties which she has to learn to cope with.

The high prevalence of psychological morbidity after surgery of breast cancer is well documented (Maguire et al, 1978; Fallowfield et al, 1986). Most breast units have a specifically designated Breast Care Nurse who is specially trained in breast cancer to provide practical advice and support. The effectiveness of the role of the Breast Care Nurse has been well researched and evaluated and has been shown to reduce the incidence of psychological morbidity (Maguire et al, 1980; Watson et al, 1988).

If there is no Breast Care Nurse in post, support may be provided by voluntary organizations such as Breast Cancer Care. A recent study comparing the effectiveness of support from a Breast Care Nurse and a voluntary organization, showed the Breast Care Nurse to be more effective in reducing psychological morbidity (McArdle et al, 1996).

ALTERED BODY IMAGE

The breast throughout history has been a symbol of womanhood. It is seen as a symbol of sexuality as well as a symbol of motherhood.

The woman should not be forced into looking at the wound before she is ready. When she feels able to look, she may or may not want her partner with her. Looking at the wound should be handled with sensitivity and understanding. A nurse should be present when this is done. A hand mirror should be available, so the woman can gradually look at the scar before seeing herself in a full-length mirror.

If a mastectomy has been performed, the woman should be fitted with a soft temporary prosthesis, sometimes called a 'Comfie' (Fig. 19.3), as soon as she wishes prior to discharge. Arrangements for fitting a permanent silicone prosthesis should be made for 4–6 weeks postoperatively when the scar has healed. The woman should be encouraged to wear her own clothes on the ward.

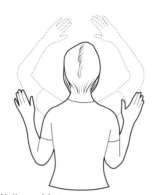

Wall reaching
With your feet apart for good balance, standing very close to, and facing a wall. Slowly 'walk' both hands up the wall, slide hands back down again and repeat

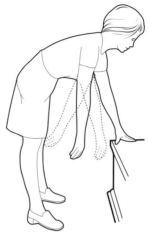

Pendular arm swing
Support yourself with your unaffected arm. Let your other arm hang loosely and swing from the shoulder. Swing forwards, backwards, side to side and in circles

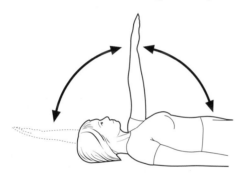

Reaching back
Lying on a firm surface, lift your affected arm to the vertical position then gently back so that it brushes past your ear

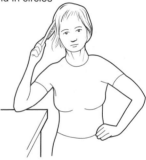

Hair-brushing
Rest your elbow on a table and sit up straight. Start by brushing your hair on one side and progress to brushing the whole head

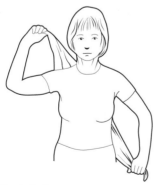

Back drying
Using a towel, practise a back drying movement

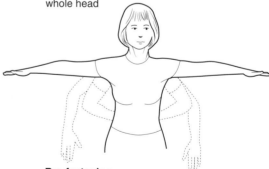

Bra-fastening
Hold your arms out level with your shoulders. Bend at the elbows and slowly reach behind your back to bra level

Figure 19.2   Arm exercises following breast surgery.

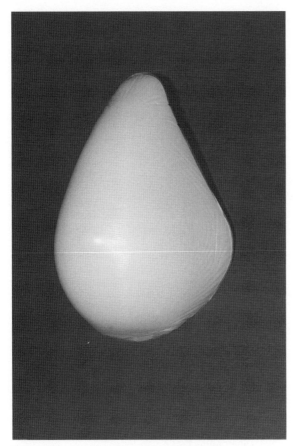

Figure 19.3   External silicone breast prosthesis.

The woman and partner may need reassurance that they can resume a sexual relationship as soon as they wish.

SUPPORT FOR THE FAMILY

This is also a very traumatic time for a partner and family. It is difficult to see someone you love suffering. The partner and family should be encouraged to take part in the care and be present at consultations. Breast Cancer Care provides a helpline for partners, so this information should be made available (see Useful addresses section).

EXAMPLE OF A NURSING CARE PLAN

Ann is a 58-year-old married woman who was referred to the breast unit by her GP after she had found a lump in her left breast. She was naturally very anxious, as her mother had died from breast cancer at the age

of 60. Unfortunately, the mammogram and the fine-needle aspiration confirmed this lump to be a breast cancer.

Ann and her husband were seen by the consultant surgeon and the Breast Care Nurse, who discussed the possible treatment options. They were given time to go away and consider these options. They returned to see the Breast Care Nurse 3 days later for the results of the staging tests, which were normal. Ann and her husband had decided that a mastectomy would be the best option for them, as Ann felt she would constantly worry about the cancer returning in that breast.

The care plan (Table 19.4) uses the Roper, Logan and Tierney model (Roper et al, 1996). It looks only at the specific nursing care for a patient undergoing a mastectomy.

DISCHARGE PLANNING AND ADVICE

Going home is going to be greeted with some pleasure but it also instils some fear into the woman, as she may feel alone and vulnerable. Her home situation should be assessed to see if any other services are required, e.g. home help.

Advice should be given on resuming normal activities. Only light housework should be undertaken for the first 4–6 weeks, until full arm movement has returned. It is advisable not to lift heavy objects with the affected arm, indefinitely. Driving can be resumed normally after 4–6 weeks, once the woman has resumed full arm movement and feels she can safely stop the car in an emergency. The woman should seek advice from her surgeon regarding resumption of sporting activities.

Information regarding voluntary organizations, e.g. Breast Cancer Care and BACUP (see Useful addresses section), should be given to the woman so she has someone she can contact if she needs to talk to someone, or to receive added written information. If a Breast Care Nurse is in post, the woman should have her contact number so she can call the nurse if she has a problem. It is, however, important to return some control to the woman, so she can develop her own coping mechanisms and not become too reliant on the Breast Care Nurse or voluntary organizations.

A follow-up appointment should be made for the following week after discharge home, so the wound can be checked and the pathology result can be given to the woman. Further treatment can then be discussed. The woman should be reassured that she will have regular follow-up appointments. The follow-up policy will vary between breast units, but on average it is usually 3-monthly for 1 year, 6-monthly until 5 years when the patient is discharged.

Table 19.4   A nursing care plan for a patient undergoing surgery for breast cancer, using the Roper, Logan and Tierney model (1996)

Assessment/ usual routine	Patient's problem	Goal	Nursing action	Evaluation
Maintaining a safe environment				
Ann's skin is healthy and intact	Potential wound infection following surgery	To prevent infection	Use an aseptic technique when dealing with the dressing and caring for the Redivac drains Record temperature 4 hourly Take the dressing down after 24 h Observe the wound for signs of infection and swelling	Ann remained apyrexial, and the wound healed well with no sign of infection
	Potential development of both seroma and haematoma formation	To minimize the risk of seroma and haematoma	Check drains for patency and measure the amount of drainage every $\frac{1}{4}$ hour for the first hour and then, if satisfactory, hourly for 24 h and thereafter twice daily	The drain remained patent and the loss was within normal limits
			Change bottle daily and record the output accurately every 24 h	The bottle was changed daily and the amount recorded
			Remove the drain on surgeon's instruction, usually when drainage under 50 mL in 24 h Offer oral analgesics prior to removal	The drain was removed 6 days postoperatively
Communication				
Ann settled into the ward well and chatted to the other women She became tearful when talking about losing her breast	Anxiety and fear about losing her breast	For Ann to be able to talk about her breast loss without being tearful	Refer to the Breast Care Nurse Allow Ann to express her feelings Offer Ann the opportunity to see photographs of mastectomy scars Provide written information Explain what to expect postoperatively	Postoperatively, Ann was much less tearful and talked to other patients about her operation
Ann expressed concern about her two daughters developing breast cancer	Fear of her daughters developing breast cancer	To be able to put her fears into perspective and to feel something is being done for her daughters	Give advice on how her daughters can be referred to a family history clinic Provide information on breast awareness	Ann's daughters had both visited their GPs, who had referred them both to family history clinics. Ann felt more positive that something was being done
Mobilization				
Ann is a very active woman who usually	Potential risk of a stiff shoulder due	To prevent a frozen shoulder	Refer to a physiotherapist for arm exercises	At discharge Ann had a good range of

(Continued)

Table 19.4 (*Continued*)

Assessment/ usual routine	Patient's problem	Goal	Nursing action	Evaluation
does all the housework with little help from the family	to axillary surgery		Encourage the use of the affected arm Encourage the family to help with the housework	movement in her arm and was encouraged to continue the exercises at home
	Potential risk of developing lymphoedema due to axillary surgery Pain due to surgery	To reduce the risk of developing lymphoedema To be pain free, or reduce pain, to allow Ann to mobilize and be comfortable and to be able perform her exercises	Give written information regarding arm care (see Box 19.1) Administer regular analgesics orally once tolerating fluids Rest affected arm on a pillow when in bed or sitting in a chair	The written information reassured Ann, and made her less anxious Ann mobilized well postoperatively and was able to perform her exercises twice a day. Her pain was well controlled with regular Co-dydramol
Work and play Ann works full time as a secretary for an accountancy firm. The firm is having some financial problems and there have been some redundancies	Ann is worried she may lose her job due to her sick leave and is considering early retirement	To return to work as soon as she is able	Encourage Ann to express her fears Refer to a social worker	The surgeon wrote a supportive letter to her boss, who in fact was very supportive and reassured Ann her job was safe
Ann attends a weekly water aerobic class	Ann is concerned the other women will stare at her	To encourage Ann to return to the class	Refer Ann to the Breast Care Nurse for advice regarding swimwear and prosthetics	As yet Ann had not returned to the class but had bought a new swimming costume
Expressing sexuality Ann and her husband have been married for 24 years. They still enjoy a sexual relationship	Ann fears Paul will not want to touch her	To resume normal sexual relations	Encourage Paul to be involved with Ann's care Inform them of the availability of counselling	At her 6-week follow-up, Ann informed the Breast Care Nurse that Paul had been supportive and they had kissed and cuddled but had not had sexual intercourse Ann felt this would come in time
	Fear of appearing different and people noticing her breast loss	To feel confident about her body image	Encourage Ann to look and touch the scar and for Paul to be present Refer to the Breast Care Nurse for fitting of a temporary prosthesis Encourage Ann to wear her own clothes Advise Ann about voluntary organizations, e.g. Breast Cancer Care Discuss the possibility of breast reconstruction	Ann left the ward wearing the same clothes she wore on admission and felt confident. An appointment had been made for fitting a permanent prosthesis

Table 19.4 (Continued)

Assessment/ usual routine	Patient's problem	Goal	Nursing action	Evaluation
Dying Devastated by the diagnosis of breast cancer, as she feels so well	Fear of dying	For Ann to have a realistic outlook	Allow Ann to express her fears and to correct any overly pessimistic views Explain more will be known once the histology result is available Explain the follow-up procedure Encourage Ann to plan for the future Refer to a counsellor if appropriate	Ann still has a fear of dying and leaving her family behind Ann was referred to a counsellor, who is exploring this fear further with her

CONCLUSION

Caring for women undergoing breast surgery is a very rewarding and challenging experience. It not only gives you the skill to look after a surgical patient but it also has many psychosocial issues involved, which adds another dimension. Any surgery to the breast may cause fear, anxiety and a fear of an altered body image. If the nurse can treat the woman with sensitivity and understanding, it can help to make the whole experience less traumatic.

Summary of key points

■ Breast cancer is a common problem affecting 1 in 9 women in the UK.

■ All women who find a lump will fear breast cancer.

■ All women should be treated in a specialist breast unit.

■ It is important to consider physical, social and psychological needs of patients undergoing breast surgery.

■ All women who have breast cancer should have access to a Breast Care Nurse.

■ Women should be encouraged to be breast aware.

Useful addresses

Breast Cancer Care
Kiln House
210 New Kings Road
London SW6 4NZ
Telephone: 020 7384 2984 (Admin.) Helpline: 0808 800 6000
http://www.breastcancercare.org.uk (accessed 14 April 2004)

Breast Care Campaign
1 St Mary Abbots Place
London W8 6LS

CancerBACUP
3 Bath Place
Rivington Street
London EC2A 3JR
Telephone: 020 7696 9003
http://www.cancerbacup.org.uk (accessed 14 April 2004)

Cancerlink
17 Britannia Street
London WC1X 9JN
Telephone: 020 7833 2818

References

Austoker, J. (1990) *Breast Cancer Screening*. Oxford: Cancer Research Campaign, NHS Breast Screening Programme.

Badger, C. (1996) The management of lymphoedema. In: Denton S (ed.) *Breast Care Nursing*. London: Chapman & Hall.

Badwe, R., Gregory, W., Chaudary, M., et al (1991) Timing of surgery during menstrual cycle and survival of pre-menopausal women with operable breast cancer. *Lancet* 337(8752): 1261–1264.

Baum, M., Saunders, C. & Meredith, S. (1994) *Breast Cancer – A Guide for Every Woman*. Oxford: Oxford University Press.

Berger, K. & Bostwick, J. (1994) *A Woman's Decision – Breast Care, Treatment and Reconstruction*. Missouri: Quality Medical Publishing.

Blamey, R. W., Wilson, A. R. M. & Patnick, J. (2000) Screening for breast cancer. In: Dixon M. (ed.) *ABC of Breast Diseases*. London: BMJ Publishing Group.

Breast Surgeons Group of the British Association of Surgical Oncology (1995) Guidelines for surgeons in the management of symptomatic breast disease in the United Kingdom. *European Journal of Surgical Oncology* 21 (Suppl. A): 1–13.

Burton, M. (1995) Guidelines for promoting breast care awareness. *Nursing Times* 91(24): 33–34.

Cancer Relief Macmillan Fund (1994) *Breast Cancer Minimum Standards of Care* [Information leaflet]. London: Cancer Relief Macmillan Fund.

Cancer Research UK (2003) *Breast Cancer Factsheet*. London: Cancer Research UK.

Dixon, J. M. (ed.) (2000) *ABC of Breast Diseases*. London: BMJ Publishing Group.

Dixon, J. M. & Mansel, R. E. (2000) Congential problems and aberrations of normal breast development and involution. In: Dixon, J. M. (ed.) *ABC of Breast Diseases*. London: BMJ Publishing Group.

Dixon, J. M. & Sainsbury, R. (1993) *Diseases of the Breast*. Edinburgh: Churchill Livingstone.

Fallowfield, L. J., Baum, M. & Maguire, G. P. (1986) Effects of breast conservation on psychological morbidity associated with diagnosis and treatment of early breast cancer. *British Medical Journal* 293(6558): 1331–1334.

Harden, J. T. & Girard, N. (1994) Breast reconstruction – using an innovative flap procedure. *AORN Journal* 60(2): 184–191.

Hughes, L. E., Mansel, R. E. & Webster, D. J. T. (1989) *Benign Disorders and Diseases of the Breast*. London: Baillière Tindall.

Independent Review Group Report (1998) *Silocone Gel Breast Implants*. Crown Copyright.

Kissin, M. W., Querchi della Rovere, G., Easton, D. & Westbury, G. (1986) Risk of lymphoedema following the treatment of breast cancer. *British Journal of Surgery* 73(7): 580–584.

Lerberg, L. & Prin, J. (1991) TRAM breast reconstruction. *Plastic Surgical Nursing* 11(2): 58–61.

McArdle, J. M., George, W. D., McArdle, C. S., et al (1996) Psychological support for patients undergoing breast cancer surgery: a randomised study. *British Medical Journal* 312(7034): 813–817.

Maguire, G. P., Lee, E. G., Bevington, D. J., et al (1978) Psychiatric problems in the first year after mastectomy. *British Medical Journal* 1(6118): 963–965.

Maguire, P., Tait, A., Brooke, M., et al (1980) Effect of counselling on the psychiatric morbidity associated with mastectomy. *British Medical Journal* 281(6253): 1454–1456.

Mortimer, P. S. (1990) Investigation and management of lymphoedema. *Vascular Medical Review* 1: 1–20.

Roper, N., Logan, W. W. & Tierney, A. J. (1996) *The Elements of Nursing*, 4th edn. Edinburgh: Churchill Livingstone.

Royal College of Nursing (1995) *Issues in Nursing and Health: Breast Palpation and Breast Awareness – Guidelines for Practice*. London: Royal College of Nursing.

Sacks, N. P. M., Barr, L. C., Allan, S. M. & Baum, M. (1994) The role of axillary dissection in operable breast cancer: an overview. In: Wise, L. & Johnson, H. Jr (eds) *Breast Cancer: Controversies in Management*. Armonk, New York: Futura.

Sainsbury, R. (2002) Early operable breast cancer – locoregional management – surgical management. In: Johnston, S. (ed.) *International Handbook of Breast Cancer*. Haslemere: Euromed Communications.

Sainsbury, R., Anderson, T. J. & Morgan, D. A. L. (2000). In: Dixon, J. M. (ed.) *ABC of Breast Diseases*. London: BMJ Publishing Group.

Watson, M., Denton, S., Baum, M. & Greer, S. (1988) Counselling breast cancer patients: a specialist nurse service. *Counselling Psychology Quarterly* 1(1): 25–34.

Wells, C. A., Ellis, I. O., Zakhour, H. P. & Wilson, A. R. (1994) Guidelines for cytology procedures and reporting of fine needle aspiration of the breast: Cytology Sub-Group of the National Co-ordinate Committee for Breast Cancer Screening Pathology. *Cytopathology* 5: 316–334.

Wilkinson, S. & Forrest, A. P. M. (1985) Fibroadenoma of the breast. *British Journal of Surgery* 72(10): 838–840.

Further reading

Denton, S. (1996) *Breast Cancer Nursing*. London: Chapman & Hall.

Fallowfield, L. & Clark, A. (1991) *Breast Cancer. The Experience of Illness Series*. London: Tavistock/Routledge.

Fentiman, I. (1990) *Detection and Treatment of Early Breast Cancer*. Cambridge: Dunitz.

Gyllenskold, K. (1982) *Breast Cancer: The Psychological Effects of the Disease and Its Treatment*. London: Tavistock.

Harmer, V. (ed) (2003) *Breast Cancer – Nursing Care and Management*. London: Whurr.

Smallwood, J. A. & Taylor, I. (1990) *Benign Breast Disease*. London: Edward Arnold.

Chapter 20

Care of patients requiring vascular surgery

Shelagh Murray

Key objectives of the chapter

On completion of this chapter the reader will be able to:

- describe the basic physiology of circulation

- discuss the process of atherosclerosis as the underlying cause of arterial vascular disease

- describe the nursing assessment of patients with peripheral vascular disease

- list the diagnostic investigations and radiological/surgical interventions required for patients with vascular problems

- describe the care requirements for patients undergoing various types of vascular surgery

- identify the care required for patients following lower limb amputation

- discuss the care required for patients with varicose veins

- describe the challenging and complex care and education required to help reduce risk factors and progression of peripheral vascular disease.

INTRODUCTION

This chapter aims to address the patterns of peripheral vascular disease, investigations, assessment and treatment. In addition, guidelines for diagnostic, pre- and postoperative nursing care will be discussed. This will include management of patients undergoing radiological intervention, arterial reconstruction and venous surgery.

Vascular disease is now a leading cause of death in Western societies. Varicose veins are the commonest disorder presenting to surgeons, and an average of 30% of district nursing time is spent caring for patients with venous leg ulceration (Laing, 1992). Most arterial vascular disease is a consequence of atherosclerosis. Epidemiological findings have shown that the prevalence of peripheral arterial occlusive disease (PAOD) is high and that it also has a high socioeconomic impact (Kannell and McGee, 1985).

Peripheral arterial occlusive disease is a debilitating chronic condition which can significantly affect quality of life, and care of these patients is both challenging and complex. It involves vigilant monitoring, early detection and treatment of the adverse effects of the underlying disease process, as well as knowledge of new developments in diagnostic, radiological and surgical procedures. A major component of care must include measures to reduce the progression of atherosclerosis, which requires a multidisciplinary team approach to achieve successful outcomes.

PHYSIOLOGY OF CIRCULATION

Blood flow is essential to human life, and blood is circulated to all areas of the body by the pumping action of the heart. Blood flows through arteries, veins and capillaries which compose the vascular bed. Arteries and veins have the same structure and are composed of three layers:

1. tunica intima – inner layer of endothelium which provides a smooth passage for blood to flow
2. tunica media – middle layer consisting of muscle and elastic tissue which regulates the diameter of the vessel by dilatation and constriction
3. tunica adventitia – outer layer of fibrous tissue which gives the vessel support to maintain its shape.

THE ARTERIAL SYSTEM

The arterial system is responsible for carrying oxygenated blood and nutrients to the body tissues. Arteries help to regulate the blood pressure by expanding with each surge of blood ejected from the heart and then resuming their original diameter.

The arteries branch off into smaller arterioles, which subdivide into the capillary network. The arterioles differ from the larger arteries in that the tunica media layer consists almost entirely of smooth muscle. Blood has to pass through precapillary sphincters before entering the capillary network. These sphincters work in conjunction with the autonomic nervous system to regulate the perfused capillary bed. The capillaries form a network to link the smallest arterioles to the smallest venules.

Capillaries are the simplest of the blood vessels; their walls consist of a single layer of endothelial cells, which have a semipermeable membrane. The capillaries make up the microcirculation, which allows the exchange of nutrients and waste products from the surrounding tissues. When the smaller arteries constrict, there is an increase in peripheral vascular resistance. This is a measure of the friction between the molecules of the blood and the radius and length of the blood vessel. The smaller the radius of the vessel, the greater the resistance to the flow of blood, so altering blood flow.

During vasodilatation of the artery, there is a decrease in diastolic blood pressure and in peripheral vascular resistance, so increasing blood flow. There is increasing evidence of the important function of the inner layer of the endothelial cells and its role in the development of vascular disease (Jones, 2001).

THE VENOUS SYSTEM

The venous system originates in the capillary beds to form venules, which are responsible for removal of waste products from the capillaries. The venules merge to form veins, which carry deoxygenated blood back to the heart.

VEINS

Veins have thinner walls, less muscle and elastic tissue, and lie closer to the skin surface than do arteries. Veins also differ in that some, mostly in the limbs and especially the lower limbs, have endothelial valves. These permit blood flow only towards the heart, preventing reflux. The return of blood to the heart is therefore reliant on three factors: patency of the veins, valve competence and contracting surrounding muscles (muscle pump). During exercise, the veins in the leg are compressed by the contracted leg muscles, which act as a 'muscle pump', so allowing blood to be returned towards the heart. Blood is returned from the lower limbs to the right side of the heart via the inferior vena cava by the pumping action of the muscles. This pumping action from the calf and foot muscles compresses the deep veins of the legs, which contain one-way valves, and pushes the blood back to the heart, with backflow being prevented by the valves. These muscular contractions allow emptying of the blood from the superficial veins into the deep veins, via the communicating vessels. The venous system of the leg comprises a superficial system in the skin and subcutaneous fat, and a deep system beneath the fascia. The main superficial leg veins are the long and short saphenous, which form a venous network with other perforating veins, which pass through the fascia to join the deep veins. These deep veins run alongside the arteries and have the same names.

LYMPHATIC VESSELS

Lymphatic vessels are thin-walled vessels which arise at the capillaries and also branch into their own circulation. Lymph capillaries, like veins, increase in size and, with the assistance of valves and muscular contractions, transport excess interstitial fluid (lymph) to the venous system via large ducts in the thoracic cavity. Through these ducts, the lymph flows into the inferior vena cava and subclavian vein and finally into the right atrium, where it is recycled into the central circulation. Lymphatic vessels are highly permeable, with large pores which allow the removal of proteins, cellular debris and fat absorption from the intestines. Lymph nodes are situated along the lymphatic system and filter debris from bacteria, viruses and other refuse from lymphatic fluid.

ARTERIAL OCCLUSIVE DISEASE

Arterial occlusive disease may occur suddenly, following an embolus or thrombus, or insidiously, as in atherosclerosis.

ATHEROSCLEROSIS

Atherosclerosis is the underlying cause of peripheral arterial occlusive disease and affects 5–10% of the population over 55 years old. It mainly affects the aorta, arteries to the lower limbs, coronary, carotid and renal arteries. Common sites include the aorto-iliac, femoral, popliteal and tibial arteries.

Atherosclerosis is a process which often begins in childhood and is not, as previously thought, a slowly progressive disease (Libby et al, 1996). Changes within the arterial wall are identified in three stages:

1. stage of fatty, lipid streak formation within the intima
2. stage of fibrous plaque formation in the subintimal layer which extends along the artery walls and then protrudes and narrows the lumen

3. stage of complication – characterized by endothelial ulceration, calcification, activation of platelets and leucocytes, leading to thrombus formation.

The process of atherosclerosis results in the arterial walls becoming thickened and hardened, with loss of elasticity and decreased blood flow. After the age of 30 years old, the atheromatous plaque formations become more pronounced, causing symptoms when the artery lumen becomes narrowed by more than three-quarters (Shah, 1997). This, in turn, may lead to thrombosis or emboli, causing ischaemia and a risk of gangrene.

Aneurysm formation may occur if a section of the artery wall becomes weakened by the spread of plaque, causing a local dilatation of the artery. This can lead to thrombosis and embolism, or the aneurysm may rupture as it grows larger and the blood vessel wall becomes thinner, resulting in severe haemorrhage. Aneurysms can occur throughout the arterial tree; the most commonly affected vessels are the aorta and iliac arteries, followed by the popliteal, femoral and carotid arteries.

Aneurysms are classified as *true* or *false*. A true aneurysm occurs when the artery wall becomes dilated and thin but remains intact (Fig. 20.1(a)–(c)). Thrombi can collect between the layers of artery, causing a local

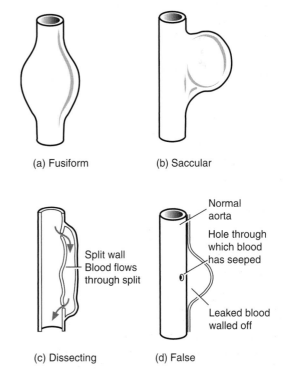

(a) Fusiform   (b) Saccular

(c) Dissecting   (d) False

Split wall
Blood flows
through split

Normal
aorta

Hole through
which blood
has seeped

Leaked blood
walled off

Figure 20.1 Types of aneurysm.

dilatation. A false aneurysm occurs, due to trauma of the three layers of artery wall, which allows blood to leak extravascularly (Fig. 20.1(d)). Clot formation occurs, and the clot becomes surrounded by periarterial connective tissue; blood then passes into the sac as it flows along the lumen of the artery (Greenhalgh, 1990).

RISK FACTORS

Risk factors for PAOD are factors which have been associated with the incidence of the disease but have not necessarily been shown to be a direct cause.

Age and gender

Symptomatic PAOD is commoner in men and also occurs earlier, the incidence being twice as high in men under 60 years old (Kannel et al, 1970). Female sex hormones are thought to account for this difference, as symptomatic disease is more common postmenopause (Sans et al, 1997).

Smoking

It is considered proven that smoking is the most preventable cause of cardiovascular morbidity and mortality. Nicotine and carbon monoxide have been shown to produce endothelial injury, leading to the development of atherosclerotic plaque in the arteries (Powell, 1991). Quitting smoking will reduce the risk of developing PAOD (Bowlin et al, 1994), and studies have shown evidence of reduction in disease progression within 3 months (Seltzer, 1989). Smoking also enhances the effect of other risk factors such as hypertension and hyperlipidaemia (Pasternak et al, 1996). Smoking should be stopped and patients informed of the harmful effects of nicotine on their condition. The majority of smokers with PAOD are nicotine addicts and require counselling and behavioural support therapy, as well as nicotine replacement therapy or bupropion on prescription in order to quit.

Hyperlipidaemia

Hyperlipidaemia and hypercholesterolaemia are recognized risk factors for atherosclerosis. A high dietary intake of saturated fat is known to contribute to a high blood cholesterol, and hyperlipidaemia is known to have a congenital factor (Oliver, 1991). In addition to a healthy low-fat diet, lipid-lowering therapy (statins) improves endothelial function. Irrespective of cholesterol levels, the Heart Protection Study strongly recommends that all patients with PAOD should be treated with a statin to reduce vascular mortality (Collins, 2002). Weight reduction will also benefit obese patients with intermittent claudication, as this reduces the workload on the lower limbs.

Diabetes

Peripheral arterial occlusive disease is a major complication of both insulin dependent and non-insulin dependent diabetes mellitus (Beach et al, 1988). Diabetics are more susceptible to atherosclerosis due to calcification of the medial lining of the arteries (Faris, 1991). Neuropathy is also common, which causes a lack of sensation, making the diabetic prone to trauma, resulting in foot injuries, infections and non-healing ulcers. Diabetic leg ulcers are usually situated on the bony prominences of the feet, resulting in necrotic wounds. Good blood glucose control reduces the risk of small vessel limb disease.

Foot care advice should be given to all patients with arterial occlusive disease, not only diabetics, to help reduce the incidence of injury and followed up with an information leaflet to aid concordance (Ley, 1993). The nurse can help educate the patient by teaching them how to perform self-assessment and foot care (Fig. 20.2). Patients should be instructed to check their feet daily or, if they are unable to do this for themselves, a relative or carer will need to be taught how to do this. The importance of contacting their nurse, doctor, foot clinic/chiropodist immediately if problems occur should be stressed.

Hypertension

Hypertension has been associated as a risk factor with generalized vascular diseases as well as peripheral occlusive disease (Kannel and McGee, 1985). Increased mechanical stress due to higher blood pressure can result in endothelial damage to the artery wall. Screening, advice and treatment to maintain blood pressure below 140/85 mmHg is recommended by the National Service Framework for Coronary Heart Disease (DoH, 2000a). Blood pressure should be taken in both arms on initial assessment. If a higher value is noted of between 10 and 15 mmHg, this may indicate an arterial stenosis on the side of the lower reading.

Hyperhomocysteinaemia

Homocysteine is a byproduct of protein metabolism, and elevated levels are linked to acceleration of atherosclerosis and increase the risk of thrombosis (Boushey et al, 1995). Elevated homocysteine levels should be checked, particularly in patients under 60 years old. Daily supplements of folic acid may help reduce the risk of developing atherosclerotic vascular disease (Hankey and Elkeboom, 1999).

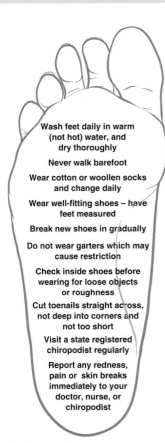

Wash feet daily in warm
(not hot) water, and
dry thoroughly

Never walk barefoot

Wear cotton or woollen socks
and change daily

Wear well-fitting shoes – have
feet measured

Break new shoes in gradually

Do not wear garters which may
cause restriction

Check inside shoes before
wearing for loose objects
or roughness

Cut toenails straight across,
not deep into corners and
not too short

Visit a state registered
chiropodist regularly

Report any redness,
pain or skin breaks
immediately to your
doctor, nurse, or
chiropodist

Figure 20.2   Foot care advice.

Alcohol

Binge drinking should be avoided and drinking kept within recommended safe limits: 21 units for men and 14 units for women a week.

Sedentary lifestyle

Physical inactivity is a major risk factor for cardiovascular disease. Regular exercise combined with weight reduction is associated with lowering cholesterol and blood pressure.

SOCIOECONOMIC FACTORS

Social deprivation also increases risk factors for developing peripheral arterial disease, as patients from lower social classes are more likely to eat an unhealthy diet, exercise less and smoke. Unemployment and high anxiety levels have been found to contribute to development of the disease (Bowlin et al, 1994).

Combination of risk factors

Vascular diseases are generally caused by a combination of risk factors. Obesity and lack of exercise are

other factors linked to its increased risk. For reasons unknown, men are also more prone to all forms of vascular disease, especially aortic aneurysms. However, women's protection diminishes with age. Over the age of 70 years old, the risks are similar for both sexes (Kannel and McGee, 1985).

Antiplatelet agents in risk factor modification

Patients with PAOD are high risk for a heart attack or thrombotic stroke. Therefore, all patients should be prescribed an antiplatelet agent such as aspirin, or clopidogrel, if aspirin cannot be tolerated, for secondary prevention to reduce viscosity of the blood and platelet aggregation.

THE PATIENT WITH CHRONIC ISCHAEMIA

CLINICAL FEATURES

A patient with chronic ischaemia may have minimal symptoms in the early stages or may develop limb pain, ulceration or gangrene. Clinical features of arterial occlusive disease occur when there is partial or complete occlusion of the artery. The primary symptom of PAOD is intermittent claudication. The term 'claudication' derives from the Latin 'claudus', meaning 'lame', which was attributed to the Emperor Claudius who walked with a limp.

Intermittent claudication

Intermittent claudication is pain induced by exercise, experienced in the foot, calf, thigh or buttock, depending on the level of arterial occlusion, when a certain distance is walked. The pain is caused by inadequate blood supply to the muscles and can vary in severity and walking distance. Walking at a brisk pace or on an incline will produce symptoms earlier. Patients frequently refer to their symptoms as an ache, heaviness or dullness of the leg muscles. Intermittent claudication may affect one or both legs, is more common in the calf and is always relieved by rest.

Patients with intermittent claudication may not experience a major handicap to their lifestyle, or their symptoms may even resolve with regular walking exercise. One study found that a patient with intermittent claudication had a 50% chance of symptoms spontaneously improving, a 30% chance of remaining unchanged, with 20% of patients deteriorating (McAllister, 1976). Although some claudicants may initially fear limb loss, only 7 of 100 patients (6 of whom had diabetes) underwent major amputation. If the

---

Box 20.1   Fontaine's classification of ischaemia

- Stage 1: asymptomatic
- Stage 2: intermittent claudication
- Stage 3: severe, persistent rest pain of the foot
- Stage 4: ulceration and/or gangrene

---

condition becomes more severe, it may lead to signs of critical ischaemia such as rest pain, ulcers and possible gangrene. In the 1950s, Fontaine classified the signs and symptoms of chronic leg ischaemia into four stages (Box 20.1). It is therefore important that patients with intermittent claudication modify their risk factors at an early stage to help prevent disease progression and also to reduce their chance of suffering a heart attack or stroke.

Rest pain

Rest pain is a chronic pain described as 'associated with a chronic pathological process which causes continuous pain' (Bonica 1990, cited in Twycross, 1994:17). As the disease progresses, the blood flow to the leg is now so reduced that pain occurs while resting rather than induced by exercise. Patients with ischaemic rest pain initially awake at night with pain in the foot and toes. Pain is continually present when the patient is immobile and prevents sleep occurring, causing rapid deterioration in the patient's morale. Temporary relief may be gained by hanging the limb out of bed or by sleeping in an armchair with the foot down.

Ulceration and/or gangrene

Arterial disease may ultimately result in tissue loss of the toes, foot or leg. Critical leg ischaemia is a condition which endangers the distal part of the limb, and there is a high risk that the patient will require toe or limb amputation. The symptoms and signs specified in the 2nd European Consensus Document on Critical Leg Ischaemia (European Working Group, 1991) are:

- persistently recurring rest pain requiring regular adequate analgesics for more than 2 weeks **or**
- ulceration or gangrene of the foot or toes **plus**
- ankle systolic pressure ≤ 50 mmHg in non-diabetics
- toe systolic pressure ≤ 30 mmHg in diabetics.

INVESTIGATIONS

A full medical history is taken, and a clinical examination performed, which will include an electrocardiogram (ECG) to determine cardiac function. An echocardiogram may be undertaken if surgical treatment is necessary. Full blood count, clotting screen, urea and electrolytes, blood glucose, HbA1c in diabetics and lipid screening will also be required, as well as routine urinalysis. Thrombophilia screen and homocysteine levels should also be undertaken in younger (<60 years old) patients. Chest X-ray and lung function tests are performed to identify potential respiratory problems prior to surgical intervention.

The limbs are observed for warmth, colour, sensation, movement and any ulceration or gangrenous changes (Figs 20.3(a)–(d)). Pallor, dusky erythema or cyanosis may be present, and absent or reduced peripheral pulses. Thin, shiny atrophic skin, thick brittle nails and hair loss on the limb may indicate poor tissue nutrition due to reduced blood supply. Capillary refill in the nails indicates perfusion time in the capillary beds; normal refill should occur within 3 seconds. The skin is prone to breakdown, especially from trauma. Tissue loss or gangrene may also be present over high areas of pressure such as metatarsal heads, dorsum of the foot and particularly the heels.

Peripheral pulses

Limb pulses are palpated to assess the adequacy and volume of the blood supply at femoral, popliteal, posterior tibial and pedal pulse sites (Fig. 20.4). The absence of pulses or a weak pulse may determine the presence of arterial disease, and require confirmation by Doppler ultrasound (Moffatt et al, 1994).

The presence of bruits (abnormal 'whooshing' sounds or murmurs) may be heard with a stethoscope. This turbulent flow, heard over major arteries, may be significant in carotid vessels which are narrowed due to atherosclerosis.

Doppler ultrasound

Doppler ultrasound is a practical non-invasive test using ultrasonic high-frequency sounds emitted from a hand-held transducer probe. It is used to assess the arterial blood supply to the lower limb by listening to the arterial sounds, and for measuring the ankle/brachial systolic pressure ratio, to aid diagnosis and detect the degree of arterial insufficiency. Doppler ultrasound can also be used to ascertain the presence of pedal pulses following intervention such as angioplasty, thrombolysis or reconstructive bypass surgery.

The highest systolic pressure in the arm at the brachial artery is compared with the highest systolic pressure in the ankle at the dorsalis pedis and the posterior tibial artery, to give an ankle–brachial pressure index:

$$ABPI = \frac{\text{highest systolic ankle pressure (mmHg)}}{\text{highest systolic arm pressure (mmHg)}}$$

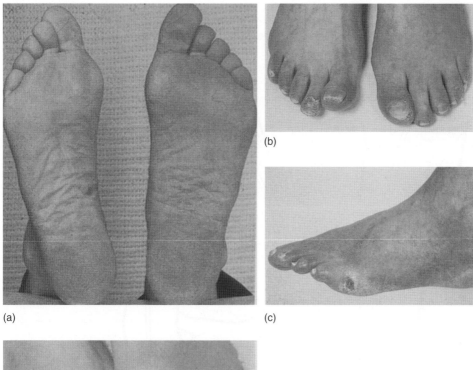

(a)

(b)

(c)

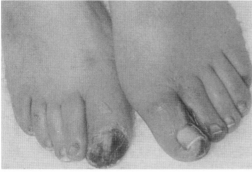

(d)

Figure 20.3 Features of critical leg ischaemia. (a) Ischaemic pallor of the sole of the foot. (b) Both feet show changes of ischaemic disease, such as hair loss, skin coarsening and ulceration. (c) Thinning and shininess of the skin around the toes, with ulceration at a pressure point. (d) Patient presenting with rest pain in both feet and gangrenous toes. (Reproduced with kind permission from Bettie Walker, on behalf of William F. Walker, from Walker (1988).)

- normal ABPI ≥1.00
- ABPI for patients with claudication = 0.5–0.9
- ABPI for patients with rest pain and critical leg ischaemia ≤0.5.

The lower the ABPI, the greater the arterial impairment. However, false high readings may be obtained in patients with diabetes, atherosclerosis and chronic renal disease as a result of calcification of the arteries, which means the sphygmomanometer cuff cannot fully compress the hardened arteries.

ABPI is also known to be a predictor of survival in vascular patients; the lower the ABPI, the higher the risk of vascular mortality (McDermott et al, 1994).

Toe pressures

Toe pressures can be performed to assess arterial blood flow in diabetics by using photoplethysmography (PPG). A special small occlusion cuff is attached to the 1st toe, and the PPG sensor uses changes in infrared light to detect blood flow. This technique is feasible because distal pedal vessels in diabetics are less calcified and incompressible than ankle vessels.

Treadmill assessment

A treadmill is useful in assessing exercise tolerance in patients with intermittent claudication. The patient is asked to walk on the treadmill until they experience

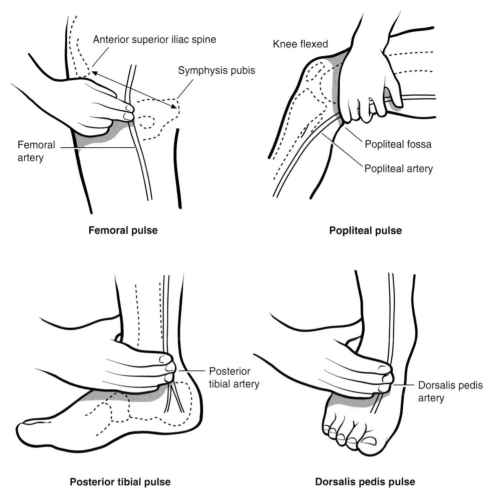

Figure 20.4 Palpation of arterial pulses in lower limb.

claudication pain, and the distance and time is noted. This test can also be combined with a pre- and post-exercise Doppler assessment of the ABPI to confirm diagnosis in patients with a normal resting ABPI. A significant drop in the ABPI after a treadmill test may indicate an arterial occlusion.

Colour duplex scan

Duplex ultrasonic scanning of the arterial tree with colour flow imaging is a non-invasive technique used to provide more accurate diagnosis of stenosis or occlusion from the aorta to the tibial vessels. The scan demonstrates the direction of arterial or venous blood flow using an ultrasonic probe and displays it as a colour. An increase in velocity of the flow and colour change occur where there is a stenosis. It is usually possible to detect whether a lesion is suitable for balloon angioplasty

and, in most centres, duplex scanning has replaced the need for more invasive diagnostic angiography.

Computerized tomography

Computerized tomography (CT) scanning uses a rotating X-ray source which allows individual slices to be obtained. Spiral CT can also be used and allows continuous rotation while the patient moves through the X-ray beam. A CT scan is useful in the diagnosis of aortic aneurysms, but the contrast medium used can cause problems in patients with impaired renal function.

Magnetic resonance angiography

Magnetic resonance angiography (MRA) is a non-invasive scan. This technique is particularly useful to more accurately detect the size and extent of atheromatous lesions and where patients may be at risk from invasive angiography. MRA is also useful to screen patients for an aortic aneurysm.

Angiography

A radio-opaque contrast medium is injected into an appropriate artery, and a series of X-rays is taken of the arteries, demonstrating filling of the vessels and any narrowing or stenosis. A femoral artery approach is normally used to investigate lower limb arteries.

Angiography is usually performed under a local anaesthetic and can be undertaken on a day case basis, depending on the age, social circumstances and clinical condition of the patient. Sedation or general anaesthesia may occasionally be required for very anxious patients. Digital subtraction angiography (DSA) allows greater clarity of the arteries (Belli and Buckenham, 1995). This is a computerized method of angiography without background information, e.g. bones and bowel.

Specific preparation of the patient prior to angiography
- The patient should be fully informed of the length of the procedure and that the injection of dye causes a sensation of heat and some discomfort.
- Fasting is not required prior to angiography. The bladder should be emptied beforehand, as the patient needs to lie very still during angiography.
- Intravenous prophylactic antibiotics will need to be given immediately prior to the procedure in patients with previous synthetic bypass grafts or stents to prevent infection.

Aftercare
- Patients are at risk from haemorrhage, haematoma formation and development of arterial occlusion. Following the procedure, pressure is applied to the puncture site to prevent haemorrhage when the catheter has been removed.
- The patient should be nursed relatively flat in bed and instructed to keep the affected limb straight for 4–6 hours post procedure, depending on the catheter size used.
- Observations of pulse and blood pressure:
  - ¼ hourly for 1 hour
  - ½ hourly for 2 hours
  - hourly for 1 hour
  - 4 hourly overnight (non-day care patients).
- Observation of foot pulse, colour, temperature, limb movement and sensation should also be made at these times and the puncture site carefully monitored for haemorrhage or signs of haematoma formation. The patient should be informed to call the nurse immediately if any bleeding occurs at the puncture site.

- The patient should be encouraged to drink at least 2 litres of fluid in order to flush out the contrast medium from the kidneys.

NURSING ASSESSMENT OF PATIENTS WITH PERIPHERAL VASCULAR DISEASE

Patients admitted to hospital will be experiencing either moderate or severe problems which may interfere with their activities of daily living. The impact of the varying stages of the disease is demonstrated within the framework of the Activities of Living model of nursing of Roper, Logan and Tierney (Roper et al, 1981). A functional assessment to identify the patient's self-care ability and lifestyle handicap is undertaken. Guidelines for these stages of the nursing process together with planning and implementing care have been included under each activity.

MAINTAINING A SAFE ENVIRONMENT

There is a potential risk of further deterioration in the blood flow to the limbs following admission. Patients with advanced arterial insufficiency are also at risk of developing breaks/ulceration to the skin's integrity, especially the sacrum and heels (Fig. 20.5). This risk is significantly increased in patients with severe ischaemic rest pain who have been immobile, and may also have been sleeping in an armchair at night to try to relieve their pain.

Initial limb assessment should be documented, and regular observations recorded for patients with severe ischaemia:

- The colour, warmth, sensation and movement of both limbs should be compared.
- The dorsalis pedis and posterior tibial pulses should be checked with a Doppler and compared with those in the other limb.

A risk assessment of the patient's skin should be undertaken within 6 hours of admission (NICE, 2001), paying particular attention to the lower limbs. The skin should be observed for dryness, infection, oedema, ulceration and gangrenous changes. Detection of any breaks or abnormalities should be reported and documented on a wound assessment chart. Skin ulceration is more commonly found on the toes, malleoli and heels in patients with advanced disease.

A reliable and valid assessment tool should be used to determine the patient's risk of developing pressure ulcers, so that an appropriate pressure-relieving mattress, seating and heel protection pads can be provided (Waterlow, 1988). Patients with rest pain may well

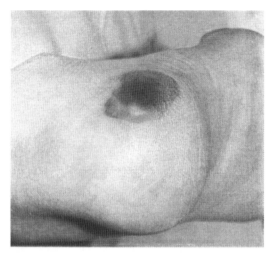

Figure 20.5   *Pressure ulceration and gangrene of heel.*

present with a high-risk score on admission. Chair nursing should be kept to a minimum and pain relief regularly reassessed to allow the patient to sleep in bed.

All patients presenting with leg ulcers must undergo a full holistic assessment and Doppler assessment to help determine the underlying aetiology of the ulcers.

COMMUNICATION

Nursing assessment should consider patients' psycho-social needs and also take account of their spiritual and ethnic requirements. Any social service requirements for home support on discharge, or advice regarding benefit/mobility allowances should be assessed and communicated to the appropriate members of the multidisciplinary team.

Patients may have fears and anxieties about any forthcoming procedures required. They may also experience varying degrees of pain which may not be adequately communicated to the nurse. Patients with severe ischaemia may also fear limb loss as a possible outcome. Social isolation is a common problem in patients with severe disease affecting their quality of life. The nurse should be aware of factors such as poor mobility, pain, smoking and drinking habits, which can contribute to a patient's isolation.

Allowing time and privacy for open discussion and providing sufficient information/explanation of proposed procedures will help to allay anxieties. It will also assist patients to make choices about their care and consider any alternatives of treatments. Evaluation of the patient's understanding of their condition is vital to ensuring informed consent and to facilitate active involvement in care and recovery. Verbal information should be reinforced where possible with leaflets on various aspects of vascular conditions and treatments.

BREATHING

Breathing may not be compromised. However, these patients are often heavy lifelong smokers, and this factor, together with restricted mobility in some, will increase the risk of developing chest infections. An increase in respiratory rate and/or production of sputum, as well as any shortness of breath on exertion, should be monitored. Baseline respiratory rate and oxygen saturation levels should be documented.

EATING AND DRINKING

Nutritional and hydration status is a high priority in assessment of vascular patients. A baseline admission weight and body mass index (BMI) should be documented. The debilitating effects of severe rest pain and consequent reduced mobility may have resulted in the patient's relying on convenience snacks at home. Heavy smokers may also have had appetite suppression, and alcohol intake should be assessed.

Patients with diabetes may require review of their dietary intake, as poorly controlled diabetes will escalate the onset of foot complications and delay postoperative wound healing. Patients who have raised blood cholesterol may also require review of their dietary intake of fat.

A full nutritional assessment by the dietitian will be needed if malnutrition is suspected, as problems such as electrolyte imbalance, delayed wound healing and sepsis can influence the morbidity and mortality of vascular patients.

ELIMINATING

Poor mobility due to severe ischaemia may prevent the patient from reaching the toilet. Routine urinalysis should be performed to check for glucose, ketones and protein. Urine output should be monitored as vascular patients frequently have renal impairment. Constipation may arise in patients with ischaemic pain having regular analgesics, particularly morphine; therefore an aperient should always be prescribed.

DRESSING AND CLEANSING

Again, limited mobility and pain may have affected the patient's ability to wash and dress independently.

CONTROLLING BODY TEMPERATURE

Temperature on admission should be checked, as elderly patients living alone who have a critically ischaemic limb may have hypothermia. Pyrexia may be an indication of chest or wound infection due to limb ulceration or cellulitis.

MOBILIZING

Pain is the main factor in reducing the patient's mobility; this is affected to a lesser or greater degree by the extent of the arterial occlusion.

Patients experiencing claudication pain on walking may have only minimal inconvenience to their normal mobility and lifestyle, whereas those affected by rest pain due to severe arterial occlusion and/or ulceration may be totally unable to bear weight on the affected leg.

The following information needs to be obtained during assessment:

- Is the pain related to exercise and is it relieved by resting?
- Does the pain occur in the foot, calf, thigh or buttock on walking, and how far can the patient walk before experiencing pain?
- Does the pain occur at rest and prevent the patient from sleeping at night?
- How has the pain been managed and what analgesics are taken?
- Has the patient had any problems with walking, and have walking aids been required?

Visual pain analogue assessment tools are essential to help establish the severity and type of pain, its effect on the patient and the effectiveness of prescribed analgesics.

Ensure that footwear is appropriate and does not cause undue pressure. This is especially important for diabetic patients, where there is an increased risk due to neuropathy. Special surgical shoes are available from appliances to help accommodate wound dressings to the foot.

WORKING AND PLAYING

Occupation or hobbies can inevitably be affected in patients with intermittent claudication, whereas reading or watching television may become a strain for those with rest pain.

SEXUALITY

A male patient with claudication may suffer impotence due to internal iliac artery occlusion, and this may also be a complication following surgical repair of an abdominal aortic aneurysm.

SLEEPING

Sleep patterns are often disturbed by severe limb pain, either by waking the patient suddenly or by preventing sleep occurring. Hanging the affected limb out of bed, or sleeping in an armchair with feet down may provide temporary pain relief but will increase leg oedema.

DYING

Some patients may express anxieties regarding proposed major surgery which may be necessary to save a critically ischaemic limb, prevent stroke or rupture of an aortic aneurysm.

MANAGEMENT OF THE PATIENT WITH CHRONIC LIMB ISCHAEMIA

There are no immediate plans for a specific National Service Framework for peripheral vascular disease; however, government initiatives have been instrumental in targeting priority areas which include heart attack, stroke prevention and diabetes (DoH, 1999, 2000a, 2000b, 2001a, 2001b). Prevention and reduction of peripheral vascular disease requires the same high profile afforded to other conditions which share similar risk factors, such as coronary artery disease and stroke. Likewise, equal emphasis for reducing the incidence of disease progression and limb amputation in patients with arterial disease, as given to diabetics, should be encouraged amongst all healthcare professionals.

Management and treatment of patients with arterial occlusive disease is based on each patient's overall health condition, age, lifestyle impairment and the severity of the disease. These factors, along with the feasibility of the procedure, will influence the decision for either radiological intervention such as angioplasty or arterial reconstructive surgery to restore blood flow. Arterial occlusive disease rarely presents in isolation, and patients will often have accompanying coronary, cerebrovascular and renal disease which must also be taken into account in their management.

Nursing this patient group is therefore complex, because of their challenging health needs. Patients may have experienced intermittent claudication and walking restrictions for many years and may have high anxiety levels about their health outcomes. Many may still be breadwinners for their family or be carers for dependent relatives. Lifestyle aspects which probably contributed to their present health problems often die hard. Advances in radiological technology and surgical techniques in the last two decades have significantly improved the prognosis for these patients, who would otherwise have faced primary amputation to alleviate rest pain and ulceration. Reconstructive bypass surgery is normally only considered for patients with critical leg ischaemia when the occluded vessel is not amenable to less-invasive procedures such as angioplasty.

MANAGEMENT OF THE PATIENT WITH INTERMITTENT CLAUDICATION

Patients with intermittent claudication need to adapt their lifestyles to comply with the risk factor modifications previously discussed. Social, environmental and lifestyle factors are known to be significant risk factors, independent of others, for development of the disease in men (Bowlin et al, 1994). Management requires an individualized and holistic approach, focusing on health education, physical and psychosocial needs. Concordance and control may depend upon a patient's social and cultural situation, which will influence their health behaviour (Ewles and Simnett, 1995).

If claudication is mild or moderate and does not severely impair the patient's lifestyle, the first line in management is now exercise and best medical therapy/risk factor modification. Intervention such as angioplasty may be indicated for more moderate to severe claudication; however, the benefits remain controversial where best medical therapy and exercise produce similar outcomes (Perkins et al, 1995).

Lifestyle and risk factor management in intermittent claudication

The role of the nurse in providing holistic care is of vital importance, as promoting a healthy lifestyle will enable patients to make lifestyle choices to try to improve their own health and quality of life. Influencing lifelong health beliefs, smoking, eating and exercise habits in this patient group provides a challenge to the nurse. The nurse, whether a novice ward nurse or an experienced nurse specialist running nurse-led services, will need to gain the patient's active participation in decision-making and actions in order to bring about change to slow disease progression. Factors affecting adherence and understanding of a patient's self-motivation are essential in effecting changed behaviour. Control of this chronic condition and prevention of complications will depend on the careful assessment of the patient's risk factors as discussed earlier, and strategies to manage them, especially smoking.

Medication concordance is vital, and patients should be advised of the importance of taking medications regularly, such as antihypertensives and diabetic, statin and antiplatelet therapy. The latter medication, such as aspirin, reduces the frequency of thrombotic events in peripheral arteries and reduces overall cardiovascular mortality in claudicants by reducing blood viscosity (Antithrombotic Trialists Collaboration, 2002).

Stress management is also important, as the body's response to life pressures and anxieties is to release adrenaline (epinephrine), which increases the heart rate, blood glucose and cholesterol levels. Consequently, the body becomes stressed, resulting in hypertension, which eventually contributes to the development of atherosclerosis. Teaching the patient stress management strategies, such as relaxation techniques, taking regular exercise and avoiding excessive alcohol or food consumption, is equally important.

Exercise therapy for intermittent claudication

Exercise is the mainstay of treatment for patients with claudication and has been shown to improve pain-free walking distance (Hiatt et al, 1991; Lungren et al, 1988; Perkins et al, 1995). It aids in the development of collateral circulation, which may help prevent ischaemia in the affected leg. The Cochrane Review recommends exercise as a key component of management of intermittent claudication (Leng et al, 2002). However, it has yet to be established what an ideal exercise programme should be, although supervised, structured programmes are more beneficial (Cheetham et al, 2004). In addition, walking exercise of 30 minutes at least 3 times a week, and walking to near-maximal pain, will achieve greatest improvement in patients (Gardner and Poehlman, 1995).

ENDOVASCULAR INTERVENTION

Percutaneous transluminal angioplasty

Percutaneous transluminal angioplasty (PTA) has become an established treatment for moderate to severe claudication, limb-threatening disease with ischaemic rest pain and to help facilitate healing of ischaemic ulcers. Angioplasty is performed under local anaesthesia and therefore carries a lower overall risk than surgery. Recent advances in technique have made day case angioplasties possible in some centres for patients with intermittent claudication (Cleveland et al, 2002).

Short stenosis or occlusion of iliac, femoral and popliteal arteries can be effectively treated by angioplasty. The procedure involves the insertion of a balloon catheter, which is passed into the lumen of the vessel, usually via the femoral artery, under local anaesthesia. The catheter is advanced to the site of the atheromatous plaque, and the balloon inflated, dilating the stricture, and hence improving the patency of the lumen of the vessel (Fig. 20.6(a)).

Other techniques such as atherectomy and insertion of stents can be combined with angioplasty. Atherectomy (Fig. 20.6(b)) uses high-speed revolving cutters to cut and remove an obstructing thrombus, whereas expandable metal stents can be inserted to prevent restenosis at the angioplasty site (Fig. 20.6(c)).

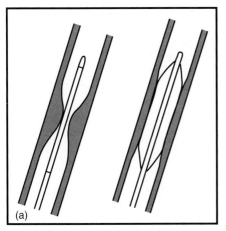

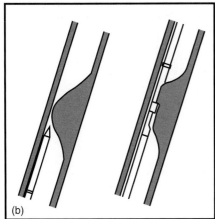

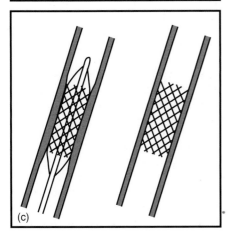

Figure 20.6   (a) Percutaneous transluminal angioplasty. (b) Atherectomy. (c) Stent insertion.

Preparation of the patient prior to percutaneous transluminal angioplasty

- Nursing care and preparation are similar to that provided prior to angiography, except that the patient should be fasted for 2–3 hours prior to the procedure in case complications arise, such as thrombosis/embolus or rupture of the vessel wall, which will require surgical intervention.

- During angioplasty, patients will be required to lie still for a long period of time and therefore will require pressure-relieving aids to prevent skin breakdown of their sacrum and heels if they have severe limb-threatening disease. Pressure on the heel, even for a short time while lying on the X-ray table, can lead to pressure ulceration and necrosis.

Aftercare

- Aftercare is also similar to that following angiography. However, the nurse must be aware of the increased risk of haemorrhage, haematoma or thrombosis, and should report any such occurrences immediately. Pedal pulses should ideally be located using the Doppler ultrasound probe.

- Continued pressure relief for sacrum and heels will be required throughout the period of bedrest in high-risk patients.

- Health education advice should be reinforced before the patient is discharged, and if necessary, advice given for self-referral to a Stop Smoking Clinic. Walking exercise should be encouraged to develop collateral circulation.

RECONSTRUCTIVE BYPASS SURGERY

Patients with ischaemic rest pain, ulceration or gangrenous lesions will require surgical intervention if less-invasive treatment is not possible, since, if left untreated, most patients with critical ischaemia will eventually require amputation.

Arterial reconstructive surgery can enhance the quality of life for patients with limb-threatening disease, although outcomes can be less predictable. It is therefore essential to be aware of the patients' expectations, as if surgical revascularisation fails an amputation will be necessary.

Revascularization methods depend on the location and extent of the stenosis/occlusion (Fig. 20.7). Restoring blood flow entails bypassing the stenosed or occluded artery using synthetic graft material or the patient's own long saphenous vein. Vein grafts are the preferred conduit as they have a superior patency rate and decrease the risk of infection (Beard and Gaines, 2001). Patency rates for prosthetic grafts used in narrower more distal arteries in the legs are poor. The operative procedure involves anastomosis of the graft from an area above to an area below the diseased vessel. A vein harvested from the arm can also be used if the leg veins are unsuitable. Due to the presence of

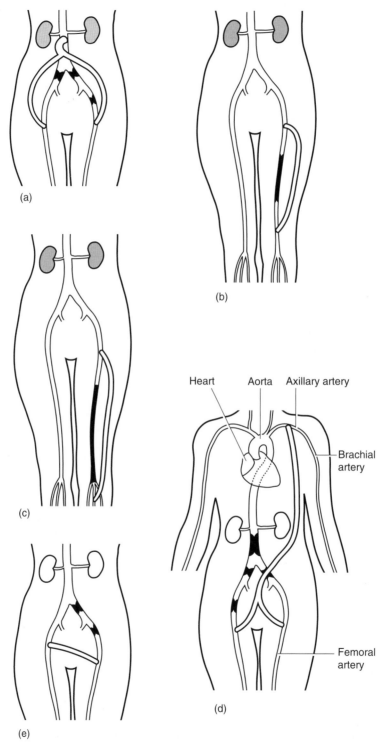

Figure 20.7   Examples of types of reconstructive surgery and types of occlusions: (a) aorto-bifemoral graft; (b) femoro-popliteal bypass; (c) femoro-distal bypass; (d) axillo-bifemoral graft; (e) femoro-femoral crossover graft.

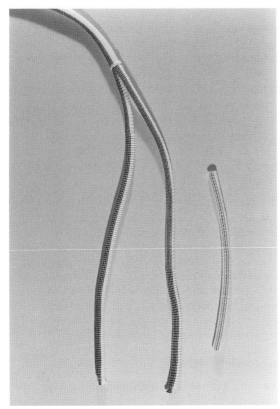

Figure 20.8 Examples of straight and bifurcated axillo-bifemoral PTFE grafts.

valves, the vein is either reversed before insertion, to enable correct direction of blood flow, or the valves are destroyed and the vein left *in situ*. Synthetic grafts made from polytetrafluoroethylene (PTFE) are now commonly used (Fig. 20.8).

Endarterectomy

This is the coring out of the atheromatous plug using a ring stripper inserted into the artery lumen; it is now more commonly used for carotid artery stenosis.

Aorto-bifemoral bypass

This bypass extends from the distal aorta to the common femoral arteries and is performed for stenosis or occlusion of the aorta or iliac vessels, using synthetic graft material. Patients with aorto-iliac disease will often present with bilateral buttock/hip claudication and impotence.

Femoro-popliteal bypass

This bypass is performed for occlusion in the superficial femoral artery.

Femoro-distal artery bypass graft

This bypass is performed for occlusion in distal vessels in patients with severe critical ischaemia who may have accompanying gangrenous lesions in the foot. The graft extends from the femoral artery to either the peroneal or tibial artery in the leg or foot. Distal bypass surgery can be a lengthy and clinically demanding procedure that may also require surgical debridement of gangrenous foot lesions at the end of the arterial reconstruction.

Extra-anatomical bypass graft

Extra-anatomical grafts may be considered for patients who are too unfit for major abdominal surgery and are at risk of limb amputation for critical ischaemia. These synthetic grafts are routed extraperitoneally through subcutaneous tissue to bypass the diseased vessel. The axillary and femoral arteries lie close to the skin surface, making the procedure more rapid and straightforward than more invasive bypassing. Although this type of bypass is less traumatic for patients, the patency rates are much lower than for aorto-iliac reconstructions (Beard, 2000).

Axillo-bifemoral graft

This graft is performed for aorto-iliac occlusion.

Crossover graft

This graft is performed for iliac artery occlusion.

Preparation of the patient for bypass surgery

Thorough multidisciplinary assessment of the patient is required. The aim of surgery with critical leg ischaemia should be a pain-free patient with a functioning limb. Primary amputation may need considering as an option if there is severe tissue necrosis which prevents weight bearing of the foot, fixed flexion deformity of the limb, or in very frail patients with severe medical problems who could not withstand a lengthy anaesthetic. Acquiring informed consent will require lengthy discussion with the patient and relatives, taking into consideration all these factors.

The patient should be fully informed of the bypass technique and the nurse will need to explain all pre- and postoperative care requirements. Due to the complexity of bypass surgery, the use of diagrams as a teaching aid may be useful for explaining the position of the intended grafts.

- Venous mapping using ultrasound technique is undertaken to determine suitability of the patient's saphenous vein as bypass material.

- Psychological support for the patient and their relatives is essential. Patients with critical limb ischaemia often experience severe pain at rest, impaired mobility, loss of independence and control. Patients may have concerns about the progression of the disease and may fear the risk of amputation (Treat-Jacobson et al, 2002).

- Relief of ischaemic rest pain by adequate analgesia will be necessary. Pain control should be a priority of care for patients awaiting revascularization to restore blood flow (Ward, 2001). Pain should be regularly assessed and analgesics administered using the WHO (1986) guidelines for pain control: by the mouth, by the clock and by the ladder. Following the ladder of analgesic choice, an oral opioid such as morphine will need to be administered 2–4 hourly, with extra doses given as required for breakthrough pain. Regular aperients will also need to be commenced to prevent constipation. Drowsiness can occur in frail patients, leading to dehydration and malnutrition.

- Nutritional status should be reviewed preoperatively as a patient with severe ischaemia may be in a malnourished state due to lack of mobility, excessive smoking, severe pain and poor diabetes control. High protein sip feeds should be regularly offered and a dietitian referral made if necessary. Blood glucose levels should be optimized in diabetics preoperatively.

- Reassessment of skin, particularly the heels and sacrum and provision of appropriate pressure-relieving mattresses should be regularly undertaken (NICE, 2001). The size, location and condition of any ulcerated lesions should be clearly documented.

- The weight of bed linen should be kept off limbs by the use of a bed-cradle, and extreme care taken to avoid accidental trauma to the ischaemic limbs. Unlike venous leg ulcers, patients with arterial leg ulceration should not have compression bandaging applied, as this will cause further impairment to the blood supply (RCN, 1998).

- Infection control measures are essential preoperatively. A culture swab should be obtained from any ulcerated lesions, and appropriate antibiotic therapy given if required, to minimize the risk of graft infection postoperatively as this can pose a catastrophic risk to the patient. Many vascular patients have prolonged hospital stays prior to surgery which will increase their risk of surgical site infections (SSIs). Patients should therefore be routinely screened for methicillin-resistant *Staphyloccocus aureus* (MRSA) and nursed in a low-risk area of the ward wherever possible. Prophylactic intravenous antibiotics are administered immediately prior to surgery to prevent graft infection. Antiseptic showers/baths are recommended to help reduce skin microbes preoperatively.

- Deep vein thrombosis (DVT) prophylaxis is usually given in the form of low molecular weight heparin and administered in the evening, to avoid the risk of dural haematoma formation if epidural anaesthesia is used. The use of anti-embolic stockings is contraindicated in patients with peripheral arterial occlusive disease.

Anaesthetic assessment

Vascular surgery patients have a high risk of cardiac complications during or following surgery (Hertzer et al, 1984). A full preoperative assessment of the patient's cardiorespiratory and renal function will be required and reviewed by the anaesthetist. The patient may need intubation and ventilation following surgery or closer monitoring for high-risk patients, which will necessitate an overnight stay postoperatively in an intensive care or high dependency unit.

Immediate aftercare

The nurse's prime responsibility for the patient after a bypass graft is the early recognition of complications. The patient should be monitored using an early warning score (EWS) system of vital signs.

- Blood pressure and pulse must be monitored half-hourly for 6 hours, then hourly for 12 hours, as hypertension may cause rupture of the anastomosis, and hypotension may reduce patency of the bypass graft.

- Urinary output should be carefully monitored. A catheter will be in situ and hourly measurements recorded as renal impairment is likely in vascular patients, particularly following aortic/iliac bypass where the renal arteries have been clamped in theatre. Depending on the patient, an output of less than 30 mL over 2 consecutive hours should be reported following the EWS protocol. The catheter is usually removed by the second or third postoperative day.

- Intravenous fluids are usually given via a central venous line to maintain hydration until the patient is able to drink adequately. Patients who have undergone aortic bypass surgery will require central venous pressure measurement hourly.

- Sliding scale insulin with 2-hourly blood glucose checks will be required for diabetics who normally take insulin or oral hypoglycaemics, until blood glucose levels are stable and they are able to return to their normal diabetic regime.

- Oxygen is administered and pulse oximetry undertaken to measure oxygen saturation levels.

- The limbs should be inspected frequently to detect early signs of ischaemia. Colour, temperature and limb movement should be observed and documented. The foot should be warm and well perfused. Sudden changes in colour, warmth, movement or sensation should be reported immediately. The patient's feet should initially be exposed with the use of a bed-cradle to aid observation, and the heels protected from skin breakdown using pressure-relieving aids. Care should be taken to ensure that the patient's limbs do not knock against the bed-cradle. Peripheral pulses should be located hourly at the dorsalis pedis or posterior tibial using a Doppler probe. The nurse should mark the location of the pulse once identified. Any loss of pulses, or a sudden increase of pain, should be reported immediately to facilitate early intervention. Graft occlusion may have occurred, and graft thrombectomy/embolectomy or further reconstruction may be required. The calf muscle should be regularly inspected, as reperfusion can occasionally lead to *compartment syndrome*, which would require a fasciotomy to relieve pressure on the microcirculation. Increased calf pain, tenderness, tenseness of the calf muscle and shiny skin accompanied by paraesthesia, or reduced sensation/foot movement should be immediately reported to the surgeons. Two skin incisions are usually made over the calf muscle to split the fascia covering the anterior, lateral and posterior compartments.

- The wounds should be inspected for bleeding or haematoma formation. Sudden increase in blood loss through the drainage tubes must also be noted and action taken, as this would indicate rupture of the graft anastomosis.

- Any indication of graft occlusion or rupture of the graft anastomosis constitutes a surgical emergency. The haste of returning the patient to theatre and increase in pain and discomfort will be alarming for the patient. The nurse should ensure that explanations of the need for returning to theatre are calmly and carefully explained to the patient and relatives to allay anxiety.

- Once haemodynamically stable, the patient can be sat upright and encouraged to deep breathe to aid lung expansion, and perform gentle foot exercises to help prevent DVT.

- Pain should be assessed and analgesics administered regularly, to enable the patient to cooperate with physiotherapy. Epidural or patient-controlled analgesia (PCA) is recommended for effective pain relief for 24–48 hours or until the patient is able to take regular oral analgesics.

- Prophylactic intravenous antibiotics will be prescribed to prevent infection of the graft.

- Paralytic ileus may be present in patients who have had aortic grafts, and therefore the stomach should be kept empty by nasogastric tube aspiration. The patient will be allowed sips of water only. Fluids and diet will be gradually reintroduced when bowel sounds return.

- A nutritious diet should be encouraged to aid wound healing, as soon as the patient is able to eat and drink. High-protein sip feeds will be required for most patients, particularly those who have undergone aortic bypass surgery who may experience temporary appetite loss.

- Mobility is encouraged 24–48 hours postoperatively, gradually increasing walking distances, although this will depend on the patient's general condition. Regular evaluation of pain relief is essential to allow early mobilization. Patients can sit out of bed after 24 hours postoperatively and should elevate their legs on a footstool following limb bypass surgery to prevent occlusion of grafts behind the knee. Elevation of feet when sitting will also help to relieve swelling, as minor reperfusion oedema following reconstructive surgery is common. Lengthy periods of chair sitting should be avoided to prevent pressure ulcer development. DVT prophylaxis with low molecular weight heparin is continued. Anti-embolic stockings should not be applied to patients following limb reconstructive surgery unless instructed by the surgeon under strict supervision: they are not recommended for patients with an ABPI of less than 0.7.

- Wound vacuum drains are normally removed 24–48 hours postoperatively.

- A non-adherent wound dressing applied in theatre can be left in situ for up to 48 hours. If the dressing becomes bloodstained or soiled, it should be replaced. Wounds should then be inspected daily for signs of inflammation. The groin wounds are particularly susceptible to infection, especially in obese patients, and there is an increased risk of graft infection in these patients. Attention to hygiene in the skin folds of the groin will help to reduce this risk. Sutures should be removed after 12–14 days. Restrictive dressings and compression bandages should not be used on wounds or ulcers on the patient's legs.

- Delayed wound healing despite successful bypass surgery can pose challenges for vascular nurses. Surgical debridement of ulcerated lesions or minor amputation of necrotic toes or tissue lesions may also be required. Frequent assessment of the wound/ulcers and the use of appropriate wound care products, as discussed in Chapter 4, will help to optimize wound healing. Many centres are enthusiastic in the use of topical negative pressure dressings to enhance healing of ulcers and cavity wounds at amputation sites, and clinical evidence for this therapy is considerable (Argenta and Morykwas, 1997). However, caution must be taken before using this type of product following revascularization to ensure there are no closely underlying grafts where the suction dressing is applied.

- Suitable footwear to accommodate dressings of foot wounds as well as ongoing chiropody and foot care advice, particularly for diabetics, should be arranged. Ongoing nutritional support and blood glucose control in diabetics is essential to aid healing of challenging wounds postoperatively.

A case study of a patient undergoing a femoral to distal popliteal bypass is demonstrated in Box 20.2.

Box 20.2   Case study of a patient undergoing femoral–distal popliteal bypass graft

Margaret is 86 years old and lives alone in a ground floor flat. She was referred by her GP to the vascular outpatient clinic with an ischaemic right leg. For 2 months Margaret had been experiencing pain at night in her right foot, requiring her to hang her leg out of bed in the dependent position. She was also having pain while resting during the day and had developed small ulcerated lesions on her right second and third toes during the last 2 weeks. For 2 years previously, Margaret had been having intermittent claudication in her right calf and her walking distance had reduced to 50 metres in the last 3 months.

Until her admission to hospital, Margaret had been able to cook for herself with the aid of her daughter, who undertook shopping for her and lived only 1 mile away. Margaret was finding this increasingly more difficult immediately prior to admission due to pain in her foot which made mobilizing more difficult. Apart from a 20-year history of hypertension treated with nifedipine and a right total hip replacement 12 years previously, her past medical history was otherwise unremarkable. She had a 30-year history of smoking but had quit in her mid fifties.

On admission, Margaret was noted to be experiencing considerable pain, which initially required dihydrocodeine 30 mg 4 hourly, and paracetamol 1 g 6 hourly. Margaret was still unable to sleep at night due to increasing pain, and was having to get out of bed to sleep in a chair. On her second night in hospital, oral morphine 10 mg was also prescribed 2–3 hourly for breakthrough pain. Margaret was then requiring 2–3 doses a day and now needed assistance to walk to the bathroom due to increasing drowsiness and unsteadiness in her gait. She had no palpable pulses below her right femoral pulse and her ABPI was 0.25 for her right leg, and 0.70 for her left leg.

A duplex scan revealed a right 50–75% stenosis of the superficial femoral artery and an occlusion of the popliteal artery, which appeared amenable to angioplasty. An angioplasty of the popliteal artery was attempted via a femoral artery approach, but an attempt to re-enter the artery beyond the popliteal occlusion was unsuccessful and the procedure was abandoned. Margaret's pain became considerably worse following the attempted angioplasty, requiring an increase in morphine to 4 doses daily in addition to regular dihydrocodeine and paracetamol. Her foot became increasingly cyanosed with onset of gangrene to the 2nd toe, indicating that urgent intervention was now required.

Margaret's case was discussed at the multidisciplinary team meeting where it was felt that reconstructive bypass surgery was the only option left to prevent limb loss. This proposed operation was discussed at length with Margaret and her daughter with the aid of diagrams. Both Margaret and her daughter agreed that surgery was urgently required the following day to restore blood flow in an attempt to reduce her pain and prevent limb amputation. They were warned that despite bypass surgery it would not be possible to save her 2nd toe. Duplex vein mapping was undertaken to assess the suitability of Margaret's long saphenous vein which would be required for the bypass graft material.

The following day Margaret underwent a 5-hour operation for a right femoral to distal popliteal bypass using in-situ long saphenous vein for the graft material. Two vacuum drains were inserted to both the femoral and popliteal wounds. Due to the length of anaesthetic, Margaret was monitored overnight on the high dependency unit. Margaret's pain control was changed to PCA and her vital signs remained stable overnight. She had no palpable pedal pulses but monophasic signals could be heard with the Doppler probe at the dorsalis pedis. Margaret was transferred back to the ward the following morning and her pain was controlled satisfactorily enough to allow her to be recommenced on regular non-opioid analgesics and the PCA stopped after 48 hours.

Margaret made excellent progress postoperatively. The drains were removed the next day and her foot became warm and well perfused. Her pain was now well controlled and she was sleeping well at night. By the 4th day following surgery, Margaret was able to mobilize independently with a walking stick and an occupational therapy assessment was undertaken and a discharge date set for 10 days postoperatively. A duplex ultrasound scan was arranged prior to discharge which confirmed the bypass graft had remained patent. The ulcerated lesion on her 3rd toe had shown signs of healing and the gangrenous 2nd toe was dry and mummified. Her wound staples were removed prior to discharge. Margaret and her daughter were warned that the gangrenous toe was expected to auto-amputate after discharge. A community nurse was arranged to dress her toes on alternate days following discharge and a follow-up outpatient appointment was made for 6 weeks. Immediately prior to her outpatient appointment, the gangrenous toe had auto-amputated, leaving healthy granulating tissue at the base, and complete healing had occurred of the 3rd toe. A repeat duplex ultrasound was arranged for 3 months following surgery.

Discharge planning

The admission assessment may have identified problems, especially in elderly patients whose mobility may temporarily be more limited after having undergone major bypass surgery.

The multidisciplinary team, in liaison with the patient's relatives or carers, should agree a provisional discharge date and inform community services. A home assessment may be required by the occupational therapist and social worker before discharge.

Health promotion and discharge advice

- Risk factor modification and lifestyle changes have previously been discussed. However, these factors, especially in relation to smoking cessation and foot care, must be re-emphasized to the patient and relatives before discharge. Explanations must be given as to why each risk factor is dangerous and that stopping smoking will increase graft patency (Wiseman et al, 1989). Walking exercise should be encouraged following discharge, as this will also help to maintain graft patency and improve collateral circulation.

- Aspirin or other antiplatelet therapy is usually prescribed to prevent platelet aggregation, improve graft patency and reduce the risk of having a heart attack or stroke. The importance of continuing to take this along with other medications, e.g. antihypertensive and statin therapy, should be explained.

- Patients should be advised to inform any dentist or doctor they may consult, that they have had an artificial graft bypass, as prophylactic antibiotic cover may be required prior to any invasive procedure.

- Information leaflets are recommended to help reinforce patient education and concordance following discharge. Contact telephone numbers should be included and the patient instructed to make contact in the event of any sudden coolness, numbness or increased pain to the limb, which may indicate graft occlusion.

- Graft surveillance using duplex scanning is recommended following discharge, for early detection of graft failure in patients who have had vein grafts (Kirby et al, 1999). The importance of this procedure needs to be explained to the patient.

SYMPATHECTOMY

Lumbar sympathectomy may be performed for patients with ischaemic rest pain who are unfit for major reconstructive surgery. The sympathetic nerve chain stimulates vascular tone and sweat glands. Chemical lumber sympathectomy is performed more frequently than surgical lumbar sympathectomy using an image intensifier and local anaesthesia, by injecting phenol into the sympathetic chain. In surgical sympathectomy, approximately 2–3 cm of sympathetic nerve chain is excised via a right or left lumbar incision or laparoscopically. Sympathectomy may be temporarily beneficial in reducing rest pain but does not improve blood flow. There is little evidence to support the value of this procedure, and any success can be short-lived (Campbell, 1988).

ACUTE LEG ISCHAEMIA

Acute leg ischaemia is common in elderly people and requires urgent diagnosis and treatment to restore blood flow to the affected leg in order to prevent limb loss. It may be difficult to differentiate between a thrombotic and embolic event. Thrombosis of a pre-existing atheromatous plaque is a more common cause of acute lower limb ischaemia than an embolus.

SIGNS AND SYMPTOMS

Classic features frequently associated with the sudden onset of acute ischaemia are the 'six Ps': pain, pallor, pulselessness, paraesthesia, paralysis and perishing cold.

DIAGNOSIS

A medical history and careful assessment may help elicit an obvious cause of acute ischaemia, although it is not always easy to determine whether acute ischaemia is embolic or thrombotic (Earnshaw, 2001). If an embolus is suspected, an ECG and urgent abdominal ultrasound may be required. An urgent angiogram or duplex ultrasound will confirm diagnosis.

THROMBOSIS

Thrombosis is the commonest cause of acute ischaemia. In situ thrombosis can occur on an athero-sclerotic stenosis in a patient with a history of claudi-cation, or in a pre-existing bypass graft. Other causes of thrombosis include patients with clotting disorders (e.g. malignancy), drug-induced thrombosis (e.g. contraceptive pill) or following radiation therapy (McPherson and Wolfe, 1992). The resulting symptoms are often less severe than from an embolic source, as collateral blood vessels may have developed.

EMBOLISM

An embolism is a thrombus which becomes detached from the left atrium, left ventricle or from an athero-matous abdominal aorta. The embolus travels in the bloodstream and eventually lodges at a major arterial bifurcation such as the common femoral or popliteal arteries. Emboli can become lodged in any vessel, but the lower limbs are more commonly affected.

MANAGEMENT OF THE PATIENT WITH ACUTE LEG ISCHAEMIA

Patients are generally categorized into two groups based on the severity of the ischaemia (Earnshaw et al, 2001):

- *Acute critical ischaemia*: no audible ankle Doppler signal *with neurosensory deficit*. These patients require very urgent treatment on the day of admis-sion, e.g. surgical embolectomy or urgent vascular opinion and angiography.

- *Acute subcritical ischaemia*: patients have ischaemic rest pain, with audible ankle Doppler signal and *no neurosensory deficit*. These patients require prompt intervention but more time is available to investigate, allowing intravenous heparinization overnight and vascular opinion/angiography the following day.

Embolectomy

Embolectomy is undertaken to remove limb-threatening occlusions and may be performed under local anaesthesia to reduce cardiac morbidity. The procedure requires insertion of a balloon-tipped Fogarty catheter after exposure of the artery at the level of obstruction. The uninflated balloon is gently passed proximally and distally within the artery and inflated. The balloon is then partially deflated and pulled through the artery to extract the embolus and any propagated thrombus via the arteriotomy. An arte-riogram should be performed to confirm that there is no remaining embolus in the vessel. Fasciotomy is frequently performed with embolectomy to prevent compartment syndrome.

Preparation of the patient

- The patient will need to be prepared for an emer-gency surgical procedure. This should be calmly and carefully explained to the patient and relatives to allay anxiety.

- Intravenous heparin will be commenced to reduce the risk of further thromboembolic episodes and may be temporarily discontinued immediately prior to surgery to prevent haemorrhage.

Regular analgesics will be required to help alleviate pain preoperatively.

Aftercare

Postoperative observations and care are similar to those for patients having bypass grafting.

- Minor leg swelling is not uncommon postopera-tively. However, severe swelling, paraesthesia, reduced/absent pedal pulses and red, glossy skin in patients without fasciotomy would indicate com-partment syndrome. If this increased pressure is not relieved, necrosis and gangrene can occur. The nurse must carefully observe for this and report any occur-rence immediately. Other signs and symptoms of compartment syndrome include increased pain when stretching the leg muscles, muscle weakness and passive dorsiflexion of the foot (McPherson and Wolfe, 1992).

- Calf fasciotomy wounds may be dressed with an algi-nate and secondary dressing until healed. However, larger wounds often benefit from skin grafting or topical negative pressure to hasten healing.

- A Roylan foot support splint can be used immedi-ately postoperatively to help prevent or correct foot drop, and regular flexion and extension exercises encouraged.

- Intravenous heparin will be recommenced and the patient will then be converted on to oral anticoagu-lants (warfarin). Activated partial thromboplastin time (APTT) levels are monitored regularly, to prevent bleeding from overadministration, or further embolism from underadministration of anticoagulants. The APTT is maintained between 1.5 and 3.5. Heparin administration should be stopped if the APTT result is >7 and the medical staff informed immediately.

- The source of the emboli will need investigation by an echocardiogram and a cardiology opinion will be sought. Long-term warfarin therapy will be reviewed after 3 months.

- A vacuum wound drain may be in situ and can be removed 24–48 hours postoperatively. Sutures will be removed 10–12 days postoperatively.

Thrombolysis

Thrombolysis can be performed intra-arterially as conservative management of an acute thrombosis with critical limb ischaemia, and to revascularize thrombosed bypass grafts (Buckenham et al, 1992). Although this technique can be used for embolism, surgical embolectomy is usually recommended (Whitman et al, 2002).

Thrombolytic therapy can be given to any patient with a recent arterial or bypass graft occlusion. The National Audit of Thrombolysis for Acute Leg Ischaemia (NATALI) database results found that over two-thirds of patients treated for acute leg ischaemia achieved complete or partial lysis with a 72.9% limb salvage rate (Braithwaite et al, 2001). The main complications reported were related to bleeding; minor haemorrhage was common but 8% had major bleeding. Stroke is the most severe complication and occurred in 2% of patients.

Thrombolysis or clot breakdown occurs through activation of plasminogen, a plasma protein. Plasminogen activators convert plasminogen into plasmin, which breaks down fibrin, resulting in clot dissolution and the production of fibrin degradation products which act as potent anticoagulants.

The agent of choice in the UK is rtPA (human tissue-type recombinant plasminogen activator), which is administered intra-arterially. Thrombolysis can be administered by low-dose infusion, or by high doses (accelerated thrombolysis) using a pulsed administrating technique of up to three 5 mg bolus doses at 10–15 minute intervals.

As successful lysis of the thrombosis usually takes 18–24 hours, thrombolysis is not recommended for patients with very severe ischaemia where muscle necrosis is likely (Whitman et al, 2002). Patients who have a history of stroke, peptic ulceration, recent surgery or any medical condition likely to cause haemorrhage are also not suitable for this treatment.

Preparation of the patient

- Preparation of the patient is similar to that provided for angiography, although the patient should be fasted for 2–3 hours prior to the procedure in case emergency surgical intervention is required.

- Prophylactic antibiotics will be required and administered intravenously if a patient has a synthetic graft or stent in situ.

- Oral morphine is the recommended choice of analgesics for patients having thrombolysis, who may be experiencing ischaemic limb.

- Informed written consent should be obtained and the patient warned of the seriousness of the condition of their leg and the potential risks of thrombolysis clearly explained, e.g. bleeding and stroke. The patient should also be forewarned of the possibility of further treatment such as angioplasty or surgery to correct other occlusive lesions.

- A pressure-relieving mattress and heel protection should be available prior to the procedure, which will require the patient to be immobile for many hours, significantly increasing the risk of developing a pressure ulcer.

Monitoring during thrombolysis

The administration of any thrombolytic agent has potential adverse side-effects, of which the nurse must be aware. These are mainly related to bleeding either locally at the puncture site or systemically (Buckenham et al, 1992). Thrombolysis should be considered as a high-risk procedure (Murray, 1992) and patients should be cared for only on wards with experienced nurses who are familiar with the care and risks involved. The care and observations are similar to those for patients post angioplasty.

Care following low-dose administration

- The patient returns to the ward from the angiography suite with a femoral arterial catheter in place, attached to a continuous infusion of the lysing agent until clot dissolution is achieved. This may vary from approximately 8 to 48 hours.

- Care must be taken to ensure that the catheter does not become dislodged or disconnected, and it should be held in place by a secure sterile dressing such as OpSite.

- Monitoring of blood pressure, pulse, catheter puncture site and pedal pulses should be continued ½ hourly for 2 hours, and then hourly for the duration of the infusion, for early detection of haemorrhage or further limb deterioration.

- Reperfusion of the limb may produce excessive swelling, resulting in compartment syndrome; therefore, the nurse should observe for any increased calf pain, tenderness, tenseness of the calf muscle and shiny skin accompanied by paraesthesia or reduced sensation/foot movement. This should be promptly reported in case a fasciotomy is required.

- The patient should be kept well hydrated and encouraged with oral fluids, and an intravenous infusion may be required. Fasting the patient is unnecessary, unless urgent surgical intervention is thought necessary.

- A urinary catheter may be advisable to monitor hydration and avoid the need for unnecessary movement to void urine, which may dislodge the arterial catheter.

- Pressure areas should continue to be observed during this period of immobility.

- Bedrest is maintained for 12 hours following removal of the femoral catheter to prevent haemorrhage or haematoma formation at the catheter entry site.

- Opioid analgesics are recommended for pain relief during lysis and should ideally be given orally on a regular basis. Intramuscular injections should not be administered due to the risk of haematoma formation.

- Check angiography will be required to confirm progress of thrombolysis and the patient will need escorting back to radiology by a qualified nurse.

- Anticoagulation with intravenous heparin is recommended once the arterial catheter is removed following thrombolysis to prevent further clot formations. This will continue for about 48 hours. Thereafter, a decision will be made whether warfarin or aspirin antiplatelet therapy, or a combination of aspirin and clopidogrel is used.

MANAGEMENT OF THE PATIENT REQUIRING LOWER LIMB AMPUTATION

Amputation of a leg is a destructive but sometimes necessary outcome for patients with critical limb ischaemia. It is essential that amputation is viewed as a positive way of improving a patient's quality of life and is often the most effective means of relieving the pain and suffering they may have been experiencing for many months. It is estimated that around 5000 major limb amputations are performed in the UK each year (Department of Health and Social Security, 1996).

Approximately 90% of these are as a result of peripheral vascular disease.

Each patient needs to be assessed individually, when a decision is made as to whether a bypass operation or amputation is the more appropriate action. The decision to amputate is based on a number of factors and would only be taken if the patient's quality of life cannot be improved by saving their leg: i.e. severe uncontrollable pain, a non-healing infected, gangrenous ulcer and immobility. The patient with peripheral vascular disease may already be in hospital following failed bypass surgery, or may have been coping at home with conservative management until amputation became necessary. Either way, the patient and relatives will probably be familiar with the health professionals involved in their care, and a rapport established. However, some patients will present as an emergency with acute leg ischaemia requiring immediate amputation, and will have been denied the time to consider the reality of their situation before amputation is performed.

Ethical issues may often arise when a decision for agreement to amputation is required (Fenech, 1993; Murphy, 1993). Giving consent to amputation requires courage, and helping the patient make an informed choice is vital at this stage. Some patients who are experiencing severe pain will readily accept the need for surgery without delay, whereas others will need more time to reach a decision. In some patients, a decision for surgery will often follow discussion with family members because the patient may be unable to make a rational decision, as a result of confusion from associated sepsis due to gangrene, or because of the effects of strong analgesics to maintain the patient's comfort. In such cases, a final decision will be the surgeon's responsibility made in collaboration with the patient's family and other members of the multidisciplinary team involved in the patient's care. Occasionally, a patient may refuse or postpone a decision to undergo amputation. The team should respect these wishes as long as the patient is fully informed of the possible risks involved in delaying surgery. Advice can be sought for symptom control and home care support from a palliative care team (Wilson, 2001).

LEVEL SELECTION FOR AMPUTATION

The level of amputation will be discussed with the patient and is determined by the extent of ischaemia, the level at which healing is likely to take place and the patient's mobility and general health (Fig. 20.9). The primary aim of amputation is to remove sufficient diseased, infected and gangrenous tissue to allow stump healing, while at the same time retaining adequate limb

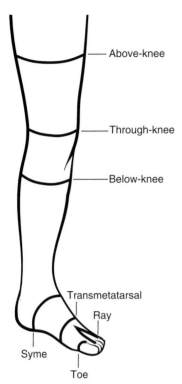

Figure 20.9   Levels of lower limb amputation sites.

length for a prosthesis. The two major amputations performed for critical ischaemia are above-knee (trans-femoral) and below-knee (transtibial). Approximately 80% of amputations performed are below-knee (Maher et al, 1994). The physiotherapist should be actively involved in this decision following assessment of functional ability. Preservation of the knee joint where possible gives far greater success for a limb prosthesis, provided that the knee joint is functional preoperatively (Donohue and Sutton-Woods, 2001).

It is of vital importance that amputations are performed by experienced vascular surgeons, as rehabilitation and prosthesis fitting can be extremely problematic if the level of amputation is not selected correctly, or the stump is not formed sufficiently (Ham and Cotton, 1991).

Below-knee

This amputation has the advantage of preserving the knee joint, which helps with mobilization and limb fitting.

Above-knee

This amputation can be performed in patients who are likely to have stump healing problems with below-knee wounds.

Through-knee

This amputation is a less traumatic procedure than above-knee amputation, when a below-knee procedure is not possible, as no bony structures need to be divided during surgery. However, this type of amputation is rarely performed, as difficulties can arise with limb fitting.

Syme's

This amputation is not commonly performed in patients with ischaemic disease. It involves a disarticulation through the ankle joint at the lower end of the tibia.

Toe, transmetatarsal and metatarsal

Toe, transmetatarsal or metatarsal (Ray) amputations can be performed for localized toe or foot gangrene (Robinson, 1992). These patients may also require an arterial bypass to increase blood flow and aid wound healing. Suturing of these wounds is usually avoided due to poor skin flap healing or infection. The wound is left to granulate and epithelialize using either an alginate cavity-filling dressing and secondary dressing, or topical negative pressure to hasten healing.

Hindquarter (hip disarticulation)

Hindquarter amputation may be indicated for severe aorto-iliac ischaemia and involves disarticulation at the hip. This procedure is generally only performed as a life-saving operation.

PREPARATION OF THE PATIENT FOR AMPUTATION

Pre- and postoperative care of the patient and their family or carers requires setting short- and long-term goals using a team approach. This will include input from nurses, surgeons, physiotherapist, occupational therapist, social worker, dietitian, prosthetist and counsellor.

Psychosocial preparation

Amputation of a limb is a stressful event for the patient, involving a major life change. Reactions will depend upon the patient's personality, cultural and life experience, and also the significance of the limb loss. A patient who may have suffered with a painful, immobile limb for many weeks or months may be able to adjust to the reality of amputation and the relief it will bring. A major responsibility of the nurse is to help the patient develop coping strategies. The loss of a limb is a crisis to the patient and can affect them in a similar way to bereavement (Murray Parkes, 1993). The patient will experience phases of adjustment to the loss of a limb (Walters, 1981).

Assessment may reveal a very positive attitude in some patients who have a supportive family, whereas another patient may have less family support and may feel very isolated and negative about the future. A preoperative visit to the local limb-fitting centre and a visit from another amputee patient may also offer some positive support.

Patients must be fully informed about what to expect after the operation as well as what to expect regarding their rehabilitation, both physically and emotionally. Allowing patients to make an informed choice is critical in helping them accept the need for amputation. A preoperative environmental visit to the patient's home by the occupational therapist is recommended if time allows, to aid discharge planning at an early stage.

Physiological preparation

Pain control

Preoperative ischaemic limb pain must be effectively controlled, as this is a risk factor for the development of postoperative phantom limb pain (Rounseville, 1992). Opioid analgesics should be administered by regular oral, epidural or patient-controlled analgesia. Phantom limb pain and sensations should be discussed with patients preoperatively, reassuring them that this is normal following amputation. These feelings may vary from tingling sensations to a more unpleasant sensation resembling the pain felt in the limb prior to amputation.

Controlling postoperative stump and phantom pain is of vital importance in allowing the patient to participate in postoperative rehabilitation, especially knee straightening exercises to prevent contracture. Early involvement of the pain team is therefore essential. There has been some evidence that good pain control prior, during and after surgery will reduce the intensity of chronic phantom pain, with a recommendation for epidural analgesia commencing 72 hours preoperatively and continuing for several days afterwards (Bach et al, 1988; Baron et al, 1998). However, a randomized prospective trial concluded that although preoperative epidural significantly reduced the severity of postoperative stump pain, there was no significant difference in reducing phantom pain (Lambert et al, 2001).

Nutritional status and pressure ulcer risk

Nutritional status and pressure ulcer risk should be reassessed due to the patient's reduced mobility and pain. High-protein drinks should be encouraged and a review of blood glucose control in diabetics.

PHYSIOLOGICAL CARE FOLLOWING AMPUTATION

- Blood pressure, pulse and respiratory rate must be regularly monitored on return from theatre, for early detection of haemorrhage or respiratory complications.

- Oxygen therapy is administered overnight and saturation levels monitored.

- Intravenous fluids are administered to prevent dehydration until the patient is able to drink adequately. Frail, elderly patients may need an infusion over a longer time period if they are unable to drink adequate amounts orally to maintain hydration over the first few days.

- Urine output is monitored to ensure the patient is adequately hydrated. A urinary catheter may be in situ until the patient is more mobile and able to use a bed pan or commode/toilet.

- The dietitian may need to see the patient, as malnutrition can prevent wound healing and development of pressure ulcers.

- Blood glucose control in diabetics is essential to aid stump healing. Intravenous sliding scale insulin regimes will be required in patients who normally have insulin or oral hypoglycaemics, until they can tolerate normal diet.

- Deep breathing exercises should be encouraged hourly to prevent chest infection, and thromboprophylaxis with low molecular weight heparin is given to prevent DVT or pulmonary embolism.

- Postoperative pain will need reassessing and appropriate analgesics administered regularly. Epidural or patient-controlled analgesia should continue until regular oral morphine is tolerated.

- Uncontrolled phantom limb pain or sensation may cause the patient some distress. These sensations of the limb still being present are often so vivid that the patient may even attempt to walk on the missing limb (Melzack, 1973). Reassurance will need to be given that these are normal sensations which will decrease or disappear; however, this may take time.

- Non-analgesic medication can also be used in conjunction with conventional analgesics such as morphine to help reduce phantom limb pain and sensation. Anticonvulsants such as sodium valproate or gabapentin, and antidepressants such as amitriptyline are commonly used.

CARE OF THE STUMP

- The stump dressing should be observed for signs of haemorrhage on return from theatre and should ideally be left undisturbed for 3 days. Severe pain or pyrexia may necessitate earlier wound inspection for signs of infection or stump ischaemia.

- Staples, sutures or steristrips or a combination of these are used for wound closure and are removed 14–21 days postoperatively.

- To facilitate fitting of the prosthesis, the ideal stump shape should be conical. Incorrect stump bandaging performed by an inexperienced nurse will lead to poor stump shape and delays in limb fitting. Tight bandages must not be used, as patients with vascular disease are especially at risk from stump ischaemia, and a poorly applied stump bandage will contribute to this. Therefore, the application of a light tubular support bandage in theatre, e.g. Tubifast, applied double over a sterile wound dressing, is recommended instead of bandaging, as this will reduce oedema and promote healing.

- A bed-cradle will help prevent bed clothes resting directly on the stump wound.

- Vacuum drains are removed 24–48 hours postoperatively.

- Prophylactic antibiotics are given to prevent wound infection.

- When the stump has healed, a Juzo stump sock can be applied by the patient to give support and reduce oedema after 2–3 weeks postoperatively.

- Longer-term stump care includes daily bathing of the stump and application of a moisturizing cream. Stump socks should be changed daily, and the patient should not wear the prosthesis if an ulcer develops, and should contact their limb-fitting centre as soon as possible.

MOBILITY AND REHABILITATION

Rehabilitation will commence on the first postoperative day to enable patients to feel more independent and self-confident at an early stage if their general condition allows. Patients are encouraged to provide as much self-care as possible to maintain their independence in daily living activities. Help and assistance with toilet or commode transfers, away from the open ward, will help to maintain patients' privacy until they can transfer independently. Patients should also be encouraged to wear comfortable day clothes as soon

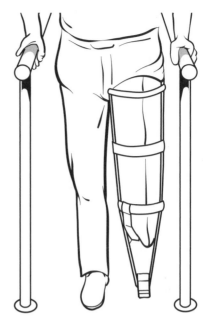

Figure 20.10   Pneumatic postamputation mobility aid.

as possible after the operation, which will help them regain their self-esteem.

Dynamic stump exercises will be taught by the physiotherapist. Patients who have had a below-knee amputation should be encouraged to exercise and completely extend the knee hourly on the first postoperative day, to help prevent a flexion contracture developing. Full hip extension exercises are also taught and encouraged, to prevent hip contracture, as the risk of muscle contracture is increased in patients who spend long periods of time lying or sitting postoperatively.

A wheelchair should be provided on the first or second postoperative day to promote independence. The patient is taught how to safely transfer to and from the wheelchair, and a slide board and monkey pole may be required. The physiotherapist and occupational therapist will assess sitting and standing balance and teach arm/leg strengthening exercises and wheelchair mobility. It is important to take patients to the gym as soon as possible following surgery to help them regain their confidence. Walking training in the parallel bars is practised daily to regain balance. Hopping with crutches is not recommended for new amputees, as this can be both unsafe and tiring for the patient. This practice can also prevent reduction of stump oedema and may also cause an abnormal gait.

It is important for the physiotherapist and occupational therapist to establish at an early stage whether the patient will be able to cope safely with mobilizing on an artificial limb, as this will require strength, free joint movement and an efficient cardiopulmonary system. This decision should be made after ascertaining what the patient's expectations of rehabilitation are and if limb fitting is a realistic option. In some vascular patients with arthritis, eyesight problems or cardio-pulmonary insufficiency, aiming for wheelchair inde-pendence is often a more realistic rehabilitation choice.

Mobilization with an early walking aid, known as a pneumatic postamputation mobility aid (Fig. 20.10), should commence after 7 days, and a temporary limb prosthesis can be fitted within 3–4 weeks.

The occupational therapist will assess and teach the patient how to regain independence with everyday activities, e.g. washing and dressing practice, bathing, kitchen activities, hobbies and work skills.

LIMB–FITTING REFERRAL

An appointment will be made with the local limb-fitting centre for prosthetic limb fitting if appropriate. The initial assessment will be made when the stump has healed, sutures have been removed and swelling has reduced, and when the patient is competent using an early walking aid. The design, construction and fitting techniques of prostheses have become very sophisticated over the last few years. The prosthesis is selected to meet the individual's requirements and can be dressed in accordance with the amputee's taste of shoes, socks or stockings, so as to look cosmetically attractive. A referral can also be made for a cosmetic prosthesis if the amputee is unsuitable for a walking prosthesis.

A patient will often experience initial discomfort with their prosthesis, and regular visits to the pros-thetist at the centre will be required until the limb fits correctly. If they are able to manage at home in a wheelchair, arrangements can be made for the patient to continue walking training on an outpatient basis, until they achieve independence with the prosthesis.

PSYCHOLOGICAL SUPPORT

Ongoing psychosocial support for the amputee and their family is required for many months following amputation. The patient may continue to express grief over the loss of their leg and will have alteration in their body image. All patients must be given adequate coun-selling, and this is particularly important for patients who have undergone an emergency amputation. The nurse has an important role to play and can assist the patient to adjust to this loss by encouraging open com-munication with the patient, relatives and health pro-fessionals. Some denial and anger may be shown by the patient towards the nurses, physiotherapist and

relatives. Postoperatively, the patient may initially wish to hide the stump under bedclothes until they feel able to cope with looking at and touching their stump. The nurse should allow the amputee opportunity to express their feelings and concerns. Praise of the posi-tive accomplishments achieved by the patient will also help them feel more positive about the future, bearing in mind that full acceptance of such a major alteration of their body image will require time.

DISCHARGE PLANNING

Discharge planning will commence immediately fol-lowing the surgery. A home assessment will be carried out by the social worker and occupational therapist. Plans can be made for discharge when the patient is wheelchair independent or safely using his prosthesis. Home adaptations, rehousing or even consideration for residential or nursing care may be necessary for some patients. Weekend leave or a day out at home, prior to discharge, may help the patient and his family adapt to the reality of leaving the protective hospital environment.

Some patients may want to return to work if appro-priate, and will need to discuss this with their GP and employer. All patients, particularly diabetics, should also be given advice on care of their remaining limb and may require chiropody or foot clinic follow-up.

Advice and support for smoking cessation and medication concordance to reduce risk factors for further complications should be reiterated. If patients wish to continue driving, their doctor will tell them when they are able to do so again. They will also need to inform DVLA of their disability, who will advise them of how to adapt the car to a satisfactory standard.

MANAGEMENT OF THE PATIENT WITH AN ABDOMINAL AORTIC ANEURYSM

An aneurysm is an abnormal dilatation of an artery. *True aneurysms* may be saccular in shape, or fusiform, where the entire circumference of the affected aorta is dilated (see Fig. 20.1).

A true aneurysm is defined as a 50% increase in the normal width of the artery (Thompson and Bell, 2000) and is the commonest type, involving all three layers of the artery wall. An aneurysm may affect any large or medium-sized blood vessel. They occur more com-monly in the aorta below the origin of the renal arter-ies (infra-renal) and often extend to the common iliac vessels. Aneurysms can also occur commonly in the thoracic, femoral, popliteal and carotid arteries.

The incidence of abdominal aneurysm is increasing in the UK and these aneurysms are responsible for 10 000 deaths each year (Scott et al, 1995). They usually affect men over 65 years of age, with a prevalence of 5%.

AETIOLOGY

It remains unclear as to the exact mechanism responsible for aneurysm formation. In the inherited disorder Ehlers–Danlos syndrome, defects in certain collagen genes result in weakening of the arterial wall, causing eventual rupture of large vessels (Krupski, 1995). There is an increased risk of abdominal aortic aneurysm formation if a first-degree relative is affected, possibly associated with elastin and collagen defects within the artery wall (Sternbergh et al, 1998). People with the inherited disorder Marfan's syndrome, due to a genetic mutation in the fibrillin-1 gene, are at high risk of developing progressive aneurysm formation (Clifton, 1977).

Although atherosclerosis may contribute to formation of aneurysms, there is some doubt that it may be a direct cause, although untreated hypertension may be a risk factor (Sternbergh et al, 1998). Rarer causes of abdominal aortic aneurysm are trauma, arteritis, syphilis and infections (mycotic).

CLINICAL FEATURES

Most patients with an abdominal aortic aneurysm will have no symptoms and may be diagnosed when they or their doctor detect a pulsatile mass, or incidentally while having routine investigations. Other patients may complain of vague abdominal and/or lumbar pain, which is more common in patients with inflammatory aneurysms.

Ultrasound screening programmes for males over 65 years old are now undertaken in many centres within the UK, and results from the Multicentre Aneurysm Screening Study (MASS) have demonstrated the benefits of screening (Ashton et al, 2002).

DIAGNOSIS

Palpation of the abdomen is insufficient for routinely diagnosing an aneurysm. It is usually confirmed by ultrasound, which gives an accurate size and position of the aneurysm. More accurate confirmation of its position to the renal arteries can be obtained by a CT scan or MRA.

RUPTURED ABDOMINAL AORTIC ANEURYSM

Rupture of an abdominal aortic aneurysm accounts for 1.4% of all male deaths over the age of 65 years old in the Western world (Fowkes et al, 1989). Less than half of patients with ruptures will reach hospital alive and around 50% of those who undergo emergency surgery will survive. Those who present as an emergency will be clinically shocked, with severe abdominal and lower back pain.

EMERGENCY SURGERY

The patient presenting with a ruptured aneurysm will usually arrive in the Accident and Emergency Department, although a rupture may occur in a patient who has already been admitted to a ward awaiting surgery. Without emergency surgery there is a 100% fatality. On diagnosis, the patient will be taken immediately for surgery. The nurse will need to provide reassurance and emotional support for the patient and their family, at the same time recognizing that this situation is a dire emergency. Only minimal physical preparation may be possible, and this should be performed calmly and competently, as the patient will be very frightened by the need for major surgical intervention. The patient will be hypovolaemic and may be semiconscious. The main priority of care will be to maintain the patient's airway, breathing and circulation, to optimize oxygen delivery and tissue perfusion. Immediate resuscitation with IV plasma substitutes if blood is not available, using a pressure infusor, will be continued during transfer of the patient to theatre.

INDICATIONS FOR TREATMENT

The decision to perform elective surgery depends on balancing the risk of aneurysm rupture against the risks of operative morbidity and mortality for the patient concerned. Abdominal aortic aneurysms above 5.5 cm are considered as an indication for surgery (Parkin et al, 2002). Patients and their relatives will be advised of the increased risk of rupture if surgery is not performed. Patients with smaller aneurysms can usually be treated by actively reducing risk factors and carrying out regular ultrasound scans to detect any increase in size.

CONVENTIONAL ELECTIVE SURGERY

The surgical procedure involves replacing the abdominal aneurysm with a straight synthetic (PTFE) tube graft or with an aorto-bifemoral graft if the aneurysm extends to the common iliac arteries (Fig. 20.11).

Preparation of patients for elective surgical aneurysm repair

- The patient is usually assessed both physically and psychologically in a preadmission clinic 1–2 weeks

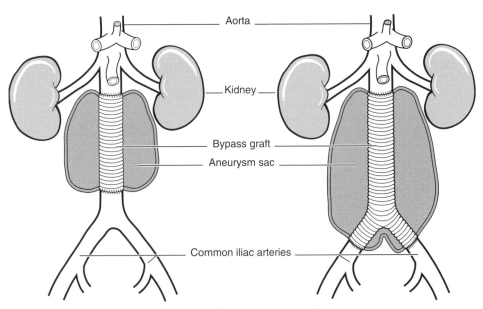

Figure 20.11 Abdominal aortic aneurysm with straight or bifurcated synthetic graft replacement.

prior to surgery. This allows the patient and their family time to be fully informed of the proposed operation, length of stay, associated risks of surgery and the care involved. It also allows time to discuss any concerns with an anaesthetist regarding any special preoperative investigations which may be needed.

- Pre-existing cardiac disease is a significant risk factor for patients undergoing surgery; therefore, a full cardiorespiratory and renal assessment is undertaken. Relevant investigations discussed under the assessment section earlier in the chapter will be needed before the patient is assessed by the anaesthetist.

- The patient is then admitted the day prior to surgery to become familiar with the ward environment and members of the multidisciplinary team.

- Infection prophylaxis is essential to minimize risk of infection of the prosthetic graft, which could pose a catastrophic risk to the patient. A routine screen for MRSA should be taken in the preadmission clinic and the patient admitted into an area of the ward where risk of contamination is low. Antiseptic showers are recommended prior to theatre to help reduce skin microbes, and prophylactic antibiotics will be commenced in theatre.

- Written consent will be obtained from the patient following several prior discussions with the vascular surgeon of the risks and benefits of the operation.

- Deep vein thrombosis prophylaxis of low molecular weight heparin is prescribed and administered in the evening to avoid the risk of dural haematoma if epidural anaesthesia is used.

- The patient and their family should be informed of the need for close monitoring on the high dependency or intensive care unit immediately following surgery.

- Anti-embolic stockings may only be worn if there is no evidence of arterial insufficiency of the lower limbs.

Postoperative care

- Immediate nursing care will be given in the high dependency or intensive care unit for continuous monitoring following prolonged anaesthesia. Most patients are extubated following surgery and will only require high dependency care for 24–48 hours. Patients requiring longer intubation/ventilation will remain in intensive care.

- The patient will be transferred back to a ward with nurses experienced in managing vascular patients when their cardiac, respiratory and renal functions are considered stable.

- A profiling bed will assist with maintaining the patient sitting upright to aid lung expansion. A pressure-relief mattress and heel protection will be required until mobility increases, as epidural analgesics will increase the risk of pressure ulcer development if the patient is unable to feel discomfort to vulnerable areas.

- An early warning observation score should be commenced on the patient's return from the unit, with support from the critical care outreach team if the score increases.

- Close monitoring of vital signs and oxygenation, initially ¼ hourly and then ½ hourly to hourly. Humidified oxygen can be given via a facemask, with arterial blood gases checked 2–3 times daily while on the unit.

- Respiratory rate is monitored hourly and is a good indicator of the onset of chest complications. Deep breathing exercises must be encouraged to ensure lung expansion, and regular physiotherapy is given.

- Blood pressure will need titrating, as hypertension can cause bleeding at the graft anastomosis and hypotension can result in multiorgan failure.

- Hourly urine output and central venous pressure observations will be required to assess hydration.

- Pain control is essential to allow adequate chest expansion, which will reduce the risk of chest infection. Epidural analgesia is recommended for 2–3 days, until the patient is able to tolerate oral analgesics.

- Limb observations should initially be undertaken 1–2 hourly to assess for warmth, colour, sensation and movement, with Doppler assessment of pedal pulses. Distal embolization ('trash foot') can occur following aortic surgery. Caution is therefore needed if antiembolic stockings are in situ, as full examination of the limb can be hindered, and onset of limb ischaemia can go unnoticed or be compounded by the stockings. Assessment of limb movement is important, as the rare complication of paraplegia following this type of surgery may be missed in acutely unwell patients or those with epidural analgesia.

- Nutritional status will be regularly assessed, as it will take several days for normal gut peristalsis to be established due to handling of the bowel during surgery. A nasogastric tube will be in situ and aspirated regularly, and the patient allowed to drink small amounts of water immediately postoperatively. This can be increased as bowel sounds return and nasogastric aspirate lessens. High calorie/protein sip feed supplements should be introduced when nasogastric tube aspirate lessens and the tube is then removed. Diet can be recommenced when free fluids are tolerated and high-protein drinks continued until appetite returns. Total parenteral nutrition will need considering if prolonged ileus occurs.

- Mobility should be encouraged at an early stage, with the patient sitting out of bed for short periods and gradually increasing walking distance.

- Patients often experience diarrhoea following aortic aneurysm repair and a stool specimen should be sent to exclude *Clostridium difficile*. If diarrhoea persists and the patient's abdomen becomes distended and tender, further investigation will be required, as bowel necrosis can occur due to the lengthy clamping of the mesenteric artery during surgery.

Health promotion and discharge advice

- Temporary loss of appetite and excessive tiredness often occurs following abdominal aortic aneurysm repair. The patient should be warned of this and advised to eat regular small nourishing meals and take regular naps initially. Full recovery will take at least 3–6 months.

- Patients should be advised not to lift anything heavier than a kettle for the first 4 weeks but should be encouraged to lead an active life, gradually increasing their activity level, and taking daily walks. Stair practice should be undertaken with the physiotherapist prior to discharge.

- Driving should not be resumed until the patient is reviewed in the outpatient clinic.

- The patient should be advised about the best way to achieve and maintain a healthy lifestyle in relation to diet and taking regular exercise. Smoking must not be resumed in patients who have smoked previously, and ongoing specialist support will be required.

- Discharge drugs will probably include aspirin, antiplatelet and statin therapy, and the importance of taking this, as well as any other prescribed medications should be explained. The patient should also be instructed to have regular blood pressure checks and to continue taking any required antihypertensive medications.

- Patients should also inform any dentist or doctor they may consult that they have an artificial graft in their aorta, as they may require prophylactic antibiotics before any procedure is undertaken.

- A follow-up appointment is required 4 weeks after discharge. The patient should be given an information leaflet with a contact phone number in case any problems are encountered following discharge.

ENDOVASCULAR REPAIR OF ABDOMINAL AORTIC ANEURYSM

Endovascular repair is a new technique for treating abdominal aortic aneurysm. It is a minimally invasive procedure in which a prosthetic stent graft is introduced usually through bilateral groin incisions into the femoral artery and positioned up into the aorta under X-ray guidance, to exclude the aneurysm from the circulation. The endovascular stent is placed into the aorta and iliac arteries, and this allows the aneurysmal sac to thrombose to prevent future rupture.

This technique is advantageous over major surgical repair, in that it is minimally invasive and requires a postoperative hospital stay of only 2–3 days, with minimal discomfort in comparison to conventional surgery. It is also preferential for patients who are unfit for conventional major surgical repair, as the rupture rate of aneurysms in these patients is substantial (Lederle et al, 2002).

However, the main disadvantage is the durability of the procedure compared to conventional open surgical repair. A quarter of patients have developed leaks (endoleak) between the stent and the aneurysm (Thompson and Bell, 2000). Longer-term results of this treatment are unknown and two multi-centred UK trials are ongoing: EVAR 1, comparing open surgery versus endovascular stent repair; and EVAR 2, comparing endovascular stent repair versus observation of the patient.

Depending on the patient's general condition, the procedure can be performed under local or general anaesthesia. A high dependency bed may be required, depending on the patient's fitness, or the patient can be closely monitored by experienced nurses on a dedicated vascular surgery ward.

Blood pressure, pulse, urine output and oxygen saturations are closely monitored overnight using an EWS. The intravenous infusion is removed the following day, as there is no restriction on oral intake. The urinary catheter and any wound drains are also removed the next day and the patient encouraged to mobilize early. Patients are normally fit for discharge 2–3 days after the procedure and instructions given for removal of sutures after 10 days. A duplex ultrasound is usually undertaken prior to discharge to check for an endoleak, and a CT scan arranged 4 weeks postoperatively with a 6-week outpatient appointment.

MANAGEMENT OF THE PATIENT REQUIRING CAROTID ENDARTERECTOMY

A stroke can leave a patient with severe physical and mental disability, making them highly dependent on family and society. Stroke accounted for 12% of deaths in the UK in 1991, and a high morbidity rate of 100 000 strokes every year (DoH, 1991). Most strokes (80%) are ischaemic, and 10% of strokes are secondary to extracranial carotid atherosclerosis.

In carotid disease, atheromatous plaques occur at the origin of the internal carotid artery in the neck. Classic symptoms of carotid disease are a sudden loss of focal cerebral function such as difficulty or loss of speech, weakness/numbness of one or both contralateral limbs, or transient ipsilateral blindness. Transient monocular blindness (*amaurosis fugax*) is described as like a blind being drawn down or across one eye. Symptoms of carotid artery disease are rarely global, such as general dizziness, unsteady gait or coma.

Sudden loss of focal cerebral function lasting less than 24 hours is referred to as a *transient ischaemic attack* (TIA). Symptoms which last for more than 24 hours are called a **stroke**.

Whereas stroke prevention has recently been afforded a high priority within the National Service Framework for Older Persons (DoH, 2001a), access to specialist fast-track diagnostic services remains variable. Prompt referral of patients to rapid access clinics is vital, as delays will significantly increase the risk of further stroke (Gasecki et al, 1994).

INVESTIGATIONS

All patients presenting for investigation of a TIA or a stroke should have a duplex ultrasound scan to identify disease and accurately measure the degree of stenosis. MRA or DSA may also be needed to confirm the extent of stenosis; however, duplex ultrasound has now become the gold standard investigation.

Carotid endarterectomy is performed for stenosis of the internal carotid artery and is a prophylactic procedure to prevent a major disabling stroke or death. Carotid endarterectomy is presently recommended for patients with severe stenosis (70–99%) who have recent symptomatic disease (European Carotid Surgery Trialists Collaborative Group, 1998; Gasecki et al, 1994). The decision to perform carotid endarterectomy therefore depends on balancing the risk of stroke occurring if surgery is not performed against the risk of perioperative or postoperative stroke occurring. These risks and benefits will need to be carefully discussed with the patient and their family, in order for them to make an informed decision about the proposed operation.

HEALTH PROMOTION AND RISK FACTOR MANAGEMENT

Even if surgery is not required, assessment of risk factors and 'best medical therapy' includes smoking cessation support, well-controlled blood pressure and cholesterol, weight and diabetes control to prevent disease progression. Antiplatelet therapy of aspirin, clopidogrel or combination therapy is recommended for all patients with stenosis, unless otherwise indicated. Statin therapy is also now routinely recommended, regardless of baseline cholesterol levels (Collins, 2002). Time permitting referral to appropriate agencies for help and support is important before admission for surgery where possible.

PREOPERATIVE PREPARATION OF THE PATIENT UNDERGOING CAROTID ENDARTERECTOMY

- Depending on the urgency for surgery, the patient will be assessed in the preadmission clinic 7–10 days before surgery. This allows time for the patient and their relatives to discuss any further anxieties and to reconfirm the indication for surgery. The clinic nurse should carefully explain the care pathway requirements and proposed discharge day to the patient and relatives to help allay anxiety. A routine screen for MRSA should be undertaken at this stage.

- Routine blood screening will be undertaken, as well as full cardiorespiratory and renal assessment. Investigations will include a chest X-ray, ECG and possible echocardiogram. A cardiology opinion may also be required for patients with cardiac symptoms.

- A review of the antiplatelet therapy with the vascular consultant surgeon or neurologist should be undertaken at this stage, as patients having combination therapy of aspirin and clopidogrel may need to have the clopidogrel stopped several days before the operation due to reports of excessive bleeding during surgery.

- The patient is admitted 12–48 hours preoperatively into an area of the ward where there is a low risk of contamination from MRSA.

- Due to the increased risk and complications of haematoma formation during and after surgery, DVT prophylaxis of low molecular weight heparin is omitted in many centres and only anti-embolic stockings provided unless contraindicated. Patients undergoing carotid endartectomy are mobilized quickly, which decreases the risk of DVT in comparison to the risk of severe haemorrhage.

- A full neurological examination is normally performed by the neurologist to identify and document any pre-existing deficit. The anaesthetist will review the patient and discuss the type of anaesthetic required, as local anaesthesia is an option for suitable patients.

- Informed written consent is obtained and the risks of a stroke occurring during or after surgery will be again explained to the patient and relatives by the surgeon. Other risks of surgery: e.g. heart attack, minor haemorrhage, temporary numbness of the face/neck, tongue and mouth weakness are also explained, which will inevitably heighten anxiety. A vein patch may be required and will be obtained from the patient's neck or leg veins, or a prosthetic patch can be used. This patch is anastomosed onto the carotid artery to widen the vessel, preventing narrowing at the incision site. The patient needs to be informed that this may occur.

- An antiseptic shower immediately prior to operation is recommended to help reduce skin microbes.

- Medications for risk factors will need to be given on the morning of surgery and these will include aspirin and antihypertensive drugs. Due to the risk of stroke immediately prior to surgery, antiplatelet therapy, including clopidogrel, should not be stopped unless specific written instructions are given to do so by the senior surgeon.

- Monitoring of the patient's cerebral function during the operation can be undertaken in an 'awake' patient having local anaesthesia, by asking the patient simple questions and testing their grip power on the contralateral hand. Transcranial Doppler monitoring is now more commonly used for both local and general anaesthesia to assess cerebral blood flow.

POSTOPERATIVE CARE

The patient will require either an extended recovery or brief high dependency stay if they are considered a high-risk patient prior to return to the vascular surgery ward for monitoring by experienced nurses.

- An early warning observation score should be commenced on the patient's return to the ward.

- Close monitoring of vital signs, oxygenation, and for recovery of consciousness, speech, facial weakness and limb function are required for early detection of any neurological deficit.

- Blood pressure should be carefully monitored. The parameters and necessary treatment to titrate blood pressure must be clearly documented in the medical notes or care pathway by the anaesthetist or surgeon before the patient leaves the recovery ward.

- Oxygen is given as prescribed for up to 24 hours and saturations recorded 1–2 hourly initially, to maintain >95%.

- Blood pressure, pulse and respiratory observations are undertaken:
  - ¼ hourly for 1 hour
  - ½ hourly for 6 hours
  - hourly for 12 hours, then 4 hourly if stable.

- The patient is observed for stridor or other signs of respiratory distress.

- Urine output is carefully observed and IV fluids administered for approximately 24 hours and removed when the patient is drinking adequately.

- Blood glucose monitoring and sliding scale insulin is required for diabetics who normally have insulin or oral hypoglycaemics until eating normally. Normal diet can be resumed as desired when the patient is awake.

- The wound, situated behind the angle of the jaw, should be observed for haemorrhage or haematoma formation. Staples are removed 5 days following surgery.

- A vacuum drain is usually inserted and removed on the first postoperative day.

- Deep breathing and leg exercises are encouraged.

- Analgesics are administered as necessary, as patients usually experience only minor discomfort following surgery.

- The patient may mobilize the following day once normotensive.

FOLLOW-UP ADVICE

- Slight numbness to the face or some tongue weakness, due to trauma of the nerves during the operation, is not uncommon following surgery. Patients need to be informed that this is quite normal and may take some weeks to disappear.

- Modification of risk factors must be re-emphasized to the patient and relatives, especially in relation to smoking, blood pressure and diet.

- Patients need to be reminded of the importance of taking their prescribed antiplatelet therapy and other medications, and should continue to have their blood pressure monitored regularly.

- A follow-up outpatient appointment is normally arranged for 6 weeks after discharge.

MANAGEMENT OF THE PATIENT WITH VARICOSE VEINS

Varicose veins is a very common condition, with over 50 000 people each year admitted to hospitals in the UK for treatment of varicose veins or their complications (Hobbs, 1991). Although varicose veins have traditionally been considered commoner in women, an Edinburgh study found the prevalence of varicose veins was 40% in men and 30% in women (Bradbury et al, 1999). Malfunctioning valves in the veins anastomosing the deep and superficial veins, called perforators, cause an increase in pressure, which leads to tortuous and dilated superficial varicose veins.

Most varicose veins are *primary* where the exact cause is unknown, but is possibly a congenital defect giving rise to valvular incompetence and weakness in the vein wall. Only a minority are *secondary* to conditions following DVT, pregnancy or pelvic tumours. The valves become damaged by increased pressure, causing back flow from the deep to the superficial veins. Risk factors for the development of primary varicose veins include increasing age, obesity and occupations which involve standing.

There are three types of superficial varicose veins:

- True or trunk varicose veins are widened, tortuous and bulging.
- Reticular veins are normal but more visually prominent superficial veins which do not usually become widened.
- Spider or thread veins (telangiectases).

SYMPTOMS

Symptoms that commonly occur are tiredness, swelling, aching, itching, throbbing and restless legs. These are made worse by standing for long periods and hot weather, and are relieved by walking. Many patients have no symptoms but will present with varicose veins because they are worried about the cosmetic appearance. Dilated, tortuous, lumpy veins can cause considerable disfigurement and give rise to cosmetic concern.

COMPLICATIONS OF VARICOSE VEINS

Complications include superficial inflammation (phlebitis) and superficial thrombosis (thrombophlebitis). Haemorrhage from a ruptured vein through the skin may result from trauma, and spontaneous rupture can also occur, particularly in elderly people with thin overlying skin.

Skin changes, particularly in the gaiter area can occur over time due to chronic venous hypertension.

These may include eczema, skin pigmentation (brown staining), atrophie blanche (white scar tissue) and lipodermatosclerosis (hard, woody, indurated skin texture) (Vowden, 1998).

If dermatitis and eczema does develop in the affected limb, causing dry, scaly and itching skin, this may predispose the patient to the development of varicose ulceration (Royle, 1992) as 70% of leg ulceration is of venous origin (Cullum and Roe, 1995).

INVESTIGATIONS

Duplex ultrasound scanning

This procedure is a non-invasive scan to accurately assess sites of valve incompetence in the deep and superficial venous systems, and is considered the gold standard method of investigation.

Venography

Venography can be performed to assess chronic venous insufficiency but has a limited role and subjects patients to unnecessary radiation. Performed under local anaesthesia, a radio-opaque contrast medium is injected into a vein on the dorsum of the foot to demonstrate the patency of deep veins, and for an indication of past or present thrombosis and valve competency.

Trendelenburg test

This test can confirm the source of venous incompetence. A tourniquet is placed around the upper thigh after raising the leg. Veins that fill slowly when the patient stands, but fill rapidly on releasing the tourniquet, have incompetent saphenofemoral valves. The test can be used with the tourniquet placed below the knee to assess the short saphenous vein.

Doppler ultrasound

Doppler ultrasound can be used to determine the presence of venous reflux in the veins behind the knee.

TREATMENT

Compression hosiery

Support hosiery will help relieve symptoms by aiding venous return and will conceal varicosities. They require correct fitting to achieve results and aid concordance. Significant arterial disease should be excluded before applying compression hosiery. The patient should also be advised to moisturize their skin well to avoid dryness.

Sclerotherapy

Sclerotherapy of trunk varicosities is associated with high recurrence rates, as it fails to correct the source of venous reflux and is therefore used with caution in patients with significant varicosities (Galland et al, 1998). Minor below-knee reticular veins and thread veins are frequently treated with this method for cosmetic reasons. A sclerosing agent (3% sodium tetradecyl/sulphate) is injected into the lumen of the prominent veins. This agent eliminates the varicosity by creating inflammation of the lumen walls, which become adherent when immediate local pressure is applied with pads. Compression bandaging or stockings should be worn for 2–3 weeks following the treatment. Prior to injection treatment for cosmetic reasons, the patient should be informed that there is a risk of developing skin pigmentation (Henry, 1992).

MANAGEMENT OF VARICOSE VEINS BY SURGERY

Although most patients with varicose veins can be managed in primary care settings, many patients will require surgical intervention if indicated. Surgery is not usually offered for cosmetic reasons but is normally performed in patients who have haemorrhaging or skin changes (eczema, lipodermatosclerosis, recurrent thrombophlebitis, ulceration), or severe symptoms with an impact on their quality of life (NICE, 2000).

During surgery, the long or short saphenous veins are stripped out distally with a wire stripper. Several small incisions may be made if it is not possible to remove the entire vein through one incision. The vessel will be ligated where it meets the perforators at the saphenofemoral junction.

Preoperative preparation

- The surgeon will mark the skin over the vein to be stripped, and the nurse should ensure that these markings are not removed prior to surgery.
- Many patients are concerned with the cosmetic appearances after surgery and may have unrealistic expectations. It is therefore important for the surgeon to explain that the small incisions made at operation will leave small scars.
- Women taking a combined oral contraception should stop taking them 4 weeks before surgery and use an alternative method.

Aftercare

- The foot of the bed is elevated on return from surgery to promote venous return.

- The incision sites should be observed for bleeding. Compression bandages will have been applied from toes to thigh. Bedrest is usually only required for 2–3 hours after day care surgery and maybe longer, depending on the extent of the surgery.

- Patients are at risk from DVT and should be encouraged to mobilize when there is no further risk of haemorrhage. DVT prophylaxis is usually prescribed for inpatients staying overnight, as their mobility may be limited if they are more elderly or have had bilateral surgery.

Discharge advice

- The patient is advised to remove the bandaging after 48 hours. Either medium-strength (Class II) elastic support stockings or anti-embolic stockings should then be worn for 10 days following surgery but can be removed at night.

- The patient is advised to keep the wounds as dry as possible. Soluble sutures are normally used for groin incisions with steristrips over the multiple avulsions, which can be peeled off after 48 hours.

- Bruising to the legs and discomfort are not uncommon and the patient should be forwarned of this.

- Walking exercise should be encouraged following surgery, and the patient's legs should be elevated while sitting to prevent swelling. To avoid recurrence of varicosities, patients should avoid standing still for long periods of time, as gravity can cause pooling of blood in the legs. Weight gain should also be avoided, as excess adipose tissue gives poor support to the venous system.

Summary of key points

- Patients with peripheral vascular disorders are increasingly requiring hospitalization for treatment by either radiological or surgical intervention.

- Care of these patients both in community and acute settings is challenging, requiring an holistic approach, vigilant monitoring and early detection and treatment to prevent onset of limb-threatening disease.

- Caring for patients within acute care environments requires a broad range of skills and expertise to encompass critical care, wound and tissue viability, nutritional, pain and diabetes management, as well as palliative care.

- Nurses must be aware of the importance of correct assessment, diagnosis and treatment of venous and arterial leg ulceration.

- Control of risk factors and education is a key component of care, requiring a team approach to enable vascular patients to increase control over and improve their own health.

References

Antithrombotic Trialists Collaboration (2002) Collaborative meta-analysis of randomised trial of antiplatelet therapy for prevention of death, myocardial infarction and stroke in high risk patients. *British Medical Journal* 324(7329): 71–86.

Argenta, L. C. & Morykwas, M. J. (1997) Vacuum-assisted closure: a new method for wound control treatment: clinical experience. *Annals of Plastic Surgery* 38(6): 563–577.

Ashton, H. A., Buxton, M. J., Day, N. E., et al (2002) The Multicentre Aneurysm Screening Study (MASS) into the effect of abdominal aortic aneurysm screening on mortality in men: a randomised controlled trial. *Lancet* 360(9345): 1531–1539.

Bach, S., Noreng, M. F. & Tjellden, N. U. (1988) Phantom limb pain in amputees during the first twelve months following limb amputation after pre-operative lumbar epidural seventy-two hours pre-operation. *Pain* 33(3): 297–301.

Baron, R., Wasner, G. & Lindner, V. (1998) Optimal treatment of phantom limb pain in the elderly. *Drugs* 12(5): 361–376.

Beach, K. W., Bedford, G. R., Bergelin, R. & Marin, D. (1988) Progression of lower extremity arterial occlusive disease in Type II diabetes mellitus. *Diabetes Care* 11(6): 464–472.

Beard, J. D. (2000) Chronic lower limb ischaemia. In: Donnelly, R. & London, N. J. M. (eds) *ABC of Arterial and Venous Disease*. London: BMJ Books.

Beard, J. D. & Gaines, P. A. (2001) Treatment of lower limb ischaemia. In: Beard, J. D. & Gaines, P. A. (eds) *Vascular and Endovascular Surgery*, 2nd edn. London: WB Saunders.

Belli, A. M. & Buckenham, T. M. (1995) Arteriography: developments in diagnostic and interventional techniques. *Imaging* 7(2): 107–113.

Bonica, J. (1990) Definitions and taxonomy of pain In: Bonica, J. (ed.) *The Management of Pain*, 2nd edn. Philadelphia: Lea & Febiger.

Boushey, C. J., Beresford, S. A. A., Omenn, G. S. & Motulsky, A. G. (1995) A quantitative assessment of plasma homocysteine as a risk factor for vascular disease. *JAMA* 274(13): 1049–1057.

Bowlin, S., Medalie J, Flocke, S., et al (1994) Epidemiology of intermittent claudication in middle-aged men. *American Journal of Epidemiology* 140(5): 418–430.

Bradbury, A., Evans, C., Allan, P., et al (1999) What are the symptoms of varicose veins? Edinburgh vein study cross sectional population survey. *British Medical Journal* 318: 353–356.

Braithwaite, B.D., Whitman, B. & Foy, C. (2001) Thrombolysis Study Group. Outcome analysis of over 1000 episodes of limb ischaemia treated by peripheral thrombolysis. *British Journal of Surgery* 88: A618.

Buckenham, T., George, C. D., Chester, J. F., et al (1992) Accelerated thrombolysis using pulsed intrathrombus recombinant human tissue-type plasminogen activator. *European Journal of Vascular Surgery* 6(3): 237–240.

Campbell, W. B. (1988) Sympathectomy for chronic arterial ischaemia. *European Journal of Vascular Surgery* 2(6): 357–364.

Cheetham, D. R., Burgess, L., Ellis, M., et al (2004) Does supervised exercise offer adjuvant benefit over exercise advice alone for treatment of intermittent claudication? A randomised trial. *European Journal of Vascular and Endovascular Surgery* 27(1): 17–23.

Cleveland, T., MacDonald, S., Morgan, R. & Gaines, P. (2002) Day case angiography and intervention. In: Beard, J. D. & Murray, S. (eds) *Pathways of Care in Vascular Surgery*. JVRG. Shrewsbury: tfm Publishing.

Clifton, M. A. (1977) Familial abdominal aortic aneurysms. *British Journal of Surgery* 64(11): 765–766.

Collins, R. (2002) The MRC/BHF Heart Protection Study: preliminary results. Conference Report. Nov 2001. *International Journal of Clinical Practice* 56(1): 53–56.

Cullum, N. & Roe, B. H. (1995) *Leg Ulcers: Nursing Management*. Middlesex: Scutari Press.

Department of Health and Social Security (1996) *Review of Artificial Limb and Appliance Centre Services*. London: HMSO.

DoH (1991) *The Health of the Nation*. London: HMSO.

DoH (1999) *White Paper on Public Health, Saving Lives: Our Healthier Nation*. London: HMSO.

DoH (2000a) *National Service Framework for Coronary Heart Disease*. London: HMSO.

DoH (2000b) *The NHS Plan: A Plan for Investment. A Plan for Reform*. London: HMSO.

DoH (2001a) *National Service Framework for Older People*. London: HMSO.

DoH (2001b) *National Service Framework for Diabetes*. London: HMSO.

Donohue, S. & Sutton-Woods, P. (2001) Lower limb amputation. In: Murray, S. (ed.) *Vascular Disease: Nursing and Management*. London: Whurr Publishers.

Earnshaw, J. J. (2001) Demography and etiology of acute leg ischaemia. *Seminars in Vascular Surgery* 14(2): 86–92.

Earnshaw, J. J., Gaines, P. A. & Beard, J. D. (2001) Management of acute lower leg ischaemia. In: Beard, J. D. & Gaines, P.A. (eds) *Vascular and Endovascular Surgery*, 2nd edn. London: WB Saunders.

European Carotid Surgery Trialists Collaborative Group (1998) Randomised trial of endarterectomy for recently symptomatic carotid stenosis: final results of the MRC European Carotid Surgery Trial (ECST) *Lancet* 351: 1379–1387.

European Working Group (1991) 2nd European Consensus Document on Critical Leg Ischaemia. *Circulation* (Suppl.) 84(4): IV-1–IV-26.

Ewles, L. & Simnett, I. (1995) *Promoting Health: A Practical Guide*, 3rd edn. London: Scutari Press.

Faris, I. (1991) *The Management of the Diabetic Foot*, 2nd edn. Edinburgh: Churchill Livingstone.

Fenech, P. (1993) Fit to consent? *Nursing Times* 89(24): 40–42.

Fowkes, F. G. R., MacIntyre, C. C. A. & Ruckley, C. V. (1989) Increasing incidence of aortic aneurysms in England and Wales. *British Medical Journal* 298(6665): 33–35.

Galland, R. B., Magee, T. R. & Lewis, M. H. (1998) A survey of current attitudes of British and Irish vascular surgeons to venous schlerotherapy. *European Journal of Vascular and Endovascular Surgery* 16(1): 43–46.

Gardner, A. W., & Poehlman, E. T. (1995) Exercise rehabilitation programs for the treatment of claudication pain. A meta-analysis. *JAMA* 274(12): 975–980.

Gasecki, A. P., Ferguson, G. G., Eliasziw, M., et al (1994) Early endarterectomy for severe carotid artery stenosis after a non-disabling stroke: results of the NASCET Trial. *Journal of Vascular Surgery* 20(2): 288–295.

Greenhalgh, R. (1990) *The Cause and Management of Aneurysms*. London: WB Saunders.

Ham, R. & Cotton, L. (1991) *Limb Amputation*. London: Chapman & Hall.

Hankey, G. J. & Elkeboom, J. (1999) Homocysteine and vascular disease. *Lancet* 354: 407–413.

Henry, M. (1992) Sclerotherapy for varicose veins. In: Bell, P., Jamieson, C. & Ruckley, V. (eds) *Surgical Management of Vascular Disease*. London: WB Saunders.

Hertzer, N. R., Bevan, E. G., Young, J. R., et al. (1984) Coronary artery disease in peripheral vascular patients: a classification of 1000 coronary angiograms. *Annals of Surgery* 199(2): 223–233.

Hiatt, W. R., Wolfel, E. & Regensteiner, J. S. (1991) Exercise in the treatment of intermittent claudication due to peripheral vascular disease. *Vascular Medicine Review* 2: 61–70.

Hobbs J. T. (1991) Varicose veins. *British Medical Journal* 303(6804): 707–710.

Jones, S. (2001) Anatomy and physiology of the vascular system. In: Murray, S. (ed.) *Vascular Disease: Nursing and Management*. London: Whurr Publishers.

Kannel, W. B. & McGee, D. L. (1985) Update on some epidemiological features of intermittent claudication: the Framingham study. *Journal of the American Geriatrics Society* 33(1): 13–18.

Kannel, W. B., Skinner, J. J., Schwartz, M. J. & Shurtleff, D. (1970) Intermittent claudication: incidence in the Framington Study. *Circulation* 41(5): 875–883.

Kirby, P. L., Brady, A. R., Thompson, S. G., et al (1999) The Vein Graft Surveillance Trial: rationale, design and methods. VGST participants. *European Journal of Vascular and Endovascular Surgery* 18(6): 469–474.

Krupski, W.C. (1995) Abdominal aortic aneurysm: defining the dilemma. *Seminars in Vascular Surgery.* 8(2): 115–123.

Laing, W. (1992) *Chronic Venous Diseases of the Leg.* London: Office of Health Economics.

Lambert, A. W., Dashfield, A., Cosgrove, C., et al (2001) Randomized prospective study comparing pre-emptive epidural and intra-operative perineural analgesia for the prevention of postoperative stump and phantom pain following major amputation. *Regional Anesthesia and Pain Medicine* 26(4): 316–321.

Lederle, F. A., Johnson, G. R., Wilson, S. E. et al (2002) Rupture rate of large abdominal aortic aneurysms in patients refusing or unfit for elective surgery. *JAMA* 287(22): 2968–2972.

Leng, G.C., Fowler, B. & Ernst, E. (2002) Exercise for intermittent claudication (Cochrane Review). *The Cochrane Library.* Issue 2, Oxford.

Ley, P. (1993) Improving communication, satisfaction and compliance. *Communicating with Patients*, 4th edn. London: Chapman & Hall.

Libby, P., Geng, Y.J., Aikawa, M., Schoenbeck, U., Mach, F., Clinton, S.K., Sukhova, G.K. & Lee, R.T. (1996) Macrophages and atherosclerotic plaque stability. *Current Opinion in Lipidology* 7(5): 330–335.

Lungren, F., Datillof, A., Lundolm, K., et al (1988) Intermittent claudication – surgical reconstruction or physical training? *Annals of Surgery* 209(3): 346–355.

McAllister, F. F. (1976) The fate of patients with intermittent claudication managed non-operatively. *American Journal of Surgery* 132(5): 593–595.

McDermott, M. M., Feinglass, J., Slavensky, R. & Pearce, W. H. (1994) The ankle-brachial index as a predictor of survival in patients with vascular disease. *Journal of International Medicine* 9: 445–449.

McPherson, G. & Wolfe, J. (1992) Acute ischaemia of the leg. In: Wolfe, J. H. (ed.) *ABC of Vascular Diseases*, 2nd edn. London: BMJ Publishing Group.

Maher, A., Addamo, S. & Shabtaie, J. (1994) Amputation and transplantation. In: Maher, A., Salmond, S. & Pellimo, T. (eds) *Orthopaedic Nursing.* London: WB Saunders.

Melzack, R. (1973) *The Puzzle of Pain.* New York: Basic Books.

Moffatt, C. J., Oldroyd, M. I., Greenhalgh, R. M. & Franks, P. J. (1994) Palpating ankle pulses is insufficient in detecting arterial insufficiency in patients with leg ulceration. *Phlebology* 9: 170–172.

Murphy, J. (1993) Ethical dilemmas in caring for a patient refusing amputation. *British Journal of Nursing* 2(21): 1072–1076.

Murray, S. (1992) Caring for patients undergoing treatment for vascular occlusion. *British Journal of Nursing* 2 (1):17–19.

Murray Parkes, C. (1993) *Bereavement Studies of Grief in Adult Life*, 2nd edn. London: Routledge.

NICE (2000) *Varicose Veins – Referral Practice-Version under Pilot.* National Institute for Clinical Excellence. London: NICE.

NICE (2001) *NICE Guidelines on Pressure Ulcer Risk Management and Prevention (Guideline B).* London. NICE. Online at: http://www.nice.org.uk/pdf.clinicalguide-linepressuresoreguidancenice.pdf (accessed 20 March 2004).

Oliver, M. F. (1991) Lipids: outstanding questions. In: Fowkes, F. G. R. (ed.) *Epidemiology of Peripheral Vascular Disease.* London: Springer-Verlag.

Parkin, D., Earnshaw, J. J. & Heather, B. (2002) Elective abdominal aortic aneurysm. In: Beard, J. D. & Murray, S. (eds) *Pathways of Care in Vascular Surgery.* JVRG. Shrewsbury: tfm Publishing.

Pasternak, R., Grundy, S., Levy, D. & Thompson, P. (1996) Taskforce 3. Spectrum of risk factors for coronary artery disease. *Journal of the American College of Cardiology* 27(5): 978–1047.

Perkins, J. M. T., Collins, J. C. & Morris, P. J. M. (1995) Angioplasty versus exercise for stable claudication: long term results of a prospective randomized trial. *British Journal of Surgery* 82: 557.

Powell, J. T. (1991) Smoking. In: Fowkes, F. G. R. (ed.) *Epidemiology of Peripheral Vascular Disease.* London: Springer-Verlag.

RCN Institute (1998) *Clinical Practice Guidelines: The Management of Patients with Venous Leg Ulcers.* London: RCN Institute.

Robinson, K. (1992) Amputations in vascular patients. In: Bell, P., Jamieson, C. & Ruckley, V. (eds) *Surgical Management of Vascular Disease.* London: WB Saunders.

Roper, N., Logan, W. & Tierney, A. (1981) *Learning to Use the Process of Nursing.* Edinburgh: Churchill Livingstone.

Rounseville, C. (1992) Phantom limb pain: the ghost that haunts the amputee. *Orthopaedic Nursing* 11(2): 67–71.

Royle, J. (1992) Treatment of primary varicose veins. In: Bell, P., Jamieson, C. & Ruckley, V. (eds) *Surgical Management of Vascular Disease.* London: WB Saunders.

Sans, S., Kestloot, H. & Kromout, D. (1997) The burden of cardiovascular disease mortality in Europe. *European Heart Journal* 18(12): 1231–1248.

Scott, R. A., Wilson, N. M., Ashton, H. A., & Kay, D. N. (1995) Influence of screening on the incidence of ruptured abdominal aortic aneurysm: 5 year results of a randomized controlled study. *British Journal of Surgery* 82(8): 1066–1077.

Seltzer, C. C. (1989) Framingham study data and 'established wisdom' about cigarette smoking and coronary heart disease. *Journal of Clinical Epidemiology* 42(8): 743–750.

Shah, P. (1997) New insights into the pathogenesis and prevention of acute coronary syndromes. *American Journal of Cardiology* 70(12B): 17–23.

Sternbergh, W. C., Gonze, M. D., Garrard, C. L. & Money, S. (1998) Abdominal and thoracicoabdominal aneurysm. *Surgical Clinics of North America* 78(5): 827–834.

Thompson, M. M. & Bell, P. R. F. (2000) Arterial aneurysms: clinical review. *British Medical Journal* 320(7243): 1193–1196.

Treat-Jacobson, D., Halverson, S. L., Ratchford, A., et al (2002) A patient-derived perspective of health-related quality of life with peripheral vascular disease. *Journal of Nursing Scholarship* 34(1): 55–60.

Twycross, R. (1994) *Pain Relief in Advanced Cancer.* Edinburgh: Churchill Livingstone.

Vowden, K. (1998) Lipodermatosclerosis and atrophie blanche. *Journal of Wound Care* 7(9): 441–443.

Walker, W. F. (1988) *A Colour Atlas of Peripheral Vascular Disease.* London: Wolfe Medical Publications.

Walters, J. (1981) Coping with a leg amputation. *American Journal of Nursing* 81(77): 1349–1352.

Ward, L. (2001) Pain management in vascular disease. In: Murray, S. (ed.) *Vascular Disease: Nursing and Management.* London: Whurr Publishers.

Waterlow, J. A. (1988) The Waterlow card for prevention and management of pressure sores, towards a pocket policy.

Care-Science and Practice 6(1): 8–12.

WHO (1986) *World Health Organization. Cancer Pain Relief.* Geneva: WHO.

Whitman, B., Parkin, D. & Earnshaw, J. J. (2002) Management of acute leg ischaemia. In: Beard, J. D. & Murray, S. (eds) *Pathways of Care in Vascular Surgery. JVRG.* Shrewsbury: tfm Publishing.

Wilson, L.M. (2001) Palliative care provision for vascular patients. In: Murray, S. (ed.) *Vascular Disease: Nursing and Management.* London: Whurr Publishers.

Wiseman, S., Kenchington, F., Dain, R., et al (1989) Influence of smoking and plasma factors on patency of femoro-popliteal vein grafts. *British Medical Journal* 299(6700): 643–647.

Further reading

Beard, J. D. & Murray, S. (2002) (eds) *Pathways of Care in Vascular Surgery. JVRG.* Shrewsbury: tfm Publishing.

Donnelly, R. & London, N. J. M. (2000) *ABC of Vascular Diseases.* London: BMJ Books.

Earnshaw, J. J. & Murie, J. A. (1999) *The Evidence for Vascular Surgery.* Shrewsbury: tfm Publishing.

Engstrom, B. & Van de Ven, C. (1999) *Therapy for Amputees.* London. Churchill Livingstone.

Faris, I. (1991) *The Management of the Diabetic Foot*, 2nd edn. Edinburgh: Churchill Livingstone.

MacVittie, B. (1998) *Vascular Surgery: Mosby's Perioperative Nursing Series.* London: Mosby.

Murray, S. (ed) (2001) *Vascular Disease: Nursing and Management.* London: Whurr Publishers.

Chapter 21

Patients requiring orthopaedic surgery

Nicola L Judge

Key objectives of the chapter

At the end of this chapter the reader should be able to:

- describe the structure and function of the musculoskeletal system

- classify bones according to their structure

- classify joints according to their structure and degree of movement

- discuss specific orthopaedic investigations

- discuss common orthopaedic conditions

- discuss the importance of pre-assessment and education in preparing the orthopaedic patient for their surgery

- demonstrate knowledge of the nursing care of patients requiring surgery to the hip, knee, foot, shoulder, forearm, hand and spine

- discuss the process of bone healing

- discuss types of fracture and how they are managed

- discuss the relevance of neurovascular observations in detecting compromise and the actions to be taken if detected

- discuss specific issues in planning a patient's discharge

- discuss the importance of patient education in rehabilitation.

INTRODUCTION

The term 'orthopaedics' is applied to all conditions affecting the musculoskeletal system. The scope of orthopaedic surgery includes the treatment, management and rehabilitation of patients with musculoskeletal conditions (Blauvelt and Nelson, 1998). A fully functioning musculoskeletal system is essential for optimal health in the human being, and disease or injury involving this system can significantly affect the individual's quality of life.

There are two types of orthopaedic surgery: trauma (emergency) and elective surgery. Trauma surgery is carried out on patients who require urgent surgery, such as following an accident. Elective orthopaedic surgery is for patients waiting planned orthopaedic procedures such as joint replacements for progressive osteoarthritis.

The field of orthopaedics and orthopaedic nursing has become extremely diverse and is changing at an unprecedented rate. Advances in surgical techniques, developments within nursing and healthcare provision in society in general are all contributing to the advancement within the speciality of orthopaedics.

One change that has affected orthopaedic nursing is the reduced time a patient now spends in hospital. Many patients now have orthopaedic surgery as a day case admission, instead of remaining in hospital overnight or for several days. Innovations such as preoperative assessment clinics and early discharge schemes, where patients are cared for in their own home earlier, also significantly reduce the length of time a patient spends in hospital.

In the context of change, orthopaedic nurses must continue to promote healing, maximize independence within the individual's capability and promote optimal rehabilitation.

This chapter will describe some of the more common disorders of the musculoskeletal system that are caused by disease and trauma, and will explain orthopaedic surgical procedures and the relevant nursing care.

THE MUSCULOSKELETAL SYSTEM

Most of the body's mass is made up of the musculoskeletal system. It comprises bones, joints, ligaments, muscles and cartilage. The musculoskeletal system performs and enables several essential functions:

- the maintenance of body shape
- the support and protection of soft tissue structures such as internal organs
- movement
- breathing
- the manufacture of red blood cells, white blood cells and platelets in the bone marrow
- the storage and main supply of reserve phosphate and calcium in bone.

BONE

Bones are classified by their shape and fall into five categories:

1. long bones
2. short bones
3. irregular bones
4. flat bones
5. sesamoid bones.

Long bones These bones are greater in length than width. Pulled by contracting muscles, they act as levers for body movement. Long bones include the femur, tibia, fibula, radius, ulna and humerus.

Short bones These bones measure approximately the same in length and width, and are irregular in shape. They are found where only limited movement is necessary, such as the carpal and tarsal bones.

Irregular bones These bones do not fit neatly in to any of the other categories. The facial bones and the vertebrae are examples of irregular bones.

Flat bones These bones are generally curved or thin. They have a protective function and facilitate muscle attachment. Flat bones include the ribs, sternum, scapulae and bones of the cranium.

Sesamoid bones These small bones are found where tendons pass over the joint of a long bone. Their key role is protection, such as the patella bone of the knee joint.

Anatomy of a long bone

A typical long bone consists of the following parts:

1. *Diaphysis* – the shaft or long part of the bone.
2. *Epiphysis* – a proximal and distal epiphysis can be found at opposite ends of the bone.
3. *Metaphysis* – separates the diaphysis from the epiphysis at either end of the bone. It is made up of the adjacent trabeculae of spongy bone.
4. *Medullary cavity* – contains fatty yellow marrow and can be found within the diaphysis.
5. *Endosteum* – the membrane that lines the internal cavities of bone.
6. *Articular cartilage* – the layer of hyaline cartilage which covers the epiphysis and allows a joint to function more effectively by reducing friction.

7. *Periosteum* – the fibrous membrane that covers the outer surface of bone that has not been covered by articular cartilage. It contains nerves, capillaries and lymphatic vessels and is essential for bone nutrition, growth and repair.

Bone tissue

Bone tissue comprises cells embedded in a matrix of ground substance, collagenous fibres and inorganic salts. The salts harden the bone, whereas the ground substance and collagenous fibres provide flexibility and strength.

The two main types of bone tissue are cancellous bone and compact bone.

Cancellous bone

- Cancellous bone consists of thin plates of bone tissue called trabeculae, and is also known as spongy bone because of its lattice-like appearance.
- Red marrow fills the spaces between the trabeculae, and within the trabeculae lie lacunae, which store osteocytes. The osteocytes are nourished through the marrow cavities from circulating blood.
- Cancellous bone stores some red and yellow marrow, and its main function is support.

Compact bone

- Compact bone is hard and contains cylinders of calcified bone known as osteons or Haversian systems. These systems are surrounded by calcified intercellular rings called lamellae.
- Centrally within the Haversian systems are Haversian canals, which contain nerves, blood vessels and lymphatic vessels. Haversian canals are longitudinal channels which generally branch into perforating canals called Volkmann's canals. The Volkmann's canals extend the vessels and nerves inward to the endosteum and outwards to the periosteum.
- Spaces called lacunae, which store osteocytes, can be found between the lamellae, and radiating from the lacunae are tiny canaliculi, which transport waste and nutrients into and out of blood vessels in the Haversian canals.
- Compact bone lies over cancellous bone and its main functions are support and protection.

Bone cells

Bone tissue contains four types of cell:

1. *Osteogenic cells* – found in the periosteum, endosteum and the Haversian and Volkmann's canals. They can be transformed into osteoblasts or osteoclasts during the healing process or at stressful times, e.g. following trauma.
2. *Osteoblasts* – found in the growing parts of bones and the periosteum. They secrete some of the organic components and mineral salts involved in bone formation, and their main function is bone building.
3. *Osteocytes* – the main cells of bone tissue. They derive from osteoblasts that have deposited bone tissue around themselves. Osteocytes keep the matrix healthy and help maintain homeostasis by assisting in the release of calcium into the blood.
4. *Osteoclasts* – giant multinuclear cells found around bone surfaces, which do exactly the opposite of osteoblasts. Their main function is in resorption (dissolved and assimilated), which is essential in bone development, growth, maintenance and repair.

Bone ossification

Bones develop through a process known as ossification (osteogenesis). This process begins during the sixth week of embryonic life.

There are two types of ossification:

1. *Intramembranous ossification*, when bone is formed by mesenchymal tissue (embryonic connective tissue cells).
2. *Endochondral ossification*, when bone develops by replacing a cartilage model.

The primary ossification centre of a long bone is in the diaphysis. As a result of cartilage degeneration, cavities merge, forming the marrow cavity, and osteoblasts lay down bone. Ossification then occurs in the epiphyses but not for the epiphyseal plate.

Homeostasis

Bone assists homeostasis (a state of inner balance and stability) by the storage and release of minerals and calcium, as required in the blood and tissues to maintain appropriate levels. Normal bone growth depends on calcium and phosphorus, and adequate levels of vitamins A, C and D are essential for bone growth and maintenance.

Effects of hormones on bone

Bones have an effect on hormone secretion and several hormones have an effect on bones. The parathyroid hormone assists in osteoclast production, increasing bone remodelling, whereas calcitonin (a hormone released by the thyroid gland) reduces the calcium level in the blood and reduces bone resorption. Other hormones such as thyroxine, growth hormone, the sex hormones from the gonads and vitamins A, C and D are significantly involved in bone maturation, with thyroxine and the growth hormones stimulating endochondral ossification.

Effects of ageing on bone

The ageing process affects bone in two key ways.

1. The loss of calcium from bone starts in the female at around 30 years of age and this loss increases as oestrogen levels decrease in the female's early 40s. By the age of 70 as much as 30% of the calcium in bone is lost, but in the male calcium loss does not generally start until the male is over 60 years old (Tortora and Grabowski, 2003).
2. There is a decrease in protein formation, which results in a decreased ability to produce the organic part of the bone matrix. This leads to osteoporotic bones in the elderly and an increased risk of fractures (Villareal et al, 2001).

CARTILAGE

Cartilage is a tough, avascular, flexible connective tissue which assists with the support systems of the body.

There are three types of cartilage:

1. *Hyaline cartilage* is firm and smooth, and is found on the articulating surfaces of synovial joints.
2. *Fibrocartilage* is tough, flexible and tension resistant, and is found between the intervertebral discs.
3. *Elastic cartilage* retains its strength while stretched, as it has more elastic fibres, and is found in the epiglottis and external ear.

JOINTS

A joint is the site at which two or more bones are united. A joint provides the mechanism that allows body movement. Based on the structure or type of tissue that connects the bones, joints are classified into three major groups: fibrous, cartilaginous or synovial.

Fibrous joints

The bones are united by fibrous connective tissue and allow very minimal movement, e.g. sutures between the bones of the skull.

Cartilaginous joints

The bones are united by a plate of hyaline cartilage (primary cartilaginous) or fibrocartilage (secondary cartilaginous) and will allow slight movement, e.g. the pubic symphysis or between the bodies of the vertebrae.

Synovial joints

Synovial joints contain a synovial (joint) cavity, articular capsule, synovial membrane and synovial fluid.

A synovial (joint) cavity is the space between two articulating bones. Articular cartilage covers the surfaces of the articulating bones but does not hold the bones together. Synovial joints are surrounded by an articular capsule, and the inner lining of the capsule is called the synovial membrane. The synovial membrane secretes synovial fluid to lubricate the joint and provides nourishment for the articular cartilage.

An extensive range of movement is possible with this type of joint. Based on the shape of the articulating surfaces and the range of movements possible, there are several different types of synovial joint: e.g. the ball and socket joint of the hip and shoulder and the hinge joint of the knee.

COMMON ORTHOPAEDIC DISORDERS

RHEUMATOID ARTHRITIS

Rheumatoid arthritis is the commonest chronic inflammatory disease of joints and affects 3% of women and 1% of men (Dandy and Edwards, 2003). The cause is unknown but the inflammation is the result of an abnormality of both cellular and humoral immunity. As it is a systemic disease, unlike osteoarthritis, rheumatoid arthritis affects structures all over the body.

Pathophysiology

The target for this disease is the synovium. In the early stages of the disease the synovial membrane is affected and the joints become warm, swollen and tender and range of movement is reduced. This disease generally presents in the small peripheral joints, usually of the hands, with the wrists and knees also being susceptible. The affected synovium contains plasma cells and lymphocytes, a reflection of the autoimmune nature of the disease, and left untreated the inflammatory reaction affects the neighbouring structures. As the disease progresses, there is joint cartilage, capsule and ligament destruction, leading to joint instability, subluxation and deformity (Solomon et al, 2001).

Although rheumatoid arthritis is mainly treated by rheumatologists, it does involve orthopaedic surgeons when conservative treatments have proved to be unsuccessful. Orthopaedic surgeons are involved when joints and ligaments require stabilization or reconstruction.

OSTEOARTHRITIS

Osteoarthritis is a degenerative 'wear and tear' process occurring in joints that are impaired by congenital defect, vascular insufficiency or previous disease or injury. It is by far the commonest variety of arthritis (Crawford Adams and Hamblen, 2001).

Osteoarthritis is defined as primary or secondary.

- *Primary osteoarthritis* has no obvious cause (Apley and Solomon, 2001), is most common in white females during their 50s and 60s and affects several joints (Dandy and Edwards, 2003).
- *Secondary osteoarthritis* has many causes and follows a demonstrable abnormality of which the commonest are obesity, malunited fractures, joint instability, genetic or developmental abnormalities, metabolic or endocrine disease, inflammatory diseases, osteonecrosis and neuropathies (Apley and Solomon, 2001; Crawford Adams and Hamblen, 2001; Dandy and Edwards, 2003).

Pain, limited mobility and a decrease in functional ability are the main clinical features. X-ray or imaging is undertaken to confirm the diagnosis of osteoarthritis.

Pathophysiology

In osteoarthritis the articular cartilage is slowly worn away, resulting in the exposure of underlying bone. The subchondral bone becomes hard and glossy (eburnated), and bone at the margins of the joint forms protruding ridges and spurs known as osteophytes. These spurs can break off, causing further restriction of movement and additional pain. It is the pain, stiffness and often deformity that force the patient to seek treatment.

Treatment can be conservative or operative. Orthopaedic surgery should not be recommended until all conservative measures have been considered.

Conservative treatment

- *Weight reduction*: if obese, the patient is encouraged to reduce weight, so that less weight is forced on to the joint. The patient needs to be informed of the problems caused by excess weight and understand that, by reducing their weight, they will assist in reducing their level of pain. This may be difficult for the patient, owing to the nature of the disease. It is therefore important to set small achievable targets and offer praise and encouragement as they achieve satisfactory weight loss.

- *Physiotherapy*: passive and active exercises can assist the range of joint movement, prevent contractures and improve coordination or balance. Heat therapy can often produce relief from pain.
- *Hydrotherapy*: the warmth and buoyancy of the water allows the patient active, pain-free movement and relieves muscle spasm.
- *The use of a walking stick*: the patient is encouraged to use the walking stick correctly, holding it in the opposite hand to the affected hip/knee.
- *Aids and appliances*: these can help the patient with activities of daily living: e.g. a helping hand to pick up dropped articles or an aid to assist with putting shoes and socks on.
- *A shoe raise*: application of a shoe raise to the shorter limb can correct the apparent shortening, relieving strain on the lumbar spine and opposite hip.
- *Drug therapy*: simple analgesics such as paracetamol or dihydrocodeine can be effective in reducing the pain caused by raw bone rubbing on bone; however, they are not useful in reducing the sinusitis of osteoarthritis. Non-steroidal anti-inflammatory drugs (NSAIDs), however, reduce the inflammatory response and many people find them useful before physical activity or at night. NSAIDs have historically been associated with gastrointestinal side-effects; however, new COX-2 specific NSAIDs such as celecoxib are now licensed for use in arthritis with less risk of these side-effects. Disease-modifying anti-rheumatic drugs, corticosteroids and immunosuppressive drugs may be used for patients with rheumatoid arthritis.
- *Intra-articular therapy*: local injection of hydrocortisone into the joint may help to restore comfort and mobility.

Operative treatment

All patients need to be carefully assessed before a decision to undertake surgery is made, because some patients will benefit from surgery more than others, according to their physical, mental and social circumstances. Only when conservative treatments have failed, should operative treatment be considered.

The following criteria are often used to decide on the need for surgery:

- pain
- radiological changes
- joint stability
- loss of function
- immobility.

The most common surgical procedures for patients with osteoarthritis and rheumatoid arthritis are synovectomy, osteotomy, arthrodesis and arthroplasty:

- *Synovectomy* involves excision of diseased synovial membrane and is performed more frequently for the patient with rheumatoid arthritis.
- *Osteotomy* involves surgically cutting across the bone. It is used to correct bone deformity or to relieve joint pain.
- *Arthrodesis* is carried out to surgically fuse a joint. It is used to stabilize a joint, or for pain relief in a joint severely damaged or diseased.
- *Arthroplasty* is replacement of the joint by an artificial component and one of the most successful operations in orthopaedic surgery (Dandy and Edwards, 2003).

NURSING ASSESSMENT OF THE ORTHOPAEDIC PATIENT

When assessing orthopaedic patients, it is important to first establish what their normal functional abilities were and then to see how their presenting complaint is decreasing this functional ability. A thorough nursing assessment is required to obtain essential information from patients about the physical, psychological, sociocultural, environmental and politicoeconomic factors affecting their activities of daily living and how they cope with these problems. Once the patients' problems have been identified, the nurse can set goals, take nursing action and evaluate any subsequent care. The Roper, Logan and Tierney model of nursing (Roper et al, 1996) is one example of a model used in the nursing management of an orthopaedic patient and an example of this can be seen in Table 21.1.

Every patient is a unique individual and the nursing assessment should be tailored to address these individual needs. The following points, however, are often discussed and assessed in an orthopaedic nursing assessment:

- Mobility
  - Is movement restricted and, if so, how restricted is the movement?
  - Is the range of movement limited?
  - Is active range of movement less than passive?
  - Does mobility improve throughout the day?
  - What is the condition of the patient's musculoskeletal system?
  - What is the neurological status of the affected limb?
  - Does the patient require aids to assist mobility?
- Pain
  - Where is the maximal site of pain?
  - Does the pain radiate away from the site of injury?
  - Does the pain change during the course of the day?
  - How would the pain be described?
  - Is there swelling or deformity?
- Sleep
  - Is sleep affected by pain?
- Sexuality
  - Has a limp, limb-shortening or a deformity altered the patient's body image?
  - Has the patient had surgery that is affecting their sexual relationship?
- Mental state
  - Is the patient anxious or depressed?
  - Does the patient suffer from dementia or poor attention span?
- Hygiene
  - Can the patient cope with their own personal cleansing and dressing?
  - Does the patient require assistance or special aids/appliances to assist with hygiene care?
- Breathing
  - Does the patient smoke?
  - Does the patient have a history of cardiovascular problems?
  - Does the patient have any sort of curvature of the spine that is affecting their respiratory system?
- Working and playing
  - Has the problem affected the patient's work and/or social activities?
  - Does the patient require assistance for household activities?

The main aim of the orthopaedic nursing assessment and subsequent care that is planned is to assist the patient to be as independent as is realistically possible.

ORTHOPAEDIC INVESTIGATIONS AND TESTS

STANDARD X–RAYS

Standard X-rays assist in the diagnosis and confirmation of the injury or disease, e.g. fractures, loss of joint space in osteoarthritis. Usually, no specific preparation is required.

COMPUTERIZED AXIAL TOMOGRAPHY

A computerized axial tomography (CAT or CT) scan combines X-rays with computer technology to show cross-sectional views (tomograms) of internal body structures. Prior to the scan, the patient is intravenously

Table 21.1 Postoperative care plan for a patient following a total hip replacement, using the Roper, Logan and Tierney model of nursing

Assessment/usual routine	Patient's problem	Goal	Nursing action	Evaluation
Maintaining a safe environment				
Uncemented hip prosthesis in correct position following anterior approach on return from operating theatre	Potential risk of dislocation of hip prosthesis	To prevent hip dislocation	Ensure Louise has a copy of the do's and don'ts on how not to dislocate her hip. Reinforce the information at regular intervals. Place affected leg in a gutter splint. Ensure Louise does not flex the hip to an angle of 90° or more. Ensure Louise uses a high toilet seat on the ward and at home for 3 months	Louise's hip prosthesis did not dislocate
Louise's skin is healthy and intact	Potential wound infection or haematoma following surgery	To prevent wound infection and haematoma	Administer prophylactic antibiotics as prescribed. Observe the wound for bleeding, swelling and excessive drainage. Use aseptic technique when dealing with dressings and drains. Record temperature ½–1 hourly then 2–4 hourly for a 24 hour period. Check drainage patency and maintenance of the vacuum drain every ¼ hour for 1 hour, then, if satisfactory, hourly for 24 hours. Remove staples on the 10th postoperative day	Louise remained apyrexial and the wound healed with no sign of infection. The drain remained patent, the loss was minimal and the drain was removed 24 hours postoperatively
	Potential risk of pressure ulcers as her mobility is reduced	To prevent pressure ulcers	Raise for pressure relief 2 hourly. Encourage Louise to use the overhead bar on the bed. Ensure her heels are kept free of the bed. Use a gutter splint, ensuring heel is hanging over the edge. Assess pressure ulcer risk using Waterlow score and use appropriate mattress if indicated. Encourage mobilization on day 1 postoperative	Louise's pressure areas remained intact
Louise's temperature was normal 37.1°C on admission to hospital	On return to the ward Louise's temperature was 35°C	To assist body temperature back to normal limits	Place a Bair hugger next to Louise's body and apply extra bed linen. Record Louise's temperature at regular intervals until it	Within 2 hours Louise's temperature had risen to 36.2°C and the Bair hugger was removed. Louise's temperature

(Continued)

Table 21.1 (Continued)

Assessment/usual routine	Patient's problem	Goal	Nursing action	Evaluation
			has returned to within normal limits	remained above 36.2°C and below 37.5°C
Mobilization				
Louise's mobilization and distance she could walk without pain prior to surgery was approximately 300 yards	Postoperatively, Louise had lack of confidence mobilizing, but her pain was under control	Louise to regain confidence mobilizing	Give explanations and reassurance prior to and when mobilizing	Louise can safely mobilize and transfer from bed to chair and bed to toilet with confidence
			Observe for signs of dislocation	
			On day 1 begin mobilizing Louise with the aid of a physiotherapist, starting with transfers from bed to chair, learning the correct way to sit in a chair and progressing on to how to use the sticks safely to avoid dislocation	
			Louise will need to mobilize partial weight bearing on the operated leg for 6 weeks	
Work and play				
Louise works as a part-time secretary for a small local firm. The firm is having some financial problems and there have been some redundancies	Louise is warned she may lose her job due to her sick leave. She likes to get out and does not wish to retire	To return to work as soon as she is able	Encourage Louise to express her fears. Refer to a social worker	The surgeon wrote a supportive letter to her employer who was very sympathetic and supportive
Louise is a keen gardener	Louise is concerned that she will not be able to return to her hobby of gardening, although she admits she has been unable to do any gardening during the 6 months prior to surgery	For Louise to return to light gardening activities	Refer Louise to the physiotherapist for advice on safe movement while gardening	As yet Louise has not returned to gardening but looks forward to doing so. She has learnt what she can do safely and accepts this
Expressing sexuality				
Louise and her husband have been married for 32 years and still enjoy a sexual relationship. This has been affected by pain in recent months, and Louise confided that her husband had offered to sleep in the spare bedroom to give her more room and to prevent her dislocating her hip when she got home	Fear of dislocating hip during sexual relations	Louise to return to sexual relations with her husband without dislocating her hip	Give Louise advice and reassurance that she can resume sexual intercourse in the passive role at approximately 6 weeks	Louise has yet to resume sexual intercourse but feels she knows how not to dislocate the hip
			Give Louise details of the association to aid the sexual and personal relationships of people with a disability (SPOD) and provide a leaflet on positions postoperatively	

Source: Roper et al (1996).

injected with a low-level radioactive tracer. The patient lies on a table and is slowly passed through a circular tunnel in the scanner, where rotation of a low-intensity X-ray beam across the width of the body takes place. Detectors opposite the X-ray beam record the degree to which the X-ray is absorbed by various body tissues and convert the modified beams into electronic signals that are fed into the computer. Changes in the X-ray beams are then analysed by the computer, and high-resolution images are shown on a monitor. These images are kept on film and examined one section at a time. This investigation is particularly useful in the diagnosis of spinal and skull disorders.

MAGNETIC RESONANCE IMAGING

Magnetic resonance imaging (MRI) is a non-invasive investigation of the body's deep structures. Prior to the MRI scan, patients may be asked to change into a gown or they may be permitted to wear their own clothes, provided they take off all metal items such as buckles, pins, hair clips, watches or badges, because of the powerful magnet in the scanner.

To produce an image with MRI, the patient is required to lie on a non-magnetic stretcher and is passed into a scanner where the body is exposed to a strong magnetic field. This magnetic field causes the body's protons to line upright in rows parallel to the field. The patient's body is then exposed to radiofrequency waves, which cause the protons to fall out of line. When the radiofrequency waves are stopped, the protons return to their previous position. Images of this movement are taken and visually displaced. Magnetic resonance imaging is particularly useful to show changes in the vascularity of bone following trauma, and degenerative changes in the ligaments and intervertebral discs (Dandy and Edwards, 2003).

Many patients who undergo an MRI scan experience anxiety or panic attacks. Nurses can help reduce the stress in patients undergoing MRI by maintaining verbal contact through an intercom and by using relaxation techniques (Carr and Grey, 2002).

THERMOGRAPHY

This technique involves the use of a thermographic camera which detects normally invisible infrared radiations, converts them into electrical impulses and then records them as thermograms. Thermograms create a pictorial representation of warm areas around a joint, which provides an indication of the blood supply and areas of inflammation or vascular disease. They are particularly useful to assess the progress of rheumatoid arthritis and its response to treatment.

RADIOISOTOPE BONE SCAN

The patient is given an intravenous injection of radioisotope substance, which is taken up in the bone. The amount of uptake reflects the bone turnover and is of value in the early detection of tumour invasion, bone death and repair.

BONE DENSITOMETRY

This technique is carried out to measure bone mineral density in patients with metabolic bone disease and may be required for the whole of the patient's body or an identified area. X-rays are produced and interpreted by a computer. This measurement assists the clinician to make an informed opinion on the most appropriate treatment for the patient.

ARTHROSCOPY

Arthroscopy is an invasive procedure which involves the introduction of an instrument called an arthroscope into a joint, most commonly the knee joint, under local or general anaesthetic. Arthroscopy enables inspection of the interior of the joint and allows manipulation of individual structures with a probe or hook; the movement of one structure on another as the joint is moved can also be observed.

LOWER LIMB ORTHOPAEDIC SURGERY

THE HIP

Total hip replacement (arthroplasty)

Total hip replacement (arthroplasty) is the most popular operation for osteoarthritis of the hip (Dandy and Edwards, 2003). In a total hip replacement, the worn acetabulum and femoral head are removed and replaced with artificial components, which can be either cemented or uncemented (Fig. 21.1).

- *Cemented*: this involves the use of a dense cup, usually polyethylene, and a metal or metal alloy femoral component. Each of these parts is secured by the compound methylmethacrylate, which has properties resembling bone. A disadvantage of the cemented prostheses is the potential bone destruction caused if the prosthesis becomes loose.
- *Uncemented*: where cement would have been placed, more cortical bone is preserved. This allows younger patients to have total hip replacement surgery with increased choice for revision surgery in the future.

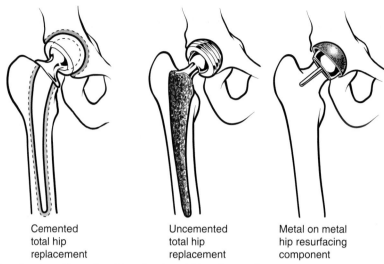

Cemented
total hip
replacement

Uncemented
total hip
replacement

Metal on metal
hip resurfacing
component

Figure 21.1   Total hip arthroplasty. (Reproduced from Dandy and Edwards, 2003.)

Metal on metal hip resurfacing

Metal on metal hip resurfacing has more recently been introduced. The resurfacing component does not use a long stem, and both the femoral and the acetabular components are metal, which decreases the amount of wear debris within the hip capsule (Dandy and Edwards, 2003). Hip resurfacing has proven to be a beneficial treatment in those younger patients with joint disease.

Preoperative assessment and care

It is recommended that patients undergoing total hip replacement attend the preoperative assessment clinic and education classes 2–3 weeks prior to surgery.

Preoperative assessment enables the multidisciplinary team to ensure that the patient is as medically fit as is possible, in order that they are not cancelled when admitted to hospital because of medical problems. This allows effective use of resources such as theatre time and hospital beds and avoids patient disappointment when their surgery is cancelled (Clinch, 1997; Smith and Rudd, 1998).

Depending on whether preoperative education classes are available, the preoperative assessment clinic may be run by a nurse practitioner alone or by a variety of members of the multidisciplinary team. The preoperative assessment will consist of:

- Routine blood tests for a full blood count, urea and electrolytes, group and save and cross-matching, and any other indicated tests, e.g. glucose, sickle cell screen.
- A urinalysis and midstream specimen of urine is sent to the laboratory for microscopy and culture to test for infection, which can be treated in advance of admission.

- Vital signs monitoring, including blood pressure, pulse, temperature, respirations and oxygen saturation levels.
- Neurovascular assessment to provide a baseline for postoperative monitoring.
- Electrocardiograph, if indicated.
- Swabs taken to ascertain methicillin-resistant *Staphylococcus aureus* (MRSA), which can be treated prior to admission.
- X-rays of the hip and chest, if indicated.
- A comprehensive health history and physical examination.

Preoperative education class   Many patients now have the opportunity to attend a preoperative education class, which is run by the multidisciplinary team alongside the patient's visit to the preassessment clinic. If education classes are not available, the multidisciplinary team will provide information at the preassessment clinic. The patient is given a detailed explanation about what the operation will involve and what they should expect postoperatively.

- Patients are often anxious about the postoperative pain they may experience. Explanations are given about the use of patient-controlled analgesia (PCA) pumps, intramuscular analgesics and distraction techniques such as deep breathing techniques and guided imagery to control their pain (Ackerman and Turkoski, 2000).

- Patients are informed that they will receive prophylactic antibiotics to prevent infection, and prophylaxis against deep venous thrombosis such as

DO'S and DON'TS after a total hip replacement

DO's

Do the exercises you have been taught twice a day, if possible

Do continue to lie flat on your back, for a short period daily (half an hour twice a day) for a couple of weeks after leaving hospital

Do use your stick(s), especially outside the house. It is advisable to use one stick for 6 weeks

Do be critical of your own posture in sitting, standing and walking

Do sleep on the side of your new hip, if you want to, and put a pillow between your legs for comfort

Do use equipment you have been given for putting on socks or stockings or shoes

Do ask advice if in doubt about any activity

DON'TS

After Hip Replacement Surgery, surrounding muscles and other tissues take time to heal and strengthen. During this time your new hip is at risk of dislocating. To minimize this risk you must take the following precautions for at least 6 weeks following your operation

Don't cross your legs

Don't sit on a low chair or toilet

Don't sleep on your unaffected side for 2 months

Don't squat or bend down to pick up things from the floor

Don't try to bend the affected leg up to your chest

Don't attempt getting in or out of the bath for 6 weeks after the operation

Don't drive until 6 weeks after the operation

Figure 21.2   Do's and don'ts following a total hip replacement.

anti-embolic stockings and anticoagulant therapy (e.g. subcutaneous injections or tablets).

- Patients are shown abduction wedges, gutter splints, vacuum drains, intravenous giving sets and catheters, as applicable, as well as the bed area, so that they are aware of the equipment when they wake up following their surgery.

- Patients are made aware of the risks of their surgery, such as dislocation of the hip, and will be taught how to prevent this during the class. A list of 'do's and don'ts' following surgery is given to the patient (Fig. 21.2).

- The physiotherapist will assess patients' gait and range of movement and will teach patients their postoperative exercises during the class so that they can practise them prior to their admission.

- The occupational therapist will carry out a daily living assessment to see what activities the patient is having difficulty with. The patient is taught how to preserve energy and adapt daily living as required. Patients are asked to bring measurements of their chair, bed and toilet to the class, where they are shown aids that will be required, e.g. raised toilet seats, and those that may help patients with their activities of daily living, e.g. sock aids, long-handled sponges and helping hands.

- The discharge coordinator or care manager will work with all members of the multidisciplinary team, to ensure that the patient has a safe home environment to be discharged to.

- Information is reinforced in the form of written documentation, which the patient can take away with them.

Postoperative care

Following total hip replacement, the patient will return to the ward with an intravenous infusion. They may also have a PCA pump and a vacuum drain, although many surgeons do not routinely use vacuum drains postoperatively as there is conflicting views regarding their benefit. To prevent neurovascular compromise, neurovascular observations of the toes and foot will be carried out and recorded at 30-minute intervals initially, progressing to 4 hourly for at least 24 hours (Fig. 21.3). Each digit of the affected limb is examined for temperature, colour, sensation and mobility. One of the patient's pedal pulses is palpated and compared with the pulse on the unaffected foot and any abnormalities are reported immediately. A pain score is also recorded.

The patient will initially return to the ward with a pressure dressing in situ, which is usually taken down after 24 hours to leave the primary dressing exposed. If a vacuum drain is in situ, it is usually removed at this time. A transparent vapour-permeable film is recommended as a primary dressing so that the wound can be inspected without the dressing being removed,

NAME		WARD		PROCEDURE/INJURY:							
CONSULTANT		NUMBER		AREA TO BE OBSERVED:							
DATE OF ADMISSION				FREQUENCY OF OBSERVATIONS:							
DATE											
TIME											
PAIN SCORE (0–5)											
VASCULAR	COLOUR	Normal									
		Pale									
		Cynotic									
		Mottled									
	WARMTH	Hot									
		Warm									
		Cold									
		Cool									
	SWELLING	Nil									
		Moderate									
		Marked									
	CAPILLARY REFILL <2 SECONDS										
	PULSE	Strong									
		Weak									
		Absent									
MOVEMENT	ANKLE DORSI-FLEXION	No active contraction detected									
		Active movement no pain									
		Active movement with pain									
		Passive movement no pain									
	ANKLE PLANTAR-FLEXION	No active contraction detected									
		Active movement no pain									
		Active movement with pain									
		Passive movement no pain									

Figure 21.3　Neurovascular chart.

MOVEMENT	TOE EXTENSION	No active contraction detected									
		Active movement no pain									
		Active movement with pain									
		Passive movement no pain									
	TOE FLEXION	No active contraction detected									
		Active movement no pain									
		Active movement with pain									
		Passive movement no pain									
SENSATION	DORSAL WEB SPACE 1st & 2nd TOE	No sensation									
		Tingling/ numbness									
		Full sensation									
	WEB SPACE 3rd & 4th TOE	No sensation									
		Tingling/ numbness									
		Full sensation									
	SOLE OF FOOT/ TOES	No sensation									
		Tingling/ numbness									
		Full sensation									
	MEDIAL ARCH OF FOOT	No sensation									
		Tingling/ numbness									
		Full sensation									
INITIALS											

Always compare with unaffected limb.
If both limbs are affected use a separate chart for each limb.
If abnormalities occur, report to the nurse-in-charge or the medical team immediately.
Document all actions taken.

Figure 21.3   (*Continued*)

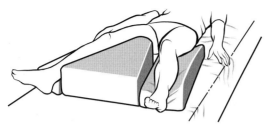

Figure 21.4 Abduction wedge and gutter splint in place to reduce the risk of dislocation of a hip prosthesis (they must be used separately and not together).

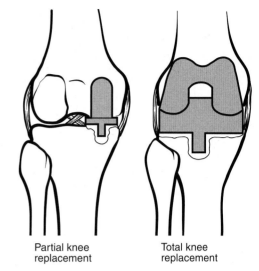

Partial knee replacement   Total knee replacement

Figure 21.5 Knee arthroplasty.

thus reducing the risk of infection. The wound is closed with either sutures or staples, which are removed between 10 and 14 days postoperatively if the wound has healed.

The patient's operated leg should remain in a gutter splint or have an abduction wedge placed between the legs for the first 24 hours (Fig. 21.4) and then at night until discharge to stop the patient crossing their legs.

Postoperative care plan The care plan given in Table 21.1 illustrates the care of Louise, a 62-year-old lady who requires a total hip replacement.

Potential postoperative complications
Deep venous thrombosis Patients are at risk of developing a DVT following surgery. To prevent this, patients receive a variety of prophylactic measures, including administration of low molecular weight heparin injections, oral anticoagulants, anti-embolic stockings and intermittent pressure devices, as well as being taught to dorsi- and plantarflex their ankles and deep breathe.

Infection Patients are at risk of bacterial infection to both bone and wound. Prophylactic intravenous antibiotics are administered and strict wound asepsis is carried out. Deep prosthetic bacterial infection after total hip arthroplasty is one of the most devastating complications in hip surgery (McPherson et al, 2002). Patients are initially treated with long-term antibiotic therapy (McPherson et al, 2002) but infection may result in removal of the prosthesis. If left without a prosthesis, the patient is left with an unstable joint (Jamieson and McFarlane, 1996).

Dislocation of the hip Dislocation following total hip replacement is an unfortunate complication that is either patient- or technique-related (Malik et al, 2002). The patient is nursed postoperatively with either an abduction wedge between the legs or with the operated leg resting in a gutter splint to reduce this risk (see Fig. 21.4), and is also given written and verbal information on how to prevent dislocation (see Fig. 21.2).

THE KNEE
Total knee replacement (arthroplasty)

Total knee replacement (arthroplasty) is generally performed to relieve patients' pain, and improve mobility and stability which have been impaired by conditions such as osteoarthritis. Total knee replacement now gives as good results as have been achieved at the hip. Excellent and durable results are now being achieved in over 90% of patients after 10 years (Crawford Adams and Hamblen, 2001).

Arthroplasty of the knee can be unicondylar (partial) or total (Fig. 21.5). Unicondylar knee arthroplasty is only suitable for early disease or disease of one compartment only. Total knee replacement is far more common.

Total knee arthroplasty involves the worn femoral and tibial surfaces being removed and replaced with metal and polyethylene components, respectively, providing gliding articular surfaces.

Preoperative care
The preoperative care for a patient undergoing a total knee replacement is much the same as for a patient undergoing a total hip replacement, with a few exceptions. At preoperative assessment, the physiotherapist teaches the patient specific leg exercises, such as static quadriceps, straight leg raising and knee bending, to help strengthen the quadriceps muscles. The patient is warned that postoperatively it is likely the leg will be painful, swollen and bruised.

- *Static quadriceps exercises*: the patient is instructed to place their hand behind the affected knee, then press

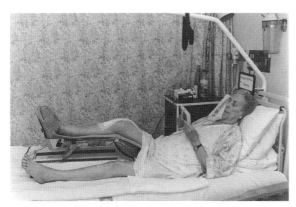

Figure 21.6   CPM machine.

their knee on to their hand and then to relax. Some patients such as those with rheumatoid arthritis of the hands have great difficulty with this, but they can generally manage to press their knee downwards into the bed.

● *Straight leg raising exercises*: the patient is instructed to tighten the thigh muscles of the affected leg, then raise the leg as high as they can.

Postoperative care

Following total knee replacement, the patient will return to the ward with an intravenous infusion, PCA pump, a vacuum drain and a pressure dressing of wool and crepe from ankle to thigh. To prevent neurovascular compromise, neurovascular observations of the toes and foot will be carried out and recorded at 30-minute intervals initially, progressing to 4 hourly until the pressure dressing is removed, which is generally 24 hours later (see Fig. 21.3). Each digit of the affected limb is examined for temperature, colour, sensation and mobility. One of the patient's pedal pulses is palpated and compared with the pulse on the affected foot, and any abnormalities are reported immediately. A pain score is also recorded.

A continual passive motion machine (CPM machine) may be used to assist the patient to flex and extend the knee joint (Fig. 21.6). Continuous passive motion may be commenced in the recovery room or when the vacuum drains and pressure dressings are removed. Some surgeons do not indicate the use of CPM unless the patient experiences particular problems in flexing and extending the joint.

The wound is closed with either sutures or staples, which are removed between 10 and 14 days postoperatively if the wound has healed.

Potential complications are similar to those for total hip replacement, e.g. DVT and infection. It is important that the patient undergoing total knee replacement

continues to flex and extend the knee in order that a range of movement is achieved and maintained, and joint contracture does not occur. For this reason, pillows should not be placed under the knee, particularly at night, leaving the knee in a fixed flexion position.

The care plan given in Table 21.2 illustrates the care of John, a 74-year-old man who requires a total knee replacement.

Discharge planning following total knee replacement

All members of the multidisciplinary team must be satisfied that the patient has achieved the defined functional milestones:

● independently mobile with an appropriate aid
● able to climb stairs (if appropriate)
● full understanding of exercises and precautions
● independent with transfers
● active knee flexion of 70–90°
● wound has healed
● medically fit

The patient is reviewed in the outpatients department 6 weeks following discharge.

KNEE INJURIES

Tears of the menisci

Tears of the menisci are common sports injuries, and are frequently found in individuals with occupations involving kneeling and crouching, such as electricians and miners, or in professional footballers with a history of repeated knee injuries (Crawford Adams and Hamblen, 1999).

Meniscus tears fall into three categories (Fig. 21.7):

● *Bucket handle tear*: complete tearing practically divides the meniscus in two, and the inner part flips over like the action of a bucket handle to create this most common tear.
● *Posterior or anterior tear*: these may only affect the posterior or anterior horns.
● *Parrot beak tear*: this is a horizontal cleavage tear that produces a flap between the condyles which resembles a parrot's beak.

These patients tend to be young males with a history of twisting a flexed knee with the weight on that leg. They experience pain and feel something tear. The knee may lock so that they cannot extend their leg; however, manipulation of the knee will cause it to unlock. There may be swelling, tenderness over the meniscus and often loss of full extension.

Table 21.2 Postoperative care plan of patient following a total knee replacement using the Roper, Logan and Tierney model of nursing

Assessment/usual routine	Patient's problem	Goal	Nursing action	Evaluation
Eliminating John occasionally has difficulty passing urine. He is concerned he may not be able to pass urine while on bedrest	Potential risk of urinary retention	To prevent urinary retention	Reassure John and try to allay anxiety Encourage at least 2 L of fluids in 24 hours Position John comfortably in the upright position in bed Sit out on commode and encourage John to mobilize out to the toilet as soon as possible Pass a catheter if indicated	All nursing actions failed John had urinary retention John was catheterized and passed 400 mL On removal of catheter John had no further problems passing urine
John opens his bowels daily	At risk of constipation while on bed rest	To prevent constipation	Encourage fluids, fruit and high-fibre diet Monitor bowel action and record daily	John opened his bowels on the second postoperative day
Mobilizing John's knee is stiff and painful and his muscles are weak	Potential risk of stiff new knee prosthesis with limited function	To achieve maximum result from knee replacement Aim for 70–90° flexion prior to discharge from hospital	Assess John's pain and administer prescribed analgesics Reassure John Encourage quadriceps and straight leg raising exercises Encourage knee flexion exercises using the CPM machine Aim for 70–90° flexion by discharge Mobilize with sticks by the 3rd postoperative day	John began to use the CPM machine 24 hours after surgery He started at 10–30° flexion. The flexion was increased daily and John achieved 90° flexion by discharge John mobilized with sticks on the 2nd postoperative day. He was discharged on day 7, mobilizing fully weight-bearing with two sticks
Maintaining a safe environment John is concerned he may not be able to do his shopping or heavy household chores when discharged	John will not be able to do his own shopping or heavy housework for up to 3 months	Ensure John has assistance with shopping and housework when discharged from hospital	Refer John to social services for assistance with shopping and housework when discharged	John was discharged with meals on wheels for 2 weeks and has a home help once a week for shopping and housework until he can manage himself

Source: Roper et al (1996).

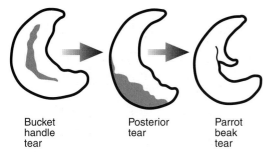

Bucket handle tear

Posterior tear

Parrot beak tear

Figure 21.7 Types of menisci tears.

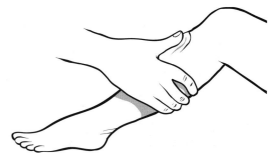

Figure 21.9 Lachman's test.

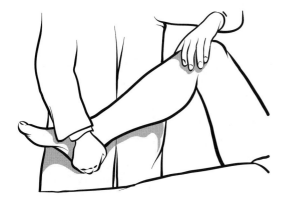

Figure 21.8 McMurrays test.

The examiner will carry out a McMurray's test as a diagnostic tool for a torn meniscus. The examiner fully flexes the patient's knee and holds the patient's heel with one hand and the affected knee with the other (Fig. 21.8). The flexed knee is then internally and externally rotated. If the meniscus is torn, a click may be felt and this may be accompanied by pain.

The knee is usually treated initially with pressure bandaging, e.g. a wool and crepe bandage from ankle to thigh, and the symptoms should gradually settle down.

When diagnosis is reached, the loose fragment should be removed and as much of the healthy meniscal tissue should be left as is possible. This procedure is commonly done arthroscopically because it allows a more precise diagnosis and careful excision. The patient is usually admitted as a day case.

Following arthroscopic day surgery, the patient is prescribed analgesics, mobilized weight-bearing as pain allows with crutches, given an exercise plan by the physiotherapist and advised to do light work 1 week after surgery and heavy work 2 weeks after surgery.

Open meniscectomy is carried out when the surgeon is unable to perform an arthroscopic meniscectomy. Although it gives a similar result, the rehabilitation period is slower and the patient is in hospital at least overnight. These patients may be unable to return to

work for as long as 3 months (Dandy and Edwards, 2003).

LIGAMENT INJURIES

The knee depends heavily on the anterior and posterior cruciate ligaments for stability. Ruptures of the cruciate ligaments are commonly found in the young adult involved in contact sports (Schoen, 2000; McRae, 2002).

Anterior cruciate rupture

The patient feels and hears a 'pop' and cannot continue the activity they were doing. The knee swells, and a haemarthrosis (blood in the joint space) is present. The presence of a haemarthrosis generally indicates a substantial injury to the joint and will cause the patient great pain (McRae, 2002). In the acute stage, investigations such as the Lachman's test are difficult to carry out because of the swelling; thus, the haemarthrosis should be aspirated first.

Lachman's test is carried out to assess the stability of the anterior and posterior cruciate ligaments. The patient lies on a couch with the knee in 90° of flexion with the foot flat and free from sliding. The amount of posterior and anterior movement is then assessed by pushing the lower leg gently backwards and forwards (Fig. 21.9).

The initial treatment is to provide the patient with analgesics and aspirate the joint to relieve pressure within the capsule. Many surgeons carry out an emergency arthroscopy to wash out the haemarthrosis. When the blood has been removed, physiotherapy is commenced to build up the muscles. The knee is then partially immobilized in a brace held at a 30–90° range of motion and the patient is mobilized with crutches. Dandy and Edwards (2003) state that one-third of patients have severe knee instability, and reconstruction of the anterior cruciate ligament may be required.

Surgical treatment

Reconstruction involves the anterior cruciate ligament being replaced with natural tissue such as the medial third of the patellar tendon or the hamstring. This complex surgery requires 3–6 months of physiotherapy and at least 6 months away from sport. The results remain satisfactory in about 80% of patients 5 years after surgery (Dandy and Edwards, 2003).

Posterior cruciate rupture

This ligament is injured less frequently than the anterior cruciate ligament, and most patients make an excellent recovery without treatment (Solomon et al, 2001; Dandy and Edwards, 2003).

Conservative treatment consists of joint aspiration or arthroscopy followed by quadriceps exercises. Surgery is only carried out if the tibial insertion of the posterior cruciate is avulsed with a block of bone and this bone can be reattached with a screw (Dandy and Edwards, 2003). Most patients manage well without a posterior cruciate ligament; therefore, conservative treatment is the best treatment and reconstruction should only be considered in extreme cases.

THE FOOT

Hallux valgus

With hallux valgus, the first metatarsal deviates medially and the great toe deviates laterally. A bunion develops over an exostosis on the first metatarsal head, and this can become inflamed and infected.

This condition may start late in childhood or in early adult life and is more common in females. Rudicel (1999) argues that forefoot problems such as hallux valgus can be prevented or relieved through the selection of proper footwear.

Conservative treatment such as chiropody, padding the bunion to relieve pressure, steroid injections and special footwear helps make the patient more comfortable but it does not correct the deformity. Pain and deformity are the main reasons why patients have surgical treatment.

Surgical treatment

More than 100 surgical techniques have been introduced for correction of hallux valgus (Torkki et al, 2001). The most common surgical procedures are as follows:

- *Bunionectomy*: the exostosis is trimmed and the bunion removed.
- *Metatarsal osteotomy*: a cut is made through the neck of the first metatarsal head, and the head is inwardly displaced and left to unite, e.g. Mitchell's osteotomy.
- *Arthroplasty*: the most common arthroplasty is the Keller's arthroplasty. This involves excision of the proximal half of the great toe first phalanx, creating

a flail joint. The position of the second toe is often affected, and this can be corrected with a Kirschner wire.

- *Arthrodesis of the metatarsophalangeal joint*: the joint is fused in slight valgus, and the great toe continues to take part in weight-bearing.

Hallux rigidus

Osteoarthritis of the first metatarsophalangeal joint is often referred to as hallux rigidus or 'stiff big toe' (Dandy and Edwards, 2003). The joint becomes painful when walking, stiffens and the toe becomes rigid.

Conservative treatment includes the use of NSAIDs and orthoses which aim to reduce the movement that produces pain (Solan et al, 2001).

Surgical treatment is by arthrodesis of the joint, as it is the most reliable procedure to give lasting pain relief, although this limits the height of a shoe heel that a woman can wear.

Mallet toe

Mallet toe is a congenital abnormality of the distal interphalangeal joint and is usually genetic. The shoe rubs against the toe, and blisters may develop. Conservative treatment such as wearing wider-fitting shoes, having regular chiropody and padding the tip of the toe to stop it rubbing against the shoe can help. Surgical treatment is by arthrodesis, or amputation of the terminal phalanx, which may be necessary if there is excessive pressure on the tip of the toe.

Hammer toe

A hammer toe consists of fixed flexion at the proximal interphalangeal joint, with hyperextension at the distal interphalangeal joint. This deformity generally involves the second toe, and a painful corn develops over the prominent head of the proximal phalanx.

Conservative treatment is by padding the corn to relieve pressure, or by strapping the toe and carrying out gentle stretching. However, this is effective in mild cases only. Surgical treatment is by arthrodesis of the joint in an extended position.

Nursing care for patients undergoing foot surgery

Preoperative care

The condition of the patient's foot is assessed for any circulatory disorders, infection or corns, and the surgeon is notified if there are any lesions or cuts. The pedal pulses should be recorded to give a baseline for postoperative monitoring, and any skin discoloration should be noted. A full explanation regarding the surgery and the type of footwear to be worn postoperatively should be given to the patient.

Postoperative care

Upon return from surgery, the patient's foot will be in either a below-knee cast or a pressure dressing; both should be closely observed for oozing or bleeding. Neurovascular observations should be recorded and the bed end should be elevated to prevent the foot swelling and aid venous return. A bed-cradle should be used to keep the weight of the blankets off the feet, particularly following a Keller's arthroplasty where a metal Kirschner wire extends through the dressing and is merely covered with a cork. Patients will experience severe pain in the early stages and will require regular analgesics when they start mobilizing. Patients are taught to walk on their heels supported by a walking aid, e.g. frame or crutches.

Discharge planning

Patients are discharged when they can safely mobilize, usually with a walking aid and often wearing a special sandal if they are not in a cast. Analgesics are also given to the patient to take home. Kirschner wires are removed at 6 weeks at the outpatients appointment.

UPPER LIMB ORTHOPAEDIC SURGERY

THE SHOULDER

Total shoulder replacement (arthroplasty)

Following the success of hip and knee arthroplasty, shoulder arthroplasty is now carried out, although it is not as common. A total shoulder arthroplasty is indicated when there is severe destruction of the joint from trauma or a disease process such as rheumatoid arthritis. The total shoulder arthroplasty replaces the humeral head with a metallic component and resurfaces the glenoid cavity (Schoen, 2000).

Preoperative care

- Preoperative tests and investigations for a patient undergoing a total shoulder arthroplasty are similar to those carried out for hip or knee arthroplasty.
- It is useful to encourage the patient to begin to use their non-dominant arm and hand if the dominant arm is being operated on.
- The neurovascular status of both arms should be recorded and used as baseline observations in the postoperative period.
- Full explanations regarding the surgery, postoperative care and recovery period should be given to the patient.

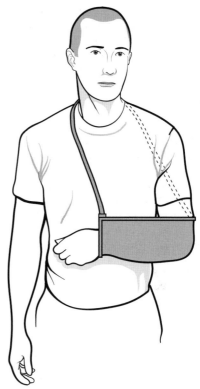

Figure 21.10   A shoulder immobiliser. (Reproduced from Schoen (2000) *Adult Orthopaedic Nursing*, 2nd edn, Figure 13.1A, with permission of Lippincott, Williams and Wilkins.)

- Patients should be taught deep breathing exercises and be made aware that these may be restricted because their arm will be in an immobilizer, which may slightly restrict chest movement (Fig. 21.10).

Postoperative care

- The patient is nursed in the supine position until they can maintain their own airway, then they are placed in the semirecumbent position with their arm in a shoulder immobilizer to prevent shoulder dislocation.
- The patient's temperature, pulse, respirations and blood pressure should be recorded ¼–½ hourly until stable, then gradually built up to 4 hourly observations for a 24-hour period.
- Neurovascular observations of the affected arm should be carried out and recorded.
- An intravenous infusion may be running and a vacuum drain in situ. Both require monitoring and recording.
- When the patient has tolerated adequate oral fluids and is hydrated, the intravenous infusion may be discontinued and a normal diet commenced. The patient will need assistance with cutting up food.

- The patient's pain is controlled with either a PCA pump or intramuscular and oral analgesics.
- Prophylactic antibiotics are administered to prevent infection.
- Sutures are generally removed 7–10 days postoperatively, unless they are self-dissolving.
- The physiotherapist will encourage the patient to do finger, wrist and hand movements and static exercises of the deltoid muscle in the early postoperative period.
- Following X-ray to confirm implant position on day 2, the patient will be encouraged to use the affected shoulder, assisted by the unaffected shoulder. Arm exercises such as walking the fingers up a wall and circulating the arm outwards and inwards (known as pendulum exercises) are encouraged.
- The patient will require assistance with hygiene care and dressing but should be encouraged to actively participate as a mode of rehabilitation.

Discharge planning

Following shoulder arthroplasty, it may take up to 6 months to 1 year before the patient has a pain-free mobile shoulder. For this reason, many patients require some social service assistance, e.g. help with cleaning and shopping.

The patient needs to be educated how not to dislocate the shoulder arthroplasty, and have a full understanding of their individual exercise regime and its importance. Exercise regimes are tailored to individual needs, but usually include movement of the shoulder using the unaffected arm, finger-walking up a wall, grasping of a gymnastic ball and pendulum exercises.

The patient is reviewed in the outpatients department 3 weeks following discharge.

Recurrent dislocation of the shoulder

Dislocation of the shoulder is a common injury, usually as a result of falling on to the hand or arm. The dislocation more often than not occurs anteriorly. The patient presents with a painful immobile shoulder that is flattened in appearance, producing a drop in the shoulder line. If this injury recurs, then surgical treatment becomes an option.

The most common operative procedures are:

1. *Putti-Platt operation*: this involves shortening of the subscapularis tendon by overlapping it, which limits external rotation.
2. *Bankart procedure*: this involves the reattachment of the capsule and glenoid labrum (Dandy and Edwards, 2003).

Postoperative care

- The arm is positioned in a shoulder immobilizer. When and how quickly the patient's shoulder is mobilized is dependent on the surgeon. The shoulder immobilizer remains in situ under clothing for 3 weeks.
- Physiotherapy starts with gentle assisted exercises only and progresses to more active exercises following the 3-week follow-up appointment.

Discharge

The patient is discharged with an individual exercise regime and analgesics, and is made fully aware that it will take several months before maximum use of the shoulder is possible. The patient is followed up in the outpatients department at 3 and 6 weeks.

THE ELBOW

Total elbow replacement (arthroplasty)

Improvements in total elbow arthroplasty during the last 20 years have resulted in clinical outcomes which are now comparable with the results of hip arthroplasty (Hargreaves and Emery, 1999). An arthroplasty of the elbow, however, is less common, but is increasingly being carried out to relieve patients with a severely painful elbow and joint destruction caused by rheumatoid arthritis and to restore stability and improve mobility of the elbow joint (Fig. 21.11).

Preoperative care

The preoperative care is similar to that for a patient undergoing shoulder arthroplasty.

Specific postoperative care

- A plaster backslab may be used over the dressings to immobilize the elbow joint for the first few days.

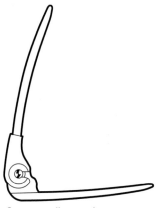

Figure 21.11 Stanmore elbow replacement.

- The arm will be elevated in a sling. An intravenous infusion will be in situ, and, depending on surgeon preference, a vacuum drain, which will usually be removed at 24 hours.
- The nurse should carefully monitor and record the neurovascular observations of the affected arm, looking for signs of ulnar nerve decompression due to elbow oedema, e.g. altered sensation in the little and ring fingers.
- Most exercises are focused on the activities of daily living, such as flexion of the elbow to brush the hair or to feed self.

Discharge

Recovery can take months, and the patient may require assistance with activities of daily living and social service support for several weeks.

THE HAND

Dupuytren's contracture

This condition occurs as a result of a thickening of the palmar fascia. The cause is unknown but it is associated with family history, liver disease, alcoholism and epilepsy (Crawford Adams and Hamblen, 2001). Dupuytren's contracture is more common in men than in women and often both hands are affected (Crawford Adams and Hamblen, 2001). There is a slow progressing flexion contracture of one or more of the fingers, which are pulled into the palm of the hand. The thickened palmar fascia tends to pucker the outlying skin (Fig. 21.12).

Surgery is the only effective treatment and involves the excision of the thickened fascia.

Postoperative care

- The hand is elevated in a Bradford sling to prevent oedema.

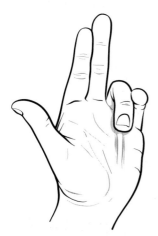

Figure 21.12   Dupuytren's contracture.

- Neurovascular observations need to be monitored and recorded, as there is a high risk of bleeding and swelling owing to the vascular nature of the palm of the hand.
- The wound needs careful observation, as haematomas are not uncommon.
- Some surgeons use a resting hand splint, whereas others prefer to leave the hand alone.
- Massage of the scar helps to decrease swelling and helps to stimulate the circulation and improve healing.

Discharge

It can take months for the hand to return to full use. Patients are sent home with a gentle exercise regime, analgesics, oils, and in some cases with silicone for hand baths.

Carpal tunnel syndrome

In this condition there is compression of the median nerve as it passes beneath the flexor retinaculum in the carpal tunnel. There may be altered sensation in half of the ring, middle and index fingers and thumb. This often affects the patient's sleep and is particularly common in young to middle-aged and pregnant women (Padua et al, 2002). Conditions such as rheumatoid arthritis or Colles' fractures which cause synovial thickening can also cause carpal tunnel syndrome (Crawford Adams and Hamblen, 2001; Dandy and Edwards, 2003).

Conservative treatments are generally tried initially, but the majority of patients require surgery in the long term. Conservative treatments include the use of rest, night splints with the wrist held in the neutral position to reduce compression within the tunnel, injection of hydrocortisone into the carpal tunnel to relieve pain, and the use of anti-inflammatory drugs to reduce inflammation.

Surgery is the only effective treatment, and involves the division of the flexor retinaculum and median nerve decompression. This surgery is generally a day case procedure.

Postoperative care

- The arm is elevated in a Bradford sling. It is important that exercises are carried out at least 4 hourly. This involves the wrist, fingers, elbow and shoulder, ensuring a full range of movement.
- Neurovascular observations require careful monitoring and recording.
- The wound needs to be observed for bleeding, and the dressing is reduced 24 hours postoperatively, with sutures being removed at 7–10 days.

- Advice is given to the patient regarding the importance of keeping the hand elevated while at rest.

Discharge

The patient is advised not to get their hands wet, and is instructed to use plastic bags to prevent this occurring. The importance of keeping the hand elevated while at rest and the continuation of exercises is reinforced, and the patient is advised to avoid heavy lifting for several weeks.

ORTHOPAEDIC SURGERY OF THE SPINE

Back pain is a common complaint. Overall, about 16.5 million people in the UK suffer from back pain in any one year, and about 3–7 million back pain sufferers are thought to consult their GP (Chambers et al, 2001). Ninety per cent of people with lower back pain have an inflammatory or mechanical spinal problem and recover within 6 weeks (Chambers et al, 2001). Backstrain is generally the result of incorrect lifting, and nurses have many opportunities in the workplace to educate patients and their families in how to avoid backstrain.

On its own, back pain is not an orthopaedic problem and is best treated conservatively (Dandy and Edwards, 2003). The majority of patients with back pain are managed conservatively with analgesics to reduce pain, anti-inflammatory drugs to reduce inflammation or corsets to give back support.

Attention to weight, avoiding heavy lifting where possible, and instruction in back care, e.g. back strengthening exercises and sleeping posture, are all helpful.

There is no scientific evidence to confirm the effectiveness of traction for back pain; however, it may be used by some therapists (Chambers et al, 2001). A back support or corset may also be used. Surgery is only considered when conservative methods have been unsuccessful, and it may be undertaken in an orthopaedic or neurosciences unit.

The criteria used to determine surgery relate to CT/MRI findings and the following:

- when conservative treatment has failed to relieve the pain
- when general health is deteriorating because of disturbed sleep caused by sciatic nerve pain
- when there is neurological disturbance, e.g. disruption of bowel and bladder control.

A variety of surgical options are available:

- *Microsurgery*: the carrying out of surgery using a microscope and miniature instruments.
- *Discectomy*: surgical removal of the protruding disc.
- *Laminectomy*: surgical removal of the protruding disc and one or more of the laminae.
- *Chemonucleolysis*: injection of chymopapain into the affected disc to reduce it (Solomon et al, 2001).
- *Spinal fusion*: fusion of the spinal vertebrae to stabilize the vertebral column.

SPECIFIC POSTOPERATIVE CARE FOR PATIENTS FOLLOWING SPINAL SURGERY

- The patient is nursed flat on a firm bed with one pillow.
- Temperature, pulse, respirations, blood pressure and neurovascular observations are monitored ½ hourly initially and gradually progressed to 4 hourly.
- The patient is log-rolled for pressure area care and observation of the wound.
- A small drain may be in situ for 24 hours, and this should be monitored and blood loss recorded.
- Sutures/staples are removed at day 10 if the wound has healed.
- Analgesics should be administered if the patient is in pain.
- An intravenous infusion requires monitoring and may be removed when the patient has tolerated adequate amounts of oral fluids.
- Urinary output should be monitored and recorded, as the patient is at risk of urinary retention due to their position in bed.
- Diet may be commenced when the patient is tolerating oral fluids, and a high-fibre diet will help prevent constipation, a complication which many back surgery patients experience.
- Deep breathing exercises, foot exercises and back strengthening exercises are encouraged.
- Following discectomy and laminectomy, a patient may be mobilized 24 hours postoperatively if pain allows. Patients following spinal fusion tend to require more time in bed, but mobility is encouraged as soon as pain allows.
- Some surgeons prefer a corset to be worn for a specified period of time.
- Patients are instructed how to safely sit, bend and stand, and given written information tailored to their individual needs to support this.

DISCHARGE

Advice on the importance of back exercises, avoiding heavy lifting and good posture is reinforced and supported with written information. If the patient has been supplied with a corset, they need to be taught

Table 21.3   Classification of fractures

Type	Definition
Complete	The bone is fractured completely into two or more pieces
Partial (incomplete)	The bone does not fracture completely
Open (compound)	The bone is fractured and breaks through the skin
Closed (simple)	The bone is fractured but does not break through the skin
Greenstick	The bone is fractured on one side and bent on the other. It is a common fracture in children
Comminuted	The bone is splintered and crushed into smaller fragments
Oblique	The bone is fractured at a 45° angle to the long bone axis
Spiral	The bone is twisted apart
Transverse	The bone is fractured at right angles to the long bone axis
Impacted	A fracture where one part of the bone is forcefully driven into another
Pathological	A fracture due to bone weakening, caused by diseases such as osteoporosis or neoplasia

how to apply and care for it. The patient is reviewed in the outpatients department 2 weeks after discharge.

FRACTURES

A fracture is a break in the continuity of bone. Fractures are classified according to the type, complexity and location of the break (Table 21.3). The stages of bone healing are illustrated in Figure 21.13.

FRACTURE MANAGEMENT

Early management is directed towards converting any contaminated wounds to clean wounds. The main aims of fracture treatment are then:

- *Reduction*: to restore normal alignment of the bone.
- *Immobilization*: to ensure the reduced position is maintained until bone union has taken place
- *Rehabilitation*: to either restore normal function or to assist the patient to cope with disability.

Reduction

Reduction may be achieved by either closed manipulation, or open reduction through a surgical procedure:

- *Closed* – involves the pulling of displaced bone fragments into their normal anatomical position, restoring alignment.

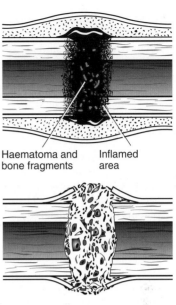

Haematoma and bone fragments   Inflamed area

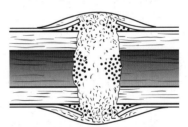

Phagocytosis of clot and debris. Growth of granulation tissue begins

Osteoblasts begin to form new bone

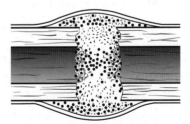

Gradual spread of new bone to bridge gap

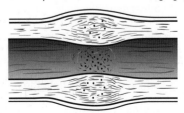

Bone healed. Osteoblasts reshape and canalize new bone

Figure 21.13   Stages of bone healing. (Reproduced from Wilson, 1990.)

- *Open* – this is achieved through a surgical incision. It is indicated when closed reduction has been unsuccessful or where it is desirable to avoid external splintage of the part, e.g. in elderly patients with fractures of the neck of femur where early immobilization is necessary.

Immobilization

Immobilization may be achieved by external or internal splintage, which comes in many forms. External splintage includes cast immobilization, skin or skeletal traction, or external fixator frames. There have been many developments in casting materials, with varying methods of application recommended by manufacturers, which should be followed.

Cast immobilization

- *Plaster of Paris* is most commonly used for patients who have just sustained their injuries, because it allows for swelling. It is less expensive than synthetic casts. The disadvantage of plaster of Paris is that it is heavy and takes 48 hours before it is completely dry.
- *Synthetic casts* allow early weight-bearing, as they dry within 20 minutes, and are ideal for the elderly patient where early mobilization is necessary. They are more expensive than plaster of Paris. Unfortunately they do not allow for swelling and therefore should not be used on patients who have just received their injuries.
- *Cast braces* can be used for fractures of the upper or lower limb. They are moulded closely to the shape of the limb and fitted with hinges to allow joint movement.

Specific care for a patient in a cast

- Limbs encased in casts should be elevated to prevent oedema and aid venous return.
- The cast should not be rested on a hard or sharp surface and must be handled using the palms of the hands to avoid denting, as this could result in pressure to the underlying skin. The signs of pressure ulcer formation include a burning pain, offensive odour and cast discoloration. A window can be cut in

---

CARE OF YOUR CAST

1. Do not allow the cast to get wet, but keep it clean and dry.

2. Do not heat the plaster as it is a good conductor and retainer of heat. Heating could cause a burn.

3. Do not scratch the skin beneath the plaster, or stick anything such as knitting needles inside the cast.

4. Move all joints out of the cast through their full range of movement, especially fingers and toes.

5. Keep the limb elevated when resting.

If any of the following occur, you should see your GP or attend the Accident & Emergency department at your local hospital at once:

1. An increase in pain in the limb.

2. Loss of normal sensation in the fingers or toes.

3. An increase in swelling.

4. Any discoloration of the fingers or toes. If it is due to the cold, cover the limb, do not heat it.

5. Fingers and toes projecting from the cast not free to move.

6. Plaster cracking or breaking.

Never try to remove the cast yourself.

Figure 21.14   Information leaflet for patients with a plaster cast.

the cast to permit treatment, but it must always be replaced so as to avoid further swelling into the space.

- The colour, sensation, temperature and mobility of all individual digits should be checked to ensure that circulation and nerve conduction are not impaired. In addition, a pain assessment should be undertaken and the cast checked for tightness at the proximal and distal regions. A digit that is cold, blanched or blue, painful and oedematous has impaired circulation.

- If signs and symptoms of neurovascular impairment are evident, the cast should be split down both sides (bivalved) immediately, the padding cut and a medical opinion sought. A tight cast can cause ischaemia of muscle compartments, which can lead to irreversible damage (see Compartment syndrome section).

Many patients go home wearing casts, and it is essential that they are given clear verbal instructions and written information on how to care for their specific cast (Fig. 21.14).

Traction

Traction is the application of a pulling force to a body part, with a counter traction force applied in the opposite direction. Traction falls into two main categories:

1. *Fixed traction*: the Thomas splint is the best example of fixed traction, with the counter force being applied to the ischial tuberosity (Fig. 21.15). Thomas splints are now rarely used, with the exception of paediatrics and during transfers.
2. *Balanced or sliding traction*: balanced traction involves the use of weights on a limb, and counter traction is achieved when the foot of the bed is elevated.

Traction can be exerted by applying skin traction in the form of strapping to the patient's affected limb (Fig. 21.16). This strapping can be adhesive or non-adhesive; however, due to the increased risk of skin deterioration, non-adhesive strapping is advised. The second method of applying traction is skeletal traction, which involves the insertion of a metal pin through a bone (Fig. 21.17). However, the use of traction has diminished with the increasing interest in internal fixation (Schoen, 2000).

Specific care for a patient in traction

- Traction equipment should be checked every shift to ensure traction and counter traction is maintained.
- Traction cords should be taut at all times and should only be untied when traction or counter traction is applied, e.g. manually.
- A bed-cradle can be used to prevent the bedclothes interfering with the traction.
- Skin traction should be removed at least daily, for limb washing and skin inspection.
- Patients with skeletal traction should be advised not to touch the pin or pin sites, and corks should be used to cover sharp pin ends to prevent the patient from injuring themselves.

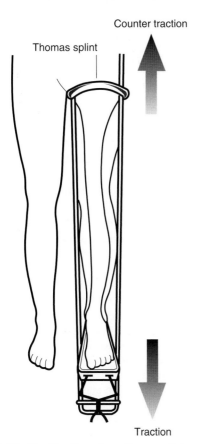

Counter traction

Thomas splint

Traction

Figure 21.15   Fixed traction using a Thomas splint.

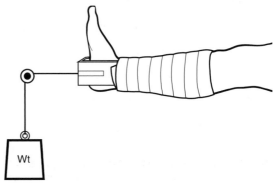

Wt

Figure 21.16   Skin traction.

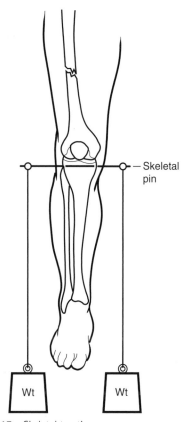

Figure 21.17   Skeletal traction.

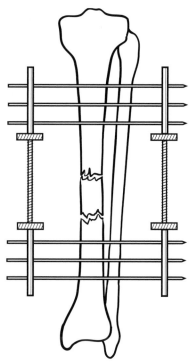

Figure 21.18   External fixation used in treatment of tibial fractures.

- Skeletal pin sites should be checked regularly for signs of infection, such as redness, warmth or oozing, and should be cleaned daily.
- The colour, sensation, temperature and movement of the extremities, and signs of pain or swelling should be observed and recorded.
- Two-hourly pressure area care is essential. The heels should rest over a Leonard's pad, and, where slings are used, areas under the edges of the slings should be observed for signs of pressure.
- Pulleys should run freely, and traction cords should run on straight lines. Weights should hang freely and not rest on the floor or chair, and should be the correct weight. Cords should be checked for fraying.
- The patient will also require general nursing care and physiotherapy to prevent deep venous thrombosis, chest infection, muscle wasting or foot drop.

External fixation

Fractures that cannot be held reduced in a cast or on traction need to be fixed externally or internally. External fixation tends to be used in fractures where there is significant bone loss or extensive soft tissue

damage. This involves the holding of bone and bone fragments by metal pins attached to an external frame (Fig. 21.18).

Specific care for a patient with an external fixator

- Observe for altered neurovascular status, as previously discussed.
- Give patients a full explanation and support in managing the external fixator, ensuring they are aware of benefits such as early assisted mobilization.
- Concordance to treatment is essential in the use of an external fixator. Patients will require a lot of reassurance and support to help them accept the unsightly external fixator frame, which may significantly alter their body image.
- The patient with an external fixator is at a high risk of developing a pin-site infection. This may be superficial and treated with simple antibiotics; however, if not treated, the infection can progress along the pin tract to the bone, which can then have devastating effects. Pin-site care should be carried out at least daily and patients should be encouraged, where possible, to undertake this themselves to help with acceptance of the fixator. Research is conflicting on pin-site protocols; however, clear

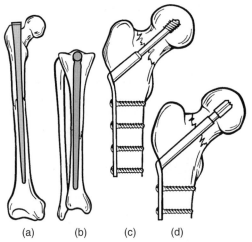

Figure 21.19   Types of internal fixation: (a) and (b) intramedullary nails; (c) compression nail for fixation of the femoral neck; (d) sliding nail fixation of the femoral neck.

Table 21.4   Complications of fractures

Immediate	Early	Late
Soft tissue damage	Infection	Malunion
Nerve injury	Neurovascular	Delayed union
Haemorrhage	compromise	Non-union
	Fat embolism	Osteoarthritis
	Pulmonary	Avascular necrosis
	embolism	
	Deep venous	
	thrombosis	
	Pressure ulcers	
	Chest infection	
	Exacerbation of	
	generalized	
	illness	

instructions should be given to the patient on discharge, with a contact number if they have any questions.

Internal fixation

There are many types of internal fixation devices, such as intramedullary nails, compression nails, plates and screws (Fig. 21.19).

Internal fixation is used in the following situations:

- when it is important to allow early limb or joint movement, or to avoid a long period of immobilization in bed, e.g. the elderly patient with a fractured neck of femur
- when sufficient reduction cannot be maintained by external fixation, e.g. fractures involving joint surfaces
- in multiple fractures where internal fixation of one or more of the fractures may assist in making the treatment of other injuries more simple
- in certain pathological fractures where the patient's life expectancy may be short, e.g. malignancy, or where union may be uncertain.

COMPLICATIONS OF FRACTURES

Patients with fractures are at risk of complications, which are described in terms of immediate, early or late complications (Table 21.4). The nurse should be observant for these complications and take preventative measures.

Compartment syndrome

One particular complication of concern to the orthopaedic nurse following a fracture or orthopaedic surgery is that of compartment syndrome. There is a progressive build up of pressure in a confined space (muscle compartment), which compromises circulation, diminishes oxygen supply and, thus, function of tissues within that space.

The onset of the symptoms can vary from as little as 2 hours to as much as 6 days after the trauma or surgery (Schoen, 2000), and should be treated as a medical emergency. If pressure is not relieved in the compartment, irreversible nerve and tissue damage will result in contractures, paralysis and loss of sensation, and in some cases amputation. If pressure is not relieved in sufficient time, a fasciotomy will be performed in which the muscle compartments are incised to relieve the pressure. The fasciotomy wounds are left open and the patient is taken back to theatre to have the ischaemic muscle debrided and in some cases the wounds skin grafted.

The orthopaedic nurse plays a vital role in detecting compartment syndrome through the assessment of the 'five P's': pain, pale, pulseless, paralysed and paraesthetic. These should be assessed and recorded on a neurovascular observation chart (see Fig. 21.3), and any changes reported immediately.

GENERAL DISCHARGE PLANNING AND ADVICE

Discharge planning commences for elective orthopaedic patients at the preassessment clinic prior to admission, or from the first day of admission for trauma patients. Many patients are discharged home to early discharge schemes where they are cared for in their own homes.

Each patient requires a systematic but individualized documented discharge plan, as the needs of orthopaedic patients vary greatly because of the wide variety of orthopaedic conditions and ages of the patients.

Patients should be actively involved in their discharge planning, and it is paramount that every member of the multidisciplinary team ensures that, through a thorough assessment, the patient is fit for a safe discharge home.

In many cases the occupational therapist visits the patient's home before the patient is discharged from hospital, to assess the home situation. Many patients require aids, appliances or adaptations to their home, such as stair rails, to assist them with their activities of daily living, or services such as Meals on Wheels, home help, or a community nurse. Some patients may require hospital transport to take them home.

Verbal and written information in the form of booklets or pamphlets should be given to the patient, with a list of contact numbers should the patient require further advice, support or information while at home.

Most patients will require a follow-up appointment with the orthopaedic surgeon, and the time period from discharge to appointment will vary depending on the patient's condition.

CONCLUSION

This chapter has outlined some of the basic principles of nursing the trauma and elective orthopaedic patient, discussing some of the more common orthopaedic conditions and surgical procedures. Orthopaedics is changing at an unprecedented rate and this chapter has introduced some of the developments in orthopaedic techniques and the speciality of orthopaedic nursing.

Summary of key points

- Orthopaedic surgery is carried out for patients with disease or injury to the musculoskeletal system. Elective orthopaedic surgery is planned surgery for patients with disease to the musculoskeletal system, such as osteoarthritis. Trauma surgery is performed as an emergency, such as following a fracture.

- It is paramount that the orthopaedic practitioner considers the physical, psychological, social and cultural needs of all elective and trauma orthopaedic patients.

- Where possible, all orthopaedic patients should be given education, advice, support and verbal and written information regarding their condition prior to admission. Where admission is as an emergency, this should be addressed as soon after admission as is possible and continue until discharge.

- Nursing care of the orthopaedic patient aims to promote healing, prevent further injury or complications, maximize independence and promote optimal rehabilitation.

Useful addresses

Arthritis Care
18 Stephenson Way
London NW1 2HD

The Association to aid the sexual and personal relationships of people with a disability:
SPOD
286 Camden Road
London N7 OBJ

Disabled Living Foundation
380–384 Harrow Road
London W9 2HU

National Osteoporosis Society
PO Box 10, Radstock
Bath BA3 3YB

RCN Orthopaedic Forum
20 Cavendish Square
London W1M 0AB

References

Ackerman, C. & Turkoski, B. (2000) Using guided imagery to reduce pain and anxiety. *Home Healthcare Nurse* 18(8): 524–530.

Apley, A. & Solomon, L. (2001) *Concise System of Orthopaedics and Fractures*, 2nd edn. London: Arnold.

Blauvelt, C. & Nelson, F. (1998) *A Manual of Orthopaedic Terminology*, 6th edn. St Louis: Mosby.

Carr, M. & Grey, M. (2002) Magnetic resonance imaging: overview, risks and safety measures. *American Journal of Nursing* 102(12): 26–33.

Chambers, R., Chambers, C., Hawksley, B. & Smith, G. (2001) *Back Pain Matters in Primary Care*. Oxford: Radcliffe Medical Press.

Clinch, C. (1997) Nurses achieve quality with pre-assessment clinics. *Journal of Clinical Nursing* 6(2): 147–151.

Crawford Adams, J. & Hamblen, D. (1999) *Outline of Fractures Including Joint Injuries,* 11th edn. Edinburgh: Churchill Livingstone.

Crawford Adams, J. & Hamblen, D. (2001) *Outline of Orthopaedics*, 13th edn. Edinburgh: Churchill Livingstone.

Dandy, D. & Edwards, D. (2003) *Essential Orthopaedics and Trauma*, 4th edn. Edinburgh: Churchill Livingstone.

Hargreaves, D. & Emery, R. (1999) Total elbow replacement in the treatment of rheumatoid disease. *Clinical Orthopaedics and Related Research* 1(366): 61–71.

Jamieson, L. & McFarlane, C. (1996) The musculoskeletal system. In: Alexander, M. F., Fawcett, J.N. & Runciman, P. J. (eds) Nursing Practice Hospital and Home. The Adult. Edinburgh: Churchill Livingstone.

McPherson, E., Woodson, C., Holtorn, P., et al (2002) Periprosthetic total hip infection: outcomes using a staging system. *Clinical Orthopaedics and Related Research* 1(403): 8–15.

McRae, R. (2002) *Clinical Orthopaedic Examination,* 4th edn. Edinburgh: Churchill Livingstone.

Malik, M., Lovell, M. & Jones, M. (2002) Patient-related factors leading to total hip replacement dislocation: a case series. *Advances in Physiotherapy* 4(2): 85–86.

Padua, L., Aprile, I., Caliandro, P., et al (2002) Carpal tunnel syndrome in pregnancy: multiperspective follow-up of untreated cases. *Neurology* 59(10): 1643–1646.

Roper, N., Logan, W. & Tierney, A. (1996) *The Elements of Nursing*, 4th edn. Edinburgh: Churchill Livingstone.

Rudicel, S. (1999) Evaluating and managing forefoot problems in women: bunions, hammer toes and lesser toe pain are often caused by bad shoe fit. *Journal of Musculoskeletal Medicine* 16(10): 562–567.

Schoen, D. (2000) *Adult Orthopaedic Nursing*. Philadelphia: Lippincott, Williams and Wilkins.

Smith, J. & Rudd, C. (1998) Streamlining pre-operative assessment in orthopaedics. *Nursing Standard* 13(1): 45–47.

Solan, M., Calder, J. & Bendall, S. (2001) Manipulation and injection for hallux rigidus: Is it worthwhile? *Journal of Bone and Joint Surgery* 83-B(5): 706–708.

Solomon, L., Warwick, D. & Nayagam, S. (2001) *Apley's System of Orthopaedics and Fractures*, 8th edn. London: Arnold.

Torkki, M., Malmivaara, A., Seitsalo, S., et al (2001) Surgery vs orthosis vs watchful waiting for hallux valgus: a randomized controlled trial. *JAMA* 285(19): 2474–2480.

Tortora, G. & Grabowski, S. (2003) *Principles of Anatomy and Physiology*, 10th edn. New Jersey: Wiley.

Villareal, D., Binder, E., Williams, D., et al (2001) Bone mineral density response to estrogen replacement in frail elderly women: a randomized controlled trial. *JAMA* 286(7): 815–820.

Wilson, K. (1990) Ross & Wilson *Anatomy and Physiology in Health and Illness*, 7th edn. Edinburgh: Churchill Livingstone.

Further reading

Biswas, S. & Iqbal, R. (1998) *Musculoskeletal System*. London: Mosby.

http://www.orthonurse.org National Association of Orthopaedic Nurses (accessed 15 April 2004).

http://www.boa.ac.uk British Orthopaedic Association (accessed 15 April 2004).

Chapter 22

Patients requiring plastic surgery

Adèle Atkinson

Key objectives of the chapter

By the end of the chapter the reader will be able to:

- define plastic surgery

- appreciate the variety of reasons why patients have plastic surgery

- be aware of some of the psychological issues when caring for plastic surgical patients

- understand why flaps and skin grafts are used in plastic surgery

- describe the physiology of graft healing

- differentiate between a graft and a flap

- understand the principles of specific nursing care of patients with skin grafts and flaps and apply these to a variety of situations

- be aware of the need to give patient/health education

- have an awareness of some of the ethical issues involved with caring for patients undergoing plastic surgery, e.g. informed consent.

INTRODUCTION

Traditionally, plastic surgery conjures up images of patients undergoing cosmetic surgery. However, this is only one part of plastic surgery. The British Association of Plastic Surgery Nurses states as one of its objectives: 'To promote the advancement of research/education for those involved/interested in the nursing care of patients undergoing plastic surgery to include burns and maxillofacial procedures' (BAPSN, 1992), which suggests that plastic surgery has a broader perspective.

Plastic surgery is derived from the Greek word *plastikos*, which means to mould or give shape (Goodman, 1988). It is also about the restoration of function and, up until the beginning of the 20th century, was more to do with reconstruction of congenital malformation or traumatic damage, rather than with cosmetic surgery (McCarthy, 1990). The author agrees with McCarthy that there is no real division between cosmetic and reconstructive surgery: for example, reduction mammoplasty (breast reduction) tends to bring with it relief from backache and gives the woman a more positive self-esteem; the removal of breasts from males who have gynaecomastia allows the boy/man to function without the psychological stigma of looking different from his peers. Both of these types of surgery may be considered as cosmetic surgery, but both allow the person to function more efficiently within society, with more positive self-esteem. Perhaps it is fair to say that plastic surgery involves using principles of reconstructive surgery and nursing care, whether this is in the treatment of congenital abnormalities, trauma or the need to reshape normal structures, to allow more positive self-esteem (Gladfelter, 1996).

The use of plastic surgical techniques is becoming more and more common on surgical wards: for example, the use of flaps in breast reconstruction following mastectomy and the use of skin grafts to help heal wounds. It is also found increasingly in hand surgery on orthopaedic wards, in some aspects of paediatric surgery and neurosurgery. This may be because in some trusts, patients are nursed on plastic surgery wards only long enough to have the operation and ensure the initial results are satisfactory, and then are either discharged home or back to the hospital ward from which they were referred. Or it may be because, with the advent of better microsurgical techniques (e.g. the free flap), there is more scope for use with other medical specialisms.

Plastic surgery covers many of the areas of anatomy and physiology discussed in other chapters – for example, wound healing and breast surgery – and so these aspects will not be discussed here.

This chapter will focus mainly on nursing issues related to caring for patients who have skin grafts and flaps, with some discussion on the use of tissue expansion, and will refer to other types of closure where appropriate.

To show application of theory to practice, patient scenarios will be used. Roy's (1976) model of nursing will be used to give structure to the assessment, planning and implementation of nursing. This particular model of nursing has been chosen because, within this specialty, the focus is adaptation, whether it be in terms of body image or physiological adaptation: for example, restoration of function.

ROY'S ADAPTATION MODEL OF NURSING

Roy believes that health is a function of adaptation to stressors – physiological, psychological and social. Successful adaptation is equated with health, and the nurse's role is to help the patient to adapt to stressors (Akinsanya et al, 1994).

The model identifies the adaptive or maladaptive behaviour in each of four modes (first-level assessment):

- physiological needs
- self-concept
- role function
- interdependence.

Problems – both potential and actual – can then be identified as well as the relevant influencing factors.

A second-level assessment assesses the stimuli that influence the behaviour, and classifies them into focal stimuli (main cause of the problem), contextual stimuli (any environmental factor which contributes to the problem) and residual stimuli (any previous experience or attitudes/beliefs that may contribute) (Akinsanya et al, 1994).

Goals can then be set, as well as the appropriate interventions.

When nursing patients requiring plastic surgery, one main theme applies throughout – body image. It is important to recognize that, for whatever reason the patient is in hospital, there will probably be an element of alteration in body image (see Ch. 6 for issues and nursing interventions regarding body image).

PSYCHOLOGICAL CONCERNS

People have plastic surgery for many reasons. Although each patient has individual needs, there are common psychological issues of which the nurse needs to be aware in order to deliver holistic nursing care (Price, 1990).

Unlike other surgical procedures, the outcome of any plastic surgical procedure is strongly influenced by how closely the result meets the patient's desires (Goin and Goin, 1981). Therefore it is important for the nurse to clarify at admission what the patient perceives the outcome will be and how long the finished result is expected to take. This will usually have been discussed with the patient by a member of the medical team beforehand. For a patient to discuss such issues with nursing staff requires a trusting relationship, so the nurse must have good communication skills and be able to spend time with the patient, especially on admission. This aids the process of informed consent. Although issues surrounding surgery and informed consent are commonly acknowledged as the responsibility of the medical staff, nurses are often involved in this process. This may be to reinforce information or clarify and answer questions (Gorney, 1985). This process is facilitated by a good, collaborative working relationship between the multidisciplinary team.

For patients having plastic surgery, hopes and fears can become focused on their abnormality (Maksud and Anderson, 1995); therefore, it is useful to assess their motivation for having the procedure. Goin and Goin (1981) found that women were more likely to be happy with augmentation mammoplasty results if they wanted to have their breasts enlarged (internal motivation), rather than because their partner wanted them to (external motivation) or because they thought their partner was having affairs because they had small breasts. This concept can be taken further to include the nurse's reactions to how the patient looks or to the type of surgery being performed. Therefore, it is important that the nurse is aware of their own body image and feelings, to allow a positive attitude to be conveyed to the patient through both verbal and non-verbal communication. Patients who believe the nurses to be concerned and caring appear to have a better postoperative recovery; they report fewer feelings of disappointment and are more satisfied with the outcome (Rankin and Mayers, 1996). This reinforces the need for patients to be adequately prepared for all stages of their stay in hospital: for example, any drains that may temporarily alter their image of themselves; how much scarring there will be; the initial appearance versus the final outcome.

Issues can be discussed first at a preadmission clinic and built upon during the patient's stay in hospital through to discharge. Photographs can be taken, preoperatively and then postoperatively, while in hospital or at an outpatient clinic. Photographs show progression of healing: alterations of appearance can easily be seen, as can the extent of any injury or deformity. If necessary, such photographs also provide evidence for any legal situations. It must be remembered that any consent (usually written) should be obtained prior to taking any photographs.

TYPES OF WOUND CLOSURE

It is useful to be aware of all the methods of wound closure, before discussing some of the principles involved in caring for patients undergoing grafts and flaps.

The surgeon will always choose the simplest way to ensure wound coverage, and nursing considerations will vary depending on the type of wound closure.

The reconstructive ladder runs from the most straightforward to the most complicated:

1. Spontaneous closure: for example, of small, uncomplicated wounds. These follow the normal manner of wound healing and are usually the sort of wounds that can be covered with a plaster.
2. Direct closure: for example, using sutures, staples or steristrips (see Ch. 4).
3. Skin grafts: for example, in burns, over some muscle flaps and over some donor sites of flaps.
4. Local flaps: for example, in pressure ulcers and some facial wounds.
5. Tissue expansion: for example in breast augmentation, and to aid removal of some congenital naevi.
6. Tube pedicle flaps.
7. Free flaps.

SKIN GRAFTS

A skin graft is a piece of skin that has been totally separated from its blood supply and is used in another area of the body to reconstruct a defect (Dinman, 1996).

TYPES OF SKIN GRAFT

There are two main types of skin graft: split skin grafts (varying thickness) and full thickness skin grafts (Wolfe grafts) (Fig. 22.1).

Split skin grafts tend to be taken from areas that can be hidden, e.g. buttock, inner thigh (Quaba, 1995), although skin can be taken from any area if necessary. They consist of skin taken from various thicknesses of the epidermis to the dermal layer, usually leaving enough epidermis behind for the skin to epithelialize. Full thickness skin grafts leave no skin structure from which regeneration can take place, and the donor site has to be closed by direct suture (Netscher and Clamon, 1994).

Split skin grafts can be meshed (Fig. 22.2) or unmeshed. Meshing allows the skin graft to be stretched

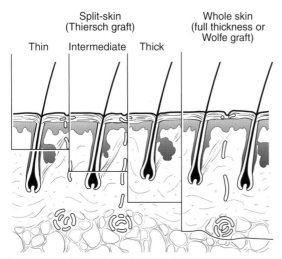

Figure 22.1 Skin graft thicknesses.

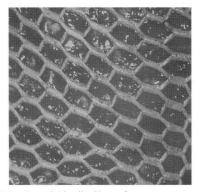

Figure 22.2 A meshed split skin graft.

and so cover a large area (rather like a string vest). It also allows exudate, which could prevent the skin graft adhering, to seep through (Quaba, 1995).

INDICATIONS FOR USE

Skin grafts can be used to replace lost tissue: in burns or traumatic injuries; when tumours have been removed leaving wide, surgical excisions; or when the rate of healing needs accelerating, for example in some ulcers or in the reconstruction of defects (Netscher and Clamon, 1994).

The disadvantage of using a split skin graft is that it contracts during healing (Goodman, 1988), and therefore its use is avoided in areas where this would be disastrous, for example on the eyelids. There is a lack of growth in the graft due to scar tissue, and this could be a problem in children. Because split skin grafts are fragile, they would not be useful in areas subjected to

a lot of wear and tear: for example, the palms of the hands or soles of the feet. In these cases full thickness grafts would be used, as they contract less: they also allow growth in children and are more durable (Quaba, 1995).

Full thickness skin grafts 'take' less readily than split skin grafts, because of their thickness. They must be fairly small because the donor area cannot regenerate and needs to be directly closed (Netscher and Clamon, 1994), and therefore they cannot be used for large areas.

Skin grafts can be taken from the patient's own skin (autograft), from another living or dead person of the same species (homograft or allograft) or from another species (xenograft), usually the pig. Allografts and xenografts tend to be more commonly used for temporary skin coverage, as a biological dressing (Wong, 1995).

Allografts tend to adhere to the wound bed and provide a physiological environment at the wound surface which prevents bacterial invasion of the wound (Wong, 1995). Although allografts are more commonly used to treat patients with burns, they have also been used successfully as dressings for venous ulcers and to cover wounds where large congenital naevi have been removed (Wong, 1995).

In recent years, in the United Kingdom, there has been a growth of skin banks which store skin. Cultured keratinocytes can be stored in liquid nitrogen and can be kept until required (Kakibuchi et al, 1996). Cadaver skin can be preserved in glycerol and kept at temperatures of 4–6°C (Piangiani et al, 2002).

Whatever type of skin graft is to be used, it is important that the patient consents to this treatment and is aware of the type of skin to be used. In the author's experience, it sometimes takes time for the patient to come to terms with cadaver skin. In this situation it may be useful to emphasize the temporary dressing nature of this type of allograft.

HEALING OF SKIN GRAFTS

For effective healing to take place, the wound site on which grafting will take place (the graft bed) must have a good, effective blood supply, be free from infection and have a healthy granulation appearance (McGregor and McGregor, 2000; Quaba, 1995). This means an holistic assessment of the patient must be undertaken, which focuses not only on the wound but on other factors which may influence healing (see Ch. 4). The graft bed can be any viable tissue – epidermis, dermis, fat, muscle, etc. – but not generally bone or tendon (Greenhalgh, 1996; McGregor and McGregor, 2000), due to the limited/lack of blood supply.

Skin grafts can be taken under general anaesthetic or under local anaesthetic, using, for example, EMLA cream (Bondville, 1994). Local anaesthetics tend to be used when small areas of skin are required, in children, and sometimes in elderly people, depending on their general health.

Excess skin is usually taken for use at a later date, in case further grafting is required. This excess skin will remain viable for up to 21 days if stored at a temperature of about 4°C (Coull, 1991a; McGregor and McGregor, 2000).

The graft can be applied either in theatre or, if the wound bed is bleeding profusely, 24–48 hours later in the ward when bleeding will have stopped. The graft may be sutured, stapled or left with just a dressing on to aid healing (depending on surgeon's preference).

To ensure viability, a split skin graft must gain a new blood supply within 2–3 days (Quaba, 1995). This process of skin graft 'take' starts as soon as the skin graft is placed on the wound bed.

Fibrin is exuded (part of the normal process of haemostasis), which allows initial adherence of the skin graft to the wound area or graft bed via weak fibrin bonds (Greenhalgh, 1996). This happens within a few hours and is called serum imbibition. At this point, nutrition to the graft is by diffusion from the plasma secreted by the graft bed (McGregor and McGregor, 2000). This is followed by a joining of the capillary networks in the skin graft to those in the graft bed. It takes approximately 24–48 hours for the endothelial cells from the blood supply within the graft bed to reach the split skin graft. This occurs in two ways: first, there is direct connection of the graft bed capillaries to the pre-existing ones in the graft (inosculation); secondly, the endothelial cells from the postcapillary venules of the graft bed migrate into the graft and form new capillaries which eventually reconnect to the arterioles in the graft bed (neoangiogenesis) (Greenhalgh, 1996). This is substantial enough to allow careful handling of the graft by about the fifth day (McGregor and McGregor, 2000). The lymphatic and nerve 'link up' happens more slowly (McGregor and McGregor, 2000). Finally, collagen bridges form across the graft bed to the graft (organization phase) (Greenhalgh, 1996) and fully stabilize the graft. Maturation occurs over many months. The adnexa, for example sweat glands, from the dermis will not be present in the grafted area (Greenhalgh, 1996) because they were left behind in the donor site and will not regenerate in the grafted area. This may cause the patient to feel itchy over the grafted area in hot weather.

If the skin graft is applied to a limb, then the limb should be elevated, to aid venous return and reduce oedema, as with any injury to a limb. Due to the slow 'link up' of the lymphatic system, the need for elevation becomes more significant.

SKIN GRAFT DRESSINGS

A non-adherent dressing such as paraffin-tulle, Mepitel or Urgotul is used to aid graft 'take'. This will ensure stability of the graft to the wound bed, while creating an appropriate environment to promote healing.

Although paraffin-tulle is described as a non-adherent dressing, it has a tendency to 'dry out' and can adhere to the wound as a result (Wilkinson, 1997), especially if the graft is exuding. This may damage epithelial tissue when removed, and the dressing may need to be soaked off to minimize trauma.

Mepitel is a non-adherent silicone dressing which is bound to a polyamide net. This open network structure allows any exudate to seep out onto a covering absorbent dressing. It adheres to healthy surrounding tissue, instead of the wound (Williams, 1995). This makes removing it pain free, and avoids trauma to the underlying tissue. Mepitel also has the advantage that it can be left in place for 7–14 days if required, allowing the secondary dressing to be changed when necessary (Williams, 1995), so avoiding trauma to the new skin graft.

Urgotul is fairly new to the UK market. It is composed of a polyester net impregnated with hydrocolloid particles and dispersed in a petroleum jelly matrix (Edwards, 2002) .The hydrocolloid and petroleum jelly combine to form a lipido-colloid interface that prevents the dressing adhering to the wound (Benbow, 2002). Exudate can drain through the open mesh but, unlike tulle, the newly formed tissue is prevented from growing into the mesh by the small diameter of the mesh (Benbow, 2002).

Topical negative pressure in the form of vacuum-assisted closure (VAC) has also been used to prepare the wound bed in order to aid skin graft 'take' on wounds which may prove difficult: for example, those in which the wound bed is heavily exuding (Mullner et al, 1997). This system works by using negative pressure to improve blood flow, promote moist healing, accelerate granulation time and reduce bacterial colonization (KCI International, 1994). More recently, the VAC dressing has been used on top of skin grafts (Argenta and Morykwas, 1997) with good results, although these grafts must be meshed to allow the exudate to be drawn through into the VAC canister. See Chapter 4 for more detail on care of the patient with a VAC dressing.

GRAFT 'TAKE'

Whatever dressing is used, its removal at first dressing change is usually linked to the physiology of skin graft healing: i.e. the graft is inspected at 5 days, at which stage it should be well established; before that, the graft would be more friable. At first dressing the graft may look like Figure 22.3. The degree of 'take' is assessed, and this is usually written as a percentage – i.e. 50% 'take' if half of the graft has survived, or, in the case of Figure 22.3, 100% 'take'. Any non-viable tissue is trimmed away, as this would provide a focus for infection. It is not unusual for the graft to be less than 100% 'take'.

There are many reasons why the graft may not 'take'. The graft bed may have been infected (common organisms include beta-haemolytic streptococcus – Lancefield group A, which digests the skin graft by fibrinolysis; and *Pseudomonas aeruginosa*, which produces a green exudate which may cause the graft to lift off). The graft itself may have 'sheared off'. The graft bed may have bled too much and prevented the graft from 'taking'; or there may have been a collection of fluid under the graft, such as a haematoma or seroma (Coull, 1991a).

If all the graft has not 'taken', then the underlying cause should be treated – e.g. antibiotics to clear an infection – before placing another skin graft to the area. If only part of the graft has taken, then healing is encouraged by use of an appropriate dressing to encourage epithelialization from the graft into the wound and granulation of the wound itself.

FULL THICKNESS SKIN GRAFTS

Full thickness skin grafts do not contract as much as split skin grafts and can be used in areas where any form of contracture would be detrimental: for example, when reconstructing eyelids. Because the graft uses all the thickness of the skin, it can also be used in areas of wear and tear: for example, on the soles of the feet. Only small areas of full thickness skin graft are taken, and the donor site is usually closed by direct closure

because this area of tissue cannot regenerate, due to the lack of epithelial tissue.

To aid full thickness skin graft 'take', the graft is sutured to the wound bed, a paraffin-tulle dressing is placed onto the graft, and a piece of foam is placed over the top as a dressing and a 'tie over pack' is created (Fig. 22.4). The first change of dressing is usually done at 5 days to ensure that graft 'take' is well established. The dressing is removed by cutting the sutures over the foam dressing and then removing the dressing. Again, any non-viable tissue is removed and the skin sutures are taken out. The principles of care are the same as for split skin grafts.

THE DONOR SITE

In a donor site of a split skin graft there remains enough epidermis (usually from the base of the hair follicles in the dermis) for healing to occur by epithelialization. Healing takes anything between 7 and 15 days, and therefore the first dressing change will be between 10 and 14 days, depending on the type of dressing used. If healing has not totally occurred, then

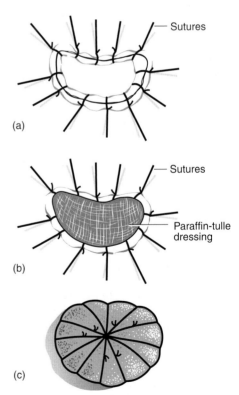

Figure 22.4 Tie-over pack: (a) sutured full thickness skin graft; (b) covered with paraffin-tulle; (c) covered with a foam dressing and sutures tied over the top.

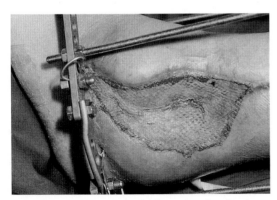

Figure 22.3 100% 'take' of split skin graft at first dressing change.

granulation is encouraged through use of an appropriate dressing. The donor site generates a lot of pain for the patient because it is a superficial wound (rather like a graze) and has plenty of exposed nerve endings. Patients often find the donor site more painful than the skin grafted area.

Wilkinson (1997) states that there are seven characteristics of an ideal donor site dressing. It should:

- retain moisture and warmth at the junction between wound bed and dressing
- remove or absorb excess exudate
- be painless to apply and remove
- inhibit multiplication of bacteria
- stay in place
- be easy to use
- be cost-effective.

Dressings that meet most or all of these requirements are:

- alginates, e.g. Kaltostat, Sorbsan
- hydrofibres, e.g. Aquacel
- hydrocolloids, e.g. Granuflex, Urgotul
- foam dressings, e.g. Lyofoam, Alleyvn
- semipermeable films, e.g. OpSite, Tegaderm.

Traditionally, paraffin-tulle, gauze padding and a crepe bandage have been used for donor site dressings. These have been found to slip down the patient's legs, thus making them uncomfortable and painful. Granulation tissue may also grow through the tulle net spaces if left undisturbed, as would be the case with a donor site dressing (Wilkinson, 1997). As previously mentioned, tulle may also be painful to remove, may dry out or, if overapplied, may cause maceration of the wound. Perhaps, for these reasons, more 'modern' dressing products should be used.

Alginates have been developed to cope with moderate or heavily exuding wounds and also have haemostatic properties. Donor site wounds have been found to heal quicker with a better cosmetic appearance using alginates, than with more conventional dressings, e.g. paraffin-tulle with gauze padding (Thomas, 1992). Once haemostasis has been achieved, it may be necessary to place another piece of the dressing over the top to allow for further absorption (Wilkinson, 1997). A secondary dressing is needed to keep the dressing in place and aid moist healing; this could either be a semipermeable film dressing or a hydrocolloid.

Alginates do not slip like conventional dressings, so they cause less pain and are more comfortable for the patient. They also cause less pain on removal than conventional dressings as they gel, so preventing adherence of the dressing to the wound bed.

There is only one hydrofibre – Aquacel (see Ch. 4 for further details). Like the alginates, Aquacel has been developed to absorb exudate from moderately or heavily exuding wounds. Morgan (2000) has found that it is capable of absorbing 50% more than the alginates and therefore would be appropriate for donor sites. Again, a secondary dressing is needed to keep the dressing in place and aid healing; this could either be a semipermeable film dressing or a hydrocolloid.

Hydrocolloids have been used to good effect on donor sites and have been found to decrease the rate of wound infection (Smith et al, 1994), but hydrocolloid wafers do not adhere well to wet wounds (Coull, 1991b), so a large margin may be required, making it less suitable for large donor areas. There is also a problem of leakage from beneath the dressing (Porter, 1991), which the patient may find distressing. However, some hydrocolloids such as Comfeel Plus now contain an alginate, making them more appropriate for small donor sites. They also cause less pain on removal than conventional dressings, due to their gelling properties. Unlike some of the other hydrocolloids, Urgotul has no adhesive layer and therefore may be an ideal alternative.

Foam dressings are hydrophilic and semiocclusive, with a low adherence to the wound bed (Wilkinson, 1997) and can be used with heavily exuding wounds. They can be cut to size and left on the donor site for several days, depending on the amount of exudate. They also cause less pain on removal than conventional dressings, as they should not 'stick' to the area.

Semipermeable films have been used in the past, but exudate tends to collect under the dressing, causing it to lift off (Coull, 1991b; Wilkinson, 1997) as it has no capacity to absorb the exudate, and therefore these dressings are inappropriate for donor sites when used alone. But, as previously mentioned, they are used as a secondary dressing with alginate and hydrofibre products.

PATIENT EDUCATION

Once the donor site has healed, it will look dry, because of the reduction of sebaceous glands which have been removed, and it will be red and itchy (Wilkinson, 1997). The area should be massaged at least three times a day with a moisturizer to keep the area hydrated and to help reduce scarring, which will eventually become paler and fade over the next year. Although the main benefit is from the massaging of the scar, the moisturizer provides a base which prevents friction and therefore prevents newly healed skin from being broken down. This applies equally to

---

Box 22.1 Example of preoperative nursing assessment, using Roy's adaptation model of nursing, of a patient who will have a skin graft applied

Mr Jones, a 38-year-old builder, is to have a malignant melanoma removed from his back. The defect will be covered with a split thickness skin graft. The donor area is his right thigh.

Mr Jones is married with two school-aged children. His wife works part time, as a helper, at the local nursery school.

The first-level assessment, on admission, is as follows:

Physiological
- Oxygenation
  - Colour good, no problems breathing. Admits to smoking 5–10 cigarettes a day
  - Blood pressure: 120/80 mmHg; pulse: 80 bpm
- Nutrition
  - Healthy appetite. No special needs
  - Weight: 70 kg
- Emination
  - No problems discussed
- Activity and rest
  - Is used to being very active. Is a member of a local gym and 'works out' three times a week. Participates in outdoor sports
  - Sleeps on his back, for about 8–9 hours a night
- Protection
  - Skin intact. Has a malignant melanoma on the middle of his back
  - Admitted for removal of malignant melanoma which will give two wounds: split skin grafted area, donor site
  - Temperature: 36.8°C
- Senses
  - Hearing: normal
  - Sight: no problems, does not wear glasses

- Fluid and electrolytes
  - Well hydrated
  - Admits to drinking 'socially' at the weekend

Self-concept
- Intrinsic
  - Concerned about his prognosis and recurrence of 'skin cancer'
  - Worries about work – will he be able to continue working outdoors

Role function
- Primary – young man
  - Concerns about leading the same active life as before the diagnosis of malignant melanoma
- Secondary – husband and father
  - Concerned about ability to contribute financially for a while
- Other – member of various clubs
  - Unable to participate in activities for a while post-operatively

Interdependence
- Describes himself as a man's man
- Has never been in hospital before and does not like people 'fussing' over him

Preoperative care will focus on concerns brought out from the assessment as well as general preoperative issues: e.g. smoking – causes vasoconstriction, which can lengthen the time a wound heals; work – malignant melanoma is a skin cancer which is increasing in incidence and is directly attributed to the sun's rays, which penetrate into the epidermis.

---

the skin grafted area. Massaging should start as soon as the skin is healed.

If the scars are unacceptable to the patient in terms of colour or body image, the patient can be referred to agencies such as the Red Cross, which will give advice on the use of cosmetic camouflage. It may be necessary to refer the patient to a support group such as Changing Faces or Let's Face It, to help the patient with coping strategies for their new body image. Specific nursing strategies are explored in Chapter 6, with regards to helping patients with their altered body image.

Advice should be given on keeping both the skin grafted area and the donor site out of the sun as much

as possible, as well as discussing the need for high factor sun creams to be used over the areas. This is because the healed skin is extremely sensitive to the sun and will burn easily.

For an example of the nursing care given to someone who has a skin graft applied, see Boxes 22.1 and 22.2 and Table 22.1.

FLAPS

The reliance on a good blood supply for split skin graft 'take' means that split skin grafts cannot be used for areas such as bone and tendon, and flaps would be

Box 22.2   Example of specific postoperative issues in the care of a patient who has had a skin graft applied

One of the main stressors for Mr Jones is that he has a split skin graft and a donor site. This appears to be one of his main focuses postoperatively.

The first and second level assessments are as follows:

Maladapted behaviour	Stimuli (F, focal; C, contextual; R, residual)
Physiological	
Protection	
Break in skin integrity	Split skin graft applied to back (F)
Unhealed wounds: potential for infection	Donor site on right thigh (F)
Temperature: 37.5°C; pulse: 85 bpm	Pain (C)
Sleep and rest	
Unable to sleep on his back	Split skin graft applied to back (F)
	Tired and anxious (C)
Reluctant to move in bed	Pain (F)
	Fear of shearing off of skin graft (C)
Regulation	
Pain: rated at 8 on a 10 point	Donor site on right thigh (F)
visual analogue scale (VAS)	Men don't complain of pain (R)
Self-concept	
Concerns expressed about	Has had a malignant melanoma removed (F)
dying and scarring	Inadequate knowledge base (C)
	Knows someone who has died of cancer (R)
Frightened what his back will look like	Has seen people with skin grafts on the TV (R)
Role function	
Concerns expressed about his job	Hospitalization (F)
and active sports life	Inadequate knowledge base (C)
Interdependence	
Feels completely dependent	Dislikes the dependence on nursing staff (F)
	Pain (C)
	Anxiety (F)
	Needs to maintain independence (R)

used instead. A flap can be defined as tissue which is moved from one part of the body to another and takes with it its own blood supply (McGregor and McGregor, 2000).

Flaps have many advantages over skin grafts: they do not contract; can be used to cover bone, tendon, etc.; can be used where vascularity is poor; can be used to 'fill' a defect; and may help to return lost function, e.g. to the hand (Netscher and Clamon, 1994; Quaba, 1995).

Because patients with flaps are now treated in a variety of clinical settings – for example, orthopaedic wards and ear, nose and throat wards, as well as plastic surgery wards (Coull and Wylie, 1990) – it is important to explore the specific nursing care these patients will require.

TYPES OF FLAP

There are various types of flap, which can be classified:

1. According to their anatomical components (Table 22.2).
2. According to the type of blood supply: for example, axial pattern or random pattern:
   - Axial pattern flaps use pre-existing arteriovenous systems which run along the length of the flap. This means the flap can be as long as the particular axial artery (McGregor and McGregor, 2000) (Fig. 22.5).
   - Random pattern flaps do not have named blood vessels running through them. This means there are strict length-to-breadth dimensions that can

Table 22.1 Example of care plan, based on problem identification from the nursing assessment, for a patient undergoing a skin graft

Problem	Aim	Nursing interventions
Potential for wounds to become infected:	To promote wound healing and skin integrity	
Split skin grafted area	Prevent infection	Leave Mepitel dressing for 5 days
		Change secondary dressing, only if 'strike-through' appears
		Observe for signs of infection, as shown by:
		• elevated temperature
		• smell
		• surrounding area feeling warm/hot pain
Donor site		Leave Kaltostat dressing for 10 days
		Observe for signs of infection
Pain	Pain assessment scale to be under 4 on visual analogue scale	Offer analgesics regularly as prescribed
		Explain all interventions as fully as possible
		Use other techniques, e.g. distraction, allowing him to participate in dressings
Difficulty in sleeping due to position of skin graft and anxiety	To promote sleeping	Encourage Mr Jones to sleep either on his side or front
		Offer milky drinks prior to bed-time
		Take time to discuss all aspects of care
Anxiety due to: Hospitalization	To reduce anxiety	Discuss all aspects of care with Mr Jones
		Show Mr Jones pictures of people who have had split skin grafts, at various stages of healing
Inadequate knowledge base	To increase knowledge on malignant melanomas	Go through various leaflets and advice sheets on malignant melanomas
		Educate Mr Jones about the sun's rays, discuss the different types of sun tan lotions and SPF numbers and which one may be most appropriate for him
		Allow Mr Jones to express fears re: his work etc. and help him to formulate coping strategies
Difficulty in accepting dependence on others	To be able to accept temporary increase in dependence	Discuss with Mr Jones all aspects of care, and the necessity of nursing and medical staff helping him
		Emphasize this dependence is transitory
		Encourage as much dependence as possible
First dressing		
Split skin graft	To promote healing	Assess percentage of graft 'take'
	To minimize scarring	Remove any dead or devitalized tissue
		Re-dress with Mepitel and change in 5 days, unless evidence of infection
		Once healed, advise Mr Jones to keep grafted area out of the sun
Donor site	To promote healing	If all healed, moisturize and encourage Mr Jones to moisturize the area
	To minimize scarring	If not all healed, cover area with a dressing such as a hydrocolloid, or a semipermeable film, and change in 5 days

be used to prevent flap necrosis (Clamon and Netscher, 1994) (Fig. 22.6). An example of this type of flap is the rotation flap, for example as used to repair a pressure ulcer.

3. According to the shape of the flap: for example, rotation, transposition, etc. (Fig. 22.7).

4. According to whether they are local or distant to the recipient area. An example of a local flap is a rotation flap (see Fig. 22.7), and examples of distant flaps are a pedicle flap and a free flap.

   • A pedicle flap is tubed and remains attached at one end by its pedicle (Clamon and Netscher,

Table 22.2 Types of flap

Tissue being used	Flap name
Skin	Cutaneous flap
Muscle	Muscle flap: e.g. trans rectus abdominis muscle (TRAM): deltopectoral
Skin and muscle	Myocutaneous flap
Bone	Osseous flap
Bone, muscle and skin	Osseomyocutaneous flap
Fascia	Fascial flap
Skin and fascia	Fasciocutaneous flap

Source: adapted from Goodman (1988).

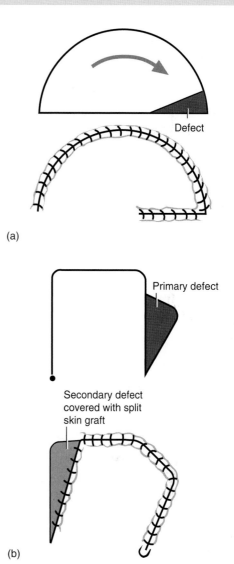

(a)

(b)

Figure 22.7 Examples of classification of flap according to shape: (a) rotation flap, pulls tissue to one side; (b) transposition flap, moves tissue into defect, and secondary defect closed by a skin graft.

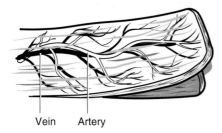

Figure 22.5 Axial pattern flap.

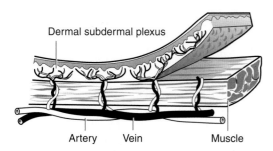

Figure 22.6 Random pattern flap.

1994), thus allowing the flap to be moved to the defect (Fig. 22.8).

- A free flap is detached totally with its artery and vein intact and reattached by microvascular techniques to the defect area (Clamon and Netscher, 1994). The free flap has, on the whole, overtaken the use of the pedicle flap because less time is spent in hospital.

For further detail about flap types and medical usage, see McGregor and McGregor (2000).

With the advent of free flaps and microsurgical techniques, a single operation is required which helps to shorten hospital stay and decrease immobility (Dinman, 1996). Even so, there are two separate sites to

heal (the difference between this and other types of flap is that areas are potentially anatomically far apart) and there is a longer operation time (Clamon and Netscher, 1994). However, the advantages far outweigh the disadvantage of longer operation time.

FLAP SURVIVAL

A flap may fail to survive because of intrinsic or extrinsic factors. Kerrigan (1983) believes that there is only one intrinsic factor – inadequate nutrient blood flow. Without a good arterial blood supply the flap will not

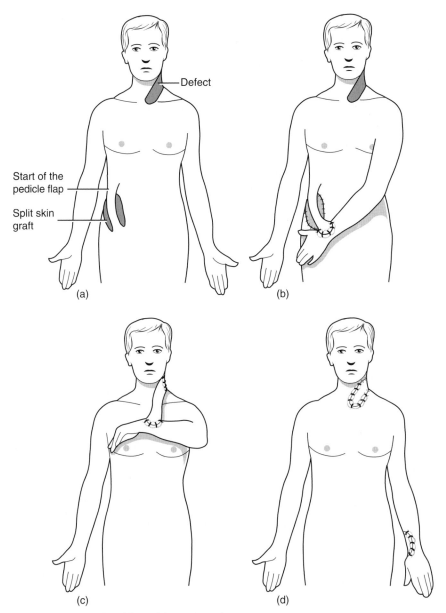

Figure 22.8 Tube pedicle being transferred from abdomen to neck.

survive, so the surgeon must ensure there is a good blood vessel anastomosis (Coull and Wylie, 1990), which will include the venous supply as well as the arterial supply. Westlake (1991) believes venous insufficiency is usually the cause of flap death and acknowledges that venous insufficiency may precipitate arterial insufficiency.

Promotion of behaviours to aid a good blood supply postoperatively should be included in the preoperative preparation of the patient. Patients should avoid drugs that cause vasoconstriction and vasospasm, such as tobacco and strong coffee (Westlake, 1991; Dinman and Giovannone, 1994). As much information as possible (about the operation and what to expect postoperatively) should also be given to the patient to reduce adrenaline (epinephrine) production from anxiety.

Extrinsic factors include pain, alteration in blood pressure, decreased fluid intake and output, marked decrease in temperature, nutrition and direct pressure on the blood supply of the flap (Coull and Wylie, 1990; Dinman and Giovannone, 1994). These factors will now be discussed in more detail.

Pain

Pain occurs from the operation itself and can be superficial (the skin is sensitive) or deep (the deeper tissues are irritated or may become ischaemic) (Gould and Thomas, 1997). Whatever the cause, the end result is the same – potential for flap death due to vasoconstriction, increased blood coagulation and raised blood pressure.

When pain is experienced, several things happen. Adrenaline (epinephrine) is secreted from the adrenal medulla which complements the sympathetic nervous system by acting on the blood vessels in the skin to cause vasoconstriction. The heart also beats faster, thus ensuring cardiac output and blood pressure increase. Aldosterone is also secreted from the adrenal cortex, which has a net effect of raising the blood pressure. The adrenal cortex also secretes cortisol, which, among other things, enhances coagulability of the blood (Gould and Thomas, 1997; Hinchliff et al, 1996) (Fig. 22.9).

Nursing assessment and interventions that are appropriate for pain are discussed in detail in Chapter 7 and include both pharmacological and non-pharmacological methods.

Alteration in blood pressure

Hypertension

The patient may already be diagnosed as hypertensive, or hypertension may be caused by pain, anxiety or excessive fluid replacement (Dinman and Giovannone, 1994). Again, this can lead to flap death if the cause is not treated. This is because, initially, blood flow through the body's tissues is increased. This leads to vasoconstriction as the body seeks to reduce the amount of blood to meet its needs (Marieb, 1998). If not treated, this can lead to decreased tissue perfusion to the flap or anastomosis rupture (Dinman and Giovannone, 1994).

Nursing interventions include blood pressure monitoring and should concentrate on trying to treat the cause, e.g. pain, or ensuring accurate monitoring of fluid input and output. If all else fails, it may be necessary for medical staff to prescribe antihypertensive drugs, such as nifedipine, that prevent vasoconstriction (Dinman and Giovannone, 1994).

Hypotension

Hypotension may be caused by haemorrhage or fluid loss. There will be a decrease in circulating blood volume, leading to a decrease in cardiac output and ultimately a decrease in tissue perfusion, which could lead to flap death.

Nursing interventions include blood pressure monitoring and accurate fluid intake and output assessments, including fluid in drains if any are present. If the

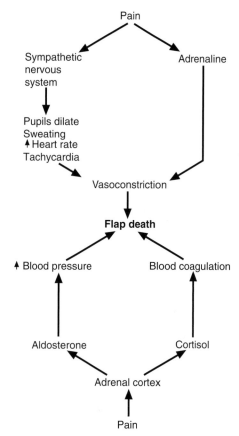

Figure 22.9   Effects of pain in relation to 'flap death'.

patient is in a negative fluid balance, intravenous fluid replacement should be considered (Dinman and Giovannone, 1994), using for example Dextran.

Decreased urinary output

If there is a decreased output, a decrease in blood flow to the flap occurs due to a decrease in tissue perfusion, which may give rise to flap death.

Nursing interventions include ensuring an adequate fluid intake, because, if the patient is hypotensive, extra fluids may be needed. If urinary output is very poor, a catheter may be inserted to ensure there is accurate monitoring of output.

Decrease in temperature (hypothermia)

When the body temperature falls, vasoconstriction occurs to conserve body heat, which decreases blood flow to the tissues. This, combined with a fresh anastomosis in the blood supply to the flap, may cause serotonin to be released. Serotonin stimulates platelet aggregation and thrombus formation at the site of the anastomosis, which could cause flap death (Dinman and Giovannone, 1994; Marieb, 1989). It is therefore important to monitor the patient's body temperature.

Nursing interventions include nursing the patient in a warm environment – a cubicle allows the room temperature to be kept warm and, if necessary, heaters can be used. A piece of gauze or 'space blanket' can be placed over the flap to help keep the peripheries warm if necessary.

Nutrition

As with any surgery, good nutrition aids the healing process, and the patient with a flap is no exception. All patients undergoing surgery will be in stress or anxious. This state of stress will cause varying degrees of hypermetabolism, and therefore a good nutritional intake is vital (see Ch. 5).

To aid flap survival, nutrients such as chocolate and other caffeine-containing products which cause vasoconstriction should be avoided.

Direct pressure on blood supply of the flap

This factor can be due to pressure (either on the anastomosis or generally), tension to the flap, haematoma or kinking of the flap. Any of these conditions will prevent an adequate blood supply to and/or from the flap. Therefore, the specific nursing care of the patient postoperatively centres on ensuring flap survival. This is done mainly by looking for indicators of vascular integrity (Westlake, 1991), such as skin colour, capillary refill, texture and temperature (Table 22.3).

If the flap is failing due to kinking or tension on the flap, then it may be possible to reposition the patient/flap, or sutures that are too tight may have to be removed.

If there is undue pressure on the flap, then the cause should be investigated: if there is pressure due to a haematoma or venous congestion, then it may be possible to use leeches to 'save' the flap (see later in chapter);

if the pressure is due to inflammation from infection, then appropriate antibiotics should be prescribed.

To try to prevent flap death, anticoagulants such as warfarin or even aspirin may be prescribed postoperatively (Westlake, 1991).

DONOR SITES OF FLAPS

Depending on how much and what tissue has been removed, the donor site may be directly closed, as in a trans rectus abdominis muscle (TRAM) flap, covered with a skin graft or allowed to heal using an appropriate dressing. The nursing care of the patient will depend on which method of closure is used. For example, if the donor area required a split skin graft to cover it, then the nursing care would relate to that, and if the donor area required direct suture, then the nursing care would link to that.

Passive drains may be used in areas where large areas of tissue are lost or if haemostasis is difficult to achieve in either the donor site or the flap area. These are usually removed after 24 hours if the drainage is under approximately 50 mL (in 24 hours).

FLAP OBSERVATIONS

It is imperative that baseline observations of colour, temperature and pulse are recorded preoperatively or immediately postoperatively in order to form parameters for flap survival. All these observations can be recorded on a flap assessment chart. Each plastic surgical unit/ward has its own flap assessment chart, one example of which can be seen in Figure 22.10.

Ideally, the same nurse should care for the patient to minimize the subjectivity of flap observations and should directly 'hand over' to another nurse at the end of their shift.

It has been suggested that flap failure occurs primarily as a result of both arterial occlusion and venous congestion, with an increased risk for arterial occlusion within 24 hours postoperatively and venous

Table 22.3   Observations for vascular integrity

	Normal	Arterial insufficiency	Venous insufficiency
Skin colour	Similar to that of donor area	Pale, mottled blue	Cyanotic blue
Capillary refill (venous return)	Approximately 3 s	Sluggish or absent	Brisk (<3 s)
Texture	Soft, firm	Spongy, prune-like	Stretched, swollen
Temperature	Warm (within normal limits); same as surrounding area	Cool	Cool

Source: adapted from Westlake (1991).

Date/time	Site	Colour	Texture	Temp.	Capillary refill	Doppler	Other/comments	Signature

Patient's details

Photograph

Temperature

Warm	-**W**
Hot	-**H**
Cool	-**C**

Colour

Use immediate postoperative photo as a baseline

1	- White
2	- Going towards white
3	- Normal
4	- Going towards blue/purple
5	- Blue/purple

Capillary refill

N	- normal
B	- brisk
S	- sluggish

Figure 22.10 Flap assessment chart.

congestion between 24 and 72 hours postoperatively (Hitchinson and Williams, 2000). Observations of the flap should be recorded half hourly for at least 36 hours, as complications may still be detected up to this time (Coull and Wylie, 1990). After this time, observations can be reduced to 4 hourly. Hitchinson and Williams (2000) suggest that half-hourly observations can be discontinued after 18 hours, but should be recorded hourly from then on up to 48 hours postoperatively.

A photograph may be taken immediately postoperatively, as this can help to minimize the subjectivity encountered when observing flaps (Dinman and Giovannone, 1994). It also gives an indication of the flap colour, which is a useful guide from which to start when later assessing colour of the flap.

Other characteristics that may also need to be recorded on the flap chart are the following.

Site

The site is useful to note if there is more than one flap or where a tube pedicle may be moved to. The donor site can also be noted on the chart.

The type of flap and the anastomosis site should be noted and can also be marked on the photograph.

Colour

Colour should be assessed in terms of the surrounding skin from the donor area (Coull and Wylie, 1990) as there may be discrepancies in colour between the recipient area and the donor area e.g. the patient may be tanned in one area but not in the other.

Assessing colour is very subjective, so a colour strip may be useful as a guide, although this could be confusing, as skin colour varies tremendously, and in the author's experience some nurses find a colour chart confusing for this very reason. A photograph taken immediately postoperatively may be useful to give a baseline.

If the flap appears white, then there may be an arterial problem; if it tends towards blue/purple, then there may be a venous problem. It is easier to assess the colour of patients with white skin, and more difficult in people with non-white skin (e.g. black or Asian people). It is important that a good light source is used when assessing the patient.

Texture

A healthy flap will be soft to touch. Any oedema, tension or haematoma will make the flap hard, swollen and stretched. If the flap feels spongy or prune-like, then there is probably an arterial occlusion or kinking of the flap (Coull and Wylie, 1990; Westlake, 1991).

Temperature

The temperature of the flap should be the same as the surrounding skin. Coull & Wylie (1990) advise that one hand should be used to assess both the temperature of the flap and the surrounding skin at the same time.

Normal temperature is noted as warm; whereas, if it is hot, this may indicate infection, and, if cool, could indicate either arterial or venous problems (venous problems tend to give a warm/hot flap initially but the flap cools as it dies). Temperature probes can be used to promote objectivity in this measurement.

Temperature alone may not be a useful guide to vascular integrity. Westlake (1991) cites a study by Jones et al (1983) where alterations in skin temperature were noted to respond slowly to vascular occlusion, and therefore skin temperature should not be used as an indicator in isolation.

Capillary refill

Capillary refill is assessed by application of gentle finger pressure to the flap, releasing it and noting how long it takes for the area to revascularize. Normal capillary refill time is approximately 3 seconds. If it is delayed or absent, then this suggests an arterial problem. If there is a brisk response, then this suggests a venous problem (Coull and Wylie, 1990; Westlake, 1991).

Doppler ultrasound

Doppler ultrasound can be used to listen to the blood flow in the flap. The arterial and venous sounds are different (Westlake, 1991; Dinman and Giovannone, 1994) and thus the Doppler is an objective way of noting vascular integrity. However, the use of Doppler ultrasound requires training, and this may not be appropriate for every clinical area. Another disadvantage with using the Doppler ultrasound is that the probe is sensitive to movement and therefore there may be difficulties in hearing blood flow, unless the operator is fairly skilled. Another type of Doppler that is also non-invasive is the laser Doppler which has been used with reasonable success in detecting problems with blood flow (Choi and Bennet, 2003). However, Dopplers should be used in conjunction with all the other observations to support clinical findings.

Other considerations

The light source should be consistent (Coull and Wylie, 1990) to decrease subjectivity, and should be noted. Any of the other observations mentioned previously, e.g. pain, should be noted, to allow a full assessment of the patient's condition, which will help towards flap survival.

USE OF LEECHES IN RECONSTRUCTIVE SURGERY

If vascular integrity is compromised, it is important to know whether there is arterial or venous insufficiency. If it is arterial, then the patient may have to go back to theatre for surgery. If it is a venous problem, then leeches (*Hirudo medicinalis* variety) can be used to suck out the congested blood from the flap and allow the flap time to re-establish a good circulation (Coull, 1993). Leeches can be used only if there is a good arterial blood supply onto which they can attach through the skin (O'Hara, 1988). Biopharm (1996) also point out that arterial insufficiency means that the patient is at greater risk from infection, including from the leech itself.

When a leech is placed upon a congested flap, it secretes an anaesthetic substance which prevents the host from feeling pain while the leech is feeding, although the patient with a flap will not feel pain initially because the nerves will not have regrown by this time (Coull, 1993). This lack of pain is an important point to emphasize to the patient, who may already be anxious about the use of leeches.

Among other substances the leech secretes are orgelase (a vasodilator), hirudin (an anticoagulant) and calin (which prevents platelet coagulation) (Coull, 1993). Hirudin allows the leech to suck out approximately 5 mL blood (Strangio, 1991) and enables the wound to ooze up to 150 mL for 10 hours or more (Biopharm, 1996). Any clots should be gently removed (Biopharm, 1996); it is important that the wound is allowed to continue to bleed, as the aim of leech therapy is to help with venous outflow. The implications of this are that the patient is at risk from infection and from the haemoglobin count dropping. When nursing patients undergoing leech therapy, it is important to observe the area around the leech bite for signs of infection, and haemoglobin levels should be checked daily if bleeding is severe. To prevent infection, the patient is given prophylactic antibiotics.

Biopharm (1996) says that, as it takes approximately 3–5 days for new blood vessels to grow around the flap margin, leech treatment should not be stopped too soon. This could mean that the patient needs several applications of leeches.

It is important to prepare the patient fully prior to using leeches. This includes gaining consent, as not everyone finds the idea of having a leech on them pleasing (Fig. 22.11).

Using leeches requires specialist nursing care which is outside the scope of this chapter, but more information can be found in Dabb et al (1992).

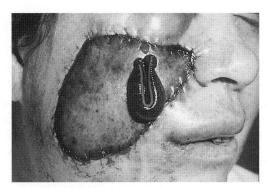

Figure 22.11   Leech applied to congested flap on face.

For an example of nursing care given to someone who is undergoing flap reconstruction, see Boxes 22.3 and 22.4 and Table 22.4.

USE OF TISSUE EXPANDERS IN RECONSTRUCTIVE SURGERY

Tissue expansion is a method for creating new tissue to reconstruct defects by gradually stretching the available tissue (Malata et al, 1995). This is usually done locally to the defect, when the defect is large and cannot be covered by a local flap, but an exact tissue match is required (Clamon and Netscher, 1994), e.g. on the scalp. The tissue expander can be likened to a balloon, which is placed under the tissue to be expanded. The 'balloon' is then filled (expanded) with sterile normal saline (0.9%) through an injection port (Fig. 22.12). This is done in stages, and patients can be seen as outpatients (usually on a weekly basis, with most patients being discharged 1 or 2 days after tissue expansion). Once full expansion has been achieved, the expander can be removed and the expanded tissue moved. This 'expanded' area can then be used as a local flap (Clamon and Netscher, 1994).

Tissue expansion is most commonly used for:

- breast reconstruction
- scalp, ear and nose reconstruction
- some post-burn contractures
- excision of large congenital naevi (Malata et al, 1995).

Extensive preoperative discussions with the patient are paramount, because the patient will have a 'balloon' under their skin for some time and may have problems coming to terms with this alteration in body image, no matter how transitory it is. Due to the discomfort that is often felt during inflation the patient may well need a lot of support from the nurse at this

Box 22.3   Example of preoperative nursing assessment of a patient who is to undergo flap reconstruction

Jane Fog is a 42-year-old teacher, married with one child, and has had a left mastectomy following breast cancer. She has been admitted for breast augmentation using a TRAM flap.

The first-level assessment, on admission, is as follows:

Physiological

Oxygenation	Colour good, no problems breathing. Does not smoke
	Blood pressure: 110/80 mmHg Pulse: 76 bpm
Nutrition	Healthy appetite. No special needs
	Weight: 57 kg
Elimination	No problems discussed
Activity and rest	Used to play squash prior to the mastectomy
	Likes reading
	Sleeps about 6 hours per night
Protection	Skin intact. Has a scar where left breast was removed.
	Has been admitted for augmentation, using a TRAM flap,
	which will leave two incisional scars
	Temperature: 36.8°C
Senses	Hearing: normal
	Sight: wears contact lenses
Fluid and electrolytes	Well hydrated
	Drinks approximately 8 units per week

Self-concept

Intrinsic	Is excited about the prospect of having a breast again.
	Has felt depressed since mastectomy
	Concerns about the operation itself

Role function

Primary – young woman	Wants to be able to look like a 'real' woman again
Secondary – mother and wife	Concerned about ability to contribute financially for a while
Other – member of squash club	Hopes she will be able to participate in squash again
Interdependence	Is independent. Very supportive family

Preoperative care will focus on concerns brought out from the assessment, as well as general preoperative issues, e.g. work.

Box 22.4   Example of specific postoperative issues in the case of a patient who has undergone flap reconstruction

The first- and second-level assessments are as follows:

Maladapted behaviour	Stimuli (F, focal; C, contextual; R, residual)
Physiological	
Protection	TRAM flap (F)
Break in skin integrity	Abdominal incision (F)
Unhealed wounds:. potential for infection; flap loss	
Temperature: 37.0°C; pulse: 80;	Pain (C)
Blood pressure: 110/60 mmHg	
Fluid and electrolytes	
Intravenous infusion (IVI) running	TRAM flap (F)
Drain in situ	Knows she needs to drink reasonable amounts (C)
Nursed in a warm cubicle: potential for dehydration	

Sleep and rest
Unable to sleep
Reluctant to move in bed

Anxious (F)
Doesn't like drips or drains (C)
Pain (F)
Frightened of splitting abdominal sutures (C)

Regulation
Pain: rated at 6 on a 10 point visual analogue scale

Surgery (F)

Self-concept
Concerns expressed about what the breast
  will look like postoperatively

Has had TRAM flap (F)
Inadequate knowledge base C)
Has been shown a variety of photographs
  preoperatively of patients with TRAM flaps (R)

Role function
Concerns expressed about her job and
  work around the house

Hospitalization (F)
Will need to take off at least 6 weeks from work (F)
Inadequate knowledge base (C)
Needs to avoid heavy lifting for some time (F)

Interdependence
Concerns expressed about how independent
  she will be able to be at home

Anxiety (F)
Needs to maintain independence (R)

Table 22.4 Example of care plan based on problem identification from the nursing assessments for a patient undergoing a flap reconstruction

Problem	Aim	Nursing interventions
Potential for altered tissue perfusion in flap	To ensure adequate tissue perfusion: – pink, warm dry flap – flap temperature to be warm, as surrounding area – flap to feel soft – capillary refill to be within normal limits	Monitor flap for colour, capillary refill, texture and temperature and record on assessment chart Monitor drainage Ensure adequate fluid intake Monitor IVI progress and take down when drinking normally
Potential for wounds to become infected: TRAM flap abdominal wound	To promote wound healing and skin integrity Prevent infection	Monitor flap as above; Observe for signs of infection – as shown by: • elevated temperature • smell • surrounding area feeling warm–hot pain Leave dressing on abdominal wound for 48 h Remove sutures/staples after approximately 10 days Observe for signs of infection
Pain	Pain assessment scale to be under 4 on the visual analogue scale	Offer analgesics regularly as prescribed and monitor effectiveness Explain all interventions as fully as possible Use other techniques, e.g. distraction, allowing her to participate in dressings
Difficulty in sleeping and moving due to surgery	To promote sleeping and moving	Encourage Mrs Fog to sleep on back with legs bent – use a pillow under knees for comfort Offer milky drinks prior to bedtime Take time to discuss all aspects of care Encourage Mrs Fog to support abdominal incision when moving or coughing Encourage Mrs Fog to walk in an upright position

(Continued)

Table 22.4 (*Continued*)

Problem	Aim	Nursing interventions

Anxiety due to:
  hospitalization
  inadequate
  knowledge base
	To reduce anxiety
	To increase knowledge
	  of TRAM flaps
		Discuss all aspects of care with Mrs Fog
		Go through photographs of people who have had TRAM flap
		  surgery, explaining the difference between initial surgery
		  and after a few months
		Explain ward advice sheet on TRAM flaps
		Allow Mrs Fog to express fears regarding work, etc.,
		  and discuss these with her

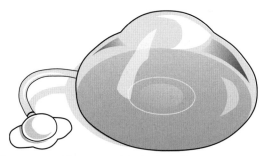

Figure 22.12   Tissue expander – basic design.

Table 22.5   Complications following insertion of a tissue expander

Possible complications	Signs/symptoms
Infection	Pain, or feels more tender than usual; rise in temperature; smell from expander site
Haematoma	Discoloration of the area; increase in tension; pain and swelling
Wound dehiscence	Wound gapes open
Exposure of expander	Tissue expander may protrude through skin or wound
Tissue ischaemia	Expanded area looks paler than the rest of the surrounding skin or may look mottled

time (Hinojosa and Layman, 1996), which may include reinforcing the positive results from expansion. Other complications/disadvantages include repeated hospital visits; some initial discomfort following each expansion; infection; haematoma; wound dehiscence; and overinflation, which causes exposure of the implant (Esposito and Dado, 1997). Therefore coping strategies need to be discussed with the patient in order to give support for this lengthy procedure. However, there are many advantages on which the nurse can encourage the patient to focus: for example, an excellent tissue match, increased likelihood of flap viability and the promise that there will be no new scars (Malata et al, 1995). Other specific nursing interventions should address prevention of infection and other complications which may arise as previously mentioned, as well as providing emotional and psychological support. Because the patient may well be treated on an outpatient basis, patient education on how to observe for signs of complications should be given (see Table 22.5), which can be reinforced through an advice sheet.

DISCHARGE PLANNING

Patients undergoing plastic surgery do not stay in hospital for long (on average about 3–5 days, in the author's experience). This means that discharge planning needs to begin at or before their admission. The initial nursing assessment can incorporate issues that may be relevant for discharge planning: for example, patients undergoing breast surgery will not have the full range of arm movements initially, so it is useful to note if they have someone at home who will be able to help with housework, etc. The use of critical pathways may help to ensure that discharge planning is undertaken in the preoperative phase, as they remind nurses of the 'best path' to take to ensure the optimal outcome (Staley and Richard, 1996).

To help prepare patients for discharge, many hospitals have developed advice sheets. One example can be seen in Figure 22.13. These can be discussed with the patient preoperatively and the information in them reinforced throughout the patient's stay. Other important issues such as care of the skin and avoidance of the sun can be reinforced as part of patient education/health education issues. These issues may also be included on advice sheets.

Community nurses will usually care for the patient's wound between hospital visits, and good communication between hospital and community staff is vital. The advent of outreach/plastic community liaison

ADVICE FOR PATIENTS UNDERGOING SKIN GRAFTING

The length of your stay will depend on the site and size of the graft and any other associated surgery being performed.

BEFORE SURGERY

Either at the pre-admission clinic or on admission to the ward a photograph will be taken for your medical notes. You may have a blood test taken to check that you are not anaemic.

Potential complications

Graft loss, either full or partial may occur as a result of :

infection – where microorganisms destroy the graft.

collection of fluid – possibly blood or serum underneath the graft preventing it from adhering to the wound.

poor blood supply – this may be due to poor circulation, pressure or through systematic disorders, e.g. diabetes.

disturbance of dressing – the dressing secures the graft and should not be removed until the specified date.

If indicated, antibiotics will be prescribed and the wound redressed until it has healed or the site prepared for another graft.

YOUR OPERATION

A sheet of skin is taken from another part of your body, usually your thigh, and placed on your wound. This area on your thigh is called your 'donor area'. The donor area is often more uncomfortable than the newly grafted area, rather like a painful graze. The graft may be secured to the wound site with stitches or staples and a dressing applied to cover it.

Sometimes the graft is applied to your wound 1–2 days after your operation, by the ward nursing staff.

AFTER YOUR OPERATION

Analgesia/painkillers are prescribed to make you more comfortable; these may be in injection, tablet or suppository form. Please tell the nursing staff if you are in discomfort.

Care of the graft site – The graft dressing will remain undisturbed for 3–5 days. The nurses will then remove the dressing to see if the graft has 'stuck' to the wound and then redress it. Further dressings will be arranged at the hospital or in your own home as determined by your circumstances.

The grafted area will be a different colour to your surrounding skin but as it matures this is likely to fade. Scarring in this area will be visible to some degree. Initially the grafted site may be indented. The extent of this defect will improve as new tissue fills in, resulting in a more acceptable contour.

Care of donor site – The donor site dressing may remain undisturbed for up to 10 days unless a large volume of fluid has collected underneath it, requiring its renewal. Subsequent dressings will be reapplied until healing has occurred. Once healed, moisturise daily with a non-perfumed cream, such as E45 or Nivea, as the new skin will be drier and may itch.

FUTURE CARE OF HEALED WOUNDS

New skin requires protection from strong sunlight as it will burn easily. Use a high factor sun-block or keep both areas covered.

The grafted area is easily traumatized. It may therefore be prudent to protect a new graft with a tubular bandage or other dressing for 3 months.

ON DISCHARGE

You will be given an out-patients appointment. If you have any problems please ring the ward from which you were discharged for advice.

If you would like to discuss your future surgery further, prior to admission, you may do so by contacting:-

Figure 22.13   Advice for patients undergoing skin grafting. (Reproduced with kind permission of Richmond, Twickenham and Roehampton Health Care NHS Trust.)

nurses, in which the plastic surgery nurse visits the patient at home, and liaises with and educates district nurses, may help to overcome any communication or specialist nursing care problems.

CONCLUSION

Surgical nurses need to know the principles of caring for patients undergoing plastic surgical procedures, because the use of such techniques is becoming more common on general surgical wards. This involves having a good knowledge base of the anatomy and physiology of structures involved in skin grafts and the different kinds of flap that may be used, as well as the principles of specialized nursing care given to patients requiring these surgical procedures.

Discharge planning should begin at or before admission in order to facilitate this process and ensure that the patient is fully conversant with their aftercare arrangements. The use of community liaison/outreach nurses can help in this process.

Summary of key points

- Plastic surgery involves using principles of nursing care that are applicable to patients requiring either reconstructive or cosmetic surgery.

- The use of plastic surgical techniques is becoming more and more common on surgical wards.

- Skin grafts are pieces of skin that have been totally separated from their blood supply and are used in other areas of the body to replace large areas of tissue, accelerate healing and reconstruct defects.

- The process of skin graft healing is in three stages: serum imbibition, revascularization and the organization phase.

- A flap is tissue which is moved from one part of the body to another and takes with it its own blood supply and can be used to cover bone, tendon, etc., where vascularity is poor; it can 'fill' a defect and may help to return lost function.

- The specialist nature of plastic surgery makes it imperative that good, understandable health/patient education is given.

References

Akinsanya, J., Cox, G., Crouch, C. & Fletcher, L. (1994) *The Roy Adaptation Model in Action*. London: Macmillan.

Argenta, L. & Morykwas, M. (1997) Vacuum-assisted closure: a new method for wound control and treatment. *Annals of Plastic Surgery* 38(6): 563–577.

BAPSN (1992) *The British Association of Plastic Surgery Nurses: Constitution and Rules*. London: BAPSN.

Benbow, M. (2002) Urgotul: alternative to conventional dressings. *British Journal of Nursing* 11(2): 135–138.

Biopharm (1996) Clinical use of leeches [online]. Available from: http://www.biopharm-leeches.com (accessed 14 March 2004).

Bondville, J. (1994) Pain-free harvesting of skin grafts with EMLA(R). *Plastic Surgical Nursing* 14(4): 231–234.

Choi, C. & Bennett, R. (2003) Laser Dopplers to determine cutaneous blood flow. *Dermatology Surgery* 29(3): 272–280.

Clamon, J. & Netscher, D. (1994) General principles of flap reconstruction: goals for aesthetic and functional outcome. *Plastic Surgical Nursing* 14(1): 9–14.

Coull, A. (1991a) Making sense of ... Split skin grafts. *Nursing Times* 87(27): 54–55.

Coull, A. (1991b) Making sense of ... Split skin graft donor sites. *Nursing Times* 87(40): 52–54.

Coull, A. (1993) Using leeches for venous drainage after surgery. *Journal of Wound Care* 2(5): 294–297.

Coull, A. & Wylie, K. (1990) Regular monitoring: the way to ensure flap healing. *Professional Nurse* 6(1): 18–21.

Dabb, R. W., Malone, J. M. & Leverett, L. C. (1992) The use of medicinal leeches in the salvage of flaps with venous congestion. *Annals of Plastic Surgery* 29(3): 250–256.

Dinman, S. (1996) Flaps and grafts for reconstruction. In: Goodman, T. (ed.) *Core Curriculum for Plastic and Reconstructive Surgical Nursing*, 2nd edn. New Jersey: ASPRSN.

Dinman, S. & Giovannone, M. (1994) The care and feeding of microvascular flaps: how nurses can help prevent flap loss. *Plastic Surgical Nursing* 14(3): 154–164.

Edwards, J. (2002) Urgotul – product focus. *Journal of Community Nursing* 16(4): 37, 40

Esposito, C. & Dado, D. (1997) The use of tissue expansion for the treatment of burn scar alopecia. *Plastic Surgical Nursing* 17(1): 11–15.

Gladfelter, J. (1996) The plastic surgery patient. In: Goodman, T. (ed.) *Core Curriculum for Plastic and Reconstructive Surgical Nursing*, 2nd edn. New Jersey: ASPRSN.

Goin, J. & Goin, M. (1981) *Changing the Body – Psychological Effects of Plastic Surgery.* London: Williams & Wilkins.

Goodman, T. (1988) Grafts and flaps in plastic surgery. *AORN Journal* 48(4): 650–663.

Gorney, M. (1985) Office staff responsibilities in the prevention of plastic surgery malpractice suits: a practical guide. *Plastic Surgical Nursing* 5(4): 147–150.

Gould, D. & Thomas, V. (1997) Pain mechanisms: the neurophysiology and neuropsychology of pain perception. In: Thomas, V. (ed.) *Pain: Its Nature and Management.* London: Baillière Tindall.

Greenhalgh, D. (1996) The healing of burn wounds. *Dermatology Nursing* 8(1): 13–23, 66.

Hinchliff, S., Montague, S. & Watson, R. (1996) *Physiology for Nursing Practice,* 2nd edn. London: Baillière Tindall.

Hitchinson, C. & Williams, K. (2000) Postoperative free flap monitoring: clinical guidelines [online]. Available at: http://www.theblackhole.co.uk/ifwh/bahnon/Professional%20Guidelines/flap%20guidelines.doc (accessed 30 September 2003).

Hinojosa, R. & Layman, A. (1996) Breast reconstruction through tissue expansion. *Plastic Surgical Nursing* 16(3): 139–145.

Jones, B., Dunscombe, P. & Greenhalgh, R. (1983) Differential thermometry as a monitor of blood flow in flaps. *British Journal of Plastic Surgery* 36(1): 83–87.

Kakibuchi, M., Hosokawa, K., Fujikawa, M. & Yoshikawa, K. (1996) The use of cultivated epidermal cell sheets in skin grafting. *Journal of Wound Care* 5(10): 487–490.

KCI International (1994) *Vacuum Assisted Closure — ProductInformation.* Oxon: KCI.

Kerrigan, C. (1983) Skin flap failure: pathophysiology. *Plastic and Reconstructive Surgery* 72(6): 766–774.

McCarthy, J. (1990) Introduction to plastic surgery. In: McCarthy, J. (ed.) *Plastic Surgery Volume: General Principles.* Philadelphia: WB Saunders.

McGregor, I. & McGregor, A. (2000) *Fundamental Techniques of Plastic Surgery,* 10th edn. Edinburgh: Churchill Livingstone.

Maksud, D. & Anderson, R. (1995) Psychological dimensions of aesthetic surgery. *Plastic Surgical Nursing* 15(3): 137–144.

Malata, C., Williams, N. & Sharpe, D. (1995) Tissue expansion: an overview. *Journal of Wound Care* 4(1): 37–44.

Marieb, E. (1998) *Human Anatomy and Physiology,* 4th edn. California: Benjamin Cummings.

Morgan, D. (2000) *Formulary of Wound Management Products,* 8th edn. Haslemere: Euromed Communications.

Mullner, T., Mrkonjic, L. & Vecsei, V. (1997) The use of negative pressure to promote the healing of tissue defects: a clinical trial using the vacuum sealing technique. *British Journal of Plastic Surgery* 50(3): 194–199.

Netscher, D. & Clamon, J. (1994) Methods of reconstruction. *Nursing Clinics of North America* 29(4): 725–739.

O'Hara, M. (1988) Leeching: a modern use for an ancient remedy. *American Journal of Nursing* 88(12): 1656–1658.

Piangiani, E., Lerardi, F., Taddeucci, P., et al (2002) Skin allograft in the treatment of TEN. *Dermatologic Surgery* 28(12): 1173–1176.

Porter, J. (1991) A review of dressing materials used for the treatment of raw areas in plastic surgery. *The Journal of Tissue Viability* 1(2): 48–53.

Price, B. (1990) *Body Image – Nursing Concepts and Care.* London: Prentice Hall.

Quaba, A. (1995) Reconstructive ladder for skin and soft tissue defects. *Surgery* 13: 126–132.

Rankin, M. & Mayers, P. (1996) Psychosocial care of the plastic surgical patient. In: Goodman, T. (ed.) *Core Curriculum for Plastic and Reconstructive Surgical Nursing,* 2nd edn. New Jersey: ASPRSN.

Roy, C. (1976) *Introduction to Nursing: An Adaptation Model.* New Jersey: Prentice Hall.

Smith, D., Thomson, P., Garner, W. & Rodriguez, J. (1994) Donor site repair. *The American Journal of Surgery* 167(1A, Suppl.): 49S–51S.

Staley, M. & Richard, R. (1996) Critical pathways to enhance the rehabilitation of burns patients. *Journal of Burn Care & Rehabilitation* 17(6, Suppl.): S12–S36.

Strangio, L. (1991) Leeches: when bleeding is exactly what you want. *RN* 54(9): 31–33.

Thomas, S. (1992) Alginates. *Journal of Wound Care* 1(1): 29–32.

Westlake, C. (1991) Commitment to function: microsurgical flaps. *Plastic Surgical Nursing* 11(3): 95–99.

Wilkinson, B. (1997) Hard graft. *Nursing Times* 93(16): 63–64, 66, 68.

Williams, C. (1995) Product focus: Mepitel. *British Journal of Nursing* 4(1): 51–55.

Wong, L. (1995) The many uses of allograft skin. *Ostomy/Wound Management* 41(4): 36–38, 40–42.

Further reading

Black, J. (1996) Surgical options in wound healing. *Critical Care Nursing Clinics of North America* 8(2): 169–182.

Changing faces (n.d.) http://www.cfac.es.demon.co.uk/default.html (accessed on 27 September 2003).

Chia, C. Stadelmann, W. (2002) *Tissue Expansion.* Accessed from: http://www.emedicine.com/plastic/topic406.htm (accessed on 27 September 2003)

Hansborough, J. (1995) Status of cultured skin replacements. *Wounds: a Compendium of Clinical Research and Practice* 7(4): 130–136.

Let's face it (n.d.) http://www.letsfaceit.force9.co.uk/ (accessed on 29 September 2003)

Walsh, M. (1997) Critical pathways. In: *Models and Critical Pathways in Clinical Nursing,* Ch. 4. London: Baillière Tindall.

Index